Understanding Autism

Understanding Autism

Edited by Paul Spencer

hayle
medical

New York

Hayle Medical,
750 Third Avenue, 9th Floor,
New York, NY 10017, USA

Visit us on the World Wide Web at:
www.haylemedical.com

ISBN: 978-1-63241-444-1

Cataloging-in-Publication Data

Understanding autism / edited by Paul Spencer.
    p. cm.
Includes bibliographical references and index.
ISBN 978-1-63241-444-1
1. Autism. 2. Autism spectrum disorder. 3. Autism--Treatment. 4. Autistic people. I. Spencer, Paul.
RC553.A88 U53 2017
616.858 82--dc23

Table of Contents

Preface...IX

Chapter 1   **Multiparametric MRI Characterization and Prediction in Autism Spectrum Disorder using Graph Theory and Machine Learning**......................................1
Yongxia Zhou, Fang Yu, Timothy Duong

Chapter 2   **Autism and Sensory Processing Disorders: Shared White Matter Disruption in Sensory Pathways but Divergent Connectivity in Social-Emotional Pathways**..........11
Yi-Shin Chang, Julia P. Owen, Shivani S. Desai, Susanna S. Hill, Anne B. Arnett, Julia Harris, Elysa J. Marco, Pratik Mukherjee

Chapter 3   **Regional Alterations in Purkinje Cell Density in Patients with Autism**......................28
Jerry Skefos, Christopher Cummings, Katelyn Enzer, Jarrod Holiday, Katrina Weed, Ezra Levy, Tarik Yuce, Thomas Kemper, Margaret Bauman

Chapter 4   **A Different View on the Checkerboard? Alterations in Early and Late Visually Evoked EEG Potentials in Asperger Observers**......................40
Juergen Kornmeier, Rike Wörner, Andreas Riedel, Michael Bach, Ludger Tebartz van Elst

Chapter 5   **Rare Mutations of *CACNB2* Found in Autism Spectrum Disease-Affected Families Alter Calcium Channel Function**......................53
Alexandra F. S. Breitenkamp, Jan Matthes, Robert Daniel Nass, Judith Sinzig, Gerd Lehmkuhl, Peter Nürnberg, Stefan Herzig

Chapter 6   **Brain Volumetric Correlates of Autism Spectrum Disorder Symptoms in Attention Deficit/Hyperactivity Disorder**......................63
Laurence O'Dwyer, Colby Tanner, Eelco V. van Dongen, Corina U. Greven, Janita Bralten, Marcel P. Zwiers, Barbara Franke, Jaap Oosterlaan, Dirk Heslenfeld, Pieter Hoekstra, Catharina A. Hartman, Nanda Rommelse, Jan K. Buitelaar

Chapter 7   **Violations of Personal Space by Individuals with Autism Spectrum Disorder**......................76
Daniel P. Kennedy, Ralph Adolphs

Chapter 8   **Altered Network Topologies and Hub Organization in Adults with Autism: A Resting-State fMRI Study**......................86
Takashi Itahashi, Takashi Yamada, Hiromi Watanabe, Motoaki Nakamura, Daiki Jimbo, Seiji Shioda, Kazuo Toriizuka, Nobumasa Kato, Ryuichiro Hashimoto

Chapter 9   **Autism-Specific Covariation in Perceptual Performances: "*g*" or "*p*" Factor?**......................101
Andrée-Anne S. Meilleur, Claude Berthiaume, Armando Bertone, Laurent Mottron

Chapter 10   **Neural Correlates of Own Name and Own Face Detection in Autism Spectrum Disorder**................114
Hanna B. Cygan, Pawel Tacikowski, Pawel Ostaszewski, Izabela Chojnicka, Anna Nowicka

Chapter 11   **Screening for Autism Spectrum Disorders with the Brief Infant-Toddler Social and Emotional Assessment**................127
Ingrid Kruizinga, Janne C. Visser, Tamara van Batenburg-Eddes, Alice S. Carter, Wilma Jansen, Hein Raat

Chapter 12   **Effect of Familiarity on Reward Anticipation in Children with and without Autism Spectrum Disorders**................135
Katherine K. M. Stavropoulos, Leslie J. Carver

Chapter 13   **Assessing the Impact of Copy Number Variants on miRNA Genes in Autism by Monte Carlo Simulation**................147
Maurizio Marrale, Nadia Ninfa Albanese, Francesco Calì, Valentino Romano

Chapter 14   **Are Maternal Social Networks and Perceptions of Trust Associated with Suspected Autism Spectrum Disorder in Offspring? A Population-Based Study in Japan**................157
Takeo Fujiwara, Ichiro Kawachi

Chapter 15   **Atypical Mismatch Negativity in Response to Emotional Voices in People with Autism Spectrum Conditions**................164
Yang-Teng Fan, Yawei Cheng

Chapter 16   **Attenuation of Typical Sex Differences in 800 Adults with Autism vs. 3,900 Controls**................174
Simon Baron-Cohen, Sarah Cassidy, Bonnie Auyeung, Carrie Allison, Maryam Achoukhi, Sarah Robertson, Alexa Pohl, Meng-Chuan Lai

Chapter 17   **High Resolution Magnetic Resonance Imaging for Characterization of the Neuroligin-3 Knock-in Mouse Model Associated with Autism Spectrum Disorder**................184
Manoj Kumar, Jeffery T. Duda, Wei-Ting Hwang, Charles Kenworthy, Ranjit Ittyerah, Stephen Pickup, Edward S. Brodkin, James C. Gee, Ted Abel, Harish Poptani

Chapter 18   **Metabolomics as a Tool for Discovery of Biomarkers of Autism Spectrum Disorder in the Blood Plasma of Children**................195
Paul R. West, David G. Amaral, Preeti Bais, Alan M. Smith, Laura A. Egnash, Mark E. Ross, Jessica A. Palmer, Burr R. Fontaine, Kevin R. Conard, Blythe A. Corbett, Gabriela G. Cezar, Elizabeth L. R. Donley, Robert E. Burrier

Chapter 19   **Views on Researcher-Community Engagement in Autism Research in the United Kingdom**................208
Elizabeth Pellicano, Adam Dinsmore, Tony Charman

Chapter 20   **Protein Interaction Networks Reveal Novel Autism Risk Genes within
GWAS Statistical Noise**..**219**
Catarina Correia, Guiomar Oliveira, Astrid M. Vicente

Permissions

List of Contributors

Index

Preface

Autism is categorized under neurodevelopmental disorders. It is commonly diagnosed in infants at an early stage by symptoms like impaired communication and interaction. This book discusses the fundamentals as well as modern approaches to understand and study this disorder. The text provides significant information of this discipline to help develop a good understanding of autism and related fields. From theories to research to practical applications, case studies related to all contemporary topics of relevance to this field have been included herein. Also, included in this book are the different techniques that are used to diagnose and treat autism like pediatric neuropathology, metabolic and neuroimaging tools to name few. This book is an invaluable source of information for researchers and experts working in this field.

The researches compiled throughout the book are authentic and of high quality, combining several disciplines and from very diverse regions from around the world. Drawing on the contributions of many researchers from diverse countries, the book's objective is to provide the readers with the latest achievements in the area of research. This book will surely be a source of knowledge to all interested and researching the field.

In the end, I would like to express my deep sense of gratitude to all the authors for meeting the set deadlines in completing and submitting their research chapters. I would also like to thank the publisher for the support offered to us throughout the course of the book. Finally, I extend my sincere thanks to my family for being a constant source of inspiration and encouragement.

Editor

Multiparametric MRI Characterization and Prediction in Autism Spectrum Disorder Using Graph Theory and Machine Learning

Yongxia Zhou[1], Fang Yu[2], Timothy Duong[2]*

1 Department of Radiology, University of Pennsylvania, Philadelphia, Pennsylvania, United States of America, 2 Research Imaging Institute, Departments of Ophthalmology, Radiology, Physiology, University of Texas Health Science Center, South Texas Veterans Health Care System, Department of Veterans Affairs, San Antonio, Texas, United States of America

Abstract

This study employed graph theory and machine learning analysis of multiparametric MRI data to improve characterization and prediction in autism spectrum disorders (ASD). Data from 127 children with ASD (13.5±6.0 years) and 153 age- and gender-matched typically developing children (14.5±5.7 years) were selected from the multi-center Functional Connectome Project. Regional gray matter volume and cortical thickness increased, whereas white matter volume decreased in ASD compared to controls. Small-world network analysis of quantitative MRI data demonstrated decreased global efficiency based on gray matter cortical thickness but not with functional connectivity MRI (fcMRI) or volumetry. An integrative model of 22 quantitative imaging features was used for classification and prediction of phenotypic features that included the autism diagnostic observation schedule, the revised autism diagnostic interview, and intelligence quotient scores. Among the 22 imaging features, four (caudate volume, caudate-cortical functional connectivity and inferior frontal gyrus functional connectivity) were found to be highly informative, markedly improving classification and prediction accuracy when compared with the single imaging features. This approach could potentially serve as a biomarker in prognosis, diagnosis, and monitoring disease progression.

Editor: Huafu Chen, University of Electronic Science and Technology of China, China

Funding: The authors reported no current external funding sources for this study.

Competing Interests: The authors have declared that no competing interests exist.

* E-mail: duongt@uthscsa.edu

Introduction

Autism spectrum disorders (ASD) are a group of polygenetic developmental brain disorders with behavioral and cognitive impairment [1]. Affected individuals exhibit stereotypical repetitive movements, restricted interests, lack of impulse control, speech deficits, impaired intelligence and social skills compared to typically developing (TD) children [2]. The underlying neurological changes and their association with the clinical manifestations remain an active area of research.

Imaging studies have been instrumental in mapping aberrant connections in the brains of ASD children. Several studies revealed both structural and functional connectivity deficits in ASD [3,4]. Structural connectivity derived from diffusion tensor imaging in ASD children demonstrate increased diffusivity and/or reduced fractional anisotropy in the long occipitofrontal fasciculus and inter-hemispheric corpus callosal (e.g., minor and major forceps) commissure [5], asymmetric and under-connected arcuate fasciculus language pathways [6,7], as well as reduced cerebellar-cortical interconnectivity [8]. Functional connectivity MRI (fcMRI) shows abnormal dis-inhibition of some subcortical circuits [9], over- or under-connectivity in the superior temporal gyrus and amygdala [10]. The caudate nucleus, which plays an important role in behavior impulsivity control, novelty seeking trait, procedural skill learning, and memory function [11], has been reported to increase in volume and its functional connectivity to the cortices is enhanced in autistic adolescents and young adults [12,13]. These abnormal caudate volume and caudate-cortical connectivity have been associated with repetitive autistic behaviors [12,13].

A key clinical manifestation of ASD is impaired learning and social interactions [14]. Mirror mechanisms in frontoparietal and sensorimotor networks are involved in the imitation of others' actions in normal subjects [15], and have been suggested to be dysfunctional in children with ASD [16,17]. In addition, neural networks underlying reflective mentalization [18] as well as emotional and interoceptive awareness [19] may be impaired in ASD. The default mode network (DMN) that consists of the medial frontal, posterior cingulate gyri and the temporo-parietal connection (which is involved in self awareness, social integration, learning and memory functions [20] and is usually deactivated under cognitive-demanded task conditions) has been found to be deficient in ASD children as well [21]. Furthermore such DMN dysfunction has been associated with decreased volumes of the structures involved [21].

The inferior frontal gyrus (IFG), which is involved in high-level memory, language production and comprehension, and learning interactions [22–24], has been reported to be abnormal in ASD children. Within the IFG, the pars opercularis plays a role in social interactions including imitation control [25], while the pars

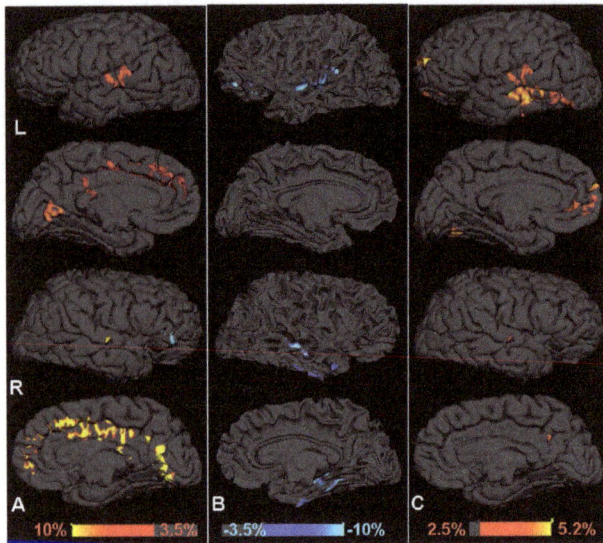

Figure 1. Regions with significant volume percentage increment (A, red color) in gray matter, and volume decrement in gray matter (A, blue color) as well as white matter volume reduction (B, blue color) in autism compared to controls (P<0.01). Significant cortical thickness increment in percentage change in autism compared to controls is shown in C with red color (P<0.01). Both medial and lateral views on sagittal surface in the left and right hemispheres of an individual control subject are shown for gray matter volume (A), white matter volume (B) and cortical thickness (C) comparison between autistic children and controls. The percentage change of volume in autism was calculated as the mean difference between volumes of two groups normalized with individual supratentorial volume and scaled by the mean normalized volume of control group.

triangularis is associated with language comprehension [26]. Task-related fMRI results have demonstrated IFG abnormalities in ASD patients, including impaired social function and affective emotion [27,28]. FcMRI shows decreased functional connectivity in IFG inhibitory circuits, consistent with disruption of mirror neurons and their projections involved in social communication and language development [29,30].

Given the large amount of anatomical and functional connectivity imaging data, a unified model integrating multiple imaging measures may be helpful to better characterize ASD and predict the phenotypic outcome [31]. Small-world network analysis based on graph theory offers some advantages in analyzing complex and multidimensional data by providing global and local inter-regional modulation information of structural and functional brain networks [32]. A potential challenge is the possibility of retrieval redundancy ("curse of dimensionality"). Principal component analysis is a feature selection method that has been widely used to reduce dimensionality by identifying essential components in the data structure, while retaining most of the data variation (i.e., information) [33]. Maximal relevance and minimal redundancy (mRMR) [34] is another feature selection algorithm to reduce dimensionality which uses filters based on mutual information and correlation to account for maximal dependency and minimal redundancy.

The goals of this study were: i) to evaluate multi-parametric functional and structural MRI of the brain in ASD versus TD children using small-world network analysis based on graph theory to derive local and global efficiency, ii) to use machine-learning algorithms to evaluate the ability of these multiparametric MRI

matrices to classify ASD versus TD groups, and iii) to employ machine-learning algorithms of these multiparametric MRI matrices to predict ASD clinical phenotypic outcomes, such as the revised autism diagnostic interview (ADI-R), autism diagnostic observation schedule (ADOS), and intelligence quotient (IQ) scores reflecting different aspects of social and learning abilities of subjects [35].

Methods

Participants and phenotypic information and MRI Imaging

Data was obtained from the multi-center Functional Connectome Project, which released MRI data of over 500 ASD patients (http://fcon_1000.projects.nitrc.org/indi/abide/). We downloaded the Autism Brain Imaging Data Exchange database from the COINS website (http://coins.mrn.org/) that hosted copies of data samples. In accordance with HIPAA guidelines and 1000 Functional Connectomes Project/INDI protocols, all datasets were de-identified. Consistent with the policies of the 1000 Functional Connectomes Project, data usage was approved for research purposes.

127 children with ASD (mean age: 13.5 ± 6.0 years, 24.1% of female), 153 age- and gender-matched control TD children (mean age: 14.5 ± 5.7 years, 24.8% of female) from the NYU/Yale/Stanford centers were selected for analyses based on age ranges. The full IQ scores were slightly lower in the ASD (104.3 ± 18.9) compared to the TD group (111.7 ± 14.4), with $P = 0.001$. Imaging data consisted of high spatial resolution 3D T1-based MPRAGE sequence (image size $= 160\times256\times256$, resolution $= 1\times1\times1$ mm^3) and resting-state (RS)-fMRI obtained using a gradient echo EPI sequence (TR $= 2000$ msec, resolution $= 3\times3\times4$ mm^3, 180 volumes) with 33 slices covering the whole cerebrum.

The corresponding clinical data from five categories were also obtained, consisting of the ADOS scores, the ADI-R, and IQ tests (full scale and sub-functionality), social responsiveness scale (SRS) and Vinland adaptive behavior scale (VABS) with five domains. Detailed information regarding the phenotypic data was outlined in previously published articles [10,14]. Briefly, the ADI-R is composed of 93 items focusing on the triadic functional domains, and administered via interview with categorical results provided. The full IQ tests evaluated both verbal IQ (VIQ) and performance IQ (PIQ). The ADOS is a semi-structured assessment of social affection and communication behaviors, using four modules to account for individual expressive language level and chronological age. The SRS rating scale measures the social ability of ASD children (including total and subdomains of cognition, communication, awareness and motivation). The VABS instrument consists of social and personal skills for everyday living, including subdomains such as interpersonal empathy and socialization.

Image Processing and Data Analysis

Preprocessing: Standard preprocessing for RS-fMRI data analysis was performed using both FMRIB Software Library (FSL) and Analysis of Functional NeuroImages (AFNI) software packages with adapted scripts (http://www.nitrc.org/projects/fcon_1000). The steps included standard realignment, spatial Gaussian smoothing with full width at half maximum (FWHM) of 6 mm, band pass temporal filtering of 0.005–0.1 Hz, co-registration with the MPRAGE images, removal of nuisance signals (motion parameters, the global signal, and signals derived from cerebrospinal fluid and white matter), and non-linear transformation to Montreal Neurological Institute (MNI) standard space. For instance, in order to control for motion artifacts, regression and

Table 1. Significant regional volume differences (P<0.01) comparing children with autism spectrum disorder (ASD) to age-matched typically developing (TD) children after supratentorial volume normalization.

Region and Location	V1- TD Children	V2- ASD Children	P value (**)	Percentage change %(Δ1)
Frontal GM				
Left inferior	0.852	0.938	0.0068	10.094%
Left superior	18.97	20.05	0.0010*	5.693%
Right superior	18.18	19.12	0.0034*	5.171%
Right medial orbital olfactory	1.204	1.104	0.0034*	−8.306%
Frontal WM–left lateral orbitofrontal	5.761	5.562	0.0090*	−3.454%
Occipital GM				
Left middle	4.941	5.292	0.0056*	7.104%
Left superior	2.623	2.902	0.0002*	10.637%
Right superior	3.279	3.582	0.0017*	9.241%
Parietal GM				
Left postcentral	3.961	4.230	0.0064	6.791%
Right superior	5.482	5.888	0.0054*	7.406%
Right postcentral	3.996	4.319	0.0020*	8.083%
Right precuneus	6.495	7.031	0.0006*	8.253%
Parietal WM				
Left postcentral	5.771	5.483	0.0074	−4.990%
Right supramarginal	7.791	7.410	0.0054*	−4.890%
Temporal WM				
Left fusiform	5.811	5.567	0.0085	−4.199%
Right inferior	5.157	4.890	0.0023*	−5.177%
Right superior	5.779	5.543	0.0058*	−4.084%

Note-Data (V1, V2) are mean brain volumes after normalization to the supratentorial volume with a scale factor of 1000, no unit.
**Calculated with two-sample t test to obtain original p-value (shown with P<0.01) between two groups, and with Bonferroni multiple region correction (x8 factor given 4 brain lobes in two hemispheres).
*Indicates a significant difference with corrected P<0.05 after Bonferroni adjustment.
Δ1 Indicates percentage change between volume of ASD children (V2) and volume of TD children (V1), calculated as Δ1 = (V2-V1)/V1*100%.

residual analyses of six motion parameters including three angular rotations (roll, pitch, and yaw in units of degrees) and three directional displacements (x,y,z in units of mm) were implemented in the preprocessing step.

Volumetry analysis

Anatomical data were processed to derive the total supratentorial volume, regional subcortical volumes (45 regions), white matter (WM) volumes (70 regions), and cortical gray matter (GM) volumes (148 regions) using Freesurfer software (version 5.1.0) [36]. Regional volume comparisons were implemented after supratentorial volume normalization. The cortical thickness of 148 cortical regions was measured automatically based on minimal communication distance between the gray and white matter ribbon of the projected cortical surface [37]. Thickness measured with Freesurfer has been shown to be especially useful in characterizing the cortical folding and cytoarchitecture shaping in different age ranges [38].

fcMRI analysis

The seed-based fcMRI was derived with seeds in the bilateral pars triangularis and opercularis regions of the IFG, the caudate, and the DMN core seed in the MNI 2 mm template space. These seed regions or networks were selected based on previously reported abnormalities in ASD [12,13,27,28]. The total number of

voxels (N) and average correlational z-value (Z) were computed from the functional connectivity map of each seed using a threshold of cluster corrected P<0.05. The statistical multiple-comparison correction was done based on Gaussian random field (GRF) theory and implemented with the FSL easythresh command using empirical minimum Z>2.3 threshold with cluster significance of P<0.05. In addition, to examine the functional interhemispheric coordination, voxel-mirrored homotopic correlations (VMHC) were derived. The global VMHC voxel number (minimum Z>2.3; cluster significance P<0.05, corrected) and average Z-value were then quantified [39].

fALFF analysis

Fractional amplitude of low frequency fluctuation (fALFF) of the fcMRI data at 0.01–0.08 Hz, which reflects spontaneous neuronal or functional activity, was analyzed with adapted scripts in FSL and AFNI [39].

Graph theory via small-world network analysis

Inter-regional correlations of individual fMRI time courses of 112 bilateral cortical and subcortical ROIs based on functional parcellation in FSL template space [40] were derived. Graph theory-based small-world network analysis for absolute and relative, local and global efficiency quantification at different connectivity sparsity levels, was then performed for each subject

Table 2. Cortical thickness increment (in a degree of 2.5–5%) comparing autism spectrum disorder (ASD) children to age-matched typically developing (TD) children (P<0.01).

Region and Location	C1- TD Children	C2- ASD Children	P value (**)	Percentage change%(Δ2)
Frontal				
Left anterior cingulum	2.908	3.031	0.0008*	4.230%
Left mid-anterior cingulum	2.875	2.985	0.0004*	3.826%
Left transverse pole	2.982	3.119	0.0083	4.594%
Occipital				
Left middle	2.795	2.939	0.0002*	5.152%
Left superior	2.341	2.453	0.0056*	4.784%
Left lingual	2.215	2.308	0.0089	4.199%
Left middle lunatus	2.118	2.220	0.0026*	4.816%
Right lingual	2.287	2.383	0.0031*	4.198%
Right calcarine	2.129	2.231	0.0023*	4.791%
Parietal				
Left inferior angular	3.036	3.166	0.0016*	4.282%
Left inferior supramar	2.987	3.107	0.0004*	4.017%
Left rectus	2.807	2.903	0.0089	3.420%
Left post-lateral fissure	2.616	2.718	0.0018*	3.900%
Left occipital junction	2.428	2.531	0.0060*	4.242%
Left postcentral	2.338	2.444	0.0036*	4.534%
Right postcentral	2.311	2.423	0.0029*	4.846%
Temporal				
Left superior	2.691	2.792	0.0009*	3.753%
Right superior	2.731	2.806	0.0089	2.746%

Note-Data (C1, C2) are mean cortical thickness in mm.
**Calculated with two-sample t test to obtain original p-value (shown with P<0.01) between two groups, and with Bonferroni multiple region correction (x8 factor given 4 brain lobes in two hemispheres).
*Indicates a significant difference with corrected P<0.05 after Bonferroni adjustment.
Δ2 Indicates percentage change between cortical thickness of ASD children (C2) and cortical thickness of TD children (C1), calculated as Δ2 = (C2–C1)/C1*100%.

[32]. Group differences of mean local and global efficiency parameters derived from in-house software were compared with a 2-sample t-test. The inter-regional correlations of group-wise cortical thickness based on 148 bilateral cortical regions and volumetry measured with Freesurfer (148 cortical regions, as well as 115 subcortical and white matter regions) were also derived, and small world network analysis based on structural measures (including relative and absolute local as well as global efficiency parameters) was then performed and compared between the two groups.

Integration model for two-group classification

To reduce possible classifier overfitting and improve generalization, feature selection was performed in two steps. First, principal component analysis was used to decompose the covariance matrix of the imaging features using the singular value decomposition program in Matlab (release 2010b; MathWorks, Natick, Mass) [33] after variance normalization. Then the number of sorted components based on singular values that contained 99% or 95% of the information from the covariance matrix of all features was determined. Finally, an advanced feature selection algorithm, based on mutual-information and integration of both mRMR criteria [34], was used to select imaging features based on the number of features (components) determined via principal component analysis.

A total of 22 quantitative local and global imaging features were generated from the structural and functional datasets based on preliminary data showing statistical differences between the two groups. These features include: i) volumes of 9 local subcortical regions (the bilateral caudate, thalami, pallidum, hippocampi and cerebellum), ii) 8 features from the fcMRI voxel number N and average Z values seeding from the bilateral caudate, bilateral IFG pars opercularis and triangularis, and DMN core seeds respectively, iii) 3 fALFF values (averaged values from the bilateral caudate, IFG pars opercularis, and IFG pars triangularis), and iv) global VMHC voxel number (corrected P<0.05) and average Z value (subtotal of 2 features).

To differentiate the two groups based on the selected imaging features, a total of 67 available classifiers, including support vector machine (SVM), Bayes network (BayesNet), radial basis function (RBF), and sequential minimal optimization (SMO) algorithms, were tested with batch-mode scripts developed in WEKA software (http://www.cs.waikato.ac.nz/ml/weka, version 3.6.7).

To evaluate each classifier, a cross validation method with different folds (numbering from 2 to 10) or percentage splits (from 10% to 90%) was applied to the training data set as well as to the whole dataset in WEKA software. After the dataset was randomly reordered and splitted into n folds of equal size, one fold was used for testing and the other n-1 folds were used for training the classifier for each iteration. The performances of these classifiers

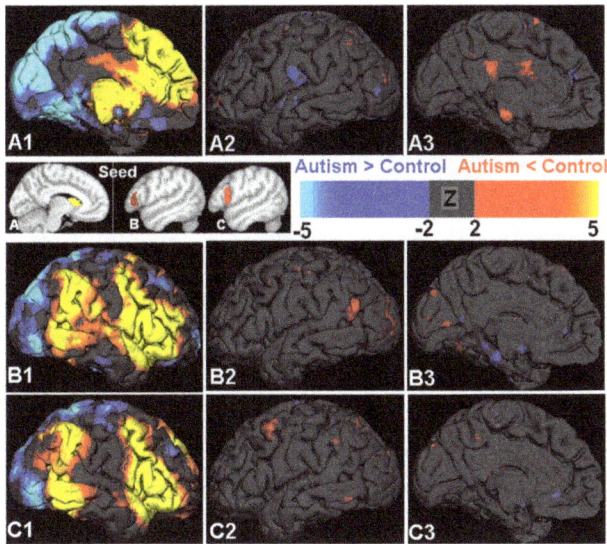

Figure 2. The functional connectivity network seeding from caudate and IFG region are demonstrated. In controls, the caudate-cortical network showed positive connections with the frontal and subcortical regions, and negative connections with the posterior visual and parietal areas (A1). The caudate-cortical network in children with ASD showed a primary reduction of cingulum and middle temporal connectivity (red color), but increased connectivity in several regions including the inferior and dorso-latero frontal areas (blue color, A2-A3). The functional connectivity network seeding from the IFG pars trianglaris in controls (B1) showed positive connections with the frontal and temporal regions and negative connections with the posterior visual and superior parietal areas. Difference of connectivity pattern comparing autism to controls seeded from pars triangularis are shown in B2 and B3, with some reductions of visual and temporal connectivity in autism (red) and increments in the regions including medial temporal areas (blue). Functional connectivity seeding from IFG pars opercularis is shown in C1–C3, with primarily decreased connectivity in autism in the superior frontal regions. Seed regions are shown in the upper left images, and all statistical results were obtained with the threshold of minimal Z>2.3; cluster significance, P<0.05, corrected.

were further assessed in WEKA by using margin curves and threshold curves to show the cumulative probability of difference between true and false positives as a function of population size.

Correlational analysis between imaging and phenotypic data

Quantitative analysis of single imaging features of regional volume, N and Z from fcMRI, as well as the combined selected imaging features were correlated with the clinical data (i.e., ADOS, ADI-R, SRS, VABS, and IQ tests including both full and sub-domain scores). Bonferroni adjustment was implemented by multiplying the original p-values with both the number of category tests (x5 in this study) and the number of sub-domain tests (e.g., x10 for ADOS, x3 for IQ, x5 for ADI-R, x7 for SRS and x15 for VABS) of each category.

Integration model of imaging data for phenotypic prediction

To improve previous phenotypic correlation with multiparametric imaging data, regression analysis in WEKA (i.e., prediction of clinical data from imaging metrics) between the imaging features and clinical data was implemented. A total of 23 available advanced regression models were evaluated. These regressors were divided into seven families: Kstar, linear and non-linear ZeroR rule-based regressors, decision stump trees, and Gaussian process classifiers for full data sets. For example, Kstar was taken as an instance or memory based classifier using entropy and similarity functions with the advantage of updating models based on relevance to the previously established database [41].

Results

Volumetry analysis

Volume and cortical thickness differences between the ASD and TD groups are shown in **Figure 1** and **Table 1**. A key finding is that the ASD group demonstrated significantly larger GM volume (with exception of the right medial orbital olfactory region) but less WM volume compared to the TD group. Consistent with GM volumetric findings, the ASD group also showed significantly increased cortical thickness (**Table 2**).

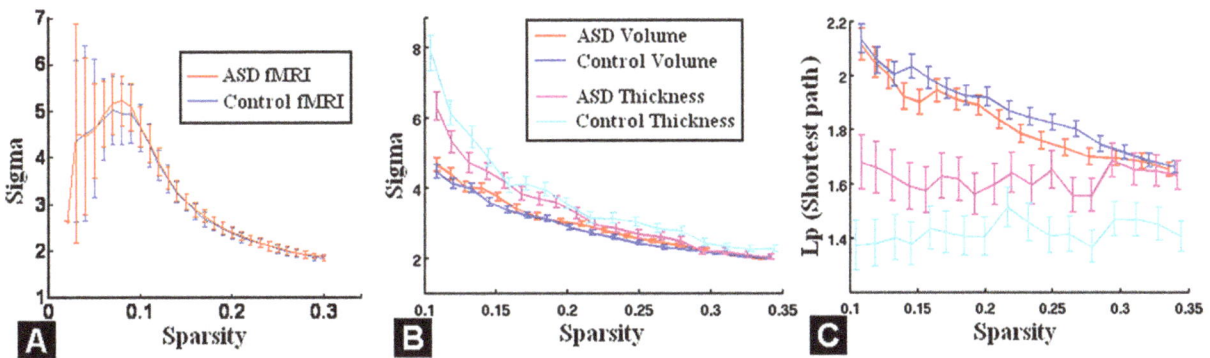

Figure 3. A: Small-world network analysis based on fMRI data showed similar efficiency (including both local and global) between children with ASD and TD controls. Small-worldness analysis based on regional volume (red and blue colors) showed no significant differences of total efficiency (B) and global efficiency (C) between children with ASD and controls neither. However, small-worldness analysis based on structural cortical thickness measure showed reduced total efficiency (B), specifically decreased global efficiency (i.e. shortest path length) (C) in ASD group (magenta color) compared to TD group (cyan color). Error bar denotes standard deviation at each sparsity level after scaling to a random network with the same number of degree.

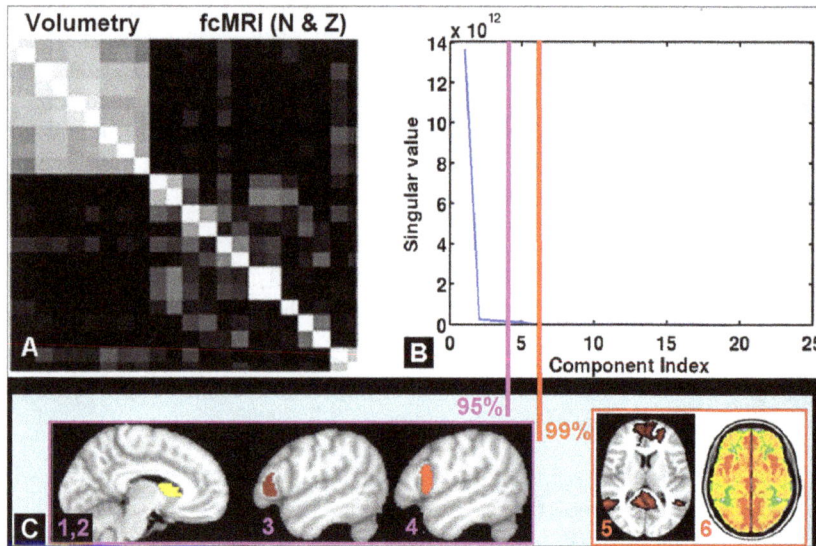

Figure 4. A: Co-variance matrix of 22 quantitative imaging features showed highly-correlated structural metrics (i.e. volumetry) of 9 regions, and strong association between average Z-value and voxel number N-value of fcMRI for each region (or global metric). B: principal component analysis decomposition of the covariance matrix showing most (>95%) data variation (information) was contained with 4 primary components (pink color) and 99% data information was contained in 6 primary components (red color). C: The four imaging features selected via mRMR criteria were right caudate volume (1), the fcMRI average Z values seeded from bilateral caudate (2), bilateral IFG pars opercularis (3) and IFG pars triangularis (4). Together with the four imaging features selected, the DMN average Z (5) and the VMHC average Z (6) were the other two imaging features selected for 99% criteria.

fcMRI analysis

With seeding in the caudate, the ASD children demonstrated reduced functional connectivity in the cingulum and middle temporal cortex compared to TD children, but increased connectivity in several regions including the inferior and dorso-lateral frontal areas (**Figure 2A**). With seeding in the IFG pars triangularis, the ASD group showed reduced fcMRI of visual and temporal regions, but increased in the medial temporal areas (**Figure 2B**). With seeding from the IFG pars opercularis, the ASD group predominantly exhibited reduced functional connectivity with the superior frontal regions (corrected P<0.05; **Figure 2C**).

Graph theory via small-world network analysis

Small-worldness analysis showed no statistically significant difference in the mean total (local and global) efficiency between ASD and TD children based on fcMRI (**Figure 3A**) and volumetric data (**Figure 3B,C**). However, there was reduced total efficiency in ASD children (**Figure 3B**) based on cortical thickness, especially in global efficiency, as indicated by increased shortest path lengths (**Figure 3C**).

Classification of ASD and TD groups

Co-variance matrix of the 22 imaging features (**Figure 4A**) showed correlated intra-module volumetry of 9 subcortical regions, as well as a strong association between the average Z-value and the voxel number of fcMRI, both regionally and globally. However, the inter-module correlation was not significant (r<0.3), suggesting volumetry and fcMRI provided complementary information. Singular value decomposition of the co-variance matrix (**Figure 4B**) found that 4 primary components accounted for >95% data variation, and 6 primary components accounted for >99% data variation. The four primary features were the right caudate volume, fcMRI Z values seeded from the bilateral caudate, IFG pars opercularis, and IFG pars triangularis; the additional two features were the mean Z score maps of the DMN and VMHC (**Figure 4C**).

For the 6 imaging features selected by the mRMR algorithm, the random tree classifier had the highest classification accuracy (100%) for correctly identifying ASD patients with the full dataset, and 70% accuracy for differentiating ASD patients from TD children using 80% percentage split cross validation. Based on the 4 imaging features, the random tree classifier also had the highest accuracy (98%) for the full dataset for two-group classification, with 68% accuracy for 10-fold cross validation. The performance of the 6-feature classifier was slightly better than that of the 4-

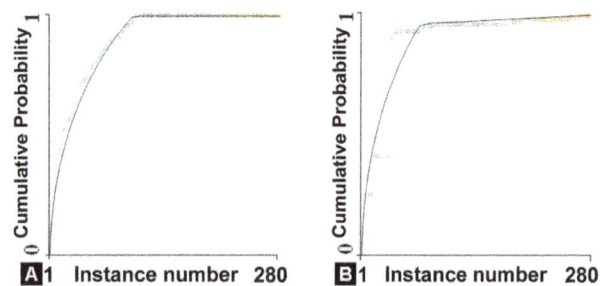

Figure 5. Margin curves showing the cumulative probability of difference between true positive (sensitivity) and false positive (1-specificity) as a function of instance number (i.e. subject number) for 4-feature classification (A) and 6-feature classification (B) based on full dataset. As expected, the 6-feature classifier performed slightly better than 4-feature classifier with faster convergence and more margins maintained.

Table 3. Significant correlations between each single MRI quantitative metric and phenotypic tests in children with autism spectrum disorder (P<0.05), adjusted with number of available patients for each test.

MRI metric	Phenotypic Test	r	p
Caudate fcMRI (N)	ADOS social affection	−0.44	0.005
	ADOS research	−0.43	0.005
	VABS socialization	0.35	<0.0001*
	VABS interpersonal skill	−0.30	<0.0001*
	IQ (full)	−0.47	0.034
Caudate fcMRI (Z)	IQ (full)	−0.47	0.034
	VABS socialization	0.35	<0.0001*
	VABS interpersonal skill	−0.44	<0.0001*
	VABS daily living standard	0.26	0.0005*
IFG triangularis fcMRI (N)	ADOS module	−0.57	0.0016
	ADOS total	−0.46	0.014
	ADOS communication	−0.47	0.04
	ADOS research	−0.47	0.04
	VABS interpersonal skill	−0.43	<0.0001*
IFG opercularis fcMRI (N)	ADOS module	−0.64	0.0002
IFG opercularis fcMRI (Z)	ADOS module	−0.50	0.007
	VABS socialization	0.34	0.0001*
	VABS interpersonal skill	−0.25	0.0006*

Note: N is the total number of voxels and Z is the average correlational z-value computed from the functional connectivity map (fcMRI) of each seed using a threshold of cluster corrected P<0.05.
*Indicates a significant difference with corrected P<0.05 after Bonferroni adjustment, with multiplication factors determined by both the number of category tests applied (x5 in this study) and the number of sub-domain tests (e.g., x10 for ADOS, x3 for IQ, and x15 for VABS) of each category.

feature classifier, with faster convergence and higher margins (i.e. better accuracy) maintained (**Figure 5**).

Correlation Analysis

Table 3 summarizes the correlation analysis of the quantitative imaging features with phenotypic scores in ASD children, with both uncorrected and multiple-comparison corrected p-values. Significant correlations were found: i) between the number of connections N based on fcMRI from the caudate and the full scale IQ in ASD children (r = −0.47, P = 0.034), ii) between caudate fcMRI N and ADOS scales (r≤−0.43, P<0.005), iii) between caudate fcMRI N and VABS social skill scores (r = 0.35, P<0.001), iv) between caudate fcMRI N and VABS interpersonal skills (r = − 0.3, P<0.001), v) between the caudate connectivity strength, Z score and the full scale IQ (r = −0.47, P = 0.034), vi) between caudate fcMRI Z and VABS scores (P<0.001), vii) between the connections (both N and Z) from the two IFG seeds and ADOS tests (r≤−0.46, P≤0.04), and viii) between the functional connections from the two IFG seeds and VABS scores (P<0.001).

Integration model for prediction

As for prediction, multiple combined imaging features in each domain showed improved correlations with clinical data compared to single imaging features for ASD children. For instance, fcMRI seeding from the pars opercularis of IFG showed a correlation coefficient of −0.64 between ADOS score and single imaging features (**Figure 6 A1–A5**). The correlation coefficient was significantly improved with four selected imaging features to predict clinical phenotypic data. The fitted score using the Kstar classifier showed tight coupling (linear slope = 1, r = 0.95, P< 0.0001) to the original ADOS module score, with only a few

outliers (**Figure 6B**). Similarly, among all regressors, Kstar also showed the best predictive power for highly correlating with other phenotypic data including full IQ test (r = 0.94, P<0.0001) and ADI-R total score (r = 0.97, P<0.0001) when using the four as well as six essential imaging features.

Discussion

We applied advanced automatic classification and machine learning algorithms to multiparametric functional connectivity and structural data (i.e., volumetry and cortical thickness) to improve characterization and prediction in autism spectrum disorders. The major findings of this study were: 1) small-world network analysis based on volumetry and fcMRI did not find differences between ASD and TD children, while small-world network analysis based on cortical thickness revealed reduced total and global efficiency in ASD, and 2) through advanced machine learning algorithms, four essential imaging features (caudate volume, caudate-cortical fcMRI and IFG pars opercularis as well as triangularis fcMRI) were able to accurately differentiate the two groups and were highly predictive of phenotypic features (e.g. IQ, ADOS and ADI scores) in ASD.

Brain volume and thickness differences

Our findings of GM volume and cortical thickness increases and WM volume decreases in ASD compared to TD group are in general agreement with prior studies [42–44]. The increased cortical thickness in multiple regions throughout the cerebrum, together with decreased WM volumes in frontal and temporal regions, may represent a reduction in long-distance pathways with accompanying local GM volume increments. These changes could

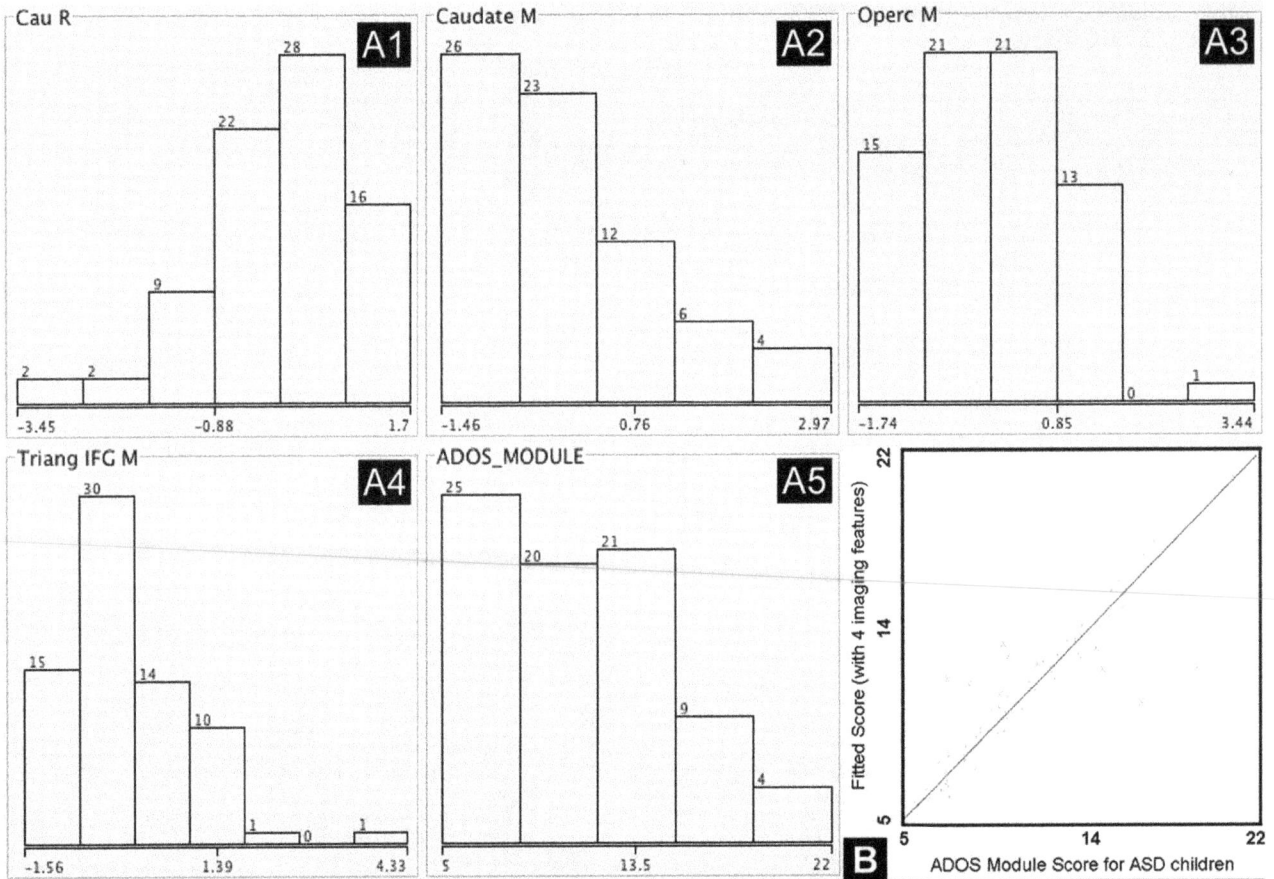

Figure 6. Kstar, an instance (similarity) based classifier for regression analysis had the greatest prediction power for ADOS module score for ASD children among all the regressors combining 4 selected imaging features. A1–A4: standardized histogram distribution showing x-axis as the z-scores of each feature and y-axis being the frequency. A1-right caudate volume, A2-average Z of caudate fcMRI, A3-average Z of IFG opercularis fcMRI, A4-average Z of IFG triangularis fcMRI. A5: phenotypic ADOS module score histogram distribution with x-axis as the original score and y-axis being the frequency. B: The correlation coefficient between integrated imaging features and ADOS module score improved largely from −0.64 based on single best imaging feature to 0.95 combining 4 imaging features. The fitted score using Kstar classifier with 4 selected imaging features showed a tight coupling (linear slope = 1; r = 0.95, P<0.0001) with the original ADOS module score with only a few outliers.

lead to a reduction in global efficiency, consistent with EEG/MEG results [45,46] supporting the hypothesis of unbalanced networks in autism [47].

Functional connectivity differences

Changes in caudate volume, caudate-cortical fcMRI, and IFG fcMRI were found to be highly predictive based on advanced machine learning algorithms. Most of the published literature on classification in autism is based on single imaging measures (such as volume, connectivity, or perfusion) [48–50]. Our integrated multiparametric model demonstrates markedly improved accuracy (i.e., sensitivity and specificity) for classification and prediction.

Consistent with task-based fMRI results [29,30], we found altered IFG functional connectivity, suggesting deficits in the mirror mechanism in autistic children. Disrupted DMN fcMRI and altered interhemispheric functional connectivity are in agreement with previously reported studies in ASD [51,52]. In addition, we found that caudate-cortical connectivity differed between ASD and TD children, and this metric correlated with full-scale IQ scores. A recent study reported aberrant functional connectivity from the caudate seed involving early developing brain areas and implicated developmental derangement of related

functional brain circuits in ASD begin at a young age (from 7–14 years old) [14].

Small-world network analysis of fcMRI could not distinguish between ASD and TD groups, suggesting there might be functional compensatory mechanism in autism, including increased regional functional connectivity and reduced global, long-distance connectivity in ASD. These plasticity changes have been reported in other functional and structural connectome studies. For example, a recent fcMRI study found that there are changes in local efficiency in the posterior cingulum associated with autistic trait accompanied with changes in local tissue integrity in ASD as measured by diffusion tensor imaging [53]. The notion of re-routing of brain structural connectivity has also been reported in less severely cognitively impaired (IQ>70) ASD patients [54]. In particular, they found that these patients utilized more visuospatial processing networks as opposed to linguistically mediated pathways.

Machine learning and prediction

Changes in caudate volume, caudate-cortical fcMRI, and IFG fcMRI were found to be highly predictive based on advanced machine learning algorithms. Most of the published literature on classification in autism has been based on single imaging measures (such as volume, connectivity, or perfusion) [48–50]. Our integrated multiparametric model demonstrates markedly improved accuracy (close to 100% sensitivity and specificity) for classification of ASD from TD groups.

The PCA and mRMR selected key features (i.e. right caudate volume, the average fcMRI Z values seeded from bilateral caudate, bilateral IFG opercularis and triangularis parts, the DMN average Z, and the VMHC average Z) are consistent with previous studies that found changes associated with ASD in each of the six imaging features. Our results based on machine learning algorithms also suggest that caudate volume and connectivity imaging features are important components in the composite score for ASD diagnosis.

Cross-validation minimizes classification error estimation bias and is thus primarily used for small sample datasets. As expected, the classification accuracy dropped from ~100% for the full dataset to ~70% with 10-fold or percentage-split cross-validation. The decreased accuracy in the cross-validation evaluation also reflected the heterogeneity of our data sample and a potential over-fitting problem. Nevertheless, the remarkable improvement in outcome prediction from multiple combined imaging features compared to any single imaging features (r≥0.94, P<0.0001) in all three phenotypic domains supports the notion that these key imaging features are reflective of the behavioral deficits in autism.

Limitations and future works

Although we used substantially large numbers of classifiers and reported the optimal one, our results were limited by the selection criteria. Incorporating other factors such as different feature and subset selection criteria besides PCA and mRMR may improve the classifier performance in the future. The current quantitative fcMRI features include local and network-based features. Further expanding the fcMRI feature space, such as using whole-brain ROI-based fcMRI and fALFF of with dual regression template model [39], may reduce ROI-selection bias. Application of recently developed deep learning algorithms [55] to prevent feature overfitting problems could provide more comprehensive

results. In order to minimize motion-related errors in RS-fMRI data, further investigation of motion parameters, such as frame displacement with dynamic temporal screening criteria, could be implemented in the future [56].

The regional parcellation with Freesurfer used in our study has been shown to be a robust method. However, the results of direct volumetry and cortical thickness could be affected by the normalization errors of projecting individual brains to a template brain, given the younger age range of our subjects compared to the averaged template. Implementing spatial normalization using age-specific templates in Freesurfer is likely important. An additional limitation is that the clinical phenotypic scales were obtained in the first years of life of participants, and not necessarily the period during which they underwent MRI scanning. This may potentially increase the possibility of mismatch between symptoms and brain features.

Conclusion

This study applied advanced automatic classification and machine learning algorithms to multiparametric structural and functional connectivity data to improve characterization and prediction in autism spectrum disorders. A major finding of this study is that the small-world network analysis based on volumetry and fcMRI did not find differences between ASD and TD children, while the small-world network analysis analysis based on cortical thickness revealed reduced total and global efficiency in ASD. Moreover, we also found caudate volume, caudate-cortical fcMRI and IFG pars opercularis as well as triangularis fcMRI to be highly predictive of phenotypic features in ASD. Graph theory and machine learning analysis of multiparametric MRI may prove useful in identifying using imaging biomarkers for disease prognosis and monitoring disease progression in ASD.

Author Contributions

Conceived and designed the experiments: YZ TD. Performed the experiments: YZ FY TD. Analyzed the data: YZ TD. Contributed reagents/materials/analysis tools: YZ TD. Wrote the paper: YZ FY TD.

References

1. Rapin I, Tuchman RF (2008) Autism: definition, neurobiology, screening, diagnosis. Pediatr Clin North Am 55: 1129-1146, viii.
2. Kang S, O'Reilly M, Rojeski L, Blenden K, Xu Z, et al. (2013) Effects of tangible and social reinforcers on skill acquisition, stereotyped behavior, and task engagement in three children with autism spectrum disorders. Res Dev Disabil 34: 739–744.
3. Uddin LQ, Supekar K, Menon V (2013) Reconceptualizing functional brain connectivity in autism from a developmental perspective. Frontiers in Human Neuroscience 7: 1–11.
4. Vissers ME, Cohen MX, Geurts HM (2012) Brain connectivity and high functioning autism: A promising path of research that needs refined models, methodological convergence, and stronger behavioral link. Neuroscience and Biobehavioral Reviews 36: 604–625.
5. Travers BG, Adluru N, Ennis C, Tromp do PM, Destiche D, et al. (2012) Diffusion tensor imaging in autism spectrum disorder: a review. Autism Res 5: 289–313.
6. Lange N, Dubray MB, Lee JE, Froimowitz MP, Froehlich A, et al. (2010) Atypical diffusion tensor hemispheric asymmetry in autism. Autism Res 3: 350–358.
7. Fletcher PT, Whitaker RT, Tao R, DuBray MB, Froehlich A, et al. (2010) Microstructural connectivity of the arcuate fasciculus in adolescents with high-functioning autism. Neuroimage 51: 1117–1125.
8. Sivaswamy L, Kumar A, Rajan D, Behen M, Muzik O, et al. (2010) A diffusion tensor imaging study of the cerebellar pathways in children with autism spectrum disorder. J Child Neurol 25: 1223–1231.
9. Langen M, Schnack HG, Nederveen H, Bos D, Lahuis BE, et al. (2009) Changes in the developmental trajectories of striatum in autism. Biol Psychiatry 66: 327–333.
10. Di Martino A, Kelly C, Grzadzinski R, Zuo XN, Mennes M, et al. (2011) Aberrant striatal functional connectivity in children with autism. Biol Psychiatry 69: 847–856.
11. Huang YY, Mei ZT (1983) [The role of the caudate nucleus in learning, memory and conditioning activity]. Sheng Li Ke Xue Jin Zhan 14: 356–358.
12. Langen M, Durston S, Staal WG, Palmen SJ, van Engeland H (2007) Caudate nucleus is enlarged in high-functioning medication-naive subjects with autism. Biol Psychiatry 62: 262–266.
13. Turner KC, Frost L, Linsenbardt D, McIlroy JR, Muller RA (2006) Atypically diffuse functional connectivity between caudate nuclei and cerebral cortex in autism. Behav Brain Funct 2: 34.
14. Di Martino A, Ross K, Uddin LQ, Sklar AB, Castellanos FX, et al. (2009) Functional brain correlates of social and nonsocial processes in autism spectrum disorders: an activation likelihood estimation meta-analysis. Biol Psychiatry 65: 63–74.
15. Hamilton AF (2013) Reflecting on the mirror neuron system in autism: a systematic review of current theories. Dev Cogn Neurosci 3: 91–105.
16. Gallese V, Rochat MJ, Berchio C (2012) The mirror mechanism and its potential role in autism spectrum disorder. DEVELOPMENTAL MEDICINE & CHILD NEUROLOGY 55: 15–22.
17. Rizzolatti G, Febbri-Destro M (2003) Mirror neurons: from discovery to autism. Exp Brain Res 2010: 223–237.
18. Frith U (2001) Mind blindness and the brain in autism. Neuron 32: 969–979.
19. Ebisch SJ, Gallese V, Willems RM, Mantini D, Groen WB, et al. (2011) Altered intrinsic functional connectivity of anterior and posterior insula regions in high-functioning participants with autism spectrum disorder. Human Brain Mapping 32: 1013–1028.
20. Fox MD, Raichle ME (2007) Spontaneous fluctuations in brain activity observed with functional magnetic resonance imaging. Nat Rev Neuroscience 8: 700–711.
21. Kennedy DP, Redcay E, Courchesne E (2006) Failing to deactivate: resting functional abnormalities in autism. Proc Natl Acad Sci U S A 103: 8275–8280.
22. Greenlee JD, Oya H, Kawasaki H, Volkov IO, Severson MA 3rd, et al. (2007) Functional connections within the human inferior frontal gyrus. J Comp Neurol 503: 550–559.

23. Nixon P, Lazarova J, Hodinott-Hill I, Gough P, Passingham R (2004) The inferior frontal gyrus and phonological processing: an investigation using rTMS. J Cogn Neurosci 16: 289–300.
24. Hsieh L, Gandour J, Wong D, Hutchins GD (2001) Functional heterogeneity of inferior frontal gyrus is shaped by linguistic experience. Brain Lang 76: 227–252.
25. Rudie JD, Shehzad Z, Hernandez LM, Colich NL, Bookheimer SY, et al. Reduced functional integration and segregation of distributed neural systems underlying social and emotional information processing in autism spectrum disorders. Cereb Cortex 22: 1025–1037.
26. Geva S, Jones PS, Crinion JT, Price CJ, Baron JC, et al. The neural correlates of inner speech defined by voxel-based lesion-symptom mapping. Brain 134: 3071–3082.
27. Bastiaansen JA, Thioux M, Nanetti L, van der Gaag C, Ketelaars C, et al. (2011) Age-Related Increase in Inferior Frontal Gyrus Activity and Social Functioning in Autism Spectrum Disorder. Biol Psychiatry 69: 8320838.
28. Depretto M, Davies MS, Pfeifer JH, Scott AA, Sigman M, et al. (2006) Understanding emotions in others: mirror neuron dysfunction in children with autism spectrum disorders. Nat Neuroscience 9: 28–30.
29. Villalobos ME, Mizuno A, Dahl BC, Kemmotsu N, Muller RA (2005) Reduced functional connectivity between V1 and inferior frontal cortex associated with visuomotor performance in autism. Neuroimage 25: 916–925.
30. Lee PS, Yerys BE, Della Rosa A, Foss-Feig J, Barnes KA, et al. (2009) Functional connectivity of the inferior frontal cortex changes with age in children with autism spectrum disorders: a fcMRI study of response inhibition. Cereb Cortex 19: 1787–1794.
31. Di Martino A, Yan C-G, Li Q, Denio E, Castellanos FX, et al. (2013) The autism brain imaging data exchange: towards a large-scale evaluation of the intrinsic brain architecture in autism. Molecular Psychiatry 2013: 1–9.
32. Zhou Y, Lui YW (2013) Small world properties in mild cognitive impairment and early Alzheimer's disease. ISRN Geriatrics 2013:542080.
33. Elliott MA, Walter GA, Swift A, Vandenborne K, Schotland JC, et al. (1999) Spectral quantitation by principal component analysis using complex singular value decomposition. Magn Reson Med 41: 450–455.
34. Peng H, Long F, Ding C (2005) Feature selection based on mutual information: criteria of max-dependency, max-relevance, and min-redundancy. IEEE Trans Pattern Anal Mach Intell 27: 1226–1238.
35. Buitelaar JK, van der Wees M, Swaab-Barneveld H, van der Gagg RJ (1999) Verbal memory and performance IQ predict theory of mind and emotion recognition ability in children with autistic spectrum disorders and in psychiatric control children. J Child Psychol Psychiatry 40: 869–881.
36. Fischl B (2012) FreeSurfer. Neuroimage 62: 774–781.
37. Fischl B, Dale AM (2000) Measuring the thickness of the human cerebral cortex from magnetic resonance images. Proc Natl Acad Sci U S A 97: 11050–11055.
38. Sowell ER, Peterson BS, Kan E, Woods RP, Yoshii J, et al. (2007) Sex differences in cortical thickness mapped in 176 healthy individuals between 7 and 87 years of age. Cereb Cortex 17: 1550–1560.
39. Zhou Y, Milham M, Zuo XN, Kelly C, Jaggi H, et al. (2013) Functional Homotopic Changes in Multiple Sclerosis with Resting-State Functional MR Imaging. AJNR Am J Neuroradiol 34: 1180–1187.
40. Stark DE, Margulies DS, Shehzad ZE, Reiss P, Kelly AM, et al. (2008) Regional variation in interhemispheric coordination of intrinsic hemodynamic fluctuations. J Neurosci 28: 13754–13764.
41. Gagliardi F (2011) Instance-based classifiers applied to medical databases: diagnosis and knowledge extraction. Artif Intell Med 52: 123–139.
42. Ecker C, Ginestet C, Feng Y, Johnston P, Lombardo MV, et al. (2013) Brain surface anatomy in adults with autism: the relationship between surface area, cortical thickness, and autistic symptoms. JAMA Psychiatry 70: 59–70.
43. Ecker C, Stahl D, Daly E, Johnston P, Thomson A, et al. (2009) Is there a common underlying mechanism for age-related decline in cortical thickness? Neuroreport 20: 1155–1160.
44. Hardan AY, Muddasani S, Vemulapalli M, Keshavan MS, Minshew NJ (2006) An MRI study of increased cortical thickness in autism. Am J Psychiatry 163: 1290–1292.
45. Khan S, Gramfort A, Shetty NR, Kitzbichler MG, Ganesan S, et al. (2013) Local and long-range functional connectivity is reduced in concert in autism spectrum disorders. Proc Natl Acad Sci U S A 110: 3107–3112.
46. Peters JM, Taquet M, Vega C, Jeste SS, Sanchez Fernandez I, et al. (2013) Brain functional networks in syndromic and non-syndromic autism: a graph theoretical study of EEG connectivity. BMC Med 11: 54.
47. Walsh CA, Morrow EM, Rubenstein JL (2008) Autism and brain development. Cell 135: 396–400.
48. van der Zande FH, Hofman PA, Backes WH (2005) Mapping hypercapnia-induced cerebrovascular reactivity using BOLD MRI. Neuroradiology 47: 114–120.
49. Wang H, Chen C, Fushing H (2012) Extracting multiscale pattern information of fMRI based functional brain connectivity with application on classification of autism spectrum disorders. PLoS One 7: e45502.
50. Duchesnay E, Cachia A, Boddaert N, Chabane N, Mangin JF, et al. (2011) Feature selection and classification of imbalanced datasets Application to PET images of children with autistic spectrum disorders. NeuroImage 57: 1003–1014.
51. Anderson JS, Druzgal TJ, Froehlich A, DuBray MB, Lange N, et al. (2011) Decreased interhemispheric functional connectivity in autism. Cereb Cortex 21: 1134–1146.
52. Assaf M, Jagannathan K, Calhoun VD, Miller L, Stevens MC, et al. (2010) Abnormal functional connectivity of default mode sub-networks in autism spectrum disorder patients. Neuroimage 53: 247–256.
53. Jakab A, Emri M, Spisak T, Szema-Nagy A, Beres M, et al. (2013) Autistic traits in neurotypical adults: correlates of graph theoretical functional network topology and white matter anisotropy patterns. PLoS One 8: 1–21.
54. Sahyoun CP, Belliveau JW, Soulieres I, Schwartz S, Mody M (2010) Neuroimaging of the functional and structural networks underlying visuospatial vs. linguistic reasoning in high-functioning autism. Neuropsychologia 48: 86–95.
55. Hinton GE, Osindero S, Teh YW (2006) A fast learning algorithm for deep belief nets. Neural Comput 18: 1527–1554.
56. Zhou Y, Lui YW, Zuo X-N, Milham MP, Reaume J, et al. (2014) Characterization of thalamo-cortical association using amplitude and connectivity of functional MRI in mild traumatic brain injury. J Magn Reson Imaging 39: 1558–1568.

Autism and Sensory Processing Disorders: Shared White Matter Disruption in Sensory Pathways but Divergent Connectivity in Social-Emotional Pathways

Yi-Shin Chang[¶1], Julia P. Owen[¶1], Shivani S. Desai[2], Susanna S. Hill[2], Anne B. Arnett[2], Julia Harris[2], Elysa J. Marco[2*], Pratik Mukherjee[1]

1 Department of Radiology and Biomedical Imaging, University of California San Francisco, San Francisco, California, United States of America, 2 Department of Neurology, University of California San Francisco, San Francisco, California, United States of America

Abstract

Over 90% of children with Autism Spectrum Disorders (ASD) demonstrate atypical sensory behaviors. In fact, hyper- or hyporeactivity to sensory input or unusual interest in sensory aspects of the environment is now included in the DSM-5 diagnostic criteria. However, there are children with sensory processing differences who do not meet an ASD diagnosis but do show atypical sensory behaviors to the same or greater degree as ASD children. We previously demonstrated that children with Sensory Processing Disorders (SPD) have impaired white matter microstructure, and that this white matter microstructural pathology correlates with atypical sensory behavior. In this study, we use diffusion tensor imaging (DTI) fiber tractography to evaluate the structural connectivity of specific white matter tracts in boys with ASD (n = 15) and boys with SPD (n = 16), relative to typically developing children (n = 23). We define white matter tracts using probabilistic streamline tractography and assess the strength of tract connectivity using mean fractional anisotropy. Both the SPD and ASD cohorts demonstrate decreased connectivity relative to controls in parieto-occipital tracts involved in sensory perception and multisensory integration. However, the ASD group alone shows impaired connectivity, relative to controls, in temporal tracts thought to subserve social-emotional processing. In addition to these group difference analyses, we take a dimensional approach to assessing the relationship between white matter connectivity and participant function. These correlational analyses reveal significant associations of white matter connectivity with auditory processing, working memory, social skills, and inattention across our three study groups. These findings help elucidate the roles of specific neural circuits in neurodevelopmental disorders, and begin to explore the dimensional relationship between critical cognitive functions and structural connectivity across affected and unaffected children.

Editor: Christophe Lenglet, University of Minnesota, United States of America

Funding: This work was funded by grants from the Wallace Research Foundation, the Gates Family Foundation and the Holcombe Kawaja Family Foundation. EJM, JPO and PM acknowledge support from the Simons Foundation. PM also acknowledges support from NIH R01 NS060776. EJM has received support from NIH K23 MH083890 and KL2 RR024130. The funders had no role in study design, data collection and analysis, decision to publish, or preparation of the manuscript.

Competing Interests: The authors have declared that no competing interest exist.

* Email: marcoe@neuropeds.ucsf.edu

¶ These authors are co-first authors on this work.

Introduction

The human brain is a sensory processor. Its core function is to perceive, integrate, interpret, and then facilitate the appropriate coordinated response to the visual, tactile, auditory, olfactory, and proprioceptive information present in the world around us. Thus it comes as no surprise that inaccurate or imprecise sensory processing and multisensory integration (MSI) can lead to impaired intellectual and social development [1]–[4]. There is a growing recognition of the crucial importance of sensory processing as it contributes to attention, learning, emotional regulation, and even social function in children affected by a wide spectrum of neurodevelopmental disorders, including autism. There is also a growing interest in studying sensory processing and cognition as dimensional traits across typically developing children and those with psychiatric labels such as autism.

Autism spectrum disorders (ASD) have traditionally been characterized by impaired communication, social interaction,

and behavioral flexibility [5]. However, individuals with ASD have also been shown to have ubiquitous challenges in sensory processing [6] with over 90% of children with autism reported to have atypical sensory related behaviors. In fact, hyper- or hyporeactivity to sensory input or unusual interest in sensory aspects of the environment is now included in the current DSM 5 diagnostic criteria for ASD [6]. There are, however, children with sensory processing disorders (SPD) who do not show primary language or social deficits but do exhibit atypical sensory reactivity and/or sensory interests to the same or greater extent as children who meet an ASD diagnosis [1]. Children with SPD remain critically underserved with regard to their developmental challenges in our society due to the lack of a diagnostic label recognized in the current DSM 5 manual. Many are instead attributed labels that better describe the sequelae of SPD, such as oppositional defiant disorder, than the root of the problem. It is therefore highly relevant to better characterize the biological bases

Table 1. Cognitive Characterization of TDC, ASD, and SPD Cohorts.

	TDC Mean ± Std	ASD Mean ± Std	Pval	SPD Mean ± Std	Pval
PRI	113.5±13.5	101.6±14.1	**0.015**	115.8±11.5	0.576
VCI	119.2±12.7	101.6±20.5	**0.007**	117.4±12.8	0.660
WMI	108.4±10.9	99.6±17.7	0.111	104.4±12.8	0.320
PSI	101.3±13.6	87.4±11.1	**0.002**	97.1±12.9	0.334

PRIs, VCIs, WMIs and PSIs for each cohort, with p values from two-tailed t-tests for differences between TDCs and each patient cohort (statistically significant p values of less than 0,05 are indicated in boldface).

of this increasingly recognized neurodevelopmental condition. In addition, the comparison of children with SPD and ASD may help to illuminate the unique neural mechanisms at the core of the ASD diagnosis: those facilitating social awareness, interest, and drive. With over 1% of children in the USA carrying an ASD label and reports of 5–16% of children in the USA having sensory processing difficulties, it is important to define the neural underpinnings of these conditions and to delineate the areas of overlap and the areas of divergence [1], [2], [7]. The advent of diffusion tensor imaging (DTI) and fiber tractography has enabled quantitative, noninvasive evaluation of white matter microstructure and connectivity. There is considerable, albeit contradictory, literature reporting altered structural connectivity in individuals with ASD using DTI [8]. There are several studies suggesting reduced connectivity via the corpus callosum [9]–[11] as well as others indicating normal or even elevated fractional anisotropy (FA), a measure of white matter tract microstructural integrity from DTI [12]. Beyond the corpus callosum, there are also reports of other white matter tracts that may show variance from typically developing controls, including the inferior fronto-occipital fasciculus (IFOF) and the uncinate fasciculus (UF). A recent meta-analysis of 25 DTI studies in individuals with autism reports decreased FA in the corpus callosum, the left UF, and the left superior longitudinal fasciculus (SLF), supporting the theory of specific underconnectivity in autism focused on tracts supporting auditory information and language processing [13]. Finally, in addition to auditory and language related tracts, there is considerable interest in tracts that mediate emotional face recognition, a pervasive deficit in children with autism. DTI studies have specifically investigated the fusiform-hippocampal and fusiform-amygdala tracts in individuals with autism and have reported variation thought to relate to atypical function [14], [15].

In comparison to DTI studies of ASD, investigation of structural connectivity in children with isolated SPD is in its infancy. We recently reported that, although children with SPD do not exhibit morphological abnormalities from structural MR imaging, they have strikingly decreased white matter microstructural integrity, especially in posterior cerebral regions [16]. These regions are implicated in unimodal sensory processing as well as MSI, and are regulated by top-down attention modulation via thalamic projections. We further showed that white matter connectivity correlates with behavioral measures of unimodal sensory behavior, multisensory integration, and inattention. White matter microstructural integrity is crucial to the speed and bandwidth of information transmission throughout the brain. Degraded connectivity of primary sensory cerebral tracts or of pathways connecting multimodal sensory association areas may thereby result in the loss of the precise timing of action potential propagation needed for accurate sensory registration and integration. These effects may be reflected in assessable metrics such as processing speed and

working memory, the latter of which has been proposed to be mediated by stereotypical time-locked spatiotemporal spike timing patterns [17].

In this study, we examine white matter tracts that we hypothesize will be atypical in children with SPD or ASD subjects relative to typically developing children (TDC). Based upon our previous work on white matter microstructure in SPD [16], and upon previous studies of white matter microstructure in ASD, we posit that both ASD and SPD subjects will have reduced structural connectivity compared to controls in parieto-occipital white matter tracts involved with sensory processing and integration, whereas only ASD subjects will have diminished structural connectivity relative to controls in temporal tracts associated with social-emotional processing. Furthermore, we posit that tract connectivity will correlate with measures reflecting sensory processing, inattention behavior, social behavior, verbal comprehension, processing speed, and working memory across groups.

Methods

The Institutional Review Board (IRB) at the University of California in San Francisco approved this study (UCSF IRB Protocol #: 10-01940). Subjects were recruited from the UCSF Autism and Neurodevelopment Program clinical sites and research database, and from local online parent board listings. Informed consent was obtained from the parents or legal guardians, with the assent of all participants.

2.1. Demographic, sensory, cognitive and behavioral data
2.1.1. General demographics. Sixteen right-handed males with SPD, fifteen males with ASD (12 right-handed, 1 left-handed, 2 ambidextrous), and 23 right-handed male TDC, all between 8 and 12 years of age, were prospectively enrolled under our IRB protocol.

Voxel-based analysis of the DTI data from the 16 SPD subjects and the 23 TDC using tract-based spatial statistics (TBSS) to investigate white matter microstructure was previously reported in [16]. Group differences in the TBSS analysis were determined in a common atlas space after inter-subject image registration. In the present study, we examine white matter connectivity using diffusion fiber tractography in each subject's native space, with the addition of an ASD cohort.

2.1.2. General cognition. All subjects were assessed with the Wechsler Intelligence Scale for Children-Fourth Edition [18] and were required to have a Perceptual Reasoning Index (PRI) score ≥70. We used PRI as our measure of cognition for inclusion, as communication deficits are part of the core diagnosis of ASD. Verbal Comprehension Index (VCI), Processing Speed Index (PSI), and Working Memory Index (WMI) were also obtained

Table 2. Sensory Profile Characterization of TDC, ASD, and SPD cohorts.

	TDC Mean ±Std	ASD Mean ±Std	SPD Mean ±Std
Auditory	33.6±3.5	*24.4±5.9	*22.7±4.9
Tactile	83.3±5.8	72.4±8.6	*62.9+8.8
Visual	41.2±3.0	35.6±6.3	32.3±7.1
Inattention	28.7±3.6	*20.3±4.4	*17.8±5.3
Total	172.3±11.0	*135.1±18.2	*128.5±15.8
Multisensory	31.3±3.1	23.7±4.5	22.2±3.7

Asterisks indicate mean scores that fall within the definite difference range. None of the mean scores fell in the probable difference range.

from this assessment. These measures are displayed in Table 1 for each cohort.

2.1.3. Sensory processing evaluation. All subjects were evaluated with the Sensory Profile [19], which is currently the most widely used parent report measure of atypical sensory related behavior. The Sensory Profile (SP) is a caregiver report questionnaire (125 items) which measures behavioral sensory differences, yielding scores within individual sensory domains and factors as well as a total score. A probable difference (PD) in sensory behavior is defined as a total score between 142 and 154, while a definite difference (DD) is a score of ≤141. Lower scores reflect more atypical behavior. We use the auditory, visual, tactile, multisensory integration, and inattention/distractibility scores to explore behavioral correlations based on findings from our prior report [16].

Inclusion in the SPD group required a community based Occupational Therapy diagnosis of Sensory Processing Disorder plus a score in the definite difference (DD) range, defined as greater than two standard deviations from the mean, of either the total or the auditory processing score of the Sensory Profile. Five of the SPD subjects scored in the DD range for total score alone, four scored in the DD range for the auditory processing score alone, and seven scored in the DD range for both the total and auditory score. Two ASD subjects scored in the DD range for the total score alone, one ASD subject scored in the DD range for the auditory score alone, and seven of the ASD subjects scored in the DD range for both the total and auditory score. The sensory profile was not obtained for one ASD individual. All of the controls scored in the normal range (Table 2).

2.1.4. Autism evaluation. All subjects were evaluated with the Social Communication Questionnaire (SCQ), a parent report ASD screening instrument [20]. All of the ASD cohort (carrying community diagnosis of ASD) as well as the SPD individuals with a score above threshold (≥15) were evaluated with the Autism

Diagnostic Inventory-Revised (ADI-R) [21], a parent history interview, and the Autism Diagnostic Observation Schedule (ADOS) [22], a structured play session. We used current diagnostic scoring for the ADOS and lifetime scoring for the ADI-R. None of the TDC cohort had an SCQ score ≥15. All participants in the ASD cohort met criteria on both the ADI-R and ADOS; all but one scored ≥15 on the SCQ.

Three of the SPD cohort scored above 15 on the SCQ and were further evaluated with the ADI-R and ADOS. One SPD participant scored above the ASD cutoff on the current diagnosis scoring of the ADOS but did not meet criteria on the ADI-R. Another SPD individual met criteria on the ADI-R but not the ADOS. Neither was considered to meet clinical criteria when evaluated by a cognitive behavioral child neurologist with expertise in autism and neurodevelopment (EJM). The third SPD participant who scored above 15 on the SCQ met neither the ADI-R nor ADOS cut-off. A supplementary analysis was performed, excluding these three SPD subjects from the study cohort (Table S2).

2.1.5. Attention deficits. On the inattention/distractibility factor of the Sensory Profile, eleven of the 16 SPD subjects scored in the definite difference range, four in the probable difference range, and one in the typical range. Of the 15 ASD subjects, seven scored in the definite difference range, five scored in the probable difference range, two in the typical range, and one was not administered the Sensory Profile. Of the 23 TDC, none scored in the definite difference range, three in the probable difference range, and twenty in the typical range. Atypical inattention/distractibility scores on the Sensory Profile do not necessarily indicate that individuals would meet clinical criteria for an attention deficit (hyperactivity) disorder (ADHD) diagnosis. Formal ADHD evaluations were not conducted as part of this study.

Table 3. Tractographical approach for temporal tracts.

White matter tract	Seed mask	Waypoint and termination mask	Exclusion mask
Fusiform - amygdala	Fusiform gyrus	Amygdala	All other gm regions
Fusiform - hippocampus	Fusiform gyrus	Hippocampus	All other gm regions
Uncinate fasciculus (UF)	Orbitofrontal cortex*	Entorhinal cortex + temporal pole	All other gm regions
Inferior longitudinal fasciculus (ILF)	Pericalcarine cortex	Inferior temporal cortex	Thalamus + all other cortical regions
Inferior frontooccipital fasciculus (IFOF)	Lingual gyrus	Orbitofrontal cortex*	Thalamus + all other cortical regions

The Freesurfer seed, waypoint, termination, and exclusion masks used in fiber tractography to delineate examined temporal tracts. *Orbitofrontal cortex was created by summing the medial orbitofrontal cortex and lateral orbitofrontal cortex.

Table 4. Tractographical approach for parieto-occipital tracts.

White matter tract	Seed mask	Waypoint and termination mask	Exclusion mask
Optic radiation	Pericalcarine cortex	Eroded thalamus	All other cortical regions
Dorsal visual stream	Pericalcarine cortex	Inferior parietal cortex	Thalamus
Splenium of the corpus callosum	Left lateral occipital cortex	Right lateral occipital cortex*	All other cortical regions
Posterior corona radiata (PCR) (occipital)	All occipital regions	Cerebral peduncle	All other cortical regions
Posterior corona radiata (PCR) (parietal)	All parietal regions	Cerebral peduncle	All other cortical regions

The Freesurfer seed, waypoint, termination, and exclusion masks used in fiber tractography to delineate examined parieto-occipital tracts. *For the tract through the splenium of the corpus callosum, a callosal waypoint mask was also used.

2.1.6. Prematurity. Three of 16 SPD boys were born prematurely, one at 32 weeks gestation and two at 34 weeks gestation. One of the 23 typically developing children was born prematurely, at 33 weeks gestation. These four subjects were found to be in the middle of the distribution for global FA and mean FA extracted from clusters of significantly affected voxels using TBSS for their respective groups, and therefore they were not considered to be outliers [16]. None of the ASD subjects were born prematurely.

2.2. Image acquisition

MR imaging was performed on a 3T Tim Trio scanner (Siemens, Erlangen, Germany) using a 12-channel head coil. Structural MR imaging of the brain was performed with an axial 3D magnetization prepared rapid acquisition gradient-echo (MP-RAGE) T1-weighted sequence (TE = 2.98 ms, TR = 2300 ms, TI = 900 ms, flip angle of 9°) with a 256 mm field of view (FOV), and 160 1.0 mm contiguous partitions at a 256×256 matrix. Whole-brain DTI was performed with a multislice 2D single-shot twice-refocused spin-echo echo-planar sequence with 64 diffusion-encoding directions, diffusion-weighting strength of b = 2000 s/mm^2, iPAT reduction factor of 2, TE/TR = 109/8000 ms, averages = 1, interleaved 2.2 mm axial slices with no gap, and in-plane resolution of 2.2×2.2 mm with a 100×100 matrix and FOV of 220 mm. An additional volume was acquired with no diffusion weighting (b = 0 s/mm^2). The total DTI acquisition time was 8.67 min.

2.3. DTI analysis

2.3.1. Pre-processing. The diffusion-weighted images were corrected for motion and eddy currents using FMRIB's Linear Image Registration Tool (FLIRT; www.fmrib.ox.ac.uk/fsl/flirt) with 12-parameter linear image registration [23]. All diffusion-weighted volumes were registered to the reference b = 0 s/mm^2 volume. To evaluate subject movement, we calculated a scalar parameter quantifying the transformation of each diffusion volume to the reference. A heteroscedastic two-sample Student's t-test verified that there were no significant differences between SPD, ASD, and TDC groups in movement during the DTI scan (p> 0.05). The non-brain tissue was removed using the Brain Extraction Tool (BET; http://www.fmrib.ox.ac.uk/analysis/research/bet). FA was calculated using the FMRIB Software Library (FSL) DTIFIT function.

2.3.2. High angular resolution diffusion imaging (HARDI) and fiber tractography. The FSL bedpostx tool was used for HARDI reconstruction of the diffusion data, modeling multiple fiber orientations per voxel, and thereby accounting for crossing fibers [24]. Probabilistic streamline tractography was performed using FSL's probtrackx2 to delineate white matter tracts of interest, using the strategies described in Tables 3–5 and illustrated in Figure S1. Seed, waypoint, termination, and exclusion masks for tractography were primarily derived from the gray-white matter boundaries (GWB) of the 82 Freesurfer cortical and subcortical regions, which were automatically segmented on the T1-weighted MR images using Freesurfer 5.1.0 [25] and registered using a linear affine transformation to diffusion space using FLIRT. The left and right cerebral peduncles were manually defined for each subject.

2.3.3 Tract delineation. Subsequent to performance of probabilistic streamline fiber tractography, tract masks for every tract described in Tables 3–5 were separately generated for each subject. Each mask was created by taking the intersection of the

Table 5. Tractographical approach for frontal tracts.

White matter tract	Seed mask	Waypoint and termination mask	Exclusion mask
Anterior thalamic radiation (ATR) (medial orbitofrontal cortex)	Medial orbitofrontal cortex	Eroded thalamus	All other gm regions
Anterior thalamic radiation (ATR) (rostral middle frontal cortex)	Rostral middle frontal cortex	Eroded thalamus	All other gm regions
Genu of the corpus callosum (medial orbitofrontal cortex)	Left medial orbitofrontal cortex	Right medial orbitofrontal cortex	All other cortical regions
Genu of the corpus callosum (rostral middle frontal cortex)	Left rostral middle frontal cortex	Right rostral middle frontal cortex	All other cortical regions
Anterior corona radiata (ACR)	All frontal regions	Cerebral peduncle	All other cortical regions

The Freesurfer seed, waypoint, termination, and exclusion masks used in fiber tractography to delineate examined frontal tracts. *For the tracts through the genu of the corpus callosum, a callosal waypoint mask was also used.

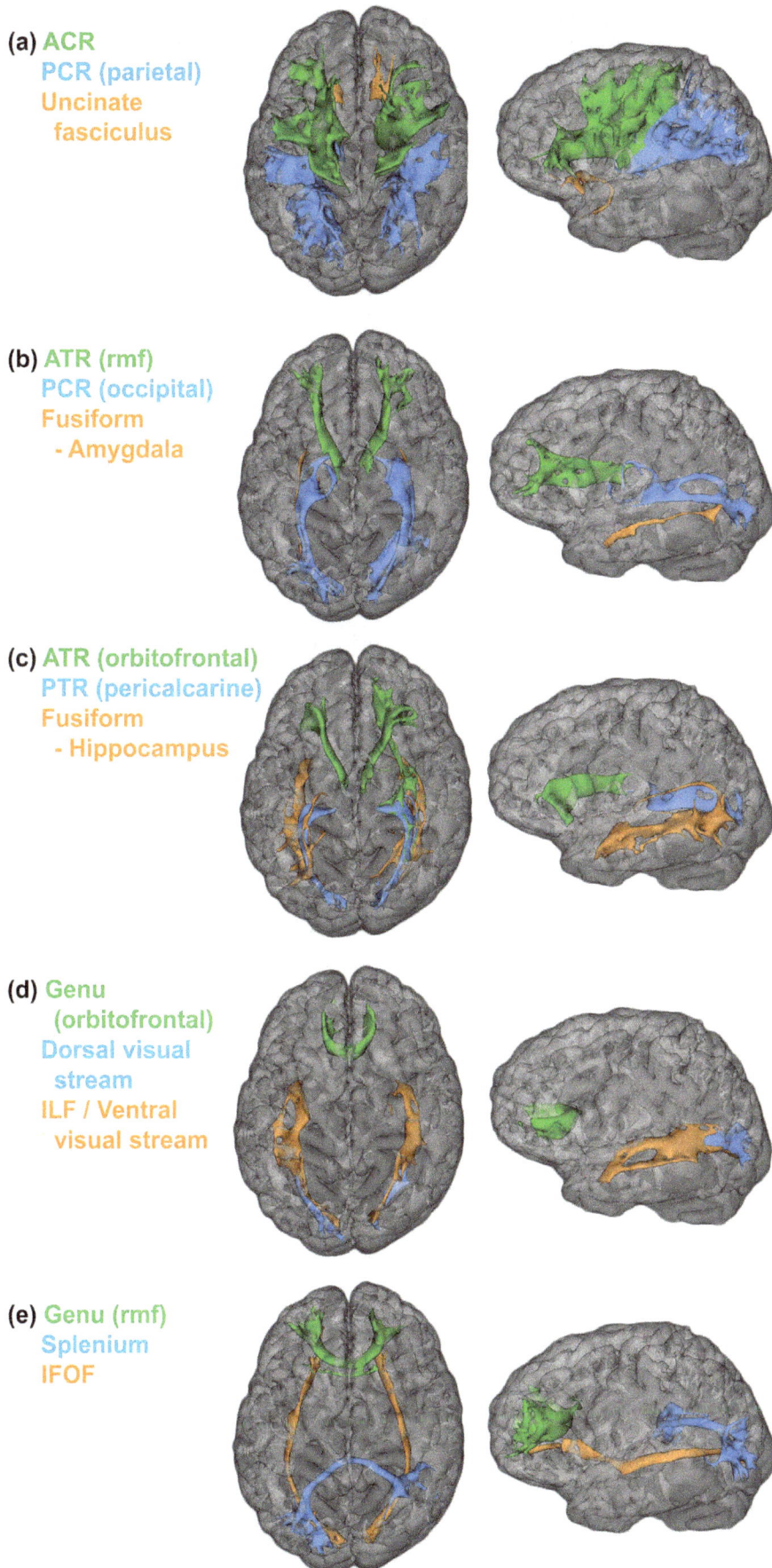

(a) ACR
PCR (parietal)
Uncinate
fasciculus

(b) ATR (rmf)
PCR (occipital)
Fusiform
- Amygdala

(c) ATR (orbitofrontal)
PTR (pericalcarine)
Fusiform
- Hippocampus

(d) Genu
(orbitofrontal)
Dorsal visual
stream
ILF / Ventral
visual stream

(e) Genu (rmf)
Splenium
IFOF

Figure 1. Examples of each delineated tract for a representative subject. Green masks represent frontal tracts, blue masks represent parietal-occipital tracts, and orange masks represent temporal tracts. The tracts are superimposed upon the T1 image, registered to diffusion space and with decreased opacity, of the representative subject.

binarized, thresholded, tractography-derived streamline map and a binary mask of FA>0.2. The streamline threshold used for binarization was separately calculated for each streamline map, and equal to 1% multiplied by the maximum number of streamlines passing through any voxel in the map. This streamline threshold was a consistent strategy of removing spurious streamlines, while retaining most voxels contained within the desired white matter tract. The FA threshold further ensured that the voxels contained within the mask were confined to white matter. Additionally, each tract mask for each subject was visually inspected to confirm that the anatomy of each target tract was accurately and consistently defined.

White matter connectivity was calculated as the average FA value within the delineated tract of interest. This measurement has been shown to be highly reproducible in cross-sectional [26] and longitudinal studies [27].

Representative examples of each of the 15 delineated tracts are displayed in Figure 1. All masks used for tractography were the GWBs of Freesurfer regions except for manually-defined cerebral peduncles and corpus callosum masks. Eroded thalamus masks refer to an eroded version of the Freesurfer thalamus which was transformed using the *fslmaths* erode filtering operation with a box kernel of width 9, a step taken to prevent the thalamic mask from overlapping the corpus callosum and resulting in spurious interhemispheric streamlines. Except for callosal connections, each tract was delineated separately in both the left and right hemispheres. Following mask extraction (after thresholding by streamlines and FA), corresponding left and right hemisphere tract masks were combined for subsequent analysis. The unilateral

tracts were individually assessed to confirm bilateral consistency and to evaluate hypothesized tract laterality.

2.4. Statistical analysis of group differences

For each tract, decreases in FA were separately assessed for the SPD and ASD cohorts relative to controls using one-tailed permutation tests (n = 10,000) (adapted from [28]). Permutation testing was utilized, as it is a nonparametric method and thereby does not assume normally distributed data. The true two-sample t statistic was calculated for control FA vs. patient FA, and a two-sample t statistic distribution was generated by permuting the control and patient labels 10,000 times, calculating a t-statistic value each time. The one-tailed p value was then calculated as the number of permuted t statistic values lying below the true t statistic, divided by the number of permutations (10,000). Group differences were assessed separately for each patient cohort relative to controls at a false discovery rate (FDR) - corrected p value threshold (from p<0.05), with FDR correction applied separately to tracts within each region (separately for the temporal, parietal-occipital, and frontal tracts). Because the perceptual reasoning index (PRI) scores were significantly lower for the ASD cohort compared to the TDC and SPD subjects, a post-hoc group difference analysis was conducted while controlling for PRI. For each tract, a general linear model (GLM) was fit to the data using PRI as a regressor, and permutation tests were performed in the same way as described above, using t statistics for the group coefficient estimates from the GLM. Differences were again assessed using FDR correction within the temporal, parietal-occipital, and frontal regions.

Group Differences in FA of Temporal Tracts

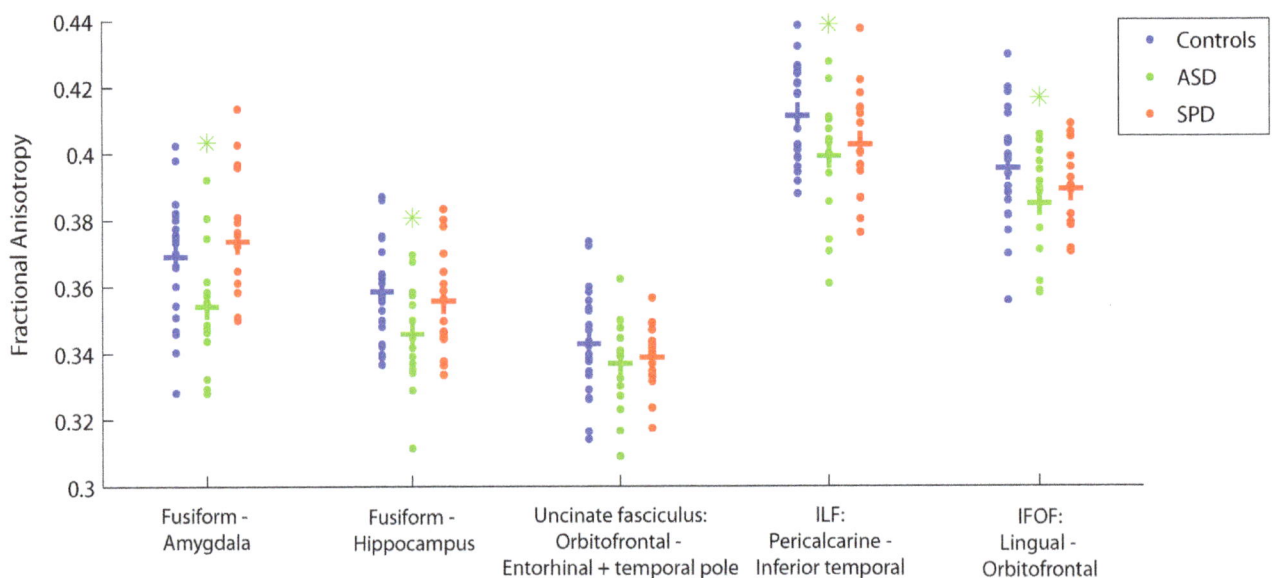

Figure 2. Group differences between TDC, SPD, and ASD subjects in average FA within different temporal tracts. Crossbars correspond to group averages. Green asterisks depict significant group differences between ASD and TDC subjects, and red asterisks depict significant group differences between SPD and TDC subjects, FDR corrected at p<0.05.

Group Differences in FA of Parietal-Occipital Tracts

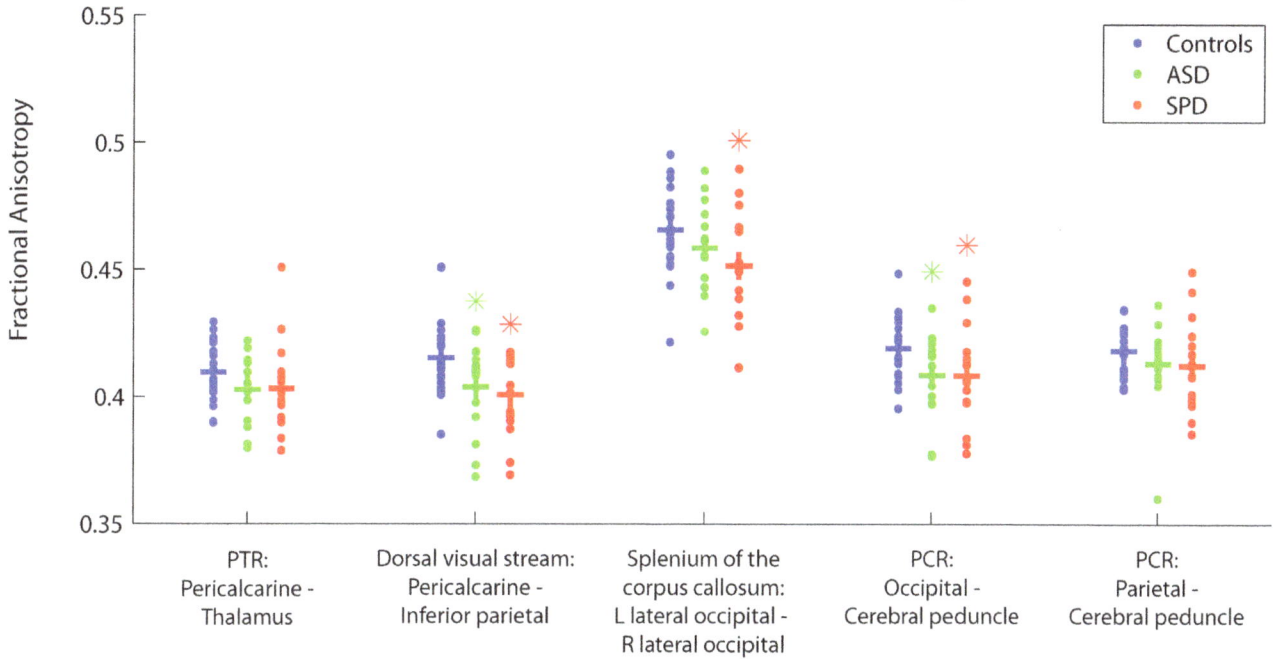

Figure 3. Group differences between TDC, SPD, and ASD subjects in average FA within different parietal-occipital tracts. Crossbars correspond to group averages. Green asterisks depict significant group differences between ASD and TDC subjects, and red asterisks depict significant group differences between SPD and TDC subjects, FDR corrected at p<0.05.

2.5. Cognitive associations

Pearson's correlations of FA in the 15 examined tracts with the VCI, PRI, WMI, PSI, the social component of the SCQ, and the five subtests of the SP (auditory, visual, tactile, inattention, multisensory integration) were investigated dimensionally across all individuals. Statistical significance was assessed at p<0.05 with

Group Differences in FA of Frontal Tracts

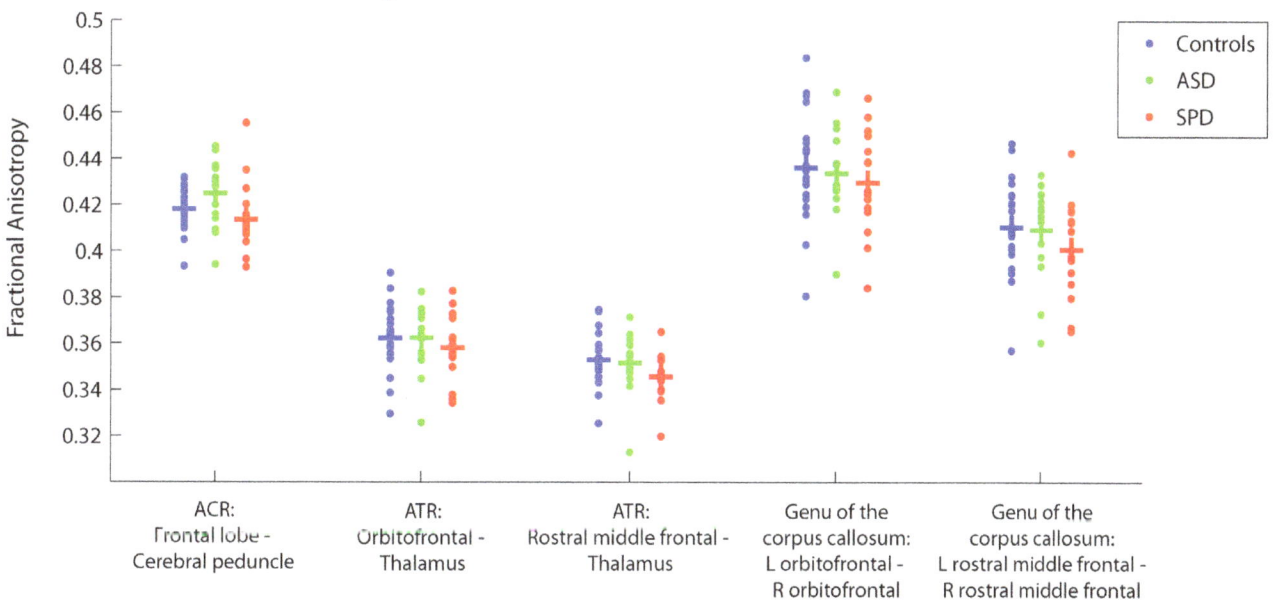

Figure 4. Group differences between TDC, SPD, and ASD subjects in average FA within different frontal tracts. Crossbars correspond to group averages. Green asterisks depict significant group differences between ASD and TDC subjects, and red asterisks depict significant group differences between SPD and TDC subjects, FDR corrected at p<0.05.

Table 6. Connectivity (FA) in all tracts.

Tract	TDC mean FA±SD	ASD mean FA±SD	P-val	SPD mean FA±SD	P-val
Fusiform - amygdala	0.3693±0.0182	0.3546±0.0177	**0.0112**	0.3738±0.0203	0.2298
Fusiform - hippocampus	0.3587±0.0146	0.3469±0.0156	**0.0078**	0.3558±0.016	0.282
Uncinate fasciculus	0.3429±0.0156	0.3375±0.0137	0.118	0.3388±0.0099	0.1886
ILF	0.4114±0.0147	0.4008±0.0192	**0.019**	0.4028±0.0164	0.0468
IFOF	0.3956±0.0171	0.3844±0.0156	**0.031**	0.3893±0.0128	0.11
PTR (optic radiations)	0.4095±0.0113	0.4029±0.0127	0.0516	0.4032±0.0175	0.0814
Dorsal visual stream	0.4155±0.0147	0.4052±0.0179	**0.0134**	0.4009±0.0156	**0.0028**
Splenium of the CC (lat occipital)	0.4658±0.0161	0.4589±0.0167	0.1012	0.4517±0.0238	**0.0164**
PCR (occipital)	0.4194±0.0123	0.4093±0.0161	**0.0144**	0.4085±0.019	**0.0198**
PCR (parietal)	0.4182±0.0093	0.4142±0.0168	0.1338	0.4124±0.0178	0.1018
ACR	0.4182±0.0091	0.4259±0.0146	0.0508	0.4136±0.0156	0.1236
ATR (orbitofrontal)	0.3623±0.0137	0.3627±0.0137	0.4984	0.3581±0.014	0.1694
ATR (rostral middle frontal)	0.3330±0.0111	0.3532±0.0143	0.3616	0.3457±0.0105	0.0238
Genu of the CC (orbitofrontal)	0.4361±0.0224	0.4338±0.0179	0.3666	0.4296±0.0218	0.1916
Genu of the CC (rostral middle frontal)	0.4105±0.0196	0.4078±0.0208	0.4306	0.4008±0.0204	0.0674

The mean and standard deviation of FA within each tract for each group, with associated p values for group differences of the TDC cohort with either the SPD cohort or the ASD cohort. Bolded p values represent significant group differences at p<0.05, FDR corrected.

FDR correction across all 15 tracts. For tracts and cognitive/behavioral metrics demonstrating significant associations across groups, post-hoc correlational analyses were conducted for the unilateral tract FA (left and right hemisphere independently) across groups, as well as unilateral and bilateral tract FA (left and right combined) for each cohort (TDC, SPD, and ASD) independently.

Results

3.1. Group differences in white matter connectivity

Figures 2–4 depict group differences of structural connectivity denoted by fractional anisotropy (FA) in tracts predominantly involving the temporal, parietal-occipital, or frontal regions. Table 6 quantitatively details these group differences. We have additionally added the results of mean diffusivity, axial diffusivity, and radial diffusivity for the three groups).

3.1.1. Group differences of connectivity in temporal tracts. Significantly impaired connectivity (lower FA) was detected for the ASD cohort alone relative to the TDC cohort in the fusiform-amygdala and fusiform-hippocampus tracts, the inferior fronto-occipital fasciculi (IFOF), and the inferior longitudinal fasciculi (ILF) (p<0.05, FDR corrected). The SPD cohort showed no significant differences in these tracts relative to the TDC cohort. There was no significant difference in connectivity of the uncinate fasciculi of either the ASD or SPD cohorts relative to the controls.

3.1.2. Group differences of connectivity in parietal-occipital tracts. The SPD group alone showed significantly decreased connectivity in the splenium of the corpus callosum relative to the TDC cohort. Both the SPD and the ASD group showed reduced connectivity relative to controls in the dorsal visual stream and the posterior corona radiata (occipital portion) (all results with p<0.05, FDR corrected).

Neither the SPD nor ASD groups demonstrated significant differences in the optic radiations (pericalcarine – thalamus PTR) or parietal PCR relative to TDC; however, there were strong trends toward lower connectivity of the optic radiations in both the ASD and SPD groups relative to TDC.

3.1.3. Group differences of connectivity in frontal tracts. Connectivity in the frontal tracts was not significantly decreased for either the SPD or ASD cohorts, although the SPD group showed trends towards decreased connectivity for all measured frontal tracts.

3.2. Unilateral versus bilateral white matter tracts

Homologous white matter tracts of the left and right cerebral hemispheres were combined for purposes of consolidation and improved statistical power. However, group differences were also computed unilaterally for each tract. In all cases, the results from bilateral tracts shown here agree with trends or statistically significant group differences from the component unilateral tracts, with no appreciable hemispheric asymmetries found.

3.3. Accounting for perceptual reasoning index variation

PRI was significantly lower in the ASD cohort compared to the TDC subjects, thus group differences in connectivity were computed while controlling for PRI scores. After controlling for PRI and including FDR correction, connectivity for the ASD cohort was no longer significantly lower in the IFOF or ILF, but still demonstrated decreased FA in the fusiform -amygdala and fusiform –hippocampus tracts. The results for the SPD subjects were unchanged when controlling for PRI, as expected since these subjects did not demonstrate differences in PRI relative to TDC.

3.4. Cognitive associations

Significant combined-group correlations were found between WMI and the bilateral optic radiations (r = 0.41, p = 0.003) as well as the bilateral PCR (occipital) (r = 0.49, p<0.001) (Figure 5). These tracts both demonstrate left lateralized associations for the combined groups. The SPD cohort alone demonstrates significant

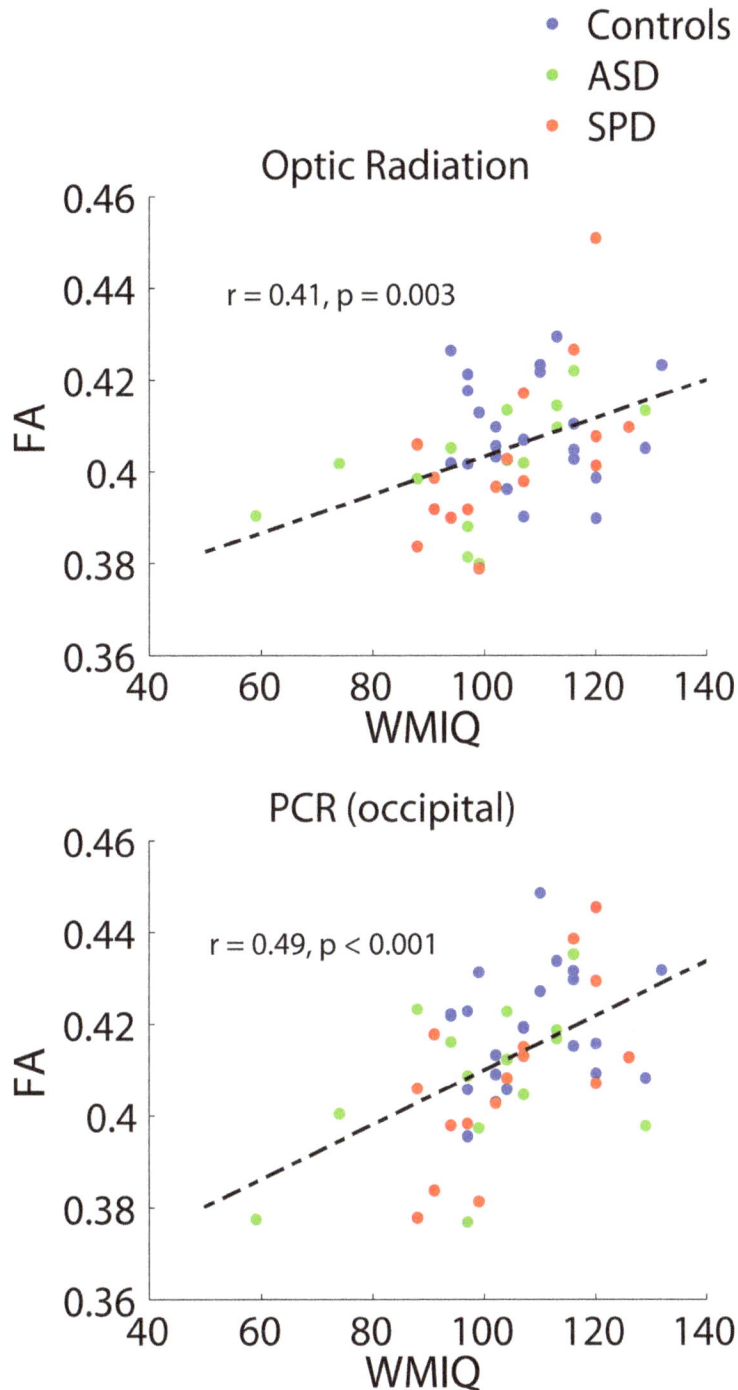

Figure 5. Combined-group associations between tract connectivity and WMI. The two bilateral tracts demonstrating significant associations between FA and WMI after FDR correction are displayed. Optic radiation: r = 0.41, p = 0.003. PCR (occipital): r = 0.49, p<0.001. Results of unilateral and individual group correlations are displayed in Table 7.

individual-group associations between WMI and FA in both of these bilateral tracts, while ASD demonstrates significant or trend-level associations (Table 7).

Significant combined-group correlations were found between the social component of the SCQ and the bilateral fusiform - amygdala (r = −0.44, p = 0.001) as well as the bilateral fusiform-hippocampus (r = −0.39, p = 0.004) (Figure 6). These tracts both demonstrate right lateralized associations for the combined groups (Table 8).

Significant combined-group correlations were found between the inattention measures of the Sensory Profile and the dorsal visual stream (r = 0.38, p = 0.006) as well as the bilateral PCR (occipital) (r = 0.46, p = 0.001) (Figure 7). There is no strong evidence of lateralization for the combined groups (Table 9). The association between inattention and FA in the bilateral PCR

Table 7. Associations between tract connectivity and WMI, for significantly associated tracts.

	r - bilateral	p - bilateral	r - left	p - left	r - right	p - right
PTR (optic radiation)						
All	0.41	*0.003*	0.36	*0.009*	0.32	*0.020*
TDC	−0.08	*0.715*	0.07	*0.753*	−0.14	*0.522*
ASD	0.54	*0.048*	0.53	*0.054*	0.25	*0.380*
SPD	0.62	*0.010*	0.35	*0.188*	0.73	*0.001*
PCR (occipital)						
All	0.49	*<0.001*	0.50	*<0.001*	0.32	*0.022*
TDC	0.22	*0.320*	0.39	*0.077*	−0.07	*0.746*
ASD	0.46	*0.101*	0.40	*0.161*	0.30	*0.299*
SPD	0.67	*0.004*	0.68	*0.004*	0.56	*0.024*

The bilateral tracts demonstrating significant combined-group associations with WMI are displayed. Correlation coefficients and p values are displayed for these tracts, along with combined group unilateral associations, individual group bilateral associations, and individual group unilateral associations.

(occipital) is consistent with our previously published findings in the combined SPD and TDC cohorts [16].

Significant combined-group correlations were found between the auditory factor of the Sensory Profile and the bilateral PCR (occipital) (r = 0.42, p = 0.004) (Figure 8). There is no strong evidence of lateralization for the combined groups (Table 10). The association between this auditory measure and FA in the PCR is consistent with our previously published findings in the combined SPD and TDC cohorts [16].

The combined groups did not demonstrate significant correlations between FA in the 15 investigated tracts and PRI, VCI, or the other subscores of the Sensory Profile after correction for multiple comparisons.

3.5. Tract overlap

Some tracts demonstrated a significant fraction of shared voxels. Figure 9 depicts the average fraction of each tract's voxels that are shared with every other investigated white matter tract. In the most extreme case, a subject average of 77% of the fusiform - amygdala tract voxels were contained within the fusiform - hippocampus tract. There were also significant spatial overlaps within the delineated parietal-occipital tracts, and between some parietal-occipital and temporal tracts. These results demonstrate that some tracts were not completely independent in the group difference results above. Sections of the fusiform-amygdala tract that were independent of the fusiform-hippocampus, and sections of the fusiform-hippocampus that were independent of the fusiform-amygdala tract, were separately assessed for group differences. Neither of the independent sections of these tracts demonstrated statistically significant group differences, suggesting that shared voxels drive the observed differences between the ASD cohort and controls.

Discussion

This study is the first to investigate white matter connectivity of both children with SPD and children with ASD relative to typically developing children. Diffusion MR fiber tracking was employed for the hypothesis-driven identification of specific white matter tracts. The results suggest both overlapping and divergent white matter microstructural pathology affecting the two clinical cohorts, with tracts traditionally associated with social emotional processing being significantly affected for the ASD cohort relative

to TDC, but relatively unaffected in SPD. While both the ASD and the SPD participants demonstrate white matter pathology in the sensory processing regions of the dorsal visual stream and the posterior corona radiata, only the SPD cohort demonstrates statistically significant differences in the splenium of the corpus callosum relative to the TDC cohort. These findings extend previous research using DTI in autism cohorts to include concurrent analysis of children that exhibit sensory processing differences, but not the language and social deficits that characterize a full ASD diagnosis.

While the most extensive white matter alterations in the SPD subjects are observed in the parieto-occipital tracts, which subserve auditory, tactile, and visual perception and integration, this cohort demonstrates trends towards decreased connectivity compared to TDC in most measured tracts. It is also worth specific comment that, while both the SPD and ASD cohorts were affected in these fundamental sensory processing tracts, the FA in all but one of these tracts trended lower for the SPD subjects relative to the ASD subjects. This difference may reflect the prominence of abnormal sensory related behaviors, which is an inclusion criterion for SPD group membership, whereas, in general, children with ASD are primarily characterized by profound social communication deficits. In this sample, 65% of children with ASD scored in the definite difference (DD) range (>2 standard deviations from the mean) on the Sensory Profile Total Score and 57% were in the DD range for the Auditory Processing Score. While many children with ASD have auditory, tactile and visuomotor processing challenges, these deficits are not as ubiquitous as in our SPD cohort. Our findings further suggest that sensory-based behavioral deficits in both groups may be predicated on atypical conduction of information from unimodal to multimodal integration regions as well as inefficient transfer of information between hemispheres via the corpus callosum for the SPD group.

Perhaps the most striking finding is that, relative to the control group, the ASD cohort shows reduced structural connectivity in the fusiform gyrus connections to the amygdala and hippocampus, whereas children with SPD do not. These white matter pathways are thought to facilitate facial emotional processing, a core feature of autism and the domain of clinical divergence for ASD versus SPD [29]. In fact, a recent study reports that infants later diagnosed with autism show reduced attention to essential facial information with declining direct eye gaze as early as 2–6 month of age [30]. The neuroanatomy of facial emotion processing has been

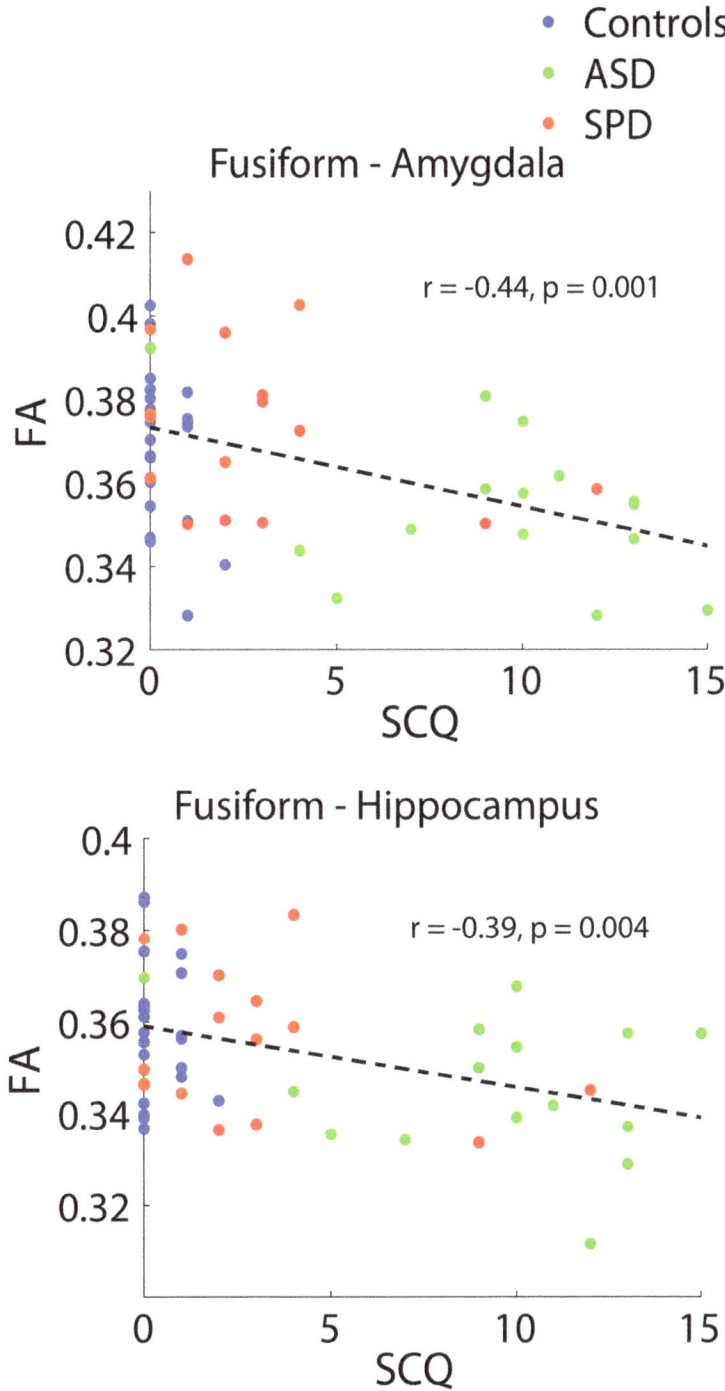

Figure 6. Combined-group associations between tract connectivity and SCQ-social. The two bilateral tracts demonstrating significant associations between FA and the social component of the SCQ after FDR correction are displayed. Fusiform-amygdala: r = −0.44, p<0.001. Fusiform-hippocampus: r = −0.39, p=0.004. Results of unilateral and individual group correlations are displayed in Table 8.

intensively studied with repeated implication of the amygdala-fusiform system. Individuals with ASD have been reported to have less activation of subcortical regions including the amygdala and fusiform gyrus during subliminal emotional face processing, a lack of expected volumetric correlation between the amygdala and fusiform gyrus, as well as behavioral deficits in face recognition that negatively correlate with left fusiform cortical thickness [31], [32]. In a DTI based analysis of adolescents and adults with

autism, the right hippocampal fusiform tract was suggested to have smaller diameter axons corresponding with slower neural transmission, which was thought to lead to secondary changes in the left amygdala-fusiform and hippocampal-fusiform pathways [16]. By contrast, a diffusion fiber tractography study of individuals with Williams syndrome (7q11.23 deletion) are reported to show elevations of FA in fusiform tracts [33]. Individuals with Williams Syndrome show a social phenotype that is in some ways opposite

Table 8. Associations between tract connectivity and the SCQ-social, for significantly associated tracts.

	r - bilateral	p - bilateral	r - left	p - left	r - right	p - right
Fusiform-amygdala						
All	−0.44	*0.001*	−0.27	*0.048*	−0.37	*0.006*
TDC	−0.39	*0.066*	−0.18	*0.423*	−0.29	*0.178*
ASD	−0.40	*0.137*	−0.34	*0.220*	−0.18	*0.515*
SPD	−0.32	*0.233*	0.03	*0.907*	−0.50	*0.049*
Fusiform-hippocampus						
All	−0.39	*0.004*	−0.25	*0.065*	−0.40	*0.003*
TDC	−0.14	*0.510*	−0.11	*0.613*	−0.15	*0.508*
ASD	−0.25	*0.370*	−0.22	*0.433*	−0.12	*0.680*
SPD	−0.27	*0.307*	−0.01	*0.979*	−0.47	*0.069*

The bilateral tracts demonstrating significant combined-group associations with the social component of the SCQ are displayed. Correlation coefficients and p values are displayed for these tracts, along with combined group unilateral associations, individual group bilateral associations, and individual group unilateral associations.

to the autism phenotype with increased attention to faces and abundant social interest and drive. It is thus worthwhile to consider social cognition, or facial emotion recognition specifically, as a continuous trait that might map directly to connectivity of the fusiform tract to limbic structures.

There are however additional farther reaching implications for fusiform connectivity disruptions with regard to language development. A theoretical model of audiovisual affective speech perception begins with input to primary auditory and visual cortex [34]. The *input module* feeds information to the fusiform gyrus as well as the *integration module* of the superior and middle temporal cortex. The primary sensory cortices as well as the fusiform gyrus are reciprocally connected to the amygdala and insula, which comprise the *emotion module* that guides emotional relevance and may facilitate the rapid recruitment of limbic brain regions by visual inputs. Additional contextual information is brought in through connections with the *memory module*, including the hippocampus and parahippocampal gyrus. This framework is useful in considering how autism social communication deficits may map to neuroanatomic networks.

In addition to the fusiform connections, our ASD group was found to have reduced FA in the ILF and the IFOF. This is in line with previous reports, although there is considerable variability in the literature, likely resulting from group heterogeneity in terms of symptom variability, severity, and age of cohort [8], [35]–[38]. The ILF, or inferior longitudinal fasciculus, has been shown to directly connect the occipital cortex to the anterior temporal lobe and the amygdala. The IFOF originates in the visual cortex runs medially to the ILF and directly connects to the inferior frontal and dorsolateral frontal cortex. In a study involving children with visual perceptional impairment, decreased FA of the ILF correlated with impaired object recognition [39]. The IFOF likely overlaps spatially and functionally with the ILF, and is thought to be a tract that is relatively new evolutionarily due to its absence in animal brains [40]. In a large lesion-based study population, the right IFOF in particular is implicated in rapid recognition of emotional facial expressions [41]. The finding of significantly reduced connectivity in ASD of the ILF and IFOF is in concordance with the reduced connectivity seen specifically in the fusiform connections. What is most revealing is the relative preservation of these connections in our SPD cohort. Clearly additional investigation to understand the relationship between the speed of information transmission in these tracts as well as the

behavioral correlates of altered connectivity is warranted. However, these findings suggest a role for neuroimaging in understanding the neural mechanisms that differentiate children with a variety of domain specific deficits, including basic sensory processing and social emotional processing. The role of development and therapeutic interventions on these systems remains an open and important question to explore in these clinical cohorts as it is unclear whether these findings are primary or represent a consequence of aberrant tract remodeling predicated on less practice of these skills from early infancy.

As can be seen from the group comparison figures, while there are clear and statistically significant group differences, there is also considerable overlap in the measurements from tracts across all three groups: ASD, SPD, and TDC. This highlights the importance of a new direction for cognitive and behavioral research based on the investigation of abilities as a continuous measure across children rather than split by exceedingly broad and overlapping clinical labels, a concept which has been formalized in the Research Domain Criteria (RDoC) Project [42]. It is in this context that we frame our investigation of associations between cognitive measures and tract connectivity across all three study groups. The fusiform-amygdala and fusiform-hippocampus tracts are the only two (out of 15) tracts to demonstrate significant associations with the social component of the SCQ across groups with correction for multiple comparisons (Figure 6, Table 8). Further investigation of laterality in these two tracts revealed that these associations are significantly right-lateralized (Table 8), an observation which is consistent with the Conturo et al. (2008) [16] finding of primary right-lateralized effects in these two tracts for ASD subjects. It is important to note that the associations between connectivity in these two tracts and the SCQ-social measure were not significant on an individual group basis. However, the individual group correlations all trended in the same (negative) direction as the combined-group correlations (Table 8). Connectivities (FA) in the optic radiation and PCR (occipital) were found to be significantly correlated with WMI after FDR correction in the combined groups. Investigation of these associations in the individual cohorts revealed strong associations with WMI for the SPD cohort bilaterally in both of these tracts. The ASD cohort alone also demonstrates significant or trend-level associations with WMI and connectivity in these tracts. Though the optic radiation and PCR (occipital) were the only two tracts that demonstrated significant associations with

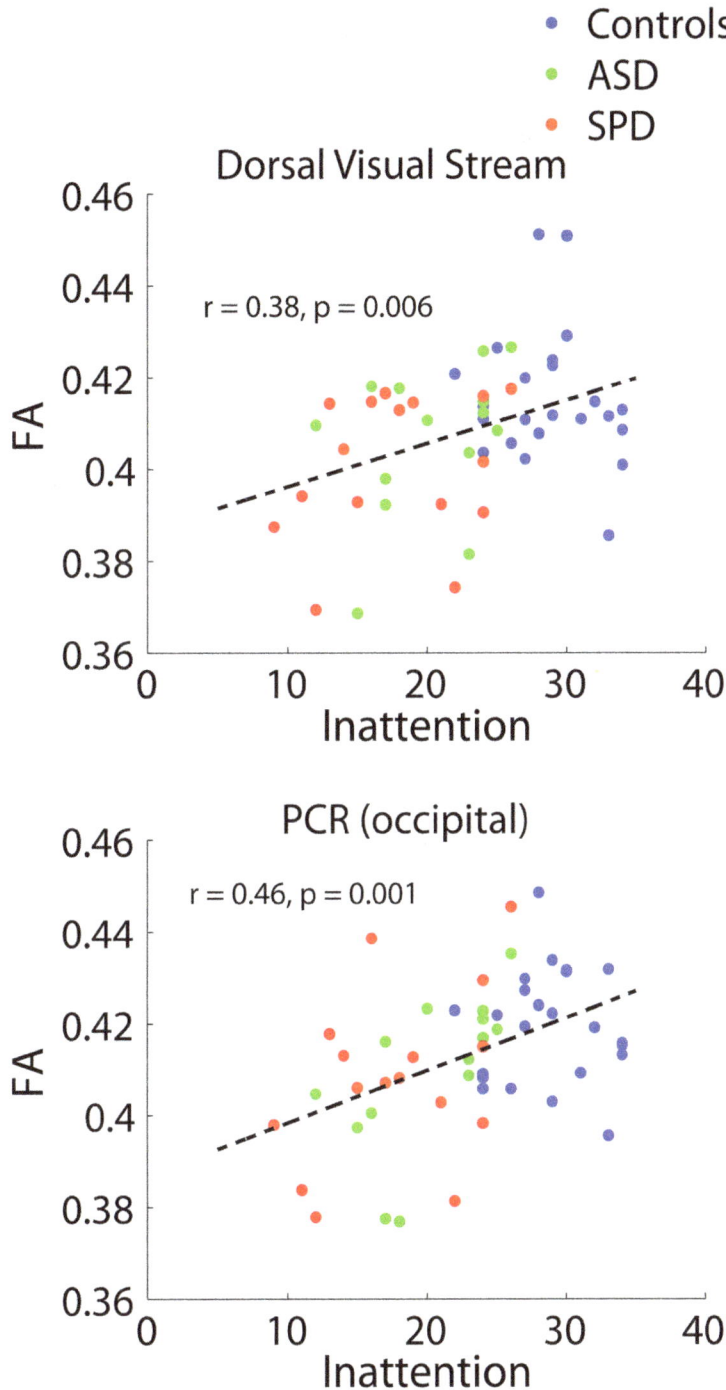

Figure 7. Combined-group associations between tract connectivity and the inattention measure of the Sensory Profile. The two bilateral tracts demonstrating significant associations between FA and the inattention measure of the Sensory Profile after FDR correction are displayed. Dorsal visual stream: r = 0.38, p = 0.006. PCR (occipital): r = 0.46, p<0.001. Results of unilateral and individual group correlations are displayed in Table 9.

WMI after FDR correction, many of the other investigated tracts (including frontal, temporal, and parietal-occipital tracts) demonstrated trend-level associations. This is consistent with reports from prior DTI studies of WMI that have found widespread associations of WMI with white matter connectivity [43], [44]. While our findings of significant associations between connectivity in the PCR (occipital) and the Sensory Profile auditory and inattention measures are consistent with our prior findings [16], we did not find significant associations with the other Sensory Profile measures after correction for multiple comparisons.

There are important limitations to note for this study, which should motivate further investigation. First, we have not determined an optimal method for characterizing the sensory subtypes and distinguishing between hypo- or hyper-sensory sensitivity, nor

Table 9. Associations between tract connectivity and the inattention factor of the Sensory Profile, for significantly associated tracts.

	r - bilateral	p - bilateral	r - left	p - left	r - right	p - right
Dorsal Visual Stream						
All	0.38	*0.006*	0.34	*0.012*	0.27	*0.052*
TDC	−0.16	*0.479*	−0.09	*0.688*	−0.19	*0.408*
ASD	0.37	*0.197*	0.04	*0.885*	0.37	*0.195*
SPD	0.25	*0.358*	0.05	*0.858*	0.40	*0.121*
PCR (occipital)						
All	0.46	*0.001*	0.37	*0.006*	0.41	*0.002*
TDC	0.00	*1.000*	0.06	*0.772*	−0.05	*0.836*
ASD	0.63	*0.015*	0.44	*0.112*	0.63	*0.017*
SPD	0.41	*0.117*	0.19	*0.488*	0.54	*0.029*

The bilateral tracts demonstrating significant combined-group associations with the inattention measure of the Sensory Profile are displayed. Correlation coefficients and p values are displayed for these tracts, along with combined group unilateral associations, individual group bilateral associations, and individual group unilateral associations.

do we have sufficient power in this study for sensory subtype group analysis. We and many sensorimotor based researchers are working to develop a phenotyping tool that maps to specific white matter tracts, and we hope to identify and characterize separate constructs of sensory deficits in larger cohorts going forward. Second, tract overlap exists in our results. A significant portion of the amygdala-fusiform tract is contained within the hippocampal-fusiform tract. In addition, the ILF is partially contained within the dorsal visual stream and the PTR is partially contained within the PCR. Despite these spatial overlaps, the group difference results are not identical between overlapping tracts and provide separately valuable information about structural connectivity in these subjects. Additional connectivity analysis, both structural and functional, will shed additional light on specific regional contributions to the neural underpinnings of sensory and emotional processing differences. Our investigation is also limited in generalizability, as all of the subjects were boys between the ages of 8 and 12 years in an effort to limit developmental confounds in

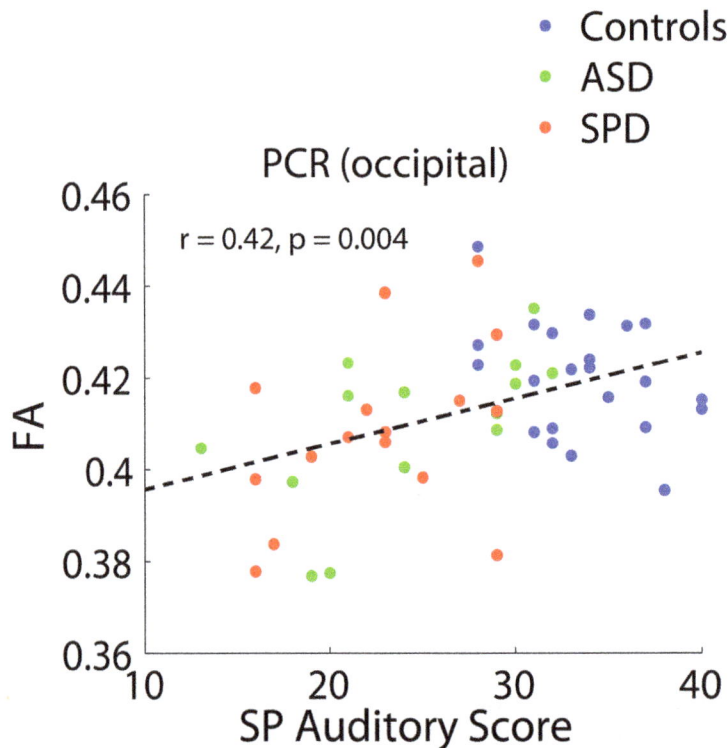

Figure 8. Combined-group associations between tract connectivity and the auditory measure of the Sensory Profile. The bilateral tract demonstrating significant associations between FA and the auditory measure of the Sensory Profile after FDR correction are displayed. PCR (occipital): r = 0.42, p = 0.002. Results of unilateral and individual group correlations are displayed in Table 10.

Table 10. Associations between tract connectivity and the auditory factor of the Sensory Profile, for significantly associated tracts.

	r - bilateral	p - bilateral	r - left	p - left	r - right	p - right
PCR (occipital)						
All	0.42	*0.004*	0.33	*0.017*	0.37	*0.007*
TDC	−0.33	*0.129*	−0.20	*0.353*	−0.27	*0.216*
ASD	0.60	*0.023*	0.38	*0.185*	0.62	*0.021*
SPD	0.41	*0.114*	0.20	*0.465*	0.49	*0.056*

The bilateral tracts demonstrating significant combined-group associations with the inattention measure of the Sensory Profile are displayed. Correlation coefficients and p values are displayed for these tracts, along with combined group unilateral associations, individual group bilateral associations, and individual group unilateral associations.

this small sample. The PRI scores of the ASD cohort were significantly lower than that of the SPD and TDC cohorts; however, the most important group differences in structural connectivity between ASD and controls remained statistically significant after regressing out the effect of PRI. Further research is

therefore needed to determine whether these findings generalize to other ages, genders, and intellectual abilities.

Future research will include investigation of functional connectivity using resting state fMRI and magnetoencephalography (MEG). The ROIs used to determine structural connectivity in this study can be used to assess differences in functional connectivity

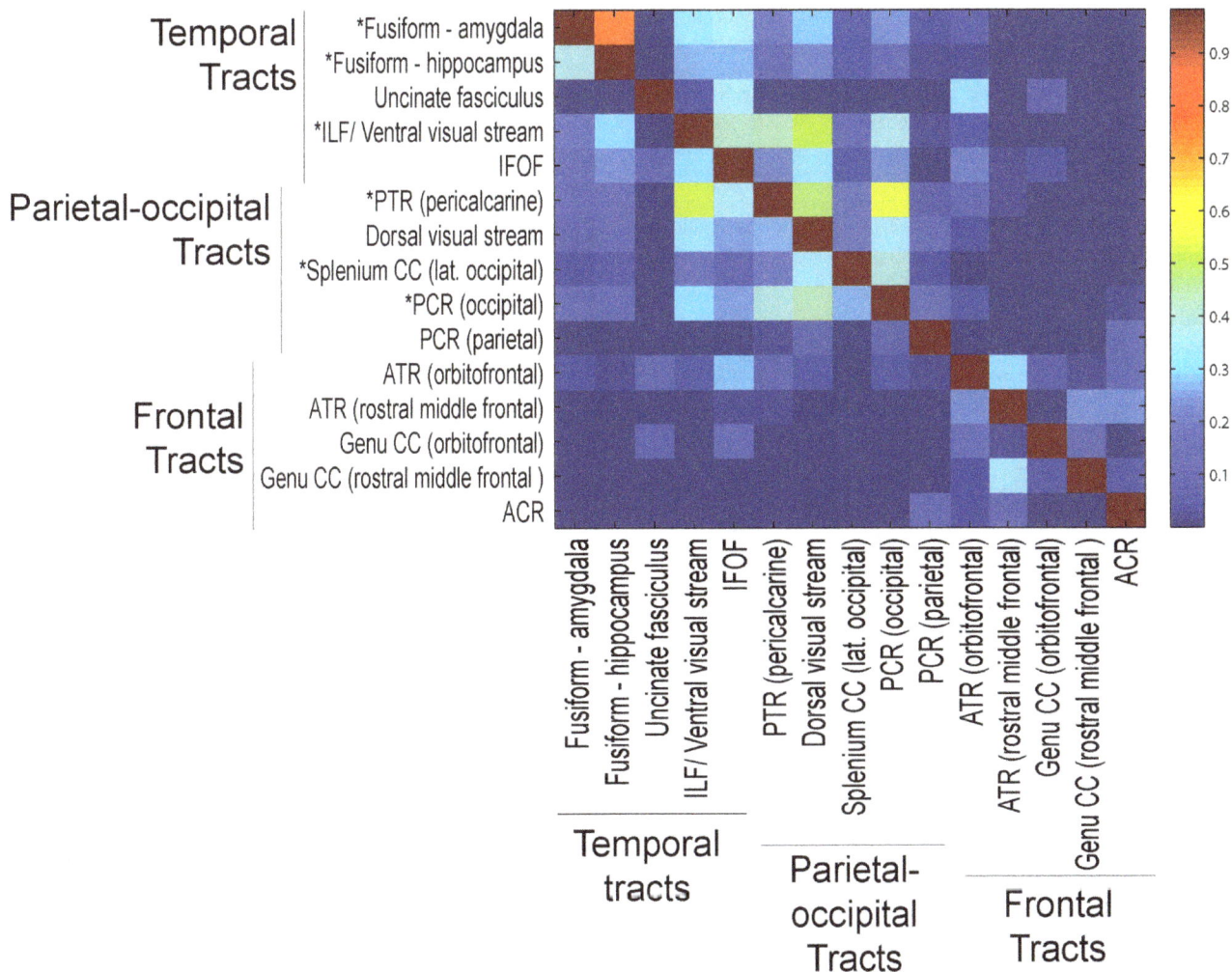

Figure 9. Average fraction of tract overlap. Color intensity corresponds to the subject average of the fraction of the voxels of the tracts on the vertical axis that are contained within the tracts on the horizontal axis. Tracts that are more than one-third contained in any other tract are indicated by an asterisk on the vertical axis.

between these same regions, with functional coupling hypothesized to be reduced where decreased structural connectivity was found in this work. While prior studies have found relationships between functional connectivity and white matter volume in ASD [45]–[47], there have been no reported associations between functional connectivity and DTI measures in SPD.

We hope that by utilizing larger sample sizes and direct assessment of auditory, tactile, visuomotor processing, we will be able to gain a deeper understanding of how neural circuitry differences map to clinically relevant challenges for individual children. The ultimate goal of this and future work is to guide personalized treatments ranging from behavioral interventions and targeted psychopharmacology to cognitive training using child-friendly video game platforms.

Supporting Information

Figure S1 Example ROIs for fiber tracking of the homotopic visual tract through the splenium of the corpus callosum. Displayed is an axial slice from the FA image of a representative subject with overlaid ROIs for probabilistic fiber tractography. The seed mask is the grey-white matter boundary of the left lateral occipital cortex, and contains voxels from which 2000 streamlines each are initiated. The termination mask is the grey-white matter boundary of the right lateral occipital cortex, and causes streamlines to terminate upon encountering the mask. The termination mask and the corpus callosum are both used as waypoint masks, indicating that streamlines need to pass through the corpus callosum and reach the termination mask in order to be retained. The exclusion mask is the union of the grey-white matter boundaries of all other cortical regions, and causes streamlines that encounter these voxels to be excluded. The displayed resultant tract is the result of probabilistic tractography under the previously described constraints and a subsequent streamline and FA threshold.

Figure S2 Group differences of MD in all tracts. Units of diffusivity are in mm²/sec. Asterisks indicate significant

differences based on two-tailed permutation tests with FDR correction for 15 comparisons.

Figure S3 Group differences of RD in all tracts. Units of diffusivity are in mm²/sec. Asterisks indicate significant differences based on two-tailed permutation tests with FDR correction for 15 comparisons.

Figure S4 Group differences of AD in all tracts. Units of diffusivity are in mm²/sec. Asterisks indicate significant differences based on two-tailed permutation tests with FDR correction for 15 comparisons.

Table S1 Group differences of FA between the ASD and SPD cohorts in ASD-affected temporal tracts. P values are derived from one-tailed permutation tests for SPD FA > ASD FA. Bolded p values indicate significant differences after FDR correction.

Table S2 Group differences of FA in all tracts, excluding SPD subjects with SCQ>15. P values are derived from one-tailed permutation tests for TDC FA > SPD FA. Bolded p values indicate significant group differences after FDR correction.

Acknowledgments

We are grateful to our participants and their families for their time and support.

Author Contributions

Conceived and designed the experiments: EJM PM JPO YSC. Performed the experiments: EJM AA SH JH SD. Analyzed the data: YSC JPO. Wrote the paper: YSC JPO EJM PM AA SH JH SD.

References

1. Ahn RR, Miller IJ, Milberger S, McIntosh DN (2004) Prevalence of parents' perceptions of sensory processing disorders among kindergarten children. American Journal of Occupational Therapy 58: 287–293.
2. Ben-Sasson A, Hen L, Fluss R, Cermak SA, Engel-Yeger B, et al. (2009) A meta-analysis of sensory modulation symptoms in individuals with autism spectrum disorders. Journal of Autism and Developmental Disorders 39: 1–11.
3. Brett-Green BA, Miller LJ, Gavin WJ, Davies PL (2008) Multisensory integration in children: a preliminary ERP study. Brain Research 1242: 283–290.
4. Bundy AC, Shia S, Qi L, Miller LJ (2007) How does sensory processing dysfunction affect play?. American Journal of Occupational Therapy 61: 201–208.
5. American Psychiatric Association (1994) American Psychiatric Association Diagnostic and statistical manual of mental disorders, Fourth Edition (DSM-IV) Washington, DC.
6. Marco EJ, Hinkley LB, Hill SS, Nagarajan SS (2011) Sensory processing in autism: a review of neurophysiologic findings. Pediatr Res. 69(5 Pt 2): 48R–54R.
7. Perou R, Bitsko RH, Blumberg SJ, Pastor P, Ghandour RM, et al. (2013) Mental health surveillance among children–United States, 2005–2011. Morbidity and mortality weekly report. Surveillance summaries (Washington, D.C.: 2002) 62 Suppl 2: 1–35.
8. Travers BG, Adluru NA, Ennis C (2012) Diffusion tensor imaging in autism spectrum disorder: a review. Autism Research 5: 289–313.
9. Alexander AL, Lee JE, Lazar M, Boudos R, DuBray MB, et al. (2007) Diffusion tensor imaging of the corpus callosum in Autism. NeuroImage 34: 61–73.
10. Kumar A, Sundaram SK, Sivaswamy L, Behen ME, Makki MI, et al. (2009) Alterations in Frontal Lobe Tracts and Corpus Callosum in Young Children with Autism Spectrum Disorder. Cerebral Cortex 20(9): 2103–2113.
11. Lo YC, Soong WT, Gau SF, Wu YY, Lai MC, et al. (2011) The loss of asymmetry and reduced interhemispheric connectivity in adolescents with

autism: a study using diffusion spectrum imaging tractography. Psychiatry research 192: 60–66.
12. Thomas C, Humphreys K, Jung KJ, Minshew N, Behrmann M (2011) The anatomy of the callosal and visual-association pathways in high-functioning autism: a DTI tractography study. Cortex 47(7): 863–73.
13. Aoki Y, Abe O, Nippashi Y, Yamasue H (2013) Comparison of white matter integrity between autism spectrum disorder subjects and typically developing individuals: a meta-analysis of diffusion tensor imaging tractography studies. Molecular autism 4(1): 25.
14. Conturo TE, Williams DL, Smith CD, Gultepe E, Akbudak E, et al. (2008) Neuronal fiber pathway abnormalities in autism: an initial MRI diffusion tensor tracking study of hippocampo-fusiform and amygdalo-fusiform pathways. J Int Neuropsychol Soc 14: 933–46.
15. Smith CD, Lori NF, Akbudak E, Sorar E, Gultepe E, et al. (2009) MRI diffusion tensor tracking of a new amygdalo-fusiform and hippocampo-fusiform pathway system in humans. J Magn Reson Imaging 29: 1248–61.
16. Owen JP, Marco EJ, Desai S, Fourie E, Harris J, et al. (2013) Abnormal white matter microstructure in children with sensory processing disorders. NeuroImage 2: 844–853.
17. Szatmary B, Izhikevich EM (2010) Spike-timing theory of working memory. PLoS Comput. Biol. 6: e1000879.10.1371.
18. Wechsler D (2003) WISC-IV: Administration and Scoring Manual. Psychological Corporation.
19. Dunn W, Westman K (1997) The sensory profile: the performance of a national sample of children without disabilities. American Journal of Occupational Therapy 51: 25–34.
20. Eaves LC, Wingert HD, Ho HH, Mickelson EC (2006) Screening for autism spectrum disorders with the social communication questionnaire. Journal of Developmental and Behavioral Pediatrics 27 (Suppl. 2): S95–S103.
21. Lord C, Rutter M, Le Couteur A (1994) Autism diagnostic interview-revised: a revised version of a diagnostic interview for caregivers of individuals with

possible pervasive developmental disorders. Journal of Autism and Developmental Disorders 24: 659–685.

22. Lord C, Rutter M, Goode S (1989) Autism diagnostic observation schedule: a standardized observation of communicative and social behavior. Journal of Autism and Developmental Disorders 19: 185–212.

23. Jenkinson M, Bannister P, Brady M, Smith S (2002) Improved optimization for the robust and accurate linear registration and motion correction of brain images. NeuroImage 17: 825–841.

24. Behrens TEJ, Berg HJ, Jbabdi S, Rushworth MF, Woolrich MW (2007). Probabilistic diffusion tractography with multiple fibre orientations: What can we gain?. Neuroimage 34: 144–155.

25. Fischl B (2012) FreeSurfer. NeuroImage 62: 774–781.

26. Wakana S, Caprihan A, Panzenboeck MM, Fallon JH, Perry M, et al. (2007) Reproducibility of quantitative tractography methods applied to cerebral white matter. Neuroimage 36: 630–44.

27. Danielian LE, Iwata NK, Thomasson DM, Floeter MK (2010) Reliability of fiber tracking measurements in diffusion tensor imaging for longitudinal study. Neuroimage 49: 1572–1580.

28. Nichols T, Holmes A (2001) Nonparametric permutation tests for functional neuroimaging: a primer with examples. Human Brain Mapping 15: 1–25.

29. Schultz RT (2005) Developmental deficits in social perception in autism: the role of the amygdala and fusiform face area. *International* Journal of Developmental Neuroscience 23 (2): 125–141.

30. Jones W, Klin A (2013) Attention to eyes is present but in decline in 2-6-month-old infants later diagnosed with autism. Nature 504(7480): 427–31.

31. Dziobek I, Bahnemann M, Convit A, Heekeren HR (2010) The role of the fusiform-amygdala system in the pathophysiology of autism. Archives of general psychiatry 67: 397–405.

32. Kleinhans NM, Richards T, Johnson LC, Weaver KE, Greenson J, et al. (2011) fMRI evidence of neural abnormalities in the subcortical face processing system in ASD. NeuroImage 54(1): 697–704.

33. Haas BW, Hoeft F, Barnea-Goraly N, Golarai G, Bellugi U, et al. (2012) Preliminary evidence of abnormal white matter related to the fusiform gyrus in Williams syndrome: a diffusion tensor imaging tractography study. Genes Brain Behav 11: 62–68.

34. Jansma H, Roebroeck A, Münte TF (2013) A network analysis of audiovisual affective speech perception. Neuroscience 256: 230–41.

35. Koldewyn K, Yendiki A, Weigelt S, Gweon H, Julian J, et al. (2014) Differences in the right inferior longitudinal fasciculus but no general disruption of white matter tracts in children with autism spectrum disorder. Proc Natl Acad Sci U S A. 111(5): 1981–6.

36. Jou RJ, Jackowski AP, Papademetris X, Rajeevan N, Staib LH, et al. (2011) Diffusion tensor imaging in autism spectrum disorders: preliminary evidence of abnormal neural connectivity. Aust. N. Z. J. Psychiatry 45: 153–162.10.3109.

37. McGrath J, Johnson K, O'Hanlon E, Garavan H, Gallagher L, et al. (2013) White matter and visuospatial processing in autism: a constrained spherical deconvolution tractography study. Autism Res. 6(5): 307–319.

38. Shukla DK, Keehn B, Muller RA (2011) Tract-specific analyses of diffusion tensor imaging show widespread white matter compromise in autism spectrum disorder. J. Child Psychol. Psychiatry 52: 286–295.

39. Ortibus E, Verhoeven J, Sunaert S, Casteels I, de Cock P, et al. (2012) Integrity of the inferior longitudinal fasciculus and impaired object recognition in children: a diffusion tensor imaging study. Dev Med Child Neurol 54: 38–43.

40. Forkel J, Thiebaut de Schotten M, Kawadler J, dell'Acqua F, Danek A, et al. (2012) The anatomy of fronto-occipital connections from early blunt dissections to contemporary tractography. Cortex dx.doi.org/10.1016/j.cortex.2012.09.005.

41. Philippi CL, Mehta S, Grabowski T, Adolphs R, Rudrauf D (2009) Damage to association fiber tracts impairs recognition of the facial expression of emotion. J Neurosci 29: 15089–15099.

42. Cuthbert BN, Insel TR (2013) Toward the future of psychiatric diagnosis: the seven pillars of RDoC. BMC Med 11: 126.

43. Tang CY, Eaves EL, Ng JC, Carpenter DC, Mai X, et al. (2010) Brain networks for working memory and factors of intelligence assessed in males and females with fMRI and DTI. Intelligence 38: 293–303.

44. Nagy Z, Westerberg H, Klingberg T (2004) Maturation of white matter is associated with the development of cognitive functions during childhood. J. Cogn. Neurosci 16: 1227–1233.

45. Cherkassky VL, Kana RK, Keller TA, Just MA (2006) Functional connectivity in a baseline resting-state network in autism. Neuroreport 17: 1687–1690.

46. Just MA, Cherkassky VL, Keller TA, Kana RK, Minshew NJ (2007) Functional and anatomical cortical underconnectivity in autism: Evidence from an FMRI study of an executive function task and corpus callosum morphometry. Cerebral Cortex 17: 951–961.

47. Kana RK, Keller TA, Cherkassky KL, Minshew NJ, Just MA (2006) Sentence comprehension in autism: Thinking in pictures with decreased functional connectivity. Brain 129(Pt 9): 2484–2493.

Regional Alterations in Purkinje Cell Density in Patients with Autism

Jerry Skefos*, Christopher Cummings, Katelyn Enzer, Jarrod Holiday, Katrina Weed, Ezra Levy, Tarik Yuce, Thomas Kemper, Margaret Bauman

Department of Anatomy & Neurobiology, Boston University School of Medicine, Boston, Massachusetts, United States of America

Abstract

Neuropathological studies, using a variety of techniques, have reported a decrease in Purkinje cell (PC) density in the cerebellum in autism. We have used a systematic sampling technique that significantly reduces experimenter bias and variance to estimate PC densities in the postmortem brains of eight clinically well-documented individuals with autism, and eight age- and gender-matched controls. Four cerebellar regions were analyzed: a sensorimotor area comprised of hemispheric lobules IV–VI, crus I & II of the posterior lobe, and lobule X of the flocculonodular lobe. Overall PC density was thus estimated using data from all three cerebellar lobes and was found to be lower in the cases with autism as compared to controls, an effect that was most prominent in crus I and II ($p<0.05$). Lobule X demonstrated a trend towards lower PC density in only the males with autism ($p = 0.05$). Brain weight, a correlate of tissue volume, was found to significantly contribute to the lower lobule X PC density observed in males with autism, but not to the finding of lower PC density in crus I & II. Therefore, lower crus I & II PC density in autism is more likely due to a lower number of PCs. The PC density in lobule X was found to correlate with the ADI-R measure of the patient's use of social eye contact ($R^2 = -0.75$, $p = 0.012$). These findings support the hypothesis that abnormal PC density may contribute to selected clinical features of the autism phenotype.

Editor: Izumi Sugihara, Tokyo Medical and Dental University, Japan

Funding: This work was supported by The Autism Research Foundation (http://www.theautismresearchfoundation.org) and Autism Speaks File Number 1391 (http://www.autismspeaks.org). The funders had no role in study design, data collection and analysis, decision to publish, or preparation of the manuscript.

Competing Interests: The authors have declared that no competing interests exist.

* E-mail: skefos@gmail.com

Introduction

Autism is a behaviorally defined neurodevelopmental disorder with core symptoms of impaired social interaction, delayed development of and qualitative abnormalities in communication, and restricted/repetitive and stereotyped behavior patterns [1]. Its wide range of additional associated symptoms and comorbidities has complicated efforts to determine the core neuropathological features of autism. Despite this clinical heterogeneity, numerous studies have described abnormalities involving the cerebellar circuitry and the limbic system [2]. Within the cerebellum, the consistently widely reported finding has been a decrease in the density of the Purkinje cells (PCs) [3–10], the large projection neurons in the cerebellar cortex. This is the first study, however, that was designed to precisely quantify regional alterations in PC density in autism and to test for association between PC density and a selection of relevant clinical behavioral measures.

In the present study, using a stereologic technique, we determined the PC densities in four cerebellar regions (Fig. 1). Two of these regions, crus I and II in the posterior lobe, were selected because previous studies have frequently noted abnormalities in these areas [3,5–9]. Crus I and II are known to reciprocally connect with prefrontal cortical networks that modulate social behavior and behavioral planning [11,12]. The third region, lobule X (the flocculonodular lobe), is associated with eye movement as well as vestibular regulation [13–18] and has

been previously reported to display pathology in a subset of postmortem autistic cases [19], some of which were included in the present study [20,21]. The fourth region, the hemispheric portion of lobules IV–VI, is a primary sensorimotor processing area that has been reported to undergo an age-dependent decline in PC density [22–24].

In an attempt to improve upon previous studies of PC density in autism, we sampled from a series of sections obtained throughout the entire cerebellum to measure PC density in regions within each of the three cerebellar lobes. In addition, the stereological methodology employed in this study significantly reduced the potential for variance in data acquisition due to subjective determinations, as compared with prior attempts to quantify PCs in autism [3–10,25,26]. With this methodology, we have attained a strong inter-rater reliability (>95% concurrence between the measurements of seven stereologists) and low variance in the data. Furthermore, the cases we have included in the autism group were selected to approximate the incidence of mental retardation (MR) and epilepsy in the overall autism population, which was not a feature of prior investigations and disallowed an assessment of the contribution of MR and epilepsy to the observation of lower PC density in autism in these studies [27,28].

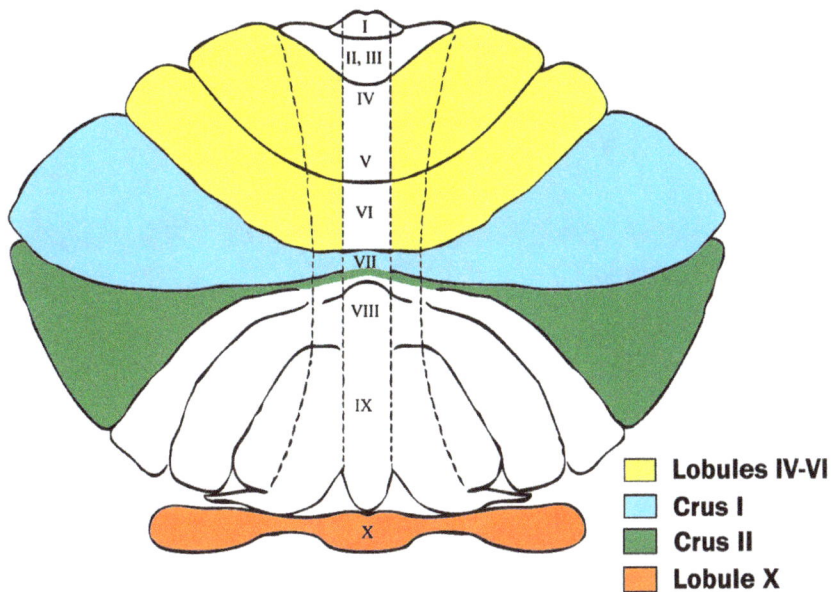

Figure 1. Cerebellar Regions Investigated. This flatmap diagram displays the four cerebellar regions of interest for our stereological assay. Hemispheric lobules IV–VI (in yellow) are bordered by the preculminate and superior posterior fissures, lateral to the fourth ventricle. Crus I (in blue) is the region bordered by the superior posterior and horizontal fissures. Crus II (in green) is bordered by the horizontal and ansoparamedian fissures. Lobule X, the flocculonodular lobe (in orange), is bordered by the posterolateral fissure. This image is an adaptation of the diagram by Larsell, 1958 [80].

Methods

Case Demographics

The cerebella were obtained from the postmortem brains of eight individuals with autism and eight gender- and age-matched controls. Six of the cases were females (age range 4 to 21 years) and ten were males (age range 7 to 56 years), thus each group had 3 females and 5 males. All individuals in the autism group met DSM-IV and ADI-R criteria for autism spectrum disorders [1,29]. The control cases had no known neurological disorder or known neuropathology. The clinical characteristics of both groups are summarized in Table 1. Postmortem interval (PMI), or time before initiating brain preservation, did not significantly differ between males and females nor between the autism and control groups. The majority of cerebella were sampled from the right hemisphere (88%), (Table 1). Three cases in the autism group were diagnosed with MR (IQ<70), ranging from mild to severe. Other symptoms in the autism group included: complications during pregnancy (38%), epilepsy (38%), delayed motor milestones (50%), delayed acquisition of verbal communication skills (88%), emotional disturbances such as depression and aggression (50%), and difficulty coordinating gaze (38%). Three cases in the autism group were reported to have suffered from developmental regression, two of whom had documented epilepsy. ADI-R scores did not significantly differ between males and females, but the male cases represented a wider age range (t = 2.35, df = 14, p = 0.036) than the female cases. The difference in average brain weight between males and females in our autism group was approximately twice the calculated difference for all autism cases cataloged in the Autism Tissue Program (ATP) database (327 vs. 186 grams) [http://www.atpportal.org], which may be a reflection of the small sample size available for this study. Based on the ATP data, cases diagnosed with autism display similar male-to-female differences in brain weight as controls, which is approximately a 10% increased fresh brain weight in males [30]. Due to this

divergence from the normative data (in which we noticed an approximate 20% difference in our samples between the male and female autism cases), we have tested our analyses of PC density for covariance with brain weight and cerebellar volume (as described below in Statistical Analyses).

Tissue Preparation

This study utilized prepared cerebellar histological sections obtained from the ATP. These sections are a component of the ATP's Brain Atlas Project, which is a multi-site collaborative investigation of an established cohort of identically processed cases that agreed to donate their brain tissue for autism research (http://www.autismtissueprogram.org).

Tissue prepared for the Brain Atlas Project was processed by the New York State Institute for Basic Research in Developmental Disabilities (NYS-IBR) following protocols approved by their Institutional Review Board [21]. Whole fresh brain weights were obtained prior to processing. Each brain was cut mid-sagittally through the corpus callosum and brainstem. One brain hemisphere was fixed in 10% buffered formalin, and the other brain hemisphere was frozen. Following at least 3 weeks of fixation, magnetic resonance imaging (MRI) scans were acquired of the fixed brain hemispheres from the cases in the autism group using a 1.5 T GE Signa Imager (General Electric, Milwaukee, USA). T1-weighted, fast gradient echo MRI was used to sample each brain in 1.5 mm-thick virtual slices in the coronal plane, perpendicular to the anteroposterior axis of the hippocampus (FOV = 25 cm, NEX = 1, matrix = 256×192, TR – 35 ms, FA = 60°). Following imaging, each fixed hemisphere was washed overnight in water and subsequently dehydrated in increasing ethanol concentrations (50% for 3 days, 70% for 4 days, 80% for 3 days, and 95% for 4 days). The tissue was then embedded in 8% celloidin [31]. Celloidin blocks were hardened in chloroform vapor for approximately 2.5 weeks, and then stored in 70% ethanol. A series of serial 200 μm sections separated by 1.2 mm increments (every 6th

Table 1. Clinical Characteristics.

Case	Diagnosis	Sex	Age	Brain Weight[a]	PMI[b]	MR[c]	Epilepsy	Regression	Cause of Death
B-6115[d]	Autism	F	17	1158	25	no	no	no	Dilated cardiomyopathy
B-6403	Autism	M	7	1610	25	no	yes	yes	Drowning
UMB-1627	Autism	F	5	1390	13.3	no	no	no	Auto trauma
IBR-93-01	Autism	M	23	1610	14	no	yes	no	Drowning
B-6276	Autism	M	56	1570	3.4	moderate MR	no	no	Arteriosclerotic heart disease
B-6212	Autism	M	36	1480	24	severe MR	no	yes	Circulatory failure, renal failure
UMB-1638	Autism	F	21	1108	50	mild MR	yes	yes	Obstructive pulmonary disease
B-5666	Autism	M	8	1570	22.2	no	no	no	Sarcoma
UMB-1843	Control	F	15	1250	9	no	no	N/A	Multiple Injuries
UMB-1846	Control	F	20	1340	9	no	no	N/A	Multiple Injuries
UMB-4898	Control	M	7	1240	12	no	no	N/A	Drowning
B-6736	Control	F	4	1530	17.0	no	no	N/A	Acute broncho-pneumonia
UMB-1646	Control	M	23	1520	6	no	no	N/A	Ruptured spleen
BTB-3983	Control	M	52	1430	12.5	no	no	N/A	Atherosclerotic cardiovascular disease
UMB-1576	Control	M	32	-	24	no	no	N/A	Compressional asphyxia
IBR-252-02[d]	Control	M	51	1450	18	no	no	N/A	Myocardial infarct

[a]Fresh brain weight (in grams) was measured prior to tissue processing.
[b]Postmortem interval.
[c]Mental Retardation.
[d]Left brain hemisphere was investigated. (All other cases were investigated from the right brain hemisphere).

section) was obtained throughout the entire brain hemisphere as well as through the brainstem and cerebellum of each case (Fig. 2a). The sections were immersed in water for 2–3 hours, after which they were Nissl-stained with cresyl violet and mounted with Acrytol. Each case was assigned a brain bank identification number to maintain donor anonymity.

Stereological Methodology

Using two cerebellar atlases [32,33], the cerebellar regions were anatomically defined as follows: crus I is bordered by the superior posterior and horizontal fissures; crus II is bordered by the horizontal and ansoparamedian fissures; lobule X includes the nodulus and flocculus which together are bordered by the posterolateral fissure; and hemispheric lobules IV–VI are bordered by the preculminate and superior posterior fissures, lateral to the fourth ventricle (Fig. 1).

To facilitate unbiased quantification of PCs within each selected cerebellar region, the optical disector probe [34], a 3D counting frame, was employed throughout the entire series of cerebellar slides (approximately 40 slides per case), such that we sampled throughout the entirety of each region of interest (Fig. 2). Each cerebellar lobule was sampled throughout the cortex and adjacent white matter (Fig. 2b). Slides were analyzed using a Nikon Eclipse 80i microscope equipped with a motorized stage (Ludl Electronic Products, Hawthorne, NY) and microcator (a positional deviation meter, Heidenhain, Schaumburg, IL) for precise navigation in the XY and Z planes of the section, respectively. The microscope was guided by a computer with the Stereoinvestigator 10 (MBF Bioscience, Williston, VT) software package calibrated to move the slide with 1 µm precision. This system ensured systematic, uniform and random sampling. Preliminary measures were taken to ensure >95% inter-rater reliability (number of stereologists = 7) and <0.07 coefficient of error (CE) for each region investigated

(Gundersen CE, m = 1. For a detailed description: [35]). Our counting object was the PC soma, which was readily identifiable with a 40× objective lens (NA = 0.75), and thus PCs were counted when the borders of the soma were in focus. Slides were viewed through the microscope eyepiece as well as on the computer monitor using an Optronics Microfire digital camera. The ATP Brain Atlas celloidin series is comprised of 200 µm sections designed to aid in volumetric analyses. However, PCs were most reliably identifiable through a depth of the first 80 µm in each section due to excessive light diffraction at greater depths. Therefore, we employed a 5 µm guard volume (to prevent counting error due to cell loss during tissue sectioning) and sampled through 75 µm below the guard volume. The computer software ensured that the 19,600 µm² counting frames were randomly imposed and evenly spaced within the region of interest on each slide (Fig. 2c). The distance between the counting frames was determined separately for each cerebellar region to ensure that optimal sampling parameters were employed. Sampling parameters were considered optimal if they minimized systematic error from oversampling, while still providing reliably reproducible estimates of PC density, as determined by the CE [36]. Using optimized parameters, a counting frame was placed every 2500 µm², 2200 µm², 400 µm², and 1400 µm² along the X and Y axes, in crus I, crus II, lobule X, and hemispheric lobules IV–VI, respectively. As a result, the mean number of counting frames for each of these four regions was: 1106, 818, 1392, and 1690, respectively. Overall, approximately 5,000 counting sites throughout the three cytoarchitectonic layers of the cortex and the associated underlying white matter were assayed in each cerebellum (Fig. 2). Using these parameters, approximately 450 PCs were counted in each cerebellar region with an average CE of 0.053.

In some cases, less than 100% of each region of interest was available, which precluded the possibility of obtaining estimates of

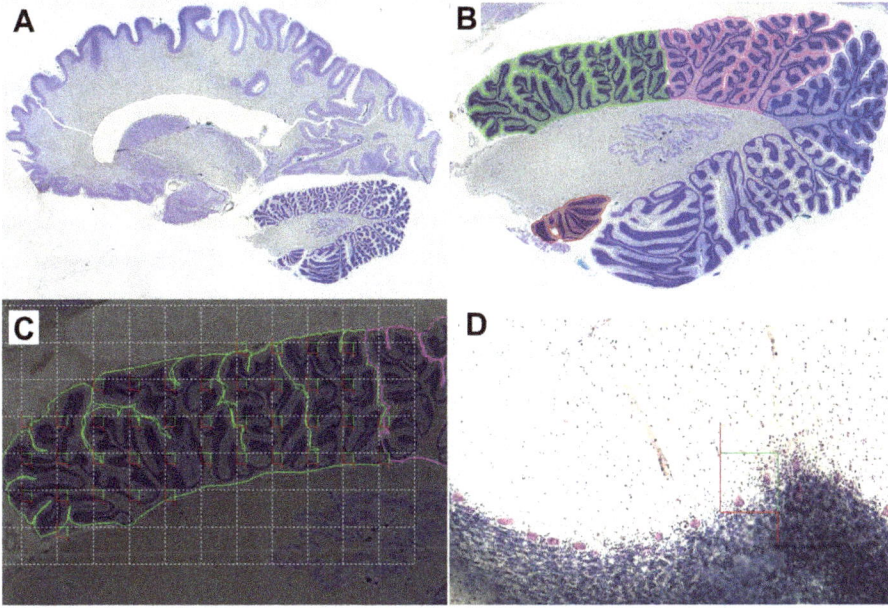

Figure 2. Stereological Assessment of PC Density. This figure depicts our stereological approach for quantifying PC density in each region of the cerebellum. 2a displays a full sagittal section of the human brain. 2b represents the positioning of contour lines used to select the boundaries around each region of interest, within which sampling occurs. Lobules IV–VI are highlighted in green, crus I is highlighted in pink, crus II is highlighted in blue, and the flocculus of lobule X is highlighted in orange at the bottom of the section. 2c displays a hypothetical placement of counting frames (optical disector probes) within lobules IV–VI. The counting frame size has been increased to aid in visualization for this example. The white dotted line displays the randomly imposed grid over the contour, which regulates the distance between counting frames along the X–Y plane of the section. A counting frame is placed in the top-left of each grid cell if it will include a portion of the region of interest as designated by the contour line. Finally, 2d displays a histological section with an imposed counting frame that includes two PCs to be counted. The use of the optical disector probe dictates that PCs are counted when within the counting frame or at all touching the green line, but never when cells intersect with the red line.

total PC number. Case notes indicated that as much as 10% of the tissue had been lost during processing. In addition, some slices demonstrated fraying at the edge of the folia. In a few instances, these complications prevented us from obtaining estimates from each target region and thus only the regions that could be completely sampled were analyzed. As a result, rather than estimating total PC number, data were analyzed as PC density measurements, calculated by dividing the total number of PCs counted in a region by the summed volume of each counting box placed in that region (Eq. 1).

$$Density_{PC} = \frac{Number_{PC}}{Volume_{sampled}} \qquad (1)$$

Additional Volumetry Using MRI

We were able to collect a measure of total cerebellar volume for each case in the autism group by performing planimetry on the MRI data obtained by the NYS-IBR using the formalin fixed brains. Tissue shrinkage during fixation ranged from 44% to 52% and did not differ significantly between the autism and control groups. Planimetry was performed with ImageJ [http://rsbweb. nih.gov/ij/] using the Yawi3D plugin [http://yawi3d.sourceforge. net], which generates an automated selection of the region of interest on each MRI slice. Following manual adjustment using a pen tablet interface (Wacom, Otone, Japan) to ensure precise delineation of cerebellar boundaries, the cerebellar area in each slice was calculated and summed. As the MRI acquisition and tissue processing protocols used in this study were standardized

across samples, it was possible to make comparisons within the autism group using the planimetric data for each case. However, since control brains in the Brain Atlas Project lacked MRI data, group comparisons were not made. Obtaining total cerebellar volume measurements for the cases in the autism group allowed for an assessment of the contribution of overall tissue volume to PC density in each region, particularly as it pertained to gender differences within the autism group, as well as the correlation between PC density and behavioral measures.

Statistical Analyses

To assess the differences between group means on the basis of gender and autism diagnosis, we performed a linear mixed model test fitted by maximum likelihood, with weighted least squares (WLS) correction based on the regional volume from which each PC density measure was obtained. To test for regional differences in PC density as an effect of gender and autism diagnosis, we repeated the test without the WLS correction. The above tests were also repeated with brain weight as a covariate to investigate the contribution of brain weight to our findings (Table 2). False discovery rate controlled t-tests [37] were then performed to inspect the interaction between gender, diagnosis, and region. The appropriate t-test was chosen based on the results of Levene's test of equality of variances between each group. PC density measures in each region were tested for correlation with the non-parametric scores in each domain of the ADI-R (communication, social interaction, and restricted/repetitive behavior), as well as with the 7 specific questions in the ADI-R recently identified by machine learning analyses to be most indicative of an autism diagnosis [Presentation by Dennis Wall, "Shortening the Behavioral Diagnosis of Autism Through Artificial Intelligence and Mobile

Health Technologies," Autism Consortium 2011 Symposium, Boston, MA]. (For a detailed description of the statistical methods used to select these specific behavioral variables, Wall et al. has recently published a similar analysis of the Autism Diagnostic Observation Schedule [38]). For all tests of correlation involving non-parametric behavioral measures, Spearman rank correlations were performed. To assess the probability of a false positive correlation, the false discovery rate procedure was performed. The effects of potentially confounding factors or clinically relevant covariables were investigated. Parametric variables such as age, brain weight, cerebellar volume, PMI, and fixation time were tested for covariance with PC density estimates using univariate generalized linear models. To test the effects of clinically relevant factors reported in the case histories of the autism group, such as epilepsy, diagnosis of MR, developmental regression, lack of verbal development, delay in attaining motor milestones, and complications during pregnancy, separate t-tests were performed for each cerebellar region. Additionally, for cases in the autism group, linear regression analysis was performed to detect potential associations between PC density and the age at which the subject first walked unaided.

Logarithmic transformation was performed on all PC density estimates to adjust for skew from a normal distribution. The significance of each finding was only marginally affected by this transformation. Because our PC measures were obtained from each lobe of the cerebellum (anterior, posterior, and flocculonodular), we generated an estimate of overall cerebellar PC density as a composite of the regional volume-weighted mean PC densities. Therefore, PC density estimates from larger cerebellar regions (crus I & II) had a greater impact on this overall PC density estimate (similar to the WLS correction in the linear mixed models described above). Cerebellar regional volumes used in this overall PC density estimate were based on planimetric measurements obtained from the histological sections during stereological PC density estimation.

All statistical tests were two-sided, with an alpha level of 0.05, and false discovery rate was used to adjust the cutoff for significance as mentioned in the Results. Confidence intervals were set at 95% for all comparisons, and for correlations, these intervals were determined using bootstrapping with 1,000 replications. Statistical computations were performed with SPSS Version 19 (IBM, Armonk, NY).

Results

Comparisons Based on Diagnosis

Autism cases demonstrate a lower overall Purkinje cell density. We pooled all PC density measurements for each case and tested for an overall difference in PC density based on autism diagnosis using a linear mixed model. The model clustered the PC density measures from each case, and weighted the significance of each region's PC density measures in proportion to the respective region's volume (thereby avoiding the overrepresentation of smaller regions in the overall analysis). The regional volume estimates utilized in this analysis were calculated from histological area measurements of each region obtained as the PCs were quantified on each slide.

Utilizing this model, we observed an effect of autism diagnosis on overall PC density (p = 0.02, Table 2, Test 1). This was reflected as an 11% lower regional volume-weighted mean PC density in the autism group. This finding was additionally corrected for covariance with each case's brain weight, which only slightly improved the significance (p = 0.01, Table 2, Test 2). Because brain weight is a correlate of brain volume [39], this finding indicates that the difference in PC density between the autism and control groups may not be due to volumetric differences but may rather reflect a difference in overall PC number. An alternative possibility is that regional volumetric changes occur in autism (that may not make a substantial impact on overall brain weight but could still affect regional PC density), but a linear mixed model designed to test this found no effect of diagnosis on regional volume (p = 0.936).

Table 2. Linear Mixed Models.[a]

		1		(2)		3		(4)	
		F	p-value	F	p-value	F	p-value	F	p-value
Variables	diagnosis	**6.050**	**0.020**	*7.515*	*0.010*	*7.407*	*0.015*	*9.583*	*0.007*
	gender	**4.802**	**0.036**	**3.697**	**0.068**	*6.373*	*0.022*	*4.423*	*0.054*
	region	*7.159*	*0.001*	*6.652*	*0.001*	**33.783**	**0.000**	**36.031**	**0.000**
Interactions	diagnosis * gender	**0.014**	**0.905**	**0.214**	**0.648**	*0.000*	*1.000*	*0.340*	*0.568*
	diagnosis * region	*0.965*	*0.418*	*1.414*	*0.253*	**0.380**	**0.768**	**0.401**	**0.753**
	gender * region	*2.281*	*0.093*	*3.171*	*0.035*	*2.093*	*0.115*	*2.291*	*0.093*
	gender * diagnosis * region	*1.615*	*0.200*	*2.013*	*0.128*	**3.946**	**0.014**	**5.078**	**0.005**
Covariables	brain weight[a]	N/A		0.372	0.551	N/A		0.311	0.585
Residual Weight		Regional volume		N/A		Regional volume		N/A	
Number of Cases		16		15		16		15	
Diagnosis & Gender	**(M/F)**	Autism (5/3) Control (5/3)		Autism (5/3) Control (4/3)[b]		Autism (5/3) Control (5/3)		Autism (5/3) Control (4/3)[b]	

[a]Cells in the table that have bold data presented designate the target results for each variable and interaction, whereas cells with italicized data designate results that are more adequately assessed by a different test presented in the table: Test 1 was designed to investigate the overall effect of gender and autism diagnosis on PC density. It incorporated cerebellar regional volume as a WLS weight to adjust the test's significance relative to the regional volume for each PC density measurement. Test 3 was designed to test the regional differences in PC density as an effect of gender and diagnosis. Tests 2 and 4 are designed to investigate the contribution of fresh brain weight (grams), as a correlate of tissue volume [39], to Tests 1 and 3, respectively.
[b]One control male case was missing brain weight information.

Purkinje cell density is more affected in crus I & II in autism. Linear mixed models were used to test for an interaction between autism diagnosis and regional PC density (Table 2, Tests 3 & 4). These tests indicated that autism did not affect any of the four regions' PC densities differentially (p = 0.768, Table 2, Test 3). Indeed, each region demonstrated a lower PC density in the autism cases compared to controls. Furthermore, we found that the densities of some of the regions were highly correlated: crus I & II exhibited the strongest correlation ($R^2 = 0.832$, $p = 1.2 \times 10^{-4}$). When the effect of gender was incorporated, however, we did observe a three-way interaction between gender, diagnosis, and region (p = 0.014, Table 2, Test 3). This indicates that autism affects each region differently in males compared to females. Figure 3 demonstrates these regional effects, and shows that in crus I & II, both males and females displayed a lower PC density in the autism group.

Our *a priori* hypothesis based on previous studies was that PC density would be most affected in crus I & II in autism [3,5–9]. To investigate this, we proceeded with *post hoc* analyses of each region's PC density with respect to autism diagnosis using t-tests controlled for false discovery rate. These tests demonstrated that the major effect of autism diagnosis on PC density was in crus I & II, which demonstrated an approximately 20% lower PC density (p = 0.039 & p = 0.032, Fig. 3, Table 3).

Age-related decline in Purkinje cell density does not differ in autism. Prior investigations have reported evidence of an age-related decline in PC density in the anterior lobe [22]. Our PC density measures from the hemispheric portions of lobules IV–VI displayed a trend in support of these previous observations that did not reach significance ($R^2 = -0.23 \pm 0.16$, p = 0.097). However, the age range of our samples did not extend as far into old age as in the prior reports. If samples from individuals with more advanced age were included in the present investigation, it is possible we would have observed a more significant correlation

Table 3. Regional Differences in Purkinje Cell Density.

Region	t	df	p-value	Austism (M/F)	Control (M/F)
Lobules IV–VI	0.677	11	0.512	6 (4/2)	7 (4/3)
Crus I	2.293	13	0.039[a]	8 (5/3)	7 (5/2)
Crus II	2.407	13	0.032[a]	8 (5/3)	7 (5/2)
Lobule X	1.44	13	0.173	8 (5/3)	7 (5/2)

[a]Met the cutoff for false discovery rate.

between age and PC density in this region. Nonetheless, we did observe an age-related decline in overall PC density ($R^2 = -0.39 \pm 0.14$, p = 0.030) (Fig. 4) that did not differ between the autism and control groups.

Flocculonodular dysplasia does not impact PC density. All of the cases in our autism group have been analyzed by neuropathologists at the NYS-IBR in a manner that was blind to diagnosis. Five cases in our study (63%) were reported to display flocculonodular dysplasia by Wegiel et al. [21]. However, we found that lobule X dysmorphology had no effect on the PC density in this region (p = 0.662).

Comparisons Based on Gender

Males have a lower overall Purkinje cell density than females. We investigated the effect of gender on overall PC density by using the same linear mixed model discussed above (Table 2, Test 1 & 2). Again, this test incorporated all PC density measures, clustered by case, and the significance of each measure was weighted by the volume of the region from which it was taken. Using this approach, we observed an effect of gender on overall PC density (p = 0.036, Table 2, Test 1). This was reflected as a

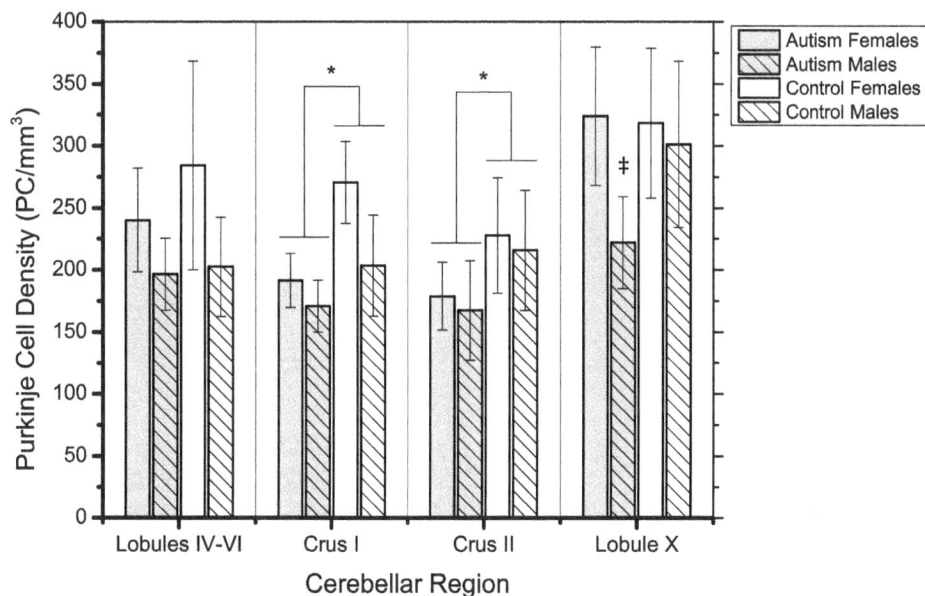

Figure 3. Regional PC Density. This graph demonstrates the findings from our linear mixed models (Table 2). Mean PC density was lower in the autism group in each region assayed, but this finding was most prominent in crus I and II (marked with *), where there was 19.8±9% and 21.7±9% lower PC densities, respectively (p = 0.039 and p = 0.032, t-test). (See the results of this test in Table 3). Lobule X PC density was lower in the males with autism (marked with ‡) than in control males (p = 0.05), and lower than female cases in the autism group (p = 0.022). Bars represent mean ± standard deviation. The number of subjects for each test from each diagnostic group and their gender are represented in the results tables (Tables 2 and 3).

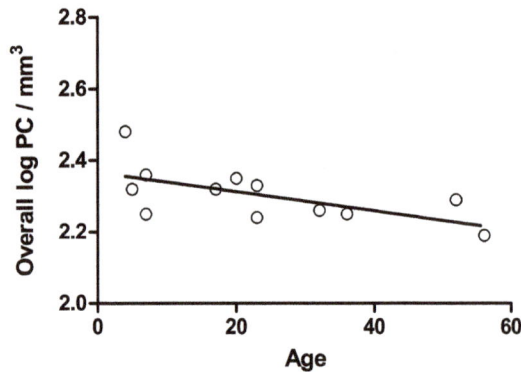

Figure 4. Overall PC Density Decreases with Age. Overall PC density obtained from the anterior, posterior, and flocculonodular lobes negatively correlates with age ($R^2 = -0.39 \pm 0.14$, p = 0.030). Some cases were missing data from an individual region (as described in Methods) and were not included: one female and one male case from the autism and control groups were not included.

21% lower regional volume-weighted mean PC density in the male cases compared to the females.

It was particularly important to correct this model for covariance with brain weight (Table 2, Test 2), because our female cases demonstrated a 13.5% lower brain weight than the male cases (t = 2.857, df = 13, p = 0.013). Doing so negatively impacted the significance of gender's effect on PC density (p = 0.068, Table 2, Test 2). However, one control male case was missing brain weight data, and by removing that case from Test 1, we were able to determine that the main difference in the significance between Test 1 and 2 was due to a loss of statistical power rather than an effect of brain weight on PC density. (Indeed, excluding this case from Test 1 resulted in a similar effect of gender, p = 0.061). Therefore, it appears that volumetric differences minimally contributed to the effect of gender on overall PC density in this investigation.

Lobule X is more affected in males with autism than females. From our linear mixed models descried above (Table 2, Tests 3 & 4), it was apparent that not all regions had similar PC densities. We further confirmed this phenomenon with an ANOVA (p = 1×10^{-4}) using Tukey's HSD *post hoc* analysis and found that lobule X differed from the other regions in terms of PC density, most substantially from crus I & II (p<0.001) and to a lesser extent from hemispheric lobules IV–VI (p = 0.036).

As demonstrated in Figure 3, we observed that males in the autism group had a lower PC density in lobule X while females' lobule X PC densities appeared to be unaffected by autism. We hypothesized this to be a crucial component of the three-way interaction between diagnosis, gender, and region identified in the linear mixed models (Table 2, Tests 3 & 4). We further analyzed this phenomenon by performing t-tests comparing the lobule X PC density in males and females in our autism and control groups. This approach demonstrated that males in the autism group had a 31.5% lower PC density than females in the autism group (t = 3.154, df = 6, p = 0.02), while there was no difference based on gender in the control group (p = 0.768). Additionally, males in the autism group had a trend towards a 26% lower PC density than control males (t = 2.312, df = 8, p = 0.05), while there was no difference between the females in the autism and control groups (p = 0.921). We must emphasize that this is a highly preliminary finding because of the low sample size, particularly with respect to female cases. Indeed, applying a univariate generalized linear

model to test for the interaction between gender and diagnosis in affecting lobule X PC density did not prove significant (p = 0.193). The observed power for this analysis was 0.24 and the effect size f was 0.36. This is a medium-sized gender by diagnosis interaction effect that would require a larger sample pool to reach significance. Further research is required to determine if this finding is reproducible in a larger study, as it may represent a unique gender-based difference in the neuropathology of autism.

We further assessed the contribution of age to our preliminary finding of a gender-based disparity in lobule X PC density in the autism group, because the females in our study were younger than the males (t = 2.35, df = 14, p = 0.036). Using generalized linear modeling with age as a covariate, we found that age only marginally affected the significance of this finding (F = 6.881, p = 0.047).

Volumetric differences may account for the observed gender difference in lobule X Purkinje cell density. The disparity between male and female brain weights in our autism group was nearly twice the expected difference (327 grams compared to 186 grams for the autism cases cataloged in the ATP database) [http://www.atpportal.org], which may be a reflection of the small sample size available for this study. Furthermore, PC density in lobule X was correlated with brain weight in the autism group ($R^2 = -0.67$, p = 0.014). Brain weight is a correlate of brain volume [39], and thus we performed a generalized linear model with brain weight as a covariate to assess its contribution to the observed gender difference in lobule X PC density. Indeed, eliminating the effect of brain weight impacted the significance of the difference between male and female lobule X PC density in the autism group (p = 0.642), as well as the difference between males with autism compared to control males (p = 0.117).

Additionally, MRI data was available for the autism cases in our study and we used these to obtain cerebellar volume measurements. Similar to what we observed with brain weight, lobule X PC density in the autism group strongly correlated with cerebellar volume ($R^2 = -0.80 \pm 0.02$, p = 0.008). After correcting the generalized linear model for covariance with cerebellar volume, we saw a similar loss of significance in the difference between male and female lobule X PC density in the autism group (p = 0.730).

In light of these findings, a gender-based disparity in lobule X volume likely contributes to the PC density differences observed in this region. This is in contrast to the findings of reduced PC density in crus I & II in autism, for which there was no observed difference in the significance following a correction for brain weight (p = 0.025 and p = 0.017). We also noticed in our linear mixed model that including brain weight as a covariate marginally increased the significance of the three-way interaction between gender, diagnosis, and region (p = 0.005, Table 2, Test 4). Therefore, this volumetric contribution to the PC density differences observed in the autism group is limited to lobule X.

Behavioral Correlation with Purkinje Cell Density

We examined our PC density estimates looking for possible correlations with behavioral measures obtained from the ADI-R. The ADI-R is comprised of 93 questions scored on an ordinal scale, which are combined into domain scores for the three core autism symptom domains (communication, social interaction, and restricted/repetitive behavior). However, these domain scores compound the intrinsic inter-rater variance of each ADI-R question, thus diminishing the power to determine relationships between neuropathological findings and specific behavioral symptoms. Therefore, we performed regression analysis on a selection of 7 specific ADI-R questions that were recently reported to associate strongly with autism diagnosis [Presentation by Dennis

Wall, "Shortening the Behavioral Diagnosis of Autism Through Artificial Intelligence and Mobile Health Technologies," Autism Consortium 2011 Symposium, Boston, MA]. We limited our regression analyses to these specific behavioral variables and performed false discovery rate analysis (as detailed in [37]) to reduce the probability of a type I statistical error.

In our initial analysis of ADI-R domain scores, we did not observe a significant association between PC density and any of the domain scores. However, in our analysis of specific questions from the ADI-R, we did identify a plausible association between lobule X PC density and social/communicative use of direct eye gaze ($R^2 = -0.75 \pm 0.04$, $p = 0.012$) (Fig. 5). Higher scores on the ADI-R correspond with increased symptom severity. Therefore, lower lobule X PC densities were associated with greater impairments in social eye contact. Utilizing false discovery rate analysis, this association failed to meet the cutoff for significance (which was $p = 0.009$); however, due to known involvement of this region in regulating eye movement [20], we feel this observation merits further investigation.

As we had done above, we utilized generalized linear models with brain weight or cerebellar volume as a covariate to determine if tissue volume contributed to the observed association between lobule X PC density and direct eye gaze. Both of these covariables were found to substantially reduce the significance of the association ($p = 0.072$ for brain weight and $p = 0.171$ for cerebellar volume). Therefore, tissue volume represents a significant component of the observed association between lobule X PC density and the social and communicative use of direct gaze.

Analyses of Clinical Covariables and Potential Confounding Factors

Potential confounding factors and clinically relevant covariables such as cerebellar hemisphere, PMI, postmortem fixation time, epilepsy, MR, developmental regression, lack of verbal development, delayed attainment of motor milestones, and complications during pregnancy were tested to determine their effects on PC density in crus I & II or lobule X, and none were found to have a significant effect. Similarly, none of these factors were found to impact the association between lobule X PC density and direct gaze.

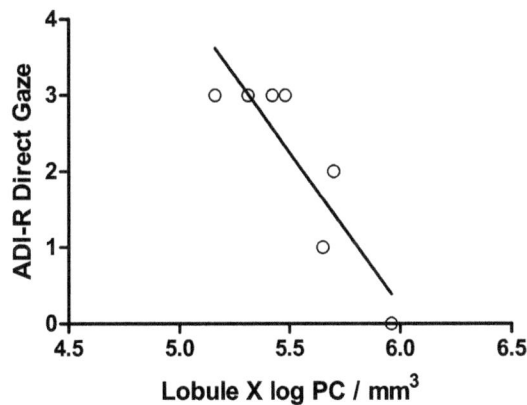

Figure 5. Lobule X PC Density is Associated with Direct Gaze. Lobule X PC density in the autism group negatively correlated with ADI-R question 50, which assessed the social and communicative use of eye contact ($R^2 = -0.75 \pm 0.04$, $p = 0.012$). Higher scores on the ADI-R correspond with increased symptom severity. One case from the autism group was lacking sufficient ADI-R data to be included in this analysis.

Discussion

Case Demographics

Cerebellar pathology was first proposed as a potential contributor to autism symptomatology in 1968 [40], and the first qualitative report of lower PC density was published in 1980 [10]. To date, PC density assessments have been reported from 45 cerebella of individuals with autism, 30 of which demonstrated a lower PC density, most prominently reported in the posterolateral hemispheres where crus I & II are located [3–10,25,26]. Apart from the most recent studies, these reports have been criticized as being semi-quantitative at best, and the sample selection has not been representative of the demographics of the overall autism population as currently defined. For example, 87.5% of cases analyzed in prior reports (for which data is available) exhibited MR compared with the recently reported 41% in the autism population [27], and 57.9% of these cases exhibited epilepsy compared with the recent estimate of 38% in the autism population [28]. Furthermore, only 6 cases were females, despite the estimated 4.5:1 male-to-female ratio of autism's prevalence [27]. This has prevented gender-based comparisons of autism neuropathology in the past. For this study, we included 3 female cases with autism and 3 female controls as a preliminary assessment of the effect of gender on PC density in autism. It is difficult to rule out the contribution of factors such as epilepsy or MR to lower PC density based on the data from prior neuropathological investigations of autism. The current study was thus designed with a sample population more representative of the overall autism population, with 38% of samples obtained from subjects with MR ranging from mild to severe, and 38% of samples having documented epilepsy.

Stereological Estimation of Purkinje Cell Density

The determination of PC density in the cerebellum is challenging, primarily due to complications in defining the anatomical boundaries of the PC layer and selecting a reference volume. A traditional approach has been to quantify PC density by drawing a line through the PC layer and counting the number of PC per unit length. Past studies using this approach have shown markedly variable density estimates in healthy controls from as little as 1.6 PC/mm to as many as 11 PC/mm [41–49]. An inherent problem in placement of this line within the PC layer is the large number of subjective determinations. Factors contributing to this subjectivity include: the variable horizontal position of the PCs within this layer, the markedly convoluted folding of the layer through which the stereologist must draw a curved line, the difficulty in determining the layer's anatomical boundaries at sites where the PCs are sparse or absent, and the changing width of the layer as viewed on obliquely cut sections (Fig. 6, 7). These considerations, along with the very narrow width of the human PC layer (1 to 2% of the width of a cerebellar folium), create problems for the accurate measurement of the PC layer volume and thus for its use as a reference volume to measure the density of PCs.

In order to obviate these issues and provide a more reliable estimate of PC density, we sampled from the entirety of each region of interest, within clear anatomical boundaries, and thus included the subcortical white matter of each region. With this strategy we were able to eliminate over 50% of the variability in our PC density estimates (compare to Whitney et el. [9]). Further, our measurements of PC/mm³ closely agree with recently published estimates obtained using a novel stereological probe designed to better assess the density of objects like PCs that are distributed within a limited and convoluted portion of the region of interest [50].

A

B

C

D

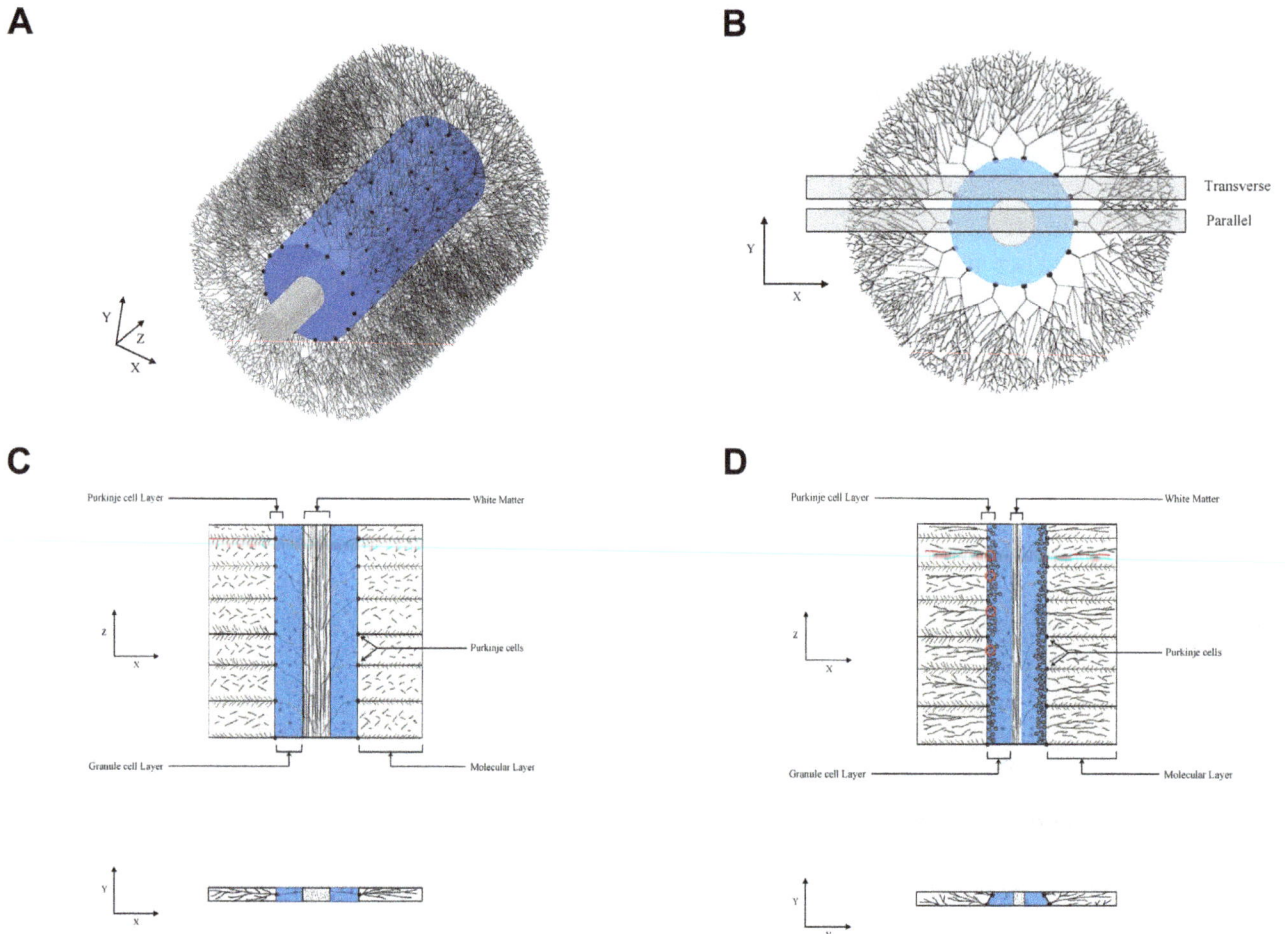

Figure 6. Models of PC Arrangement. These figures represent the importance of estimating PC density in 3-dimensional space rather than along a 1-dimensional line (PC/mm^3 rather than PC/mm). 7a and 7b display two views of a 3-dimensional model of a cerebellar folium, in which PCs (black) are arranged in a monolayer apposed to the granule cell layer (blue) that surrounds a central white matter tract (white). 7b displays two slices, one perfectly parallel to a plane of PCs, and the other, more realistically, transverse to this plane. 7c and 7d are cartoons demonstrating the PC arrangement within the parallel and transverse slice, respectively. Notice in 7d the PC layer is thicker, the degree to which depends on the slice position. Also notice that the selection of which PCs lie perfectly along a line is ambiguous (a few examples have been circled in red). This ambiguity introduces human error when performing an estimate of PC/mm that is eliminated in 3-dimensional estimates of PC/mm^3 as are utilized in this study.

Neuronal density is an important morphometric measure in neuropathology, despite the inherent variability that occurs as a consequence of differential tissue shrinkage in each case. In this study, tissue shrinkage resulting from tissue processing varied only marginally from 44% to 52% according to the pathologists' reports and did not differ between groups. An alternative stereological strategy is to quantify total neuronal number using the Optical Fractionator probe, but this requires 100% of the assayed region to be pristinely represented in the sampled slides [34]. Neuronal density measures are distinct from estimates of total number however, in that they reflect the spacing of neuronal somas and neuropil in a tissue, a property that has a number of physiological implications [51,52].

Implications of Cerebellar Neuropathology in Autism

The results of the present investigation corroborate prior reports of lower PC density in autism, and using a more precise and thorough method of quantification, demonstrate that lower PC density is most prominent in crus I and II, which constitute lobule VIIa of the posterior lobe. Lobule VIIa is intimately involved with numerous neocortical areas and has been directly implicated in

non-motor functions in humans. In a report of 156 patients with cerebellar damage, 100% of patients with crus I lesions presented with attention impairments, and 100% of patients with crus II lesions presented with impairments in visuospatial memory and verbal memory (with some overlap between the two regions' functions) [53]. Further, a recent fMRI study demonstrated involvement of lobule VII in auditory working memory in nonhuman primates [54]. Anatomical and comparative anatomical studies have demonstrated a strong relationship between lobule VII and the cerebral cortex. Comparative studies highlight a relationship between the volume of the prefrontal cortex and that of lobule VII, with a pronounced elaboration of VIIa in human evolution in concert with frontal cortical expansion [55]. Lobule VIIa is reciprocally connected with the prefrontal cortex, an executive function/working memory area, as well as the posterior parietal cortex, a multimodal processing area [12,56,57]. Recent studies employing resting state fMRI have further demonstrated functional connectivity between lobule VIIa and these cortical areas [58,59]. These prefrontal and posterior parietal cortices comprise a Frontoparietal Attention Network (FAN), which is postulated to play an important role in processing

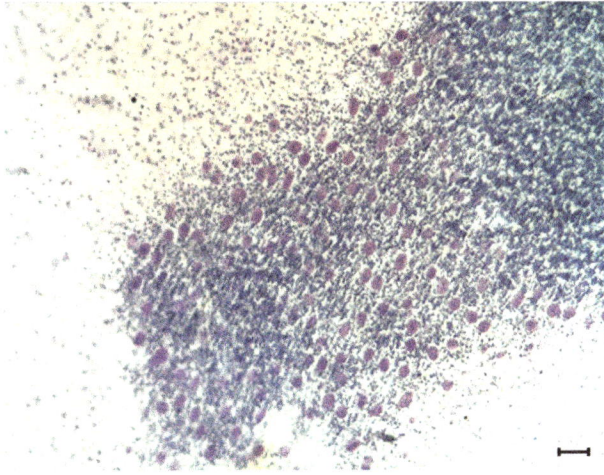

Figure 7. Photomicrograph of Transverse Section. This photomicrograph is an illustrative example of the arrangement of PCs on a transverse section. The PCs (purple) go out of focus to the left as the PC layer curves through the depth of the tissue section. The granule cell layer (blue) is visible below the PC layer, the molecular layer surrounds the PC layer (seen here as sparsely stained space), and the white matter tract is out of view to the right. Nissl-stained section from the celloidin collection used in this study, reference bar = 100 μm.

the salience of environmental cues [60]. The prefrontal cortex is involved in a variety of working memory and executive functions that have shown impairment in individuals with autism [61–65]. Further, it is important to note that in normal brain development, lobule VII displays unique features that distinguish it from other cerebellar lobules [66–69]. An example of the distinct developmental trajectory of lobule VII neurons was demonstrated in a mouse model of immune activation at mid-gestation, in which a specific reduction in PC density in lobule VII was observed but neighboring regions were unaffected [70].

We have also identified a potential sexually dimorphic effect within lobule X. Lobule X has been associated with vestibular regulation as well as coordination of gaze [13–18]. The lobule X PC density was found to be lower in males with autism as a result of increased tissue volume (Fig. 3). Furthermore, this effect appeared to correlate with the ability to properly employ social and communicative use of eye gaze, as assessed by the ADI-R (Fig. 5). This correlation between lobule X PC density and social eye gaze failed to reach the cutoff for significance imposed by false discovery rate analysis, but in light of the role of lobule X in modulating eye movement, the association is plausible [20]. These preliminary findings will require further investigation as this is the first report of the association between lobule X PC density and social employment of eye contact. Further, we recommend that future investigations analyze the flocculus and nodulus within lobule X separately, as these regions have functional distinctions [71] and may display different pathologies.

The mechanism of the alterations in PC density noted in this study remains unexplained. As the cerebellum develops in close coordination with many other networks within the central nervous system [72–76], it is possible that altered PC density represents a compensatory mechanism or downstream effect of an earlier developmental pathology. In the present study, the degree to which PC density diminished with age did not differ between the autism and control groups over the age span studied (from 4 to 56

years). This lack of a notable age-related decline in PC density in the autism cases argues against a lifelong progressive loss of PCs in this disorder. The initial neuropathological studies from members of our group predicted that the decreased density of PCs observed in the cerebella of autistic individuals may be due to the loss of these neurons during the late prenatal period [5]. This prediction was based on the observation that the inferior olivary neurons in the brain stem of individuals with autism are preserved despite reduced PC densities. The intimate relationship between inferior olivary neurons and PCs is established in late gestation, and the loss of PCs in term and older aged infants is typically associated with inferior olivary degeneration. In a follow-up investigation, Whitney et al. noted in the autistic brain that there was a preservation of basket and stellate cells in areas with decreased PCs, which indicates that the PCs in these regions established their usual relationship with these interneurons in late gestation and were subsequently lost [77].

Comments, Limitations, and Future Directions

Neuronal density can be affected by both changes in tissue volume as well as neuronal number. Therefore, we have demonstrated that the contribution of tissue volume to a subset of our findings is indeed significant.

Our study was limited by a small sample size, but each case was systematically analyzed using precise methods that allowed for the identification of consistent and potentially behaviorally relevant alterations in regional PC density in autism. Fewer female cases than would be ideal in making gender comparisons were available and thus these comparisons should be viewed as strictly preliminary. Additionally, the age range of the study was not as wide as in prior studies that identified an age-related decline in PC density. Therefore, future analyses in older patients may demonstrate a different trajectory of age-related PC decline in the autism population. Furthermore, due to the age range of our study, it was not possible to assess the early developmental processes that are believed to be crucial in understanding autism development but that occur prior to the age at which autism can be diagnosed. For a better understanding of early development, we may need to rely on animal models, as well as further advancements in *in utero* longitudinal bioimaging techniques and efforts to identify clinically relevant prenatal biomarkers [78,79]. To better understand the relationship between neuropathology and behavioral symptomatology in autism, it will be necessary to obtain more detailed qualitative as well as quantitative behavioral measures from tissue donors.

Current investigations are underway to determine biochemical differences in crus I and II that distinguish these regions from other cerebellar regions in an attempt to better characterize the pathophysiology of autism.

Acknowledgments

We gratefully acknowledge the tissue contributions made by families to the Autism Speaks' Autism Tissue Program (ATP), which provided the material for this study.

Author Contributions

Conceived and designed the experiments: MLB JS TLK. Performed the experiments: JS TY KE CC EL KW JH. Analyzed the data: JS TLK MLB. Contributed reagents/materials/analysis tools: MLB TLK. Wrote the paper: JS TLK MLB.

References

1. American Psychiatric Assotiation (1994) Diagnostic and statistical manual of mental disorders: DSM-IV. Washington DC: American Psychiatric Association.

2. Amaral DG, Schumann CM, Nordahl CW (2008) Neuroanatomy of autism. Trends in Neurosciences 31: 137–145.

3. Bailey A, Luthert P, Dean A, Harding B, Janota I, et al. (1998) A clinicopathological study of autism. Brain 121: 889–905.

4. Fehlow P, Bernstein K, Tennstedt A, Walther F (1993) [Early infantile autism and excessive aerophagy with symptomatic megacolon and ileus in a case of Ehlers-Danlos syndrome]. Pädiatrie Und Grenzgebiete 31: 259–267.

5. Kemper TL, Bauman ML (1993) The contribution of neuropathologic studies to the understanding of autism. Neurologic Clinics 11: 175–187.

6. Lee M, Martin-Ruiz C, Graham A, Court J, Jaros E, et al. (2002) Nicotinic receptor abnormalities in the cerebellar cortex in autism. Brain 125: 1483–1495.

7. Ritvo ER, Freeman BJ, Scheibel AB, Duong T, Robinson H, et al. (1986) Lower Purkinje cell counts in the cerebella of four autistic subjects: initial findings of the UCLA-NSAC Autopsy Research Report. The American Journal of Psychiatry 143: 862–866.

8. Vargas DL, Nascimbene C, Krishnan C, Zimmerman AW, Pardo CA (2005) Neuroglial activation and neuroinflammation in the brain of patients with autism. Annals of Neurology 57: 67–81.

9. Whitney ER, Kemper TL, Bauman ML, Rosene DL, Blatt GJ (2008) Cerebellar Purkinje cells are reduced in a subpopulation of autistic brains: a stereological experiment using calbindin-D28k. Cerebellum (London, England) 7: 406–416.

10. Williams RS, Hauser SL, Purpura DP, DeLong GR, Swisher CN (1980) Autism and Mental Retardation: Neuropathologic Studies Performed in Four Retarded Persons With Autistic Behavior. Archives of Neurology 37: 749–749.

11. Ito M (2008) Control of mental activities by internal models in the cerebellum. Nat Rev Neurosci 9: 304–313.

12. Schmahmann JD (2010) The Role of the Cerebellum in Cognition and Emotion: Personal Reflections Since 1982 on the Dysmetria of Thought Hypothesis, and Its Historical Evolution from Theory to Therapy. Neuropsychology Review 20: 236–260.

13. Balaban CD (2004) Projections from the parabrachial nucleus to the vestibular nuclei: potential substrates for autonomic and limbic influences on vestibular responses. Brain Research 996: 126–137.

14. Brauth SE (1977) Direct accessory optic projections to the vestibulo-cerebellum: a possible substrate for oculomotor control systems. Experimental Brain Research Experimentelle Hirnforschung Expérimentation Cérébrale 28: 73–84.

15. Cohen B, Wearne S, Dai M, Raphan T (1999) Spatial orientation of the angular vestibulo-ocular reflex. Journal of Vestibular Research: Equilibrium & Orientation 9: 163–172.

16. Pakan JMP, Graham DJ, Wylie DR (2010) Organization of visual mossy fiber projections and zebrin expression in the pigeon vestibulocerebellum. The Journal of Comparative Neurology 518: 175–198.

17. Schmahmann JD (1996) From movement to thought: anatomic substrates of the cerebellar contribution to cognitive processing. Human Brain Mapping 4: 174–198.

18. Straka H, Beck JC, Pastor AM, Baker R (2006) Morphology and physiology of the cerebellar vestibulolateral lobe pathways linked to oculomotor function in the goldfish. Journal of Neurophysiology 96: 1963–1980.

19. Bauman ML, Kemper TL (2005) Neuroanatomic observations of the brain in autism: a review and future directions. International Journal of Developmental Neuroscience: The Official Journal of the International Society for Developmental Neuroscience 23: 183–187.

20. Wegiel J, Kuchna I, Nowicki K, Imaki H, Wegiel J, et al. (2013) Contribution of olivofloccular circuitry developmental defects to atypical gaze in autism. Brain Res 1512: 106–122.

21. Wegiel J, Kuchna I, Nowicki K, Imaki H, Wegiel J, et al. (2010) The neuropathology of autism: defects of neurogenesis and neuronal migration, and dysplastic changes. Acta Neuropathologica 119: 755–770.

22. Andersen BB, Gundersen HJG, Pakkenberg B (2003) Aging of the human cerebellum: a stereological study. The Journal of Comparative Neurology 466: 356–365.

23. Itō M (2012) Cerebellum the brain for an implicit self. Upper Saddle River, N.J. : FT Press.

24. Stoodley CJ, Valera EM, Schmahmann JD (2012) Functional topography of the cerebellum for motor and cognitive tasks: An fMRI study. NeuroImage 59: 1560–1570.

25. Fatemi SH, Halt AR, Realmuto G, Earle J, Kist DA, et al. (2002) Purkinje cell size is reduced in cerebellum of patients with autism. Cellular and Molecular Neurobiology 22: 171–175.

26. Guerin P, Lyon G, Barthelemy C, Sostak E, Chevrollier V, et al. (1996) Neuropathological study of a case of autistic syndrome with severe mental retardation. Developmental Medicine and Child Neurology 38: 203–211.

27. Centers for Disease Control and Prevention (2009) Prevalence of autism spectrum disorders - Autism and Developmental Disabilities Monitoring Network, United States, 2006. MMWR Surveillance Summaries: Morbidity and Mortality Weekly Report Surveillance Summaries/CDC 58: 1–20.

28. Danielsson S, Gillberg IC, Billstedt E, Gillberg C, Olsson I (2005) Epilepsy in young adults with autism: a prospective population-based follow-up study of 120 individuals diagnosed in childhood. Epilepsia 46: 918–923.

29. Lord C, Rutter M, Le Couteur A (1994) Autism Diagnostic Interview-Revised: a revised version of a diagnostic interview for caregivers of individuals with possible pervasive developmental disorders. J Autism Dev Disord 24: 659–685.

30. Dekaban AS (1978) Changes in brain weights during the span of human life: relation of brain weights to body heights and body weights. Annals of Neurology 4: 345–356.

31. Heinsen H, Arzberger T, Schmitz C (2000) Celloidin mounting (embedding without infiltration) - a new, simple and reliable method for producing serial sections of high thickness through complete human brains and its application to stereological and immunohistochemical investigations. Journal of Chemical Neuroanatomy 20: 49–59.

32. Angevine J, Mancall E, Yakovlev P (1961) The human cerebellum: An atlas of gross topography in serial sections. Boston, MA: Little, Brown.

33. Schmahmann JD (2000) MRI atlas of the human cerebellum. San Diego: Academic Press.

34. Gundersen HJ, Bagger P, Bendtsen TF, Evans SM, Korbo L, et al. (1988) The new stereological tools: disector, fractionator, nucleator and point sampled intercepts and their use in pathological research and diagnosis. APMIS: Acta Pathologica, Microbiologica, Et Immunologica Scandinavica 96: 857–881.

35. Gundersen HJ, Jensen EB, Kieu K, Nielsen J (1999) The efficiency of systematic sampling in stereology-reconsidered. J Microsc 193: 199–211.

36. Mouton PR (2002) Principles and practices of unbiased stereology : an introduction for bioscientists. Baltimore: Johns Hopkins University Press. x, 214 p. p.

37. Curran-Everett D (2000) Multiple comparisons: philosophies and illustrations. Am J Physiol Regul Integr Comp Physiol 279: R1–8.

38. Wall DP, Kosmicki J, DeLuca TF, Harstad E, Fusaro VA (2012) Use of machine learning to shorten observation-based screening and diagnosis of autism. Translational Psychiatry 2: e100–e100.

39. Witelson SF, Beresh H, Kigar DL (2006) Intelligence and brain size in 100 postmortem brains: sex, lateralization and age factors. Brain 129: 386–398.

40. Ornitz EM, Ritvo ER (1968) Neurophysiologic mechanisms underlying perceptual inconstancy in autistic and schizophrenic children. Archives of General Psychiatry 19: 22–27.

41. Fukutani Y, Cairns NJ, Rossor MN, Lantos PL (1996) Purkinje cell loss and astrocytosis in the cerebellum in familial and sporadic Alzheimer's disease. Neuroscience Letters 214: 33–36.

42. Karhunen PJ, Erkinjuntti T, Laippala P (1994) Moderate alcohol consumption and loss of cerebellar Purkinje cells. BMJ (Clinical Research Ed) 308: 1663–1667.

43. Kume A, Takahashi A, Hashizume Y, Asai J (1991) A histometrical and comparative study on Purkinje cell loss and olivary nucleus cell loss in multiple system atrophy. Journal of the Neurological Sciences 101: 178–186.

44. Lohr JB, Jeste DV (1986) Cerebellar pathology in schizophrenia? A neurometric study. Biological Psychiatry 21: 865–875.

45. Matsumoto R, Nakano I, Arai N, Oda M, Yagishita S, et al. (1998) Loss of the dentate nucleus neurons is associated with torpedo formation: a morphometric study in progressive supranuclear palsy and dentatorubro-pallidoluysian atrophy. Acta Neuropathologica 95: 149–153.

46. Phillips SC, Harper CG, Kril J (1987) A quantitative histological study of the cerebellar vermis in alcoholic patients. Brain: A Journal of Neurology 110 (Pt 2): 301–314.

47. Sjöbeck M, Englund E (2001) Alzheimer's disease and the cerebellum: a morphologic study on neuronal and glial changes. Dementia and Geriatric Cognitive Disorders 12: 211–218.

48. Torvik A, Torp S, Lindboe CF (1986) Atrophy of the cerebellar vermis in ageing. A morphometric and histologic study. Journal of the Neurological Sciences 76: 283–294.

49. Wegiel J, Wisniewski HM, Dziewiatkowski J, Badmajew E, Tarnawski M, et al. (1999) Cerebellar atrophy in Alzheimer's disease-clinicopathological correlations. Brain Research 818: 41–50.

50. Agashiwala RM, Louis ED, Hof PR, Perl DP (2008) A novel approach to non-biased systematic random sampling: a stereologic estimate of Purkinje cells in the human cerebellum. Brain Research 1236: 73–78.

51. Cullen DK, Gilroy ME, Irons HR, Laplaca MC (2010) Synapse-to-neuron ratio is inversely related to neuronal density in mature neuronal cultures. Brain Research 1359: 44–55.

52. Ivenshitz M, Segal M (2010) Neuronal Density Determines Network Connectivity and Spontaneous Activity in Cultured Hippocampus. Journal of Neurophysiology 104: 1052–1060.

53. Tedesco AM, Chiricozzi FR, Clausi S, Lupo M, Molinari M, et al. (2011) The cerebellar cognitive profile. Brain: A Journal of Neurology 134: 3669–3683.

54. Hayter AL, Langdon DW, Ramnani N (2007) Cerebellar contributions to working memory. NeuroImage 36: 943–954.

55. Balsters JH, Cussans E, Diedrichsen J, Phillips KA, Preuss TM, et al. (2010) Evolution of the cerebellar cortex: The selective expansion of prefrontal-projecting cerebellar lobules. NeuroImage 49: 2045–2052.

56. Schmahmann JD, Pandya DN (1997) The cerebrocerebellar system. International Review of Neurobiology 41: 31–60.

57. Xiong G, Hiramatsu T, Nagao S (2002) Corticopontocerebellar pathway from the prearcuate region to hemispheric lobule VII of the cerebellum: an

anterograde and retrograde tracing study in the monkey. Neuroscience Letters 322: 173–176.

58. Habas C, Kamdar N, Nguyen D, Prater K, Beckmann CF, et al. (2009) Distinct Cerebellar Contributions to Intrinsic Connectivity Networks. The Journal of Neuroscience 29: 8586–8594.

59. O'Reilly JX, Beckmann CF, Tomassini V, Ramnani N, Johansen-Berg H (2010) Distinct and overlapping functional zones in the cerebellum defined by resting state functional connectivity. Cerebral Cortex (New York, NY: 1991) 20: 953–965.

60. Ptak R (2011) The Frontoparietal Attention Network of the Human Brain: Action, Saliency, and a Priority Map of the Environment. The Neuroscientist: A Review Journal Bringing Neurobiology, Neurology and Psychiatry.

61. Christ SE, Kester LE, Bodner KE, Miles JH (2011) Evidence for selective inhibitory impairment in individuals with autism spectrum disorder. Neuropsychology 25: 690–701.

62. Holdnack J, Goldstein G, Drozdick L (2011) Social perception and WAIS-IV Performance in adolescents and adults diagnosed with Asperger's Syndrome and Autism. Assessment 18: 192–200.

63. Poirier M, Martin JS, Gaigg SB, Bowler DM (2011) Short-term memory in autism spectrum disorder. Journal of Abnormal Psychology 120: 247–252.

64. Taylor MJ, Donner EJ, Pang EW (2012) fMRI and MEG in the study of typical and atypical cognitive development. Neurophysiologie Clinique = Clinical Neurophysiology 42: 19–25.

65. Yerys BE, Wallace GL, Jankowski KF, Bollich A, Kenworthy L (2011) Impaired Consonant Trigrams Test (CTT) performance relates to everyday working memory difficulties in children with autism spectrum disorders. Child Neuropsychology: A Journal on Normal and Abnormal Development in Childhood and Adolescence 17: 391–399.

66. Altman J, Bayer SA (1996) Development of the Cerebellar System: In Relation to Its Evolution, Structure, and Functions. Boca Raton, FL: CRC-Press.

67. Ozol K, Hayden JM, Oberdick J, Hawkes R (1999) Transverse zones in the vermis of the mouse cerebellum. The Journal of Comparative Neurology 412: 95–111.

68. Rogers JH, Ciossek T, Menzel P, Pasquale EB (1999) Eph receptors and ephrins demarcate cerebellar lobules before and during their formation. Mechanisms of Development 87: 119–128.

69. Vastagh C, Víg J, Hámori J, Takács J (2005) Delayed postnatal settlement of cerebellar Purkinje cells in vermal lobules VI and VII of the mouse. Anatomy and Embryology 209: 471–484.

70. Shi L, Smith SEP, Malkova N, Tse D, Su Y, et al. (2009) Activation of the maternal immune system alters cerebellar development in the offspring. Brain, Behavior, and Immunity 23: 116–123.

71. Pakan JM, Graham DJ, Iwaniuk AN, Wylie DR (2008) Differential projections from the vestibular nuclei to the flocculus and uvula-nodulus in pigeons (Columba livia). J Comp Neurol 508: 402–417.

72. Araujo E, Pires CR, Nardozza LMM, Filho HAG, Moron AF (2007) Correlation of the fetal cerebellar volume with other fetal growth indices by three-dimensional ultrasound. Journal of Maternal-Fetal and Neonatal Medicine 20: 581–587.

73. Herculano-Houzel S (2010) Coordinated scaling of cortical and cerebellar numbers of neurons. Frontiers in Neuroanatomy 4: 12–12.

74. Larsell O, Von Berthelsdorf S (1941) The ansoparamedian lobule of the cerebellum and its correlation with the limb-muscle masses. The Journal of Comparative Neurology 75: 315–340.

75. Limperopoulos C, Soul JS, Gauvreau K, Huppi PS, Warfield SK, et al. (2005) Late Gestation Cerebellar Growth Is Rapid and Impeded by Premature Birth. Pediatrics 115: 688–695.

76. Rubia K, Smith AB, Taylor E, Brammer M (2007) Linear age-correlated functional development of right inferior fronto-striato-cerebellar networks during response inhibition and anterior cingulate during error-related processes. Human Brain Mapping 28: 1163–1177.

77. Whitney ER, Kemper TL, Rosene DL, Bauman ML, Blatt GJ (2009) Density of cerebellar basket and stellate cells in autism: evidence for a late developmental loss of Purkinje cells. Journal of Neuroscience Research 87: 2245–2254.

78. Saksena S, Husain N, Das V, Pradhan M, Trivedi R, et al. (2008) Diffusion tensor imaging in the developing human cerebellum with histologic correlation. International Journal of Developmental Neuroscience 26: 705–711.

79. Van Kooij BJM, Benders MJNL, Anbeek P, Van Haastert IC, De Vries LS, et al. (2011) Cerebellar volume and proton magnetic resonance spectroscopy at term, and neurodevelopment at 2 years of age in preterm infants. Developmental Medicine and Child Neurology.

80. Larsell O (1958) Lobules of the mammalian and human cerebellum. Anatomical Record 130: 329–330.

A Different View on the Checkerboard? Alterations in Early and Late Visually Evoked EEG Potentials in Asperger Observers

Juergen Kornmeier[1,2]*, Rike Wörner[3], Andreas Riedel[4], Michael Bach[2], Ludger Tebartz van Elst[4]

1 Institute for Frontier Areas of Psychology and Mental Health, Freiburg, Germany, 2 Eye Center, Albert-Ludwigs-University of Freiburg, Freiburg, Germany, 3 PPD Germany GmbH & Co Kg, Karlsruhe, Germany, 4 Section for Experimental Neuropsychiatry, Clinic for Psychiatry & Psychotherapy, Albert-Ludwigs-University of Freiburg, Freiburg, Germany

Abstract

Background: Asperger Autism is a lifelong psychiatric condition with highly circumscribed interests and routines, problems in social cognition, verbal and nonverbal communication, and also perceptual abnormalities with sensory hypersensitivity. To objectify both lower level visual and cognitive alterations we looked for differences in visual event-related potentials (EEG) between Asperger observers and matched controls while they observed simple checkerboard stimuli.

Methods: In a balanced oddball paradigm checkerboards of two checksizes (0.6° and 1.2°) were presented with different frequencies. Participants counted the occurrence times of the rare fine or rare coarse checkerboards in different experimental conditions. We focused on early visual ERP differences as a function of checkerboard size and the classical P3b ERP component as an indicator of cognitive processing.

Results: We found an early (100–200 ms after stimulus onset) occipital ERP effect of checkerboard size (dominant spatial frequency). This effect was weaker in the Asperger than in the control observers. Further a typical parietal/central oddball-P3b occurred at 500 ms with the rare checkerboards. The P3b showed a right-hemispheric lateralization, which was more prominent in Asperger than in control observers.

Discussion: The difference in the early occipital ERP effect between the two groups may be a physiological marker of differences in the processing of small visual details in Asperger observers compared to normal controls. The stronger lateralization of the P3b in Asperger observers may indicate a stronger involvement of the right-hemispheric network of bottom-up attention. The lateralization of the P3b signal might be a compensatory consequence of the compromised early checksize effect. Higher-level analytical information processing units may need to compensate for difficulties in low-level signal analysis.

Editor: Sam Gilbert, University College London, United Kingdom

Funding: This study was supported by the Deutsche Forschungsgemeinschaft (KO 4764/1-1 & TE 280/8-1). The funders had no role in study design, data collection and analysis, decision to publish, or preparation of the manuscript.

Competing Interests: RW is employed by PPD Germany GmbH & Co. There are no patents, products in development or marketed products to declare.

* E-mail: juergen.kornmeier@uni-freiburg.de

Introduction

Patients with Autism Spectrum Disorder (ASD) are characterized by lifelong routines, circumscribed interests and deficits in social cognition and communication, e.g. [1]. The prevalence in the general population is estimated to be above 1% [2]. ASD results in significant socioeconomic consequences with up to 50,000 € annual costs per patient in particular due to secondary psychiatric problems and early retirement [3]. This illustrates the need for further etiological and therapeutic research.

High Functioning Autism as a Possibly More Homogenous Autistic Subcategory

Traditionally, autism has been conceptualized as a severe form of neurodevelopmental disorder, which is associated with mental retardation, and severe deficits of intelligence and language in the majority of cases [4]. However, recent research has indicated that there is a broad variety of different severities and phenotypes of ASD including those with normal or even above average intelligence [5]. Secondary and syndromal forms of ASD which often go along with subnormal IQ and learning disabilities are increasingly distinguished from primary familial but probably not mono- or oligogenetic forms [4,5,6]. Theoretical considerations as well as clinical observations support the assumption that the subgroup of "primary" autism might more often be associated with normal or even above average intelligence scores [5,7]. We thus concentrated on patients with Asperger syndrome ("AS") with normal or above average IQ in order to get a more homogenous sample and thus to minimize the number of confounding factors [8].

So far clinical diagnostics have been mainly based on behavioral variables. Physiological markers are rare and related findings inconsistent, e.g. [9,10,11]. Further, the definitions of AS and ASD in general are primarily determined by cognitive, especially social symptoms whereas specificities in lower level sensory processing have only recently been integrated in the diagnostic criteria of DSM-V (www.dsm5.org). Still, it has long been recognized that such lower level perceptual and in particular visual abnormalities in autism might well be linked to the core pathophysiology of autism. Related reports range from abnormalities in the contribution of magnocellular pathways to face perception, e.g. [12], to alterations in processing of motion, e.g. [13], contrast, e.g. [14], or spatial frequency, e.g. [15]. Simmons et al. provided a comprehensive review about psychophysical and physiological indicators of altered visual processing in autistic observers [10].

The focus in the present EEG study was thus on the question of whether this higher visual sensitivity of Asperger observers for small object details may be visible in early visual stimulus-dependent EEG signatures and whether potential findings from lower-level processing correlate with EEG signatures related to higher-level/cognitive processing.

Spatially periodic stimuli like checkerboards are well-established visual stimuli in clinical electrodiagnostics (EEG), their reversal evoking a reliable modulation of early visual event related potential (ERP) amplitudes as a function of spatial frequency, e.g. [16]. In the present study we analyzed checkerboard onset ERPs and focused on the amplitude difference between the negative N2 component and the positive P2 component, e.g. [16]. The amplitude difference between N2 and P2 (sometimes also labeled as C2 and C3) is known to vary as a function of the stimulus' size (or "dominant spatial frequency" in technical terms),

with maximal values at intermediate spatial frequencies, e.g. [17,18]. In the following sections we will call this amplitude modulation as a function of checksize the "*ERP checksize effect*". In our experiment we presented checkerboards with two different checksizes and looked for differences in the ERP checksize effect between AS and control observers.

The second focus of the current study was on the P3b ERP component, which is well-known as a cognitive component and has recently been discussed in the context of conscious versus unconscious perception, e.g. [19]. The P3b typically occurs between 250 ms and 600 ms after onset of an infrequent task-relevant target stimulus or infrequent omissions of a periodical stimulus (so called "oddball paradigm"). Its amplitude is negatively correlated with the target stimulus' frequency and positively correlated with stimulus' discriminability. P3b latency and reaction times are negatively correlated with stimulus discriminability (for recent reviews see [20,21]). The P3b is labeled as "cognitive" because its amplitude is modulated by the frequency and task-relevance of a stimulus, but not by the modulation of visual features (given a certain level of visibility). This behavior is in contrast to early "visual" ERP signatures that show amplitude and latency modulation as a function of lower-level stimulus features like luminance or size as in the present study but typically not as a function of the task.

In a balanced oddball paradigm we presented fine and coarse checkerboard stimuli both as rare targets and frequent non-targets in separate experimental runs and compared P3b amplitudes and latencies between AS and control participants. We further asked whether a potential lower-level modulation of the ERP checksize effect in AS participants would correlate with a higher-level P3b amplitude and/or latency modulation.

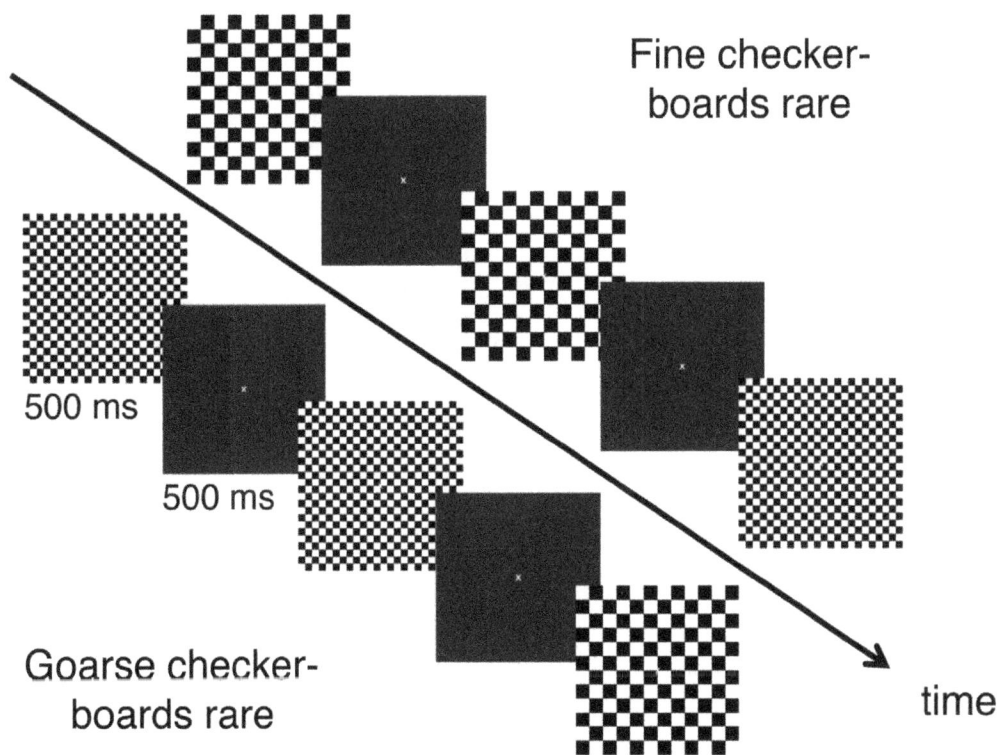

Figure 1. Experimental Paradigm. During one experimental block, checkerboards with two different checksizes were presented in random order with different frequencies (20% and 80%). Each checkerboard was presented for 500 ms and was followed by a grey screen for 500 ms. Participants had to count the occurrences of the rare checkerboards and to report the final number at the end of each experimental block.

Table 1. Number of averaged EEG trials.

	Asperger Observers				Controls			
	Fine Cb		Coarse Cb		Fine Cb		Coarse Cb	
	Freq	Rare	Freq	Rare	Freq	Rare	Freq	Rare
Mean	175.7	33.6	167.1	39.6	168.4	35.8	159.9	38.8
SD	26	1.1	46.8	7.2	30.4	12.2	42.5	8.3
Max	211	49	205	49	194	50	203	46
Min	92	10	53	17	102	6	53	38.8

Number of EEG trials per condition and observer group (SD = standard deviation) that entered ERP averaging. Cb: checkerboard; Freq: frequent Cbs.

Methods

Participants

21 Asperger (AS) participants and 17 healthy control participants were tested in this EEG-study. Control participants were selected to match the AS participants in age (±3 years) and gender. All participants had German school education comparable to junior high school or high school. Due to technical reasons only 19 AS participants (mean age = 41.3, SD = 10.7; 6 females) and 16 controls (mean age = 38.8, SD = 11.5, 6 females) entered the analysis. This resulted in 13 matched pairs (4 female) of AS observers (mean age: 39 years, SD = 10.6) and control observers (mean age 38.3, SD = 10.9).

All participants completed the autism-spectrum questionnaire "AQ" [22] and the empathy questionnaire "EQ" [23]. In the AQ, AS observers scored above 34 (Mean = 43.1; SD = 5) and the control observers scored below 28 (Mean = 15.1; SD = 5.5). The EQ scores showed the reverse picture – high scores in the control group (Mean = 43.3; SD = 8.2; Min = 29) and low scores in the AS group (Mean = 14.2; SD = 6.3; Max = 28).

All participants had a normal visual acuity. All participants gave their informed written consent. The study was performed in accordance with the ethical standards laid down in the Declaration of Helsinki [24] and was approved by the ethics board of the Albert-Ludwigs-Universität Freiburg, Germany.

Clinical Diagnostics

At the Division of Psychiatry and Psychotherapy, University Medical Center Freiburg, the clinical diagnosis of autism spectrum disorders and AS is established as a consensus diagnosis of a multiprofessional team following the recommendations of the draft version of the NICE guidelines (National Institute for Health and Clinical Excellence: Autism in Adults: full guideline DRAFT (December 2011; http://www.nice.org.uk/nicemedia/live/12339/57402/57402-.pdf)). According to these guidelines "a number of key components […] should form the basis of any comprehensive assessment of an adult with possible autism, as follows: the core symptoms of autism include social interaction, communication and stereotypical behavior; a developmental history spanning childhood, adolescence and adult life; the impact on current functioning including personal and social functioning, educational attainment and employment" (NICE 2012 page 134/135). At the center named above, the diagnostic principles are realized in a structured way. The clinical diagnosis includes a thorough history of the patient following the above principles, a history of carriers (parents, partners, siblings etc.) and behavioral observations in a diagnostic process that usually takes several sessions. Psychometric tools like AQ [19], EQ [20], Australian Scale for Asperger's Syndrome (ASAS) [32], SRS [22], BVAQ [33], AAA [34]), and BDI [35] are obtained in a routine procedure prior to clinical assessment and are used also for differential diagnostics. Additionally, instruments like ADI-R [36] and ADOS [37] are applied in selected and unclear cases. The same is true for additional neuropsychological tests assessing executive and theory-of-mind capacities. The multiprofessional diagnostic team consists of three experienced senior consultant psychiatrists and two fully qualified senior psychologists. The final consensus diagnosis is made by all persons involved in the diagnostic process, which will invariably include at least two experienced consultant psychiatrists or psychologists.

Stimuli

The stimuli consisted of fine and coarse checkerboards with checksizes of 0.6° and 1.2° visual angle and a grey screen following

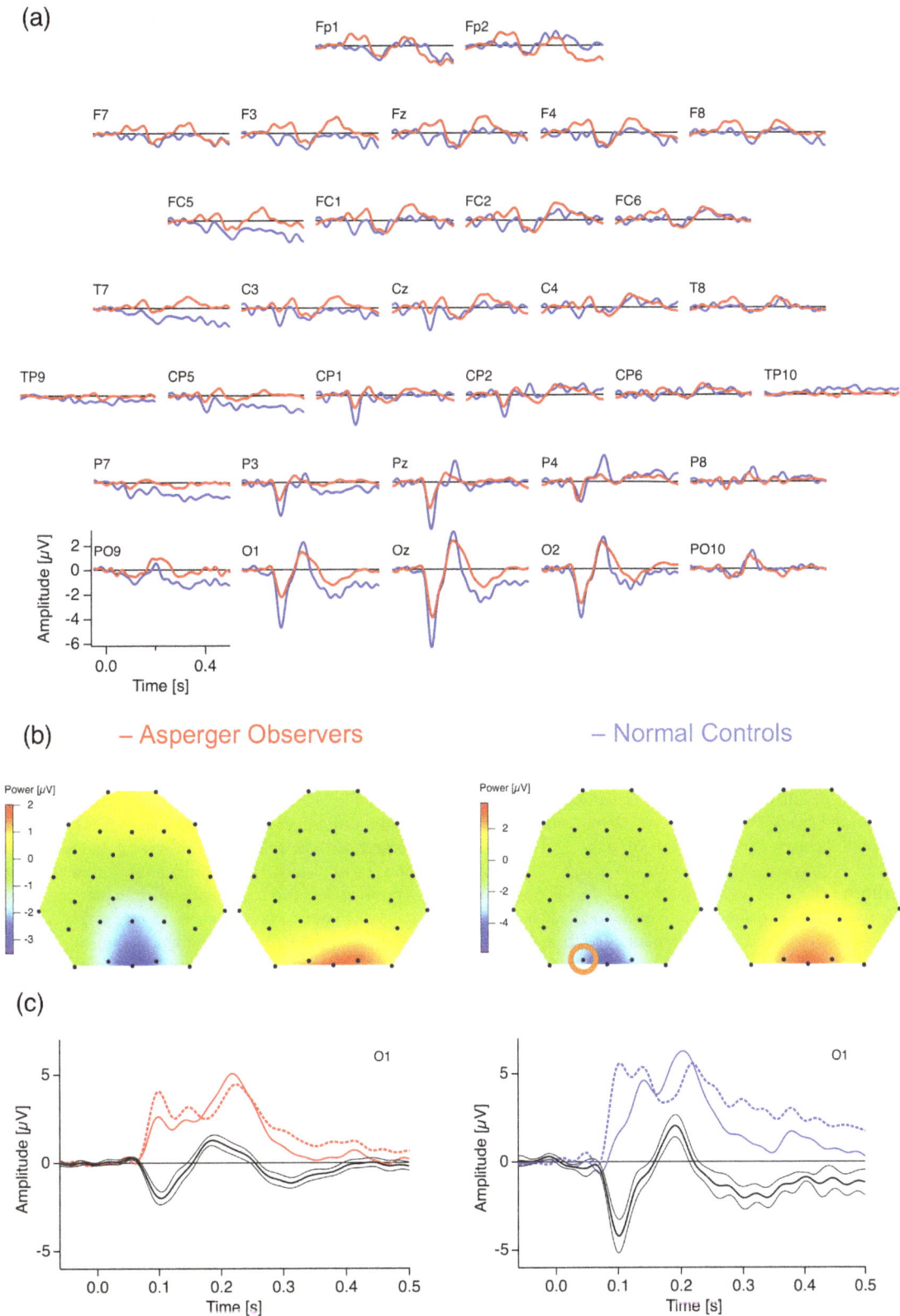

Figure 2. ERP checksize effect. (a) Grand mean ERP difference traces (fine minus coarse checkerboards) from AS observers (red) and controls (blue). Largest effects (negativity at 100 ms and positivity at 200 ms) occur at occipital electrodes. (b) Voltage maps with the spatial distribution of both the negativity (first and third voltage maps from left) and the positivity (second and fourth voltage map from left). Notice different scaling of the voltage maps between observer groups (c) Enlarged difference traces from the O1 electrode (indicated by the orange circle in (b)) ± SEM together with the underlying raw grand mean ERP traces (continuous lines for fine and dashed lines for coarse checkerboards).

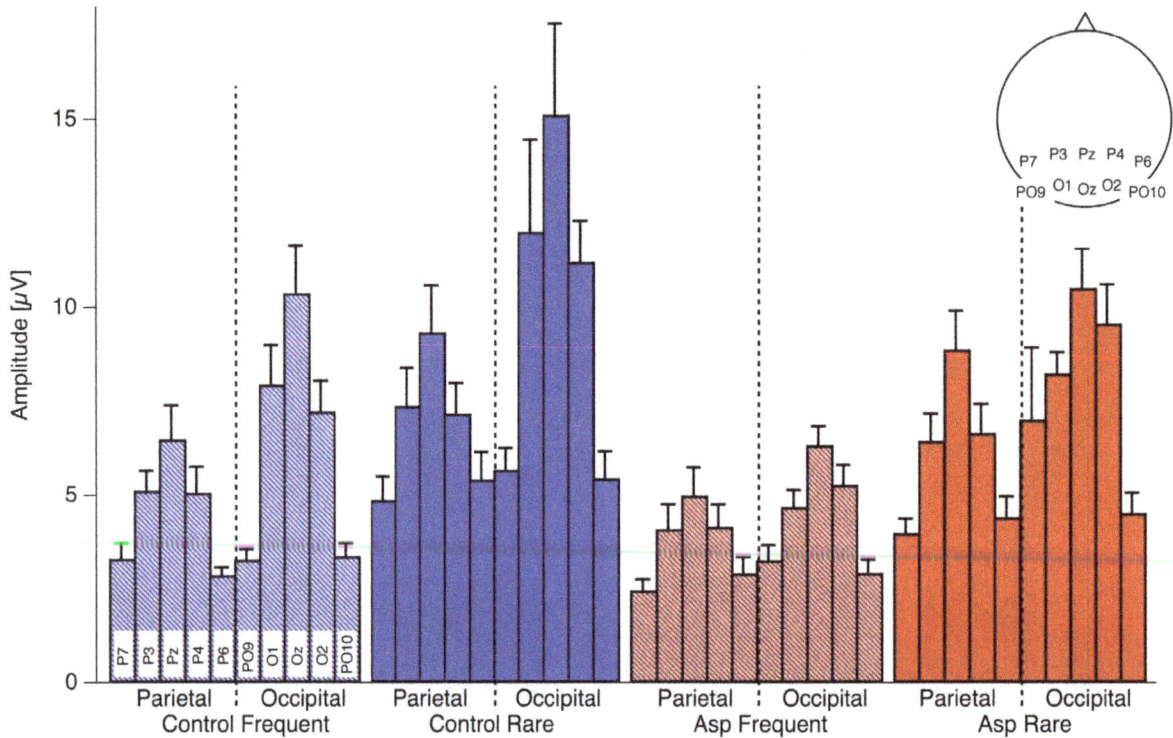

Figure 3. Grand Mean amplitudes (+SEM) of the individual checksize effect values at selected occipital and parietal electrodes (see scalp schema on the right top), separately for frequent non-target checker-boards (light colors) and rare target checkerboards (dark colors) and for AS (red) and control observers (blue). Dominance of midline occipital electrodes and smaller amplitudes for AS compared to Control observers can be observed.

each checkerboard presentation. Checkerboards and grey screen subtended a field of $13.25°$ (width)$\times 14.25°$ (height) visual angle. Luminance of the white and black checks was 220 cd/m^3 and 1.55 cd/m^3. Luminance of the grey screen was 110 cd/m^3.

Experimental Paradigm

The checkerboards were presented for 500 ms in an oddball paradigm, where rare stimuli occurred pseudo-randomly with a probability of $p = 0.2$. Each checkerboard was followed by a grey screen for 500 ms. From one checkerboard presentation to the next dark and white checks were exchanged ("reversal with interleaved grey", Fig. 1). Participants were instructed to count occurrences of the rare target checkerboards, ignore the frequent non-target checkerboards as well as the grey screens and to fixate a central fixation cross which was continuously present. The experiment consisted of two conditions with either the fine checkerboards or the coarse checkerboards as rare target stimuli. Each of the two conditions (fine checkerboard rare and coarse checkerboard rare) consisted of 240 checkerboard presentations

Table 2. Checksize-effect: Post-hoc permutation tests.

Electrodes	p-values	Cohen's D
P7	0.017	0.7
P3	0.11	0.43
Pz	0.11	0.43
P4	0.21	0.29
P8	0.35	0.2
PO9	0.17	0.32
O1	**0.0038***	**1**
Oz	0.011	0.81
O2	0.037	0.63
PO10	0.2	0.32

Post-hoc permutation tests of diffe-rences in the checksize effect for the frequent checkerboards between Asperger and control observers.
*indicates re-maining significance after Bonferroni-Holm correction.

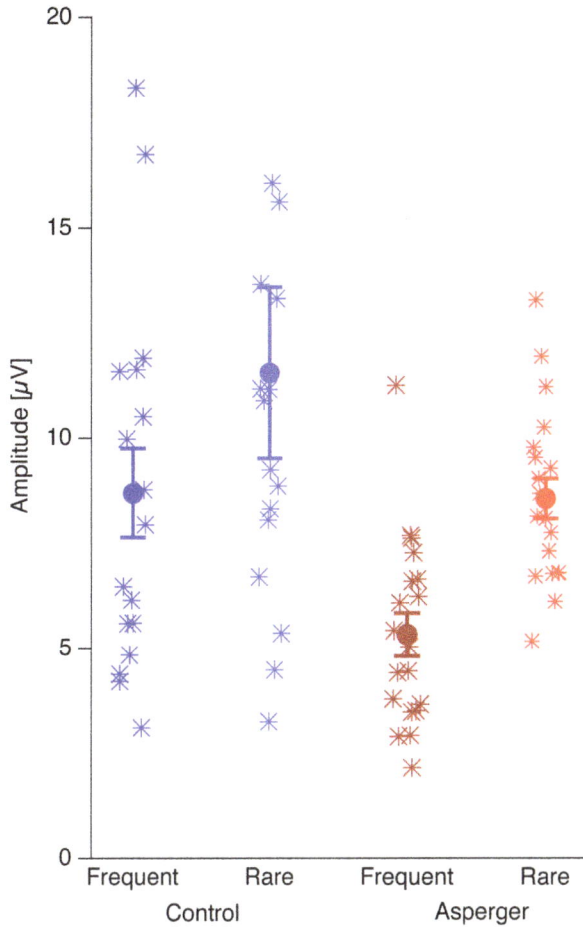

Figure 4. Individual (stars) and grand mean checksize effect data (circles ± SEM) at the right occipital O1 electrode. Here, the dark colors represent data from the frequent checkerboards and the light colors data from the rare checkerboards. Red colors represent data from the Asperger observers and blue colors represent data from the control observers. The data from the Asperger observers show both lower values and lower variance than those from the control observers.

over four minutes with 80% (192) frequent and 20% (48) rare checkerboard sizes in a pseudo-randomized order.

The stimuli were generated by a Mac mini (1.5 GHz Power PC G4) and presented on a Philips Monitor GD 402 monochrome CRT screen with a refresh rate of 85 Hz. A control screen for the investigator was placed outside the experimental room.

EEG Measurement and Processing

EEG signals were measured with the "Brain Vision" EEG system and referenced to a central midline electrode. Electrode locations were based on the extended 10–20 system [25]. Impedances were below 10 kΩ. The EEG signals were amplified with a factor of 1000, digitalized with a sampling rate of 500 Hz and streamed to disc.

Offline pre-processing of the EEG data included re-referencing to averaged mastoid electrodes and removal of single EEG trials containing artificial amplitude excursions above ±150 µV.

Currently we have no established repository for data related to the clinical electrophysiology. We will therefore archive the data locally and make them available to other researchers upon request together with information about the file format. This will be facilitated by keeping the EEG data and associated metadata strictly separate from any personal data that would make identification of the participants possible.

Data Analysis

For each participant the checkerboard EEG trials were sorted with respect to stimulus size (spatial frequency) and stimulus frequency and selectively averaged to ERPs. The ERPs were digitally filtered with a latency-neutral low-pass filter with a cut-off at 25 Hz. Table 1 lists the minimal, maximal and mean number of trials per condition entering the ERP calculation.

Analysis of the ERP checksize effect. For each participant and channel we calculated the difference ERP traces (dERPs) between the *fine and coarse checkerboard ERPs* separately for the rare target stimuli and the frequent non-target stimuli, resulting in rare and frequent dERPs. This calculation isolated the *ERP checksize effect*, i.e. the ERP difference between fine and coarse checkerboards and reduced the inter-individual variance. We determined the amplitude of the ERP checksize effect for each participant as the amplitude difference between the maximal negative excursion

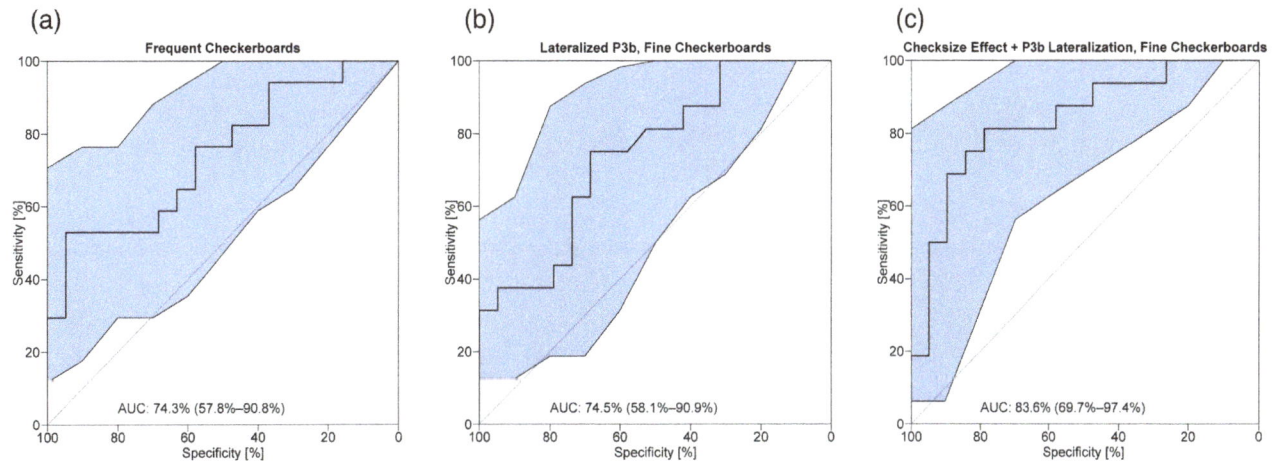

Figure 5. ROC curves of (a) the ERP checksize effect (b) the P3b lateralization effect and (c) a linear combination of both effects. The blue shaded areas indicate 90% confidence intervals based on bootstrap calculations (N = 10.000). AUC = area under curve (±90% confidence interval).

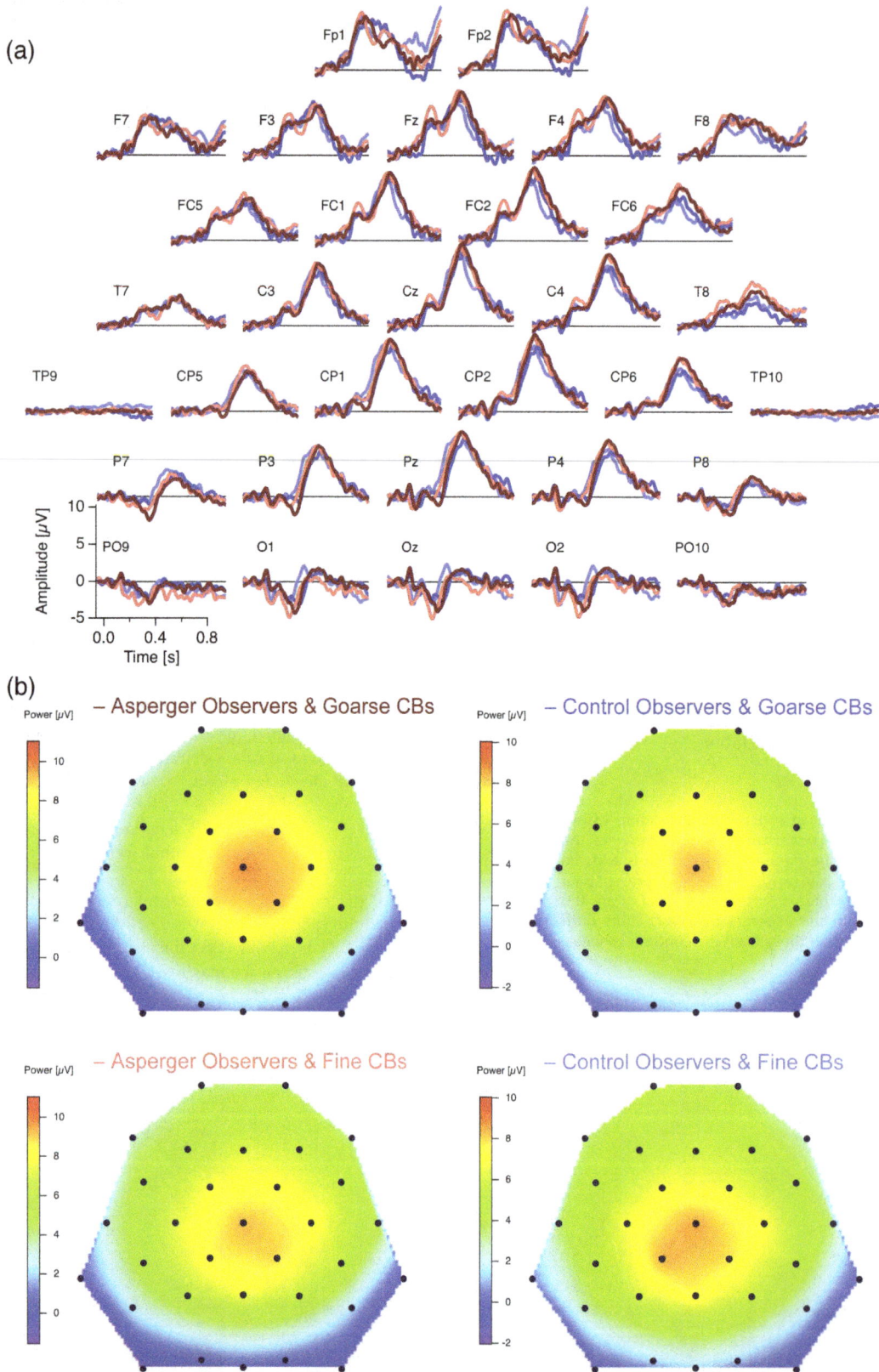

Figure 6. P3b lateralization effect. (a) Grand mean difference traces (dERPs, rare minus frequent checkerboards) separated for the AS (red) and control observers (blue) and for coarse (dark colors) and fine (light colors) checkerboards. (b) Voltage maps of the P3b 500 ms after stimulus onset. AS observers (left voltage maps) show similar amplitude and latency but a stronger right-hemispheric lateralization of the P3b at the central electrodes compared to control observers (right voltage maps).

Table 3. P3b post-hoc permutation tests.

Electrodes	Asperger observers		control observers	
	p-values	Cohen's D	p-values	Cohen's D
P3 vs. P4	0.006	0.25	0.16	0.13
C3 vs. C4	0.001*	0.46	0.39	0.031
F3 vs. F4	0.001*	0.35	0.27	0.076

p-value results from post-hoc permutation tests to compare the P3b amplitudes between hemispheres separately for Asperger and control observers. *indicates remaining significance after Bonferroni-Holm correction.

in a predefined temporal region of interest (ROI) between 60 ms and 250 ms after checkerboard onset and the subsequent positive excursion for each electrode of a predefined spatial ROI involving the five occipital (PO9, O1, Oz, O2, PO10) and the five parietal (P7, P3, Pz, P4, P8) electrodes. Amplitude and latency of the ERP checksize effect were then analyzed with a mixed model ANOVA with the within factors TASK (2 steps: rare targets vs. frequent non-targets), CHANNEL (10) and HEMISPHERE (2 steps: left- vs. right-hemispheric electrodes) and the between factor GROUP (2 steps: AS vs. control observers) where all 35 participants entered. The factor SIZE, reflecting the different checksizes, disappeared by calculating the ERP difference traces as described above.

Since our results indicated also differences in amplitude variance between Asperger and control observers we also calculated post-hoc Barlett-Tests for homogeneity of variance.

Analysis of the ERP P3b Effect

For each participant and channel we calculated the difference ERP traces between the rare and frequent checkerboard ERPs, separately for the fine and coarse checkerboards, in order to isolate the ERP oddball P3b and reduce the inter-individual variance. We determined the P3b amplitudes and latencies for each individual participant from the peaks in a temporal ROI between 250 ms and 600 ms after checkerboard onset for each electrode of our predefined spatial ROI involving three parietal (P3, Pz, P4), three central (C3, Cz, C4) and three frontal (F3, Fz, F4) electrodes.

Amplitude and latency of the P3b effect were then analyzed in a mixed model ANOVA with the within factors SIZE (2, fine vs. coarse checkerboards), CHANNEL (9) and HEMISPHERE (2, left- vs. right-hemispheric electrodes) and the between factor GROUP (2, AS vs. control observers).

Notice that the factor TASK, reflecting the frequent non-target stimuli and rare target-stimuli disappeared by calculating the ERP difference traces between frequent and rare stimuli, as described above. Where necessary, we conducted post-hoc randomization tests [26].

Finally we calculated Receiver Operating Characteristics (ROC) separately for the two effects and for their linear combination. A ROC curve displays the performance of a binary classifier. It depicts the classifiers' sensitivity (proportion of correctly classified positives) and specificity (proportion of correctly classified negatives) as a function of changing output threshold [27]. We calculated the area under the ROC curve ("AUC", in % of the maximal possible area) as a measure for the predictive power of the respective effect. An AUC of 50% indicates no discriminatory power, whereas 100% indicates optimal discriminatory power. In this case, the classifier would detect all true but no false positives.

In order to calculate the discriminatory power of the combination of the two effects we first calculated z-transformations for both data sets (the amplitude values of the checksize effect for the frequent checkerboards at electrode O1 and the P3b amplitude differences between electrode C4 and C3). We then added the P3b z-scores to the checksize effect z-scores and calculated a ROC analysis on these linear combination values. For a similar approach see [28].

Results

Psychophysical Results

The hit rate of the counting task was above 98% for both AS observers and normal controls without any group difference (p = 0.41 and p = 0.56 for fine and goarse checkerboards, based on permutation tests [26]).

ERP Checksize Effect

Figure 2a shows the grand mean target- (light colors) and non-target- (dark colors) dERPs (fine minus coarse checkerboards) from both AS (red) and control observers (blue) for all 32 electrodes, arrayed according to their position on the scalp. A prominent ERP checksize effect can be observed at the occipital and parietal electrodes (see also the voltage maps in Fig. 2b). It consists of a sharp negative deflection at about 100 ms after stimulus onset and a subsequent sharp positive excursion roughly 100 ms later. Amplitudes of both components are larger for fine than for coarse checkerboards. Figure 2c shows the underlying raw ERP traces (continuous traces for fine and dashed traces for coarse checkerboards) together with the resulting differences (black traces, fine minus coarse checkerboards ± SEM) at the electrode O1 for AS (left, red) and control (right, blue) observers. Figure 3 shows the grand means of the individual amplitudes at parietal and central electrodes separately for AS and control observers and for frequent and rare checkerboards.

For the variable amplitude, the mixed-model ANOVA indicates (1) a strong effect of the factor GROUP ($F(1,670) = 19.99$, $p = 9.2*10^{-06}$), reflecting the difference between Asperger and control observers, (2) a strong effect of the factor TASK ($F(1,670) = 88.11$, $p = 2.2*10^{-16}$) reflecting larger amplitudes for the rare target checkerboards compared to frequent non-targets, and (3) a strong effect of the factor CHANNEL ($F(9,670) = 34.36$, $p = 2.2*10^{-16}$) reflecting the dominance of the occipital midline electrodes, as can be seen in Fig. 3. The mixed-model ANOVA indicates further (4) an interaction between the factors GROUP and CHANNEL ($F(9,670) = 1.95$, $p = 0.043$) reflecting a larger difference of the ERP checksize effect between observer groups at central electrodes (Figs. 2 and 3). Uncorrected Post-hoc randomization tests [26] of differences between Asperger and control observers for frequent checkerboards are listed in Table 2. After

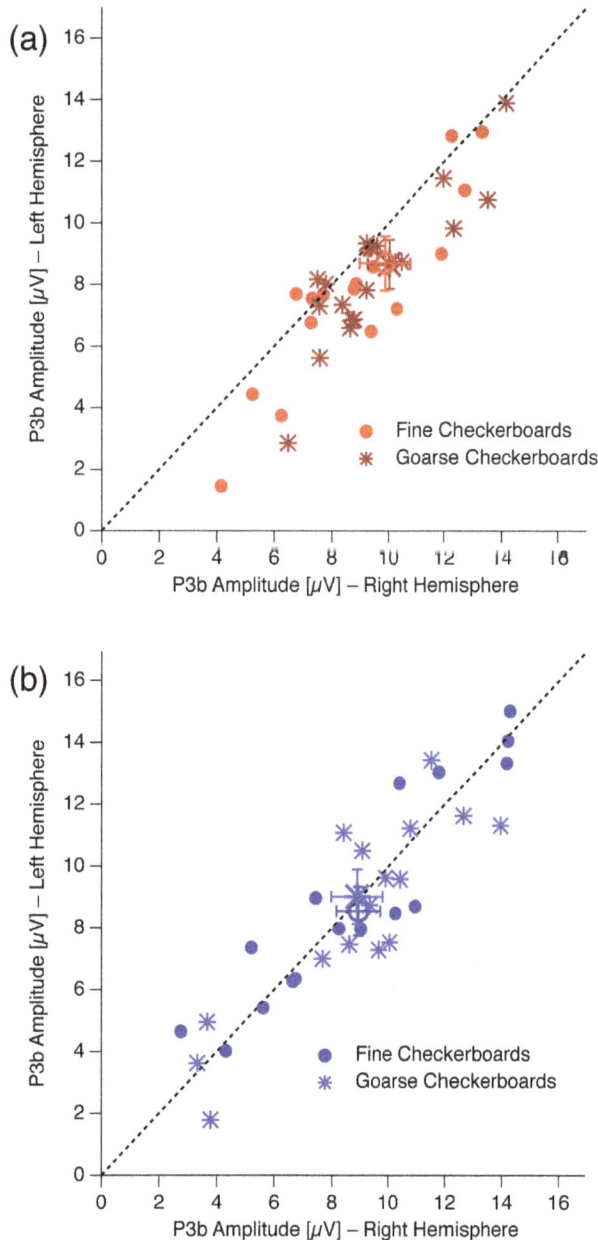

colors data from the rare checkerboards. Red colors represent data from the Asperger observers and blue colors represent data from the control observers. The data from the Asperger observers show both lower values and lower variance than those from the control observers (Barlett's Test for equal variances: p<0.01 for the frequent checkerboards and p<0.05 for the rare checkerboards).

Figure 5a depicts the receiver operating characteristic (ROC) of the checksize effect for the frequent checkerboards. The area under the ROC curve can be regarded as the probability that the checksize effect identifies a randomly chosen participant correctly as either an Asperger or a Non-Asperger person and its value is 74.3% (57.8% –90.8% for a 95%-confidence interval).

P3b Effect

Figure 5a shows the grand mean dERPs (rare minus frequent) for the fine (light colors) and coarse (dark colors) checkerboards from both AS (red) and control observers (blue) for all 32 electrodes, arrayed according to their position on the scalp. A huge oddball P3b can be observed roughly 500 ms after checkerboard onset with maximal amplitudes at parietal and central midline electrodes (see also the voltage maps in Fig. 6b). For the variable amplitude, the mixed model ANOVA indicates a significant effect for the factor CHANNEL ($F(8,264) = 11.6$, $p = 4.2*10^{-14}$), reflecting the parietal and central midline dominance of the P3b effect as indicated by the voltage maps in Fig. 6b. The ANOVA further indicates an effect for the factor HEMISPHERE ($F(1,33) = 9.7$, $p = 0.0038$), with a slight right-hemispheric dominance of the P3b. This hemispheric asymmetry is more pronounced in AS observers than in controls, which is reflected in an interaction between GROUP and HEMISPHERE ($F(1,33) = 8.3$, $p = 0.007$) and which is also indicated in the voltage maps (Fig. 6b).

Table 3 provides the uncorrected results from post-hoc randomization tests. We collapsed the data from the two different checkerboard sizes and compared amplitudes from left-hemispheric and right-hemispheric electrodes at parietal, central and frontal sites. After Bonferroni-Holm correction for multiple testing [29] the central and frontal electrode pairs from the Asperger observers showed a significant right-hemispheric lateralization of the P3b ($p = 0.005$ and $p = 0.006$). No significant P3b-lateralization remained in the control observers.

Fig. 7 shows individual P3b data to demonstrate the difference in hemispheric asymmetry of the P3b between Asperger (Fig. 7a) and control observers (Fig. 7b). Each individual icon represents amplitude values from the C3 electrode (left central hemisphere) on the ordinate and respective values from the C4 electrode (right central hemisphere) on the abscissa. Asymmetric distributions of icons, away from the bisection line indicate an asymmetric distribution of the P3b on the scalp. As can be seen easily, the data from the Asperger observers are much more lateralized to the right hemisphere than the control observer's data. Circles (dark colors) and stars (light colors) represent data from the coarse and fine checkerboards respectively. Open circles and the larger stars represent the respective grand mean values (± SEM).

Figure 5b depicts the receiver operating characteristic (ROC) of the P3b effect for the frequent checkerboards. The area under the ROC curve can be regarded as the probability that the P3b effect identifies a randomly chosen participant correctly as either an Asperger or a Non-Asperger person and its value is 74.3% (57.8% –90.8% confidence interval).

Figure 5c depicts the ROC curve of the linear combination of both effects (Checksize effect+P3b effect). Discriminatory power increases to 83.6% (69.7% –97.4% for a 95%-confidence interval).

Figure 7. Individual P3b data to demonstrate the difference in hemispheric asymmetry of the P3b between Asperger (Fig. 7a) and control observers (Fig. 7b). Each individual icon represents amplitude values from the C3 electrode (left central hemisphere) on the ordinate and respective values from the C4 electrode (right central hemisphere) on the abscissa. Asymmetric distributions of icons, away from the bisection line indicate an asymmetric distribution of the P3b on the scalp. As can be easily seen, the data from the Asperger observers are much more lateralized to the right hemisphere (below the bisection line) than the control observer data. Stars (dark colors) and circles (light colors) represent data from the coarse and fine checkerboards respectively. Open circles and the larger stars represent the respective grand mean values (± SEM).

Bonferroni-Holm correction for multiple testing [29] significance remained for the left occipital O1 electrode with $p = 0.037$.

Fig. 4 shows individual (stars) and grand mean data (circles ± SEM) at the right occipital O1 electrode. Here, the dark colors represent data from the frequent checkerboards and the light

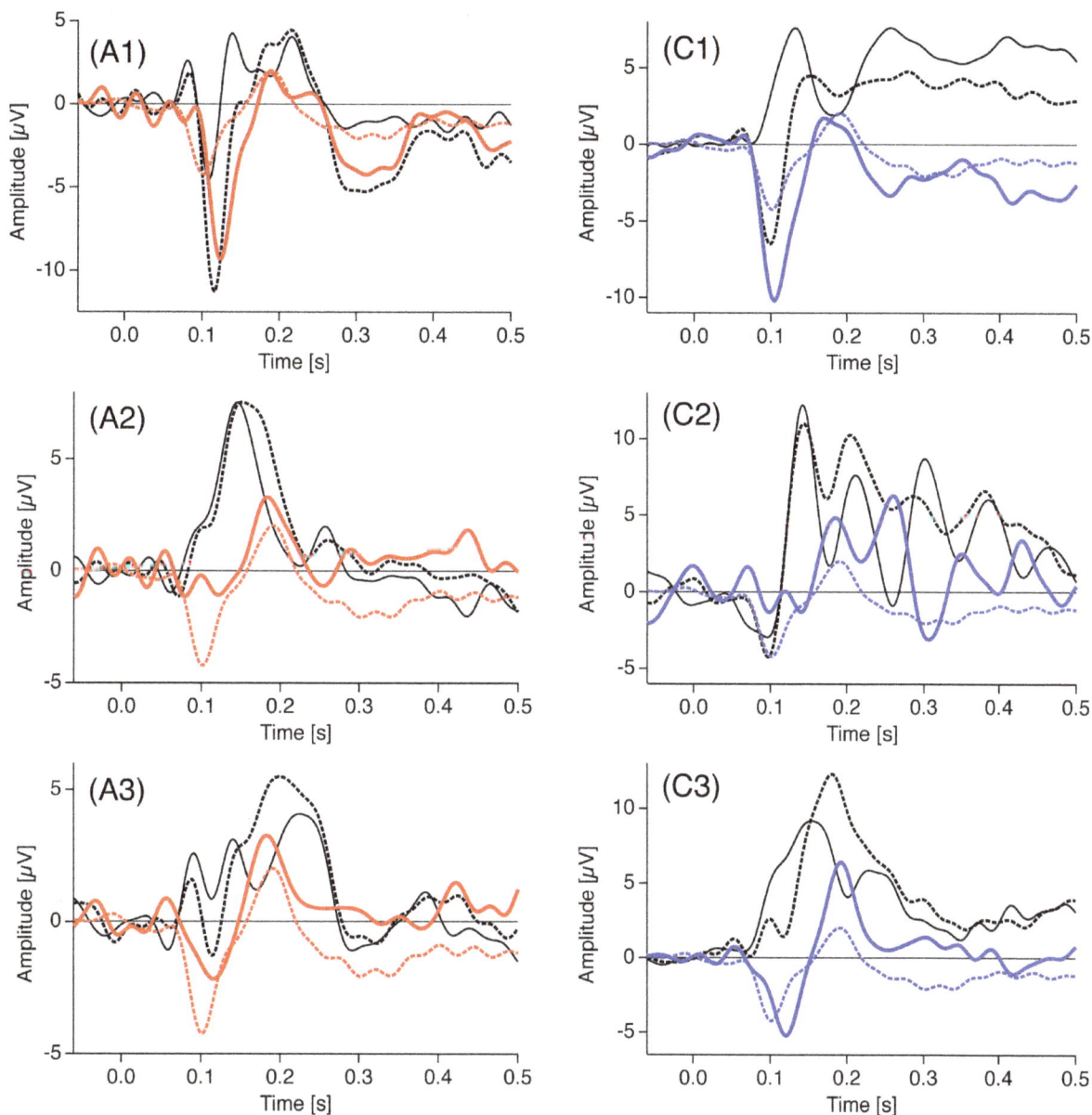

Figure 8. Individual examples of the ERP checksize effect at electrode O1. Black traces represent the raw ERP traces for fine (dashed traces) and coarse (continuous traces) checkerboards. Bold red (Asperger, "A") and bold blue (Control observers, "C") continuous traces show the individual differences (dERPs, fine minus coarse checkerboards). The red dashed traces represent the grand mean dERPs. The individual difference traces are less variable than the raw ERP traces (thus more similar to the grand means) but some variability remains. The chosen examples show observers with the effect mainly at the negativity (A1 and C1), mainly at the subsequent positivitiy (A2 and C2) or on both components (A3 and C3). All graphs are scaled for individual maxima and minima.

Discussion

In the current EEG study we presented checkerboards with two different checksizes in a classical oddball paradigm and compared both the low-level visual ERP checksize effect and the higher-level oddball P3b between AS observers and matched controls. We found a smaller checksize ERP effect and smaller amplitude variance for AS than for control observers at occipital electrodes. This effect showed a discriminatory power of roughly 74%. We further found a right-hemispheric lateralization of the oddball P3b, which was more prominent in the AS than in the control observers. This P3b lateralization showed a discriminatory power

of about 75%. A linear combination of both effects increased the discriminatory power to about 84%.

The Early ERP Checksize Effect

In the last few years a number of studies focused on differences in EEG correlates of early visual processing between AS observers and controls. Milne et al. [15] presented sinusoidal gratings of different spatial frequencies (from 0.5 cpd [= cycles per degree] to 8 cpd) in the pattern-onset mode [16] to autistic children and matched controls. They analyzed the EEG data with an independent component analysis and compared the identified components between autistic participants and matched controls.

Some striate and extrastriate components around 100 ms after stimulus onset showed smaller power in autistic children than in controls. Boeschoten et al. [30] presented horizontal square-wave gratings and compared early visual ERP effects of varying spatial frequency (0.75 cpd –6 cpd) between autistic and control children. They found weaker effects on the N80 and P130 peaks in the autistic children compared to the matched controls. Jemel et al. [31] presented vertical sinusoidal gratings in a pattern-reversal mode with varying spatial frequencies and contrasts to adult ASD observers and matched controls. They found differences in the contrast tuning functions of the N80 and P100 for mid (2.8 cpd) and high (8 cpd) spatial frequencies. Most interestingly for the current study, their data indicate a smaller difference between their low and medium spatial frequency stimuli in ASD observers compared to controls (see their Figs. 2C and 3C).

The studies cited above differ in various parameters, like participants' age, stimulus type, presentation mode, stimulus luminance, range of spatial frequencies, and the type of the focused EEG variables. Despite these differences all studies found weaker spatial frequency effects for ASD observers compared to control observers in early visual areas between 80 ms and 130 ms after stimulus onset.

EEG effects of spatial frequency from visual areas are well known in the literature and even belong to the standard diagnostic tools in clinical diagnostics, e.g. [16]. The timing of those EEG effects strongly depend on the range of spatial frequencies used. Early visual effects (N80 and P130) are known to be large with high spatial frequencies between 4 and 15 cpd, whereas strongest effects in the range of 200 ms after stimulus onset occur with intermediate values between 1 and 2 cpd (see for example Figure 5 in [18]). The studies cited above reported exclusively on early differences in spatial frequency EEG effects between AS and control observers. Our data show that similar differences are also present later, in the 200-ms-range.

Some authors tried to infer basic differences in early visual processing steps between observers with autism and controls from specific ERP components that are affected by the stimulus' spatial frequency, i.e. whether the N80 or the P130 is more affected, e.g. [30,31]. Such interpretations are fascinating; they stimulate more focused follow-up experiments and they may help replacing pure self-reported, phenomenological description of the perceptual differences between autistic and normal observers by objectively measurable signals and possibly pathophysiological description and understanding of this mental perceptual phenomenon.

However, such inferences are most informative if they can be made on the level of single participants. Unfortunately, effects identifiable at the single participant level are rare because of the large inter-individual variability in general and particularly with the present data, as can be seen in Fig. 8 (black traces). We reduced the inter-individual variability in checkerboard ERP-responses considerably by calculating the difference between the ERPs to fine and coarse checkerboards (dERPs, blue and red traces in Fig. 8). The resulting pattern including a dERP negativity and a subsequent dERP positivity (blue and red dashed traces) is visible in all example participants but still with some inter-individual variance. Interpreting each single deflection in the context of autism-specific visual processing would necessitate to subdivide our participants into four groups with either an effect (1) mainly at the earlier negativity (Fig. 8 A1 and C1), (2) mainly at the later positivity (Fig. 8 A2 and C2), (3) at both components (Fig. 8 A3 and C3) and (4) a group without an evident effect. A cluster analysis, however, would need much more participants. It may be promising for future studies to test a broader range of spatial frequencies and therewith perhaps increase the discrimi-

natory power of the ERP checksize effect. With optimal spatial frequencies at hand the basic paradigm would be very cheap, easy and fast and may be applied routinely in diagnostics to collect much more data and then do the above mentioned cluster analysis. In this context the following should be mentioned: The size of our coarse checkerboards (0.6° visual angle) can be translated to a spatial frequency of 1.18 cpd and is thus near to the critical spatial frequency of 2.2 cpd, which is reported to be important for face processing, e.g. [32,33]. It has been shown, that autistic observers show differences in the visual processing of faces compared to normal controls [10]. These high-level differences in face processing, the here-presented lower-level differences in spatial frequency processing and the earliest visual differences cited above may be causally related. For a similar line of reasoning see [31]. Further research in this direction may be promising to understand functional relations.

The Late P3b Effect

The P3b is one of the most prominent cognitive ERP components. It occurs with all sensory modalities and it seems to be composed by several neural processes around 300 ms after stimulus onset, e.g. [20]. It is labeled as cognitive because its amplitude is most dependent on the given experimental task and the frequency of occurrence (or absence) of a certain task-relevant stimulus and less on the lower-level stimulus features like size or spatial frequency, as can be observed in the present data. Interpretations of the functional role of the P3b range from context/working memory updating, e.g. [34], mediating between perceptual analysis and response initiation [35] or inhibitory processes during focused attention, e.g. [21]. The P3b has recently been discussed as one of the most reliable markers to distinguish unconscious (P3b absent) and conscious (P3b present) processing [19] although its generality and the large number of probably contributing brain sources make its relation to a specific cognitive function difficult, e.g. [20]. But see [36] for a more specific speculation.

Several P3b oddball studies have been performed with autistic and normal observers. The results are heterogeneous, with findings of smaller and larger amplitudes of the P3b in autistic observers compared to control observers or with no P3b difference at all. For reviews see [9,11]. To our knowledge the evidence for an asymmetry of the P3b amplitude has only rarely been reported, e.g. [21,37]. And we are particularly unaware of any report about differences in hemispheric symmetry of the P3b amplitude between autistic and normal observers.

One potential explanation of our P3b findings may be related to the observation that attention to the target stimulus is a necessary precondition for the P3b to occur: It is obvious and well documented that our attention system has limited capacities, e.g. [38]. There is evidence that this attention capacity is even more limited in certain subtypes of autism, like high functioning autism, e.g. [9]. It also might be possible that the attention capacity in AS is chronically overloaded by over-detailed and irrelevant information and more effort is necessary to deliberately change attention. Our data show a right-hemispheric lateralization of the P3b, which is more pronounced in the AS compared to control observers. It is well known that stimulus-induced attention capture also shows a right-hemispheric lateralization. And like the P3b this effect occurs across modalities, e.g. [39,40]. Thus the degree of lateralization of the P3b may reflect – at least in the present paradigm – the amount of attentional resources employed in the task and may explain our finding of stronger lateralization in AS compared to the control observers. This speculation could be easily tested by studying the relation between P3b lateralization and attentional load in both AS and control observers (for attentional load paradigms see [41]). An optimal degree of task complexity may then increase the discriminatory power of this lateralization effect.

Some Speculations on the Relation between the Early ERP Checksize and Late P3b Effects in Autism

Our main findings are that of a smaller checksize ERP effect and a more lateralized P3b effect in AS observers compared to controls. One might speculate that the smaller checksize ERP effect in the AS group represents alterations in low-level visual information processing in the primary occipital visual cortex of autistic observers. This might well relate to the common descriptions of altered visual experience of these people. Currently we do not know how to interpret smaller variance of the checksize effect for Asperger compared to control observers.

The lateralization of the P3b signal in the AS group might reflect the sequels of difficulties in early visual contextual information analysis which might result in a higher load of consciously driven top-down fronto-occipital analytical work load or work load of the global neuronal workspace system, e.g. [19]. Thus, the lateralization of the P3b signal might be seen as a compensatory consequence of the compromised early checksize signal in that higher degrees of conscious analytical information processing compensate for difficulties in low-level signal analysis. While speculative such interpretations relate well to clinical phenomenological observations and theoretical concepts. Clinically, particularly highly intelligent ASD-patients often report that they have learned to deliberately regulate their attention (i.e. to focus on social interaction) and are used to apply more conscious effort to focus on the requested task in a specific situation, which may be reflected by the stronger P3b lateralization. Theoretically, for example Shalom [42] has put forward the hypothesis that loss of or reduced integration of primary sensory stimuli in ASD might induce a higher degree of compensatory conscious analysis which in turn might cause other mental problems, like for example cognitive slowing and perceptual and/or attentional over-loads. These issues can be empirically tested in further research. A functional relation between the early ERP checksize effect and the later P3b lateralization effect should be reflected in their high correlation, which we did not find. The reason may be that early visual ERP responses and particularly onset responses are highly variable between participants, e.g. [16,43]. This may be caused by large inter-individual variability in brain anatomy, e.g. cortical

folding. Thus, similarities in functional processing not necessarily come along with similarities in surface EEG potentials. But optimizing stimulation parameters sometimes helps to increasing signal-to-noise ratio and thus increasing the number of participants that show both effects concurrently.

Summary

The difference traces (dERPs) between fine and coarse checkerboards show a sizable effect of checksize (or spatial frequency) at occipital electrodes and thus probably in visual areas. This effect is smaller in AS observers compared to their matched controls with a discriminatory power of about 74%. Our findings fit well with recent results from the literature and even extend them from early visual steps around 100 ms to intermediate steps around 200 ms after stimulus onset. The fine checkerboards we used have a dominant spatial frequency close to the critical values for face processing, which is also known to differ between AS and normal observers. Potential causal relations between early visual and higher level specificities in AS and more general autistic observers may be identifiable in future experiments.

In addition to these lower-level visual effects we found a stronger right-hemispheric lateralization of the late P3b ERP component in AS than in control observers with a discriminatory power of about 75%. This P3b lateralization difference may be related to a difference in attentional resources between autistic and normal people. Combination of the two effects increases the discriminatory power to about 84%. For both effects it may be possible to increase effect sizes and thus the discriminatory power by optimizing checkerboard sizes (spatial frequencies) and task complexity (addressing attentional resources). In this case the two effects may be promising candidates for physiological markers in clinical diagnostics of Asperger's syndrome and other autistic disorders.

Acknowledgments

Assistance by Dr. T. Fangmeier is gratefully acknowledged.

Author Contributions

Conceived and designed the experiments: JK RW LTvE. Performed the experiments: JK RW. Analyzed the data: JK RW AR MB. Contributed reagents/materials/analysis tools: JK MB. Wrote the paper: JK RW AR MB LTvE.

References

1. Happé F (1999) Autism: cognitive deficit or cognitive style? Trends Cogn Sci 3: 216–222.
2. CDC (2012). Atlanta, USA: National Center on Birth Defects and Developmental Disabilities Center for Disease Control and Prevention.
3. Jarbrink K (2007) The economic consequences of autistic spectrum disorder among children in a Swedish municipality. Autism 11: 453–463.
4. Levy SE, Mandell DS, Schultz RT (2009) Autism. Lancet 374: 1627–1638.
5. Moreno-De-Luca A, Myers SM, Challman TD, Moreno-De-Luca D, Evans DW, et al. (2013) Developmental brain dysfunction: revival and expansion of old concepts based on new genetic evidence. Lancet Neurol 12: 406–414.
6. Cohen D, Pichard N, Tordjman S, Baumann C, Burglen L, et al. (2005) Specific genetic disorders and autism: clinical contribution towards their identification. J Autism Dev Disord 35: 103–116.
7. Tebartz van Elst L (2013) Asperger-Syndrom und Autismusbegriff: historische Entwicklung und moderne Konzepte. In: Tebartz van Elst L, editor. Das Asperger-Syndrom im Erwachsenenalter und andere hochfunktionale Autismus-Spektrum-Störungen. Berlin: Medizinisch Wissenschaftliche Verlagsgesellschaft. 412.
8. Tebartz van Elst L, Pick M, Biscaldi M, Fangmeier T, Riedel A (2013) High-functioning autism spectrum disorder as a basic disorder in adult psychiatry and psychotherapy: psychopathological presentation, clinical relevance and therapeutic concepts. Eur Arch Psychiatry Clin Neurosci 263 Suppl 2: S189–196.
9. Marco EJ, Hinkley LB, Hill SS, Nagarajan SS (2011) Sensory processing in autism: a review of neurophysiologic findings. Pediatr Res 69: 48R–54R.
10. Simmons DR, Robertson AE, McKay LS, Toal E, McAleer P, et al. (2009) Vision in autism spectrum disorders. Vision Res 49: 2705–2739.
11. Jeste SS, Nelson CA, 3rd (2009) Event related potentials in the understanding of autism spectrum disorders: an analytical review. J Autism Dev Disord 39: 495–510.
12. McCleery JP, Allman E, Carver LJ, Dobkins KR (2007) Abnormal magnocellular pathway visual processing in infants at risk for autism. Biol Psychiatry 62: 1007–1014.
13. Sutherland A, Crewther DP (2010) Magnocellular visual evoked potential delay with high autism spectrum quotient yields a neural mechanism for altered perception. Brain 133: 2089–2097.
14. Jackson BL, Blackwood EM, Blum J, Carruthers SP, Nemorin S, et al. (2013) Magno- and Parvocellular Contrast Responses in Varying Degrees of Autistic Trait. PLoS One 8: e66797.
15. Milne E, Scope A, Pascalis O, Buckley D, Makeig S (2009) Independent component analysis reveals atypical electroencephalographic activity during visual perception in individuals with autism. Biol Psychiatry 65: 22–30.
16. Odom JV, Bach M, Brigell M, Holder GE, McCulloch DL, et al. (2010) ISCEV standard for clinical visual evoked potentials (2009 update). Doc Ophthalmol 120: 111–119.

17. Parker DM, Salzen EA (1977) The spatial selectivity of early and late waves within the human visual evoked response. Perception 6: 85–95.

18. Plant GT, Zimmern RL, Durden K (1983) Transient visually evoked potentials to the pattern reversal and onset of sinusoidal gratings. Electroencephalogr Clin Neurophysiol 56: 147–158.

19. Dehaene S, Changeux JP (2011) Experimental and theoretical approaches to conscious processing. Neuron 70: 200–227.

20. Linden DE (2005) The P300: where in the brain is it produced and what does it tell us? Neuroscientist 11: 563–576.

21. Polich J (2007) Updating P300: an integrative theory of P3a and P3b. Clin Neurophysiol 118: 2128–2148.

22. Baron-Cohen S, Wheelwright S, Skinner R, Martin J, Clubley E (2001) The autism-spectrum quotient (AQ): evidence from Asperger syndrome/high-functioning autism, males and females, scientists and mathematicians. J Autism Dev Disord 31: 5–17.

23. Baron-Cohen S, Wheelwright S (2004) The empathy quotient: an investigation of adults with Asperger syndrome or high functioning autism, and normal sex differences. J Autism Dev Disord 34: 163–175.

24. Association WM (2000) Declaration of Helsinki: ethical principles for medical research involving human subjects. JAMA 284: 3043–3045.

25. American Clinical Neurophysiology Society (2006) Guideline 5: Guidelines for standard electrode position nomenclature. J Clin Neurophysiol 23: 107–110.

26. Edgington ES, Onghena P (2007) Randomization Tests. Boca Raton, FL, USA: Chapman & Hall/CRC.

27. Robin X, Turck N, Hainard A, Tiberti N, Lisacek F, et al. (2011) pROC: an open-source package for R and S+ to analyze and compare ROC curves. BMC Bioinformatics 12. 77.

28. Preiser D, Lagreze WA, Bach M, Poloschek CM (2013) Photopic negative response versus pattern electroretinogram in early glaucoma. Invest Ophthalmol Vis Sci 54: 1182–1191.

29. Holm S (1979) A simple sequentially rejective multiple test procedure. Scand J Statist 6: 65–70.

30. Boeschoten MA, Kenemans JL, van Engeland H, Kemner C (2007) Abnormal spatial frequency processing in high-functioning children with pervasive developmental disorder (PDD). Clin Neurophysiol 118: 2076–2088.

31. Jemel B, Mimeault D, Saint-Amour D, Hosein A, Mottron L (2010) VEP contrast sensitivity responses reveal reduced functional segregation of mid and high filters of visual channels in autism. J Vis 10: 13.

32. Nasanen R (1999) Spatial frequency bandwidth used in the recognition of facial images. Vision Res 39: 3824–3833.

33. Tieger T, Ganz L (1979) Recognition of faces in the presence of two-dimensional sinusoidal masks. Percept Psychophys 26: 163–167.

34. Donchin E, Coles MGH (1988) Is the P300 component a manifestation of context updating? Behav Brain Sci 11: 355–372.

35. Verleger R, Jaskowski P, Wascher E (2005) Evidence for an Integrative Role of P3b in Linking Reaction to Perception. J Psychophysiol 19: 165–181.

36. Kornmeier J, Bach M (2009) Object perception: when our brain is impressed but we do not notice it. J Vis 9: 7 1–10.

37. Alexander JE, Porjesz B, Bauer LO, Kuperman S, Morzorati S, et al. (1995) P300 hemispheric amplitude asymmetries from a visual oddball task. Psychophysiology 32: 467–475.

38. Ophir E, Nass C, Wagner AD (2009) Cognitive control in media multitaskers. Proc Natl Acad Sci U S A 106: 15583–15587.

39. Corbetta M, Shulman GL (2002) Control of goal-directed and stimulus-driven attention in the brain. Nat Rev Neurosci 3: 201–215.

40. Fox MD, Corbetta M, Snyder AZ, Vincent JL, Raichle ME (2006) Spontaneous neuronal activity distinguishes human dorsal and ventral attention systems. Proc Natl Acad Sci U S A 103. 10046–10051.

41. Lavie N (2005) Distracted and confused?: selective attention under load. Trends Cogn Sci 9: 75–82.

42. Shalom DB (2009) The medial prefrontal cortex and integration in autism. Neuroscientist 15: 589–598.

43. Bach M (1998) Electroencephalogram (EEG). In: von Schulthess GK, Hennig J, editors. Functional Imaging. Washington: Lippincott-Raven. 391–408.

5

Rare Mutations of *CACNB2* Found in Autism Spectrum Disease-Affected Families Alter Calcium Channel Function

Alexandra F. S. Breitenkamp[1], Jan Matthes[1], Robert Daniel Nass[1], Judith Sinzig[2,3], Gerd Lehmkuhl[3], Peter Nürnberg[4], Stefan Herzig[1,5]*

1 Department of Pharmacology, University of Cologne, Cologne, Germany, 2 Department of Child and Adolescent Psychiatry and Psychotherapy, LVR-Klinik Bonn, Bonn, Germany, 3 Department of Child and Adolescent Psychiatry and Psychotherapy, University of Cologne, Cologne, Germany, 4 Cologne Center for Genomics, University of Cologne, Cologne, Germany, 5 Center for Molecular Medicine, University of Cologne, Cologne, Germany

Abstract

Autism Spectrum Disorders (ASD) are complex neurodevelopmental diseases clinically defined by dysfunction of social interaction. Dysregulation of cellular calcium homeostasis might be involved in ASD pathogenesis, and genes coding for the L-type calcium channel subunits $Ca_V1.2$ (*CACNA1C*) and $Ca_V\beta2$ (*CACNB2*) were recently identified as risk loci for psychiatric diseases. Here, we present three rare missense mutations of *CACNB2* (G167S, S197F, and F240L) found in ASD-affected families, two of them described here for the first time (G167S and F240L). All these mutations affect highly conserved regions while being absent in a sample of ethnically matched controls. We suggest the mutations to be of physiological relevance since they modulate whole-cell Ba^{2+} currents through calcium channels when expressed in a recombinant system (HEK-293 cells). Two mutations displayed significantly decelerated time-dependent inactivation as well as increased sensitivity of voltage-dependent inactivation. In contrast, the third mutation (F240L) showed significantly accelerated time-dependent inactivation. By altering the kinetic parameters, the mutations are reminiscent of the *CACNA1C* mutation causing Timothy Syndrome, a Mendelian disease presenting with ASD. In conclusion, the results of our first-time biophysical characterization of these three rare *CACNB2* missense mutations identified in ASD patients support the hypothesis that calcium channel dysfunction may contribute to autism.

Editor: Michael Edward Zwick, Emory University School Of Medicine, United States of America

Funding: This study was supported by the "Koeln Fortune" program (KF 20/2006 and KF 93/2007) and DFG, the German Research Foundation, (He 1578 15-1). The funders had no role in study design, data collection and analysis, decision to publish, or preparation of the manuscript.

Competing Interests: The authors have declared that no competing interests exist.

* E-mail: stefan.herzig@uni-koeln.de

Introduction

Autism spectrum disorder (ASD) is defined by dysfunction of social interaction and communication, stereotypic behavior and sensory integration problems. It is a complex neuro-developmental disease, which might result from an altered brain ontogenesis or altered neural homeostasis. According to the Centers for Disease Control and Prevention (CDC) the prevalence of ASD in the US population is 1:88 [1]. Until now, genetic explanations for ASD are limited to rare chromosomal abnormalities like copy number variations or very rare single gene disorders. A first hint to unravel pathophysiological pathway of ASD came from the identification of the mutation p.G406R found in the L-type calcium channel pore-forming subunit ($Ca_V1.2$) gene *CACNA1C* in patients with Timothy Syndrome (TS) [2]. Whole-cell patch clamp recordings showed that the TS-mutation leads to a decelerated and incomplete inactivation of the calcium inward current. The phenotype of TS demonstrates the consequences of inadequate inactivation behavior of voltage gated calcium channels (VGCC) in different biological contexts, like heart, brain, and the immune system. Calcium channel inactivation is a key mechanism by which cells are able to tightly control intracellular calcium levels

and therefore the activity of excitable cells. Of note, calcium channel inactivation is not exclusively controlled by the channel pore, but also depends on auxiliary subunits, namely $Ca_V\beta$ and $Ca_V\alpha2\delta$ [3,4]. The assembly of the subunits and their specific isoforms determines the distinctive behavior of VGCCs for the neuronal function. The number of permutations of calcium channel complexes with their subunits, isoforms and splice-variants paves the way for fine-tuned calcium channel function adapted for information processing. There are transcripts of ten pore-forming $Ca_V\alpha1$-subunit genes (CACNA1A to CACNA1I and CACNA1S), which undergo extensive alternative splicing and in concert with auxiliary subunits exhibit different biophysical properties and expression profiles as well as distinct subcellular targeting [5].

Particularly $Ca_V\beta$-subunits have been shown to impact surface expression and modulation of channel activity and kinetics, leading to an increased L-type calcium channel activity, as revealed in whole-cell [6,7] and single-channel recordings [8]. A wide variation of inactivation behavior has been described for the splice variants of the β2-subunit [4]. Even slight structural differences within the $Ca_V\beta$-subunit can strongly modify the gating behavior of L-type calcium channels [8–10]. Interestingly, the expression of distinct $Ca_V\beta$-subunits within the brain is dependent on the stage of neuronal development [11]. Since the discovery of the TS-mutation and its effect on inactivation of the L-type calcium channel, additional calcium channel genes or loci have been associated with ASD, e.g. the genes for the pore-forming subunits *CACNA1D* [12], *CACNA1F* [13], *CACNA1G* [14], *CACNA1H* [15] and the auxiliary subunit *CACNB1* [14]. These studies emphasize the importance of calcium channel activity, inactivation and calcium signaling in a broader sense for the pathophysiology of ASD. Interestingly, the activity and kinetics of several pore-forming subunits of L-type ($Ca_V1.1$–1.4) and Non-L-type ($Ca_V2.1$–2.3) channels [2,12,13,16] are regulated by $Ca_V\beta$-subunits. Moreover, they are involved in various signaling pathways [2,17,18], all of which have been linked to ASD pathophysiology previously. Nevertheless, studies considering the role of calcium channels in ASD have focused on the pore-forming subunits of the calcium channel complex, even though gene clusters of interacting proteins participating in linear signaling pathways would have a similar chance of being involved in the etiology of ASD [19].

Based on our previous studies showing that current and gating kinetics profoundly depend on the particular $Ca_V\beta$-subunit isoform or splice variant associated with the channel pore [8,9], we hypothesized that $Ca_V\beta$-subunit mutations might lead to electrophysiological phenotypes similar to that observed in TS. Though all four $Ca_V\beta$-subunit genes (*CACNB1–CACNB4*) are expressed within the brain [20] we chose *CACNB2* because of positional evidence from a meta-analysis of linkage data [21]. Here, Trikalinos and colleagues showed genome-wide suggestive significance for a designated bin 10p12–q11.1, which embraces a large genomic region including the *CACNB2* gene in autistic siblings. Recently, *CACNB2* was found as a risk locus for five major psychiatric disorders including ASD [22] and thus is regarded as a susceptibility gene.

In our current study, we searched for mutations in the β2-subunit gene that might affect gating behavior of voltage-dependent calcium channels. In a mutation screening, 155 patients with ASD were sequenced and the results were filtered for most promising candidates. We included only missense variants, which were not present in our cohort of 259 matched controls and located in highly conserved regions of the protein as an indicator of functional importance. Furthermore, the mutations had to be unknown or potentially damaging according to in-silico predictions.

Here, for the first time, we present three missense mutations located in conserved regions of the calcium channel *CACNB2* gene found in three families affected by ASD. In electrophysiological

analyses of recombinant channels, these missense mutations were found to differentially alter current kinetics. Though our data do not prove an association between these *CACNB2* mutations and ASD, our findings support the idea of Cavβ2 variants being of functional relevance for ASD pathophysiology.

Materials and Methods

Ethics Statement

Procedures were approved by the Institutional Review Board (application number 04-223) of the medical faculty of the University of Cologne.

Subjects

gDNA samples were available from 259 healthy controls and 155 patients with Autistic Spectrum Disorder (ASD), each are ethnically matched groups of Caucasians of west-European origin. The cases were elicited from three different sources: Twenty patients were recruited by the Department of Child & Adolescent Psychiatry and Psychotherapy, University of Cologne. These patients meet diagnostic criteria for 'broad ASD' (e.g. Aspergers's) based on interview for DSM-IV-R. A written informed consent was obtained from the parents or legal guardians of the minors using the consent form approved by the I.R.B. of the University of Cologne (Germany). Ten cases were included from Autism Tissue Program (www. atpportal.org) from the Maryland National Institute of Child Health and Human Development (NICHD) Brain Tissue Center and the Harvard Brain Tissue Resource Center (USA), published e.g. in [23]. 125 cases were provided by the Autism Genetic Resource Exchange (AGRE) Consortium (http://research.agre.org/program/descr.cfm). All AGRE-Patients met diagnosis for 'autism' and each family was ascertained on the condition that at least two individuals were diagnosed with ASD [24], where diagnostic tests included autism diagnostic interview-revised (ADI-R) [25] and the autism diagnostic observational schedule (ADOS) [26]. Regulatory review, approval, and oversight of AGRE's human subject research is provided by Western IRB (title: AUTISM GENETIC RESOURCE EXCHANGE). In order to find new sequence variations with a putative function-altering effect, all exons and their flanking intronic sequences of *CACNB2* were sequenced in 155 ASD patients. The number of sequenced cases enabled the detection of rare SNPs (f = 0.01) with a probability of 96% to detect it once and 81% to detect it twice. The power calculation was made according to Glatt et al. [27]. To assure a strong genetic background, patients from multiplex families with a severe phenotype were selected.

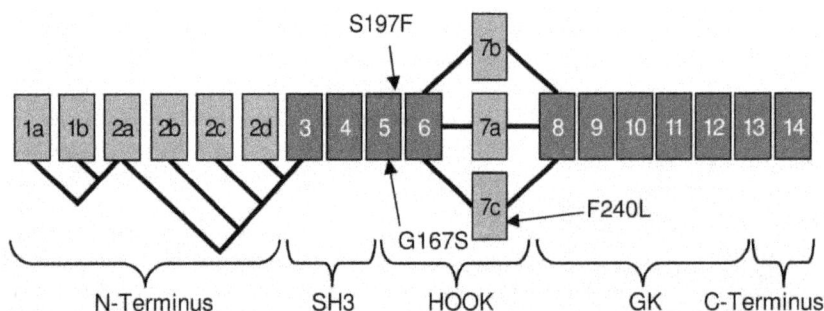

Figure 1. Splice scheme of human *CACNB2* resulting in 9 splice variants of the Ca_Vβ2-subunit with the localization of the three mutations. Spliced exons are shown in light grey and conserved exons in dark grey. All nine splice variants express the mutation-carrying exon 5, while three of variants contain the localization of the third mutation in exon 7c [10].

Table 1. Clinical Features of ASD patients with rare mutations in *CACNB2*.

Description	Patient 1	Patient 2	Patient 3
	(AU062603)	(AU1338304)	(AU066204)
Mutations	*c.334G>A*	*c.425C>T*	*c.553T>C*
(# NM_201597.2)	p.G167S	p.S197F	p.F240L
Genotype	+–	+–	+–
Gender	M	M	F
Epilepsy	Yes	Unknown	No
Type	Complex partial	–	–
Autism			
ADI-R	Autism	Autism	Autism
ADOS	Autism	Autism	Autism
Brain Imaging			
MRI	normal	Unknown	Normal

ADI-R, Autism Diagnostic Interview-Revised; **ADOS**, Diagnostic Observation Schedule-Generic; **MRI,** magnetic resonance imaging.

The control group consisting of 259 matching controls was kindly provided by Dr. Heusch and Dr. Brodde, published in [28]. Based on the gender-dependent frequency of ASD [1], we chose an appropriate male to female ratio for both groups of about 5:1.

Genotypic and DNA Sequence Analyses

Oligonucleotides to all known exons of the *CACNB2* gene were designed according to genomic sequences found in the Celera data base using Primer3. PCR amplification of DNA samples was carried out with GoTaq (Promega) according to the manufacturer's protocol; annealing temperature was chosen according to Primer3. Mutational analyses were carried out with Mutation Surveyor. PCR fragments were purified using ExoI and SAP (NEB), and sequencing was performed with an ABI 3730 automated DNA sequencer.

DNA Constructs and Site-directed Mutagenesis

For functional analysis, mutations p.G167S and p.S197F were introduced in human β_{2d}cDNA (NM_201596.2) and the mutation p.F240L was introduced in β_{2d_E7c} (NM_201597.2) by site-directed mutagenesis (Stratagene QuikChange Kit) and verified by sequencing.

EGFP was used as reporter gene, which was coexpressed together with the β2-subunit by the bicistronic pIRES2-EGFP vector (Clontech). G167S forward primer 5'-gatagggcgattggtaaaagaaagctgt-gaaatcggattc-3'; G167S reverse primer 5'-gaatccgatttcacagctttctttaccaatcgccctatc-3'; S197F forward primer 5'-cagagagccaagcaagggaaattctacttcagtaaatcaggaggaaattcatcatcc-3'; S197F reverse primer 5'-ggatgatgaatttcctcctgatttactgaagtagaatttcccttgcttggctctctg-3'; F240L forward primer 5'-ggaaaactgcaggcttgctttggcggtttactaca; F240L reverse primer 5'-tgtagtaaaccgccaaagcaagcctgcagttttcc.

Cell Culture

In brief, HEK-293α1c cells stably expressing $Ca_v1.2$ subunit (GeneBank accession #NM_000719) cloned from human heart [29] were grown in Petri dishes in Dulbeccos modified Eagle medium (PAA, Germany) supplemented with 10% FBS (PAA, Germany), penicillin (10 U/ml), and streptomycin (10 μg/ml; PAA, Germany). Cells were selected by geneticin (G418) (PAA, Germany) at a final concentration of 500 μg/ml. Cells were

routinely passaged twice a week and incubated at 37°C under 6% CO_2 growth conditions. HEK-293 α1c cells were transfected using SuperFect reagent (Qiagen). For whole-cell recordings, cells were transfected with a 2:3 ratio of either human WT or mutant β_{2d}-subunit and human $\alpha_2\delta_1$-subunit [30].

Electrophysiology

Whole-cell recordings in EGFP-positive cells were obtained 48–72 h after transfection. Immediately prior to recording, cells kept in 35-mm culture dishes were washed at room temperature (19–23°C) with bath solution. For constructs based on human β_{2d}cDNA (NM_201596.2) the bath solution contained (in mM) 20 $BaCl_2$, 1 $MgCl_2$, 10 HEPES, 40 TEA-Cl, 10 dextrose, and 65 CsCl (pH 7.2 with TEA-OH) and pipette solution (in mM) 105 CsCl, 25 TEA-Cl, 11 EGTA, and 10 HEPES (pH 7.2 with CsOH). Holding potential was −100 mV. For constructs based on human β2d_E7c cDNA (NM_201597.2) the bath solution contained (in mM) 5 $BaCl_2$, 1 $MgCl_2$, 10 HEPES, 40 TEA-Cl, 10 dextrose, and 92 CsCl (pH 7.2 with TEA-OH). Patch pipettes made from borosilicate glass (1.7 mm diameter and 0.283 mm wall thickness, Hilgenberg GmbH, Malsfeld, Germany) were pulled using a Sutter Instrument P-97 horizontal puller and fire-polished using a Narishige MF-83 microforge (Narishige Scientific Instrument Lab, Tokyo, Japan). Pipette resistance was 2–4 MΩ.

Currents were elicited by applying test potentials of −40 mV to +60 mV from a holding potential of −100 mV using Clampex software pClamp 5.5 and an Axopatch 1D amplifier (Axon Instruments, Foster City, CA, USA). Voltage dependence of Ba^{2+} current inactivation in HEK cells was determined with a two-pulse protocol. For β_{2d}cDNA (NM_201596.2) constructs the conditioning first pulse (stepped from −100 mV to +40mV) was held for 5s and the second pulse (of +10mV) for 125 ms; for β_{2d_E7c}cDNA (NM_201597.2) constructs the conditioning pulse was stepped from −75 mV to +5 mV for 1 s and the second pulse (of +10 mV) was held for 125 ms. For both steady-state inactivation protocols the relative magnitude of inward current elicited during the second pulse was plotted as a function of the voltage of the conditioning first pulse.

Data were analyzed using pCLAMP6 (Axon Instruments) and GraphPad 5 Prism. Currents were filtered at 2 kHz. Data were fitted to a Boltzmann function to obtain the half point (V0.5) and

(A)

Patient 1(AU062603) c.334G>A; p.G167S	Patient 2(AU1338304) c.425C>T; p.S197F	Patient 3(AU066204) c.553T>C; p.F240L

	K165 E166 G167 C168	**F195 Y196 S197 splice**	**G238 L239 F240 W241**
WT	A A A A G A A G G C T G T G	T T C T A C T C C A G GTA	G G C T T G T T T T G G C G
MT	A A A A G A A A G C T G T G	T T C T A C T T C A G GTA	G G C T T G C T T T G G C G

(B)

(C)

Human	VKEGCEI	Human	QGKFYSS	Human	GLFWRFT
Rat	VKEGCEI	Rat	QGKFYSS	Rat	-----------
Dog	VKEGCEI	Dog	QGKFYSS	Dog	GLFWRFT
Mouse	VKEGCEI	Mouse	QGKFYSS	Macaca	GLFWRFT
Horse	VKEGCEI	Horse	QGKFYSS	Horse	GLFWRFT
Chicken	VKEGCEI	Chicken	QGKFYSS	Chicken	-----------
Dolphin	VKEGCEI	Dolphin	QGRFYSS	Dolphin	-----------
ASD_G167S	VKE**S**CEI	ASD_S197F	QGKFYS**F**	ASD_F240L	GL**L**WRFT
Consensus	**VKEGCEI**	**Consensus**	**QGKFYSS**	**Consensus**	**GLFWRFT**

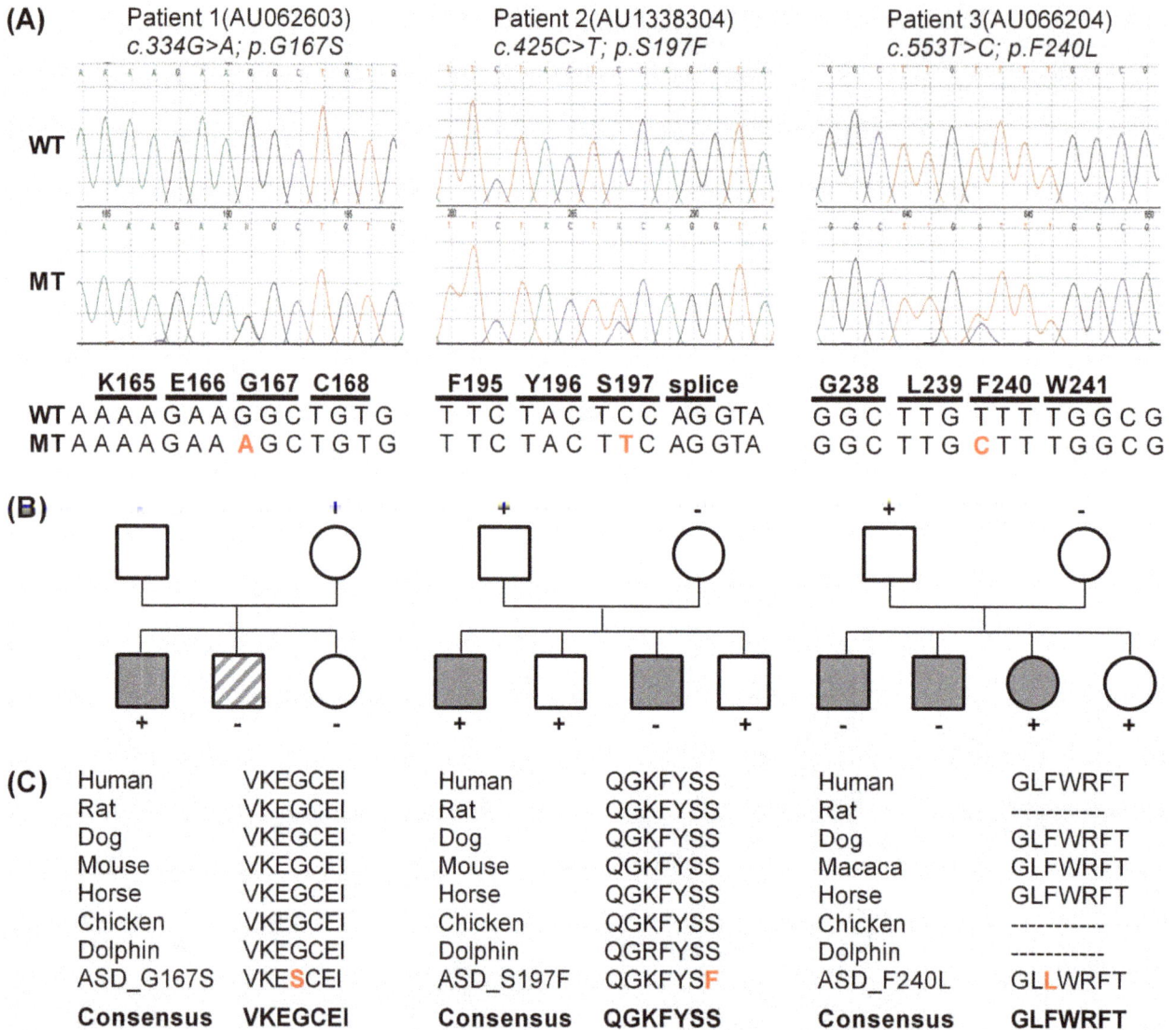

Figure 2. (a) Chromatogram showing point mutations for patient 1–3. **(b)** The pedigrees show the occurrence of the disease phenotype and the inheritance of missense mutations in *CACNB2*. Circles and squares indicate females and males, respectively. *Filled* symbols denote diagnosis of autism; *partially filled* symbols denote individuals that are diagnosed within a broad spectrum of pervasive developmental disorders. **(c)** Alignments show conservation among different species for p.G167S, p.S197F and p.F240L suggesting an importance for the topology and function.

slope factor (dV) for the voltage dependence of inactivation; Fits were performed after subtracting the offset from the peak values of the steady-state inactivation data. Offset was defined as a deviation from zero at the end of a fully inactivating current (after a 5000ms prepulse followed by a 125ms test pulse at +10mV). For voltage dependence of activation data were fitted by combined Ohm and Boltzmann relation $I(V) = (V - V_R) \times \dfrac{G_{max}}{\left(1 + \exp^{\frac{(V - V_{0.5})}{dV}}\right)}$ according to [31].

Statistical Analysis

Student's unpaired two-tailed t-test (GraphPad Prism 5, GraphPad Software, San Diego, CA) was used to compare electrophysiological parameters gained with the several CACNB2 mutations and their corresponding wildtypes. $P < 0.05$ was considered significant. All p-values are listed in table S2. Data are presented as mean ± SEM.

Results

We performed a screening for mutations in *CACNB2* by sequencing all 19 exons and their flanking intronic regions from 155 patients with ASD. All variants found are listed in table S1. We filtered for variants causing non-synonymous substitutions, frameshifts, or splice site changes and identified six missense mutations. Since two of them occurred at similar frequencies in our patient cohort, our control cohort, and the NCBI database of short genetic variations (dbSNP), they were not further considered. One substitution ("New11" in tabl S1.) is likely to be benign according to the prediction of polymorphism phenotyping tool (PolyPhen2); also the amino acid exchange of the minor allele is prevalent in other species (data not shown). Three non-synonymous mutations were located in conserved domains of the protein (Fig. 1) and subsequently analyzed for functional effects. They were detected in three different patients who all were heterozygous

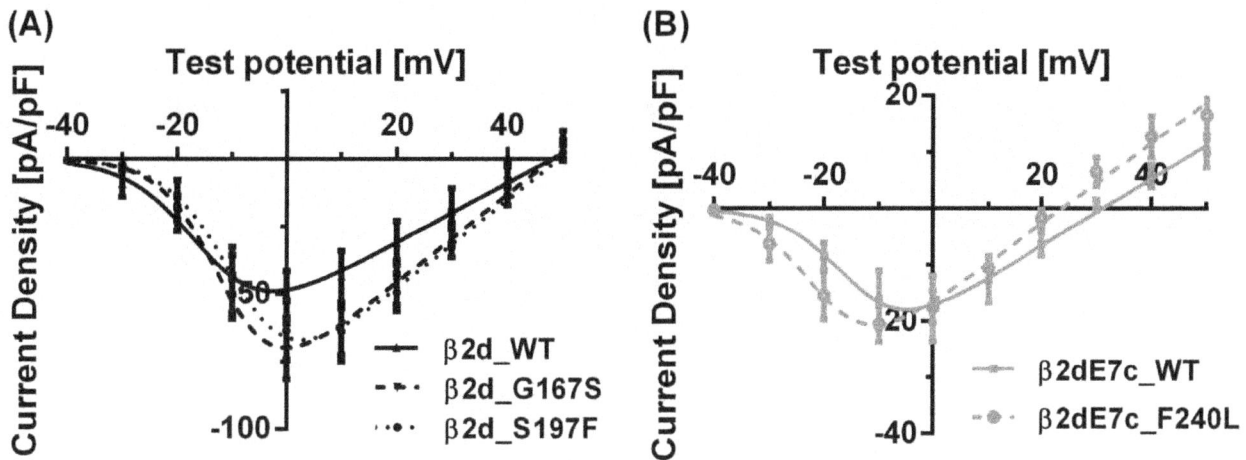

Figure 3. I–V relationships. Currents were elicited from −40 to +60 mV in 10 mV increments with 5 mM or 20 mM Ba^{2+}, respectively. The holding potential was −100 mV. Current density of the variants p.G167S (N = 11) and p.S197F (N = 8) in (a) and p.F240L (N = 5) in (b) were compared with their respective WTs (β2d_WT: N = 9 and β2dE7c_WT: N = 5).

carriers (Fig. 2a). The mutations were absent from 259 healthy controls.

Patient 1 showed a variation at cDNA position 334 from guanine to adenine resulting in an amino acid exchange from glycine to serine (p.G167S, referring to NM_201596.2). The substitution is not annotated in dbSNP and according to the PolyPhen2 prediction 'probably damaging' for the $Ca_V β2$ function. Patient 2 had the cytosine at position 425 changed to thymine resulting in a substitution of phenylalanine for serine (p.S197F). This mutation is an annotated rare variant and shows a 'possibly damaging' PolyPhen2 score. The third affected patient had the transition c.T553C which results in a phenylalanine-to-leucine change (p.F240L, referring to NM_201597.2). The missense mutation is not annotated and PolyPhen2 predicts a 'benign' phenotyping score. The mutations p.G167S and p.S197F were found by analyzing the fifth exon, which is expressed in all splice isoforms; p.F240L was found in the alternative exon 7c (nomenclature according to Foell et al. [32]). All patients were diagnosed with autism by both ADI-R and ADOS. The clinical features of the patients are compiled in table 1.

The subsequently performed cosegregation analysis showed a low penetrance. Two variants showed incomplete segregation since some siblings, who were not obviously affected, were carriers of the mutation (Fig. 2b). Since complex-genetic disorders manifest depending on multiple factors, a low penetrance and incomplete cosegregation can be expected. In the literature, it has been suggested that pathogenic variants might be masked by epigenetic marks and thus are less penetrant [33] or that pathogenic variants follow an oligogenic pattern of inheritance, resulting in more severe or different phenotypes or are modified by the presence of additional variants [34]. Accordingly, unaffected carriers of a mutation might be possibly influenced by unknown genetic and epigenetic mechanisms [35] or might be subclinically affected.

As members of the membrane-associated guanylate kinase (MAGUK) protein family [8–10], β-subunits are comprised of two highly conserved central (GK and SH3) domains, flanked and interspersed by more variable N- and C-termini and a central HOOK domain (Fig. 1). The β2-subunit is subject to extensive alternative splicing of the N-terminus and within the central HOOK domain, comprising the alternative exons 7a-c (Fig. 1) [36]. All three mutations are located within the HOOK domain

(Fig. 1), which is known to modulate calcium channel inactivation [37,38]. The wildtype sequence of all three missense mutations revealed full conservation across species (Fig. 2c) indicating functional relevance.

To investigate the effect of the mutations on calcium channel function, we heterologously expressed WT and mutant forms of the human β2 together with human α2δ1 and EGFP in HEK-293 cells stably expressing a human $Ca_V 1.2$ pore-forming subunit, followed by whole-cell patch-clamp recordings. There are nine splice-variants of $Ca_V β2$, with different inactivation kinetics [4]. The mutations p.G167S and p.S197F are present in all these $Ca_V β2$ splice forms, and there is no predominant splice form in the brain. In accordance with our hypothesis and deductions from the TS-channel model, we expect a reduction of the channels inactivation rate. To evaluate this effect in the mutations we performed whole-cell experiments using Ba^{2+} as charge carrier, since the TS-mutation selectively decelerates time-dependent inactivation and spares or even accelerates calcium-dependent inactivation [39]. For the quantification of mutants' influence on channel inactivation behavior we chose the β2d splice variant as a suitable reference isoform, because of its relatively fast inactivation kinetics [4,8]. We compared the WT with the mutations p.G167S and p.S197F and the mutation p.F240L was analyzed separately with an appropriate WTE7c including its alternative exon 7c. The respective splice forms β2d (NM_201596.2) and β2dE7c (NM_201597.2) are – according to the GNF Expression Atlas 1 and 2 - expressed in fetal brain and in various adult brain regions.

Peak current densities tended to be enhanced in the mutants β2d_G167S and β2d_S197F compared to β2d_WT. These mutations also caused a slight, non-significant shift of the I-V relationships towards more positive test potentials (Fig. 3a). Conversely, for the mutation of the β2dE7c_WT (β2dE7c_F240L), the I-V relationship revealed a trend towards enhanced channel activity at negative test potentials (Fig. 3b).

Steady-state inactivation was examined using two-pulse protocols. Data and Boltzmann fits are depicted in Fig. 4a and 4b. The voltage of half-maximal inactivation ($V0.5_{inact}$) did not differ significantly between the three mutant channel complexes and their respective controls (Fig. 4c). However, a significant flattening of the Boltzmann curves was observed for β2d_G167S and

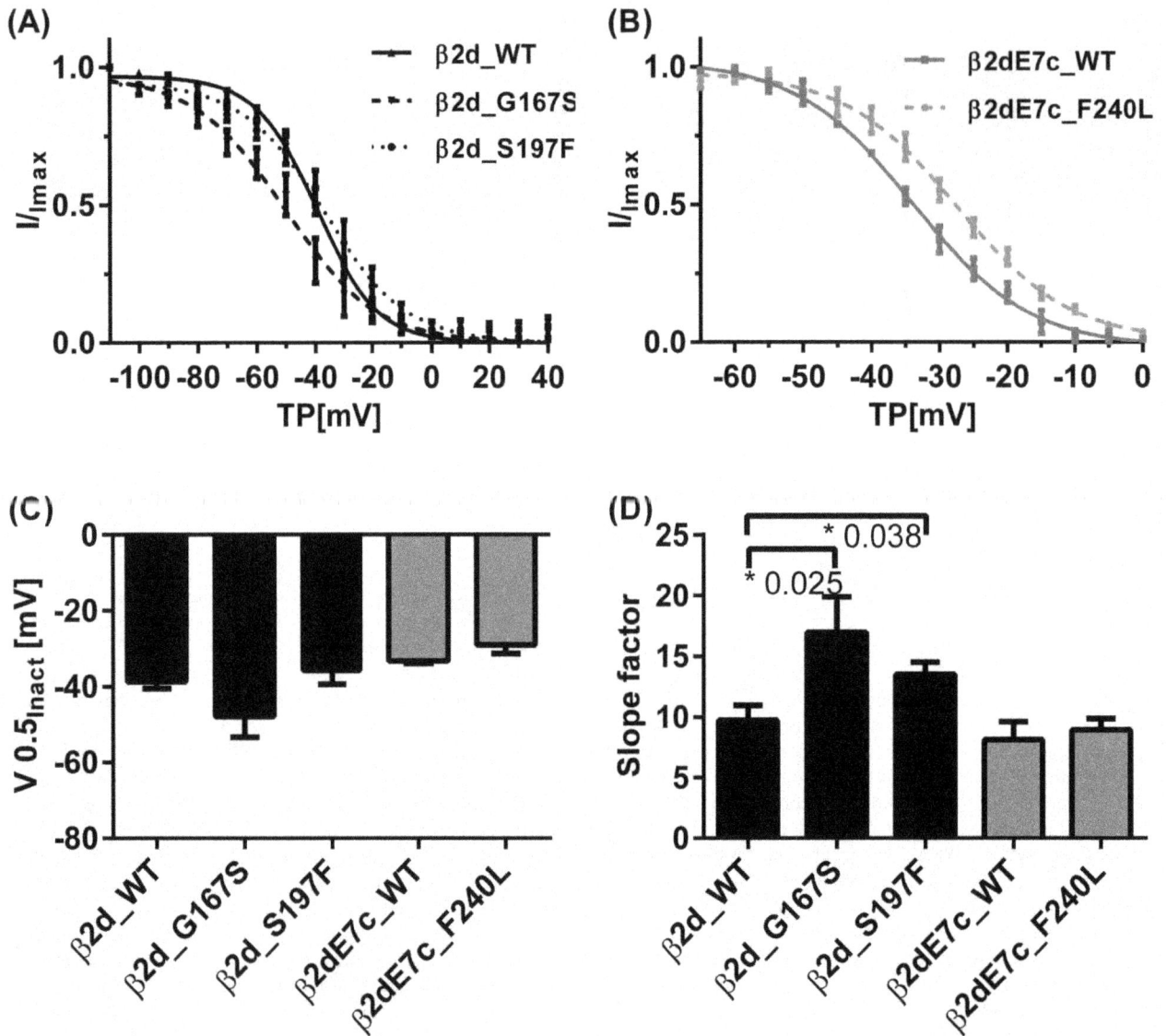

Figure 4. Voltage-dependent steady-state inactivation (a, b) of Ba^{2+} currents through L-type calcium channels. The ASD mutants p.G167S (N = 4) and p.S197F (N = 6) showed a significantly flattened slope of voltage-dependent inactivation compared to β2d_WT (N = 7). The third mutation β2dE7c_F240L. (N = 5) did not obviously differ from its corresponding β2dE7c_WT (N = 2). Half-inactivation potentials (V0.5$_{inact}$) (**c**) and the slope factors dV (**d**) were obtained from the fits of individual experiments using the Boltzmann equation and averaging the results. Asterisk (*) marks a statistical significance (P<0.05) compared to the respective WT.

β2d_S197F, as indicated by the slope factor dV (Fig. 4d). Numeric values are compiled in table 2.

As described previously for the Timothy Syndrome, the most notable differences between mutants and WT were observed in the time course of whole-cell Ba^{2+} currents. The mutant β2d_G167S and β2d_S1967F subunit induced a decelerated time-dependent inactivation of the channel complex within a 150ms test pulse (Fig. 5a). The WT with the alternative exon 7c inactivated more slowly than the WT with exon 7a. It was therefore examined using an extended test pulse duration (see scale bars in Fig. 5a). Compared with the adequate β2dE7c_WT the mutant β2dE7c_F240L showed an accelerated time-dependent inactivation. The mutants and the WT with Exon 7a were recorded with 20mM Ba^{2+} (compare [9]) and those with exon 7c were recorded with 5mM Ba^{2+} because of insufficient voltage-control with 20 mM Ba^{2+} and prolonged test pulse protocols (500ms). We

analyzed the extent of time-dependent inactivation as the percentage of current that has inactivated after 150ms of depolarization (% inactivation). As expected from the representative whole-cell current traces, the currents inactivated significantly more slowly for all test potentials in case of β2d_S197F and at − 20mV in case of β2d_G167S (Fig. 5b). In contrast, the mutant β2d_F240L led to faster, more pronounced inactivation compared to its corresponding WT (Fig. 5c). After 1000ms the currents of β2d_WT, β2d_G167S and β2d_S197F showed a comparable extent of inactivation of 94±1%, 99±2% and 96±3% at 0mV test potential.

Discussion

The complex genetic principle of origin underlying ASD is still to be elucidated [40]. So far, genome-wide association and linkage

Table 2. Current and voltage parameters (mean ± SEM) of the constructs tested.

	−β2d	β2d_WT	β2d_G167S	β2d_S197F	β2dE7c_WT	β2dE7c_F240L
	N = 3	N = 9	N = 11	N = 8	N = 5	N = 5
Peak Current Density [pA/pF]	−1.2	−56.5	−72.3	−68.8	−17.8	−21.1
	±1.0	±8.6	±10.3	±9.7	±5.8	±3.6
$V0.5_{act}$ [mV]	–	−11.9	−9.8	−6.3	−13.6	−18.7
		±2.0	±1.2	±2.5	±0.36	±2.5
Steady-state Inactivation		N = 7	N = 4	N = 6	N = 2	N = 5
$V0.5_{inact}$ [mV]		−38.7	−47.9	−35.7	−33.3	−28.2
		±1.8	±5.6	±3.7	±0.7	±1.9
dV		9.7	16.9 *	13.5 *	8.1	8.8
		±1.2	±2.9	±1.0	±1.5	±0.7

V0.5$_{act}$, Voltage of half-maximal activation; **V0.5$_{inact}$,** half-maximal inactivation voltage, dV, slope factor; **−β2d,** mock transfected cells; *indicates P<0.05 versus corresponding WT.

studies presented inconsistent loci, reflecting a broad etiological heterogeneity and suggesting the influence of rare variants weighted by common susceptibility alleles. To put the spectrum and the genes into a pathophysiological context, an oligogenic model with epistasis has been assumed [41,42]. It describes - based on their level of biological function - a combination of multiple interacting genes resulting in ASD phenotypes.

Until now, few potential pathophysiological mechanisms have been postulated [43,44]. The role of impaired calcium channel inactivation for ASD was revealed by Splawski and colleagues with the TS-mutation (CACNA1C: p.G406R) [2]. In more general terms, calcium signaling was found by a gene pathway analysis based on the 'Kyoto Encyclopedia of Genes and Genomes' (KEGG) as one of the three most significant pathways for ASD [45]. The concept is further supported by the association of mutations in various calcium channel genes with non-idiopathic ASD [2,13–16]. The activity and regulation of all L-type and some non-L-type calcium channels are dependent on their auxiliary β-subunit; therefore, the highly differentiated β-subunit function is expected to be crucial for proper function of the calcium channel complex and homeostasis in the nervous system.

Here, we present for the first time rare substitutions in highly conserved residues of the calcium channel subunit β2 in three out of 155 individuals with ASD, all of which were absent from 259 matching controls. According to the exome variant server (http://evs.gs.washington.edu/EVS), 100 variations (35 of which are missense, splice or frame-shift mutations) are known for European Americans in CACNCB2. Thus, a statistical proof of an elevated frequency of rare variants in the CACNCB2 gene in ASD patients was considered not feasible. We did not test for differences in the mutation frequency between ASD patients and controls. Instead, we searched for most promising candidates of putative causal variants. Subsequently, by using patch clamp, the variants were tested for putative impairment of the function of the channel complex. Electrophysiological analyses in HEK-cells by whole-cell patch-clamp recordings demonstrate that all three missense mutations significantly alter the kinetics of the currents carried by the Ca$_V$1.2 complex. Two mutations in the Ca$_V$β2-subunit lead to deceleration of time-dependent inactivation of Ba^{2+} currents as well as altered sensitivity of voltage-dependent inactivation. The third mutation shows a non-significant hyperpolarizing shift in current-voltage relation and an accelerated time-dependent inactivation. Of note decelerated time-dependent inactivation

and incomplete voltage-dependent inactivation behavior are the biophysical hallmarks of the TS-mutation p.G406R in CACNA1C [2,17,39].

We observed a low penetrance of the three mutations in the ASD families under investigation, indicating the influence of other factors on the full expression of the condition. However, rare variants might contribute to the complex genetics and clinical heterogeneity of ASD. For comparison, an analogous sequencing approach studying CACNA1H as a candidate gene for ASD in 461 patients revealed six non-synonymous mutations in conserved domains, all showing a low penetrance and incomplete segregation [15]. Expression of complex genetic disorders depends on multiple factors, therefore a low penetrance of causal variants is quite common. Unaffected carriers might be subclinically affected, other risk factors might have contributed to the phenotype in the affected individuals, or the described mutations may only act as modifiers of the phenotype. Even for the Timothy syndrome - one of the most penetrant monogenic forms of autism - ASD has a penetrance of ~75% only [46].

The putative effects of the Ca$_V$β2-mutations are ample as the β-subunit also plays an essential role as an interaction partner with intracellular signaling machineries. For instance, Krey et al. have recently demonstrated a new pathway involving the TS-mutation which leads to a calcium channel activity-dependent and conformation-dependent dendrite retraction via Gem-induced RhoA-signaling [18]. Here, the Ca$_V$β-subunits might be involved in two ways: firstly they are known to regulate the channel activity, but secondly the interaction of Ca$_V$1.2 with Gem, mediated through the β-subunit is important for the ability of the channel to control activity-dependent dendritic arborization [18]. In summary, the role of the Ca$_V$β2-subunit as a risk factor for ASD can not only be attributed to its interaction with diverse ASD-associated pore-forming Ca$_V$α1-subunits, but also because the Ca$_V$β2-subunit acts as a signaling hub and can link together different ASD pathways.

The mutations presented here appear to follow a similar but milder mechanism of action that occurs in TS. TS presents with a multi-organ dysfunction, possibly indicating the consequences of a dramatic elevation of the intracellular calcium concentration. Mutations resulting in an even larger effect would likely abort the organism's development [47]. Thus the mutation of the TS can be viewed as an extreme of the viable spectrum of mutations within the calcium signaling pathway. Compared to this, the mutations

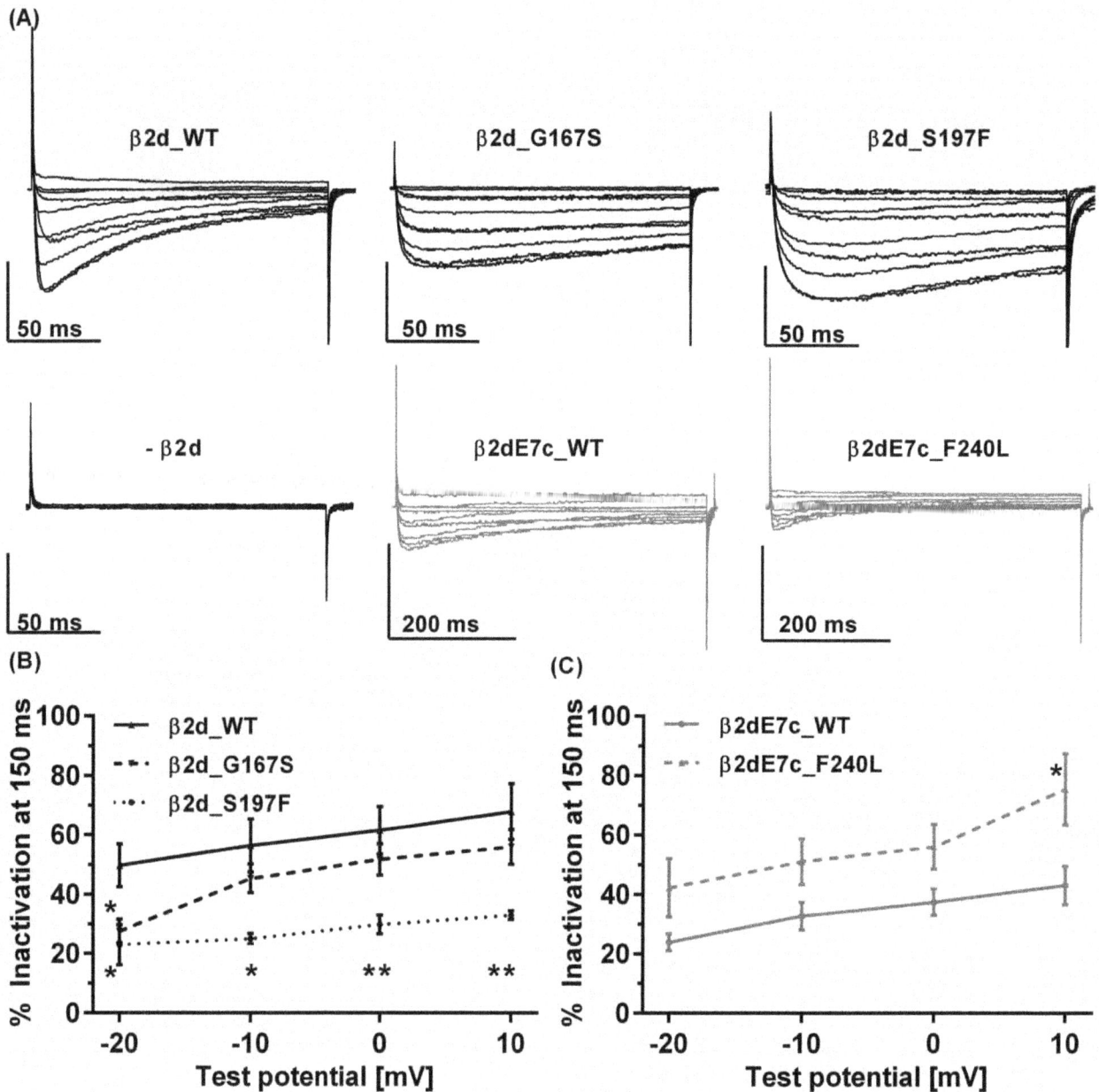

Figure 5. Time-dependent inactivation. Representative whole-cell Ba^{2+} current traces (a) of $Ca_V1.2/\alpha2\delta1$ co-expressed with β2d_WT -subunit or co-expressed with the ASD mutants β2d_G167S, β2d_S197F or the β2dE7c_WT or its variant β2dE7c_F240L. The currents were elicited from a holding potential of -100 mV by 150 ms (or 500ms) step depolarization of -40 to $+50$ mV with 20 mM Ba^{2+} (for β2d variants) or 5 mM Ba^{2+} (for β2dE7c variants), respectively. Analysis of the extent of time-dependent inactivation. (**b, c**) % Inactivation was analyzed as the remaining fraction of whole-cell current that has not inactivated after 150 ms of depolarization. β2d_WT (N = 12), β2d_G167S (N = 8), β2d_S197F (N = 11) (**c**) Similar analysis for β2dE7c variants β2dE7c_WT (N = 5), β2dE7c_F240L (N = 6). Asterisk (*) marks a statistical significance (P<0.05) compared to the respective WT, (**) marks P<0.01.

β2d_G167S, β2d_S197F and β2d_F240L exhibited rather moderate effects on channel gating that nonetheless might suffice to unbalance neuronal calcium channel function.

Because private and rare mutations seem to play a role in the predisposition to ASD [44], the discovery of rare variants with putative functional relevance might contribute to our understanding of the disorder's etiology. Integrating the data from TS [2], the meta-analysis of psychiatric disorders [22], and functional studies on auxiliary β-subunits, we propose that inappropriate function of different components of the voltage-gated calcium channel complex can result in or may contribute to autism spectrum disorder. More detailed biophysical and cell-biological studies under physiological conditions are warranted for all such mutations.

Supporting Information

Table S1 All found variants in the exons and flanking intronic regions of CACNB2 in autistic patients.

Table S2   Current and voltage parameters (mean ± SEM) of the constructs tested. P-values stem from individual Student t-tests of the indicated channels.

Acknowledgments

We gratefully acknowledge the resources provided by the Autism Genetic Resource Exchange (AGRE) Consortium and the participating AGRE families. The Autism Genetic Resource Exchange is a program of Autism Speaks and is supported, in part, by grant 1U24MH081810 from the National Institute of Mental Health to Clara M. Lajonchere (PI). We further acknowledge the Autism Tissue Program, New York Institute for Basic Research in Developmental Disabilities and Harvard Brain Tissue Resource Center for providing tissue-derived gDNA used in this study. Antonio M. Persico is acknowledged for providing the genomic DNA samples through the genomic DNA collection of the Autism Tissue Program. We are indebted to Prof. Dr. Heusch and Prof. Dr. Brodde, who kindly supplied gDNA from 259 population controls of West-European ancestry, to Dr. F. Lehmann-Horn for providing pcDNA3.1/Hygro-CACNA2D1 (Department of Applied Physiology, Ulm University, Germany) and to Dr. G. Varadi for providing us with HEK293-α1c cells (stably expressing pore-forming (α1c)subunit). We gratefully acknowledge the assistance by Dr. Wanchana Jangsangthong, Annika Häuser and Dr. Andreas Lazar.

Author Contributions

Conceived and designed the experiments: AFSB JM PN SH. Performed the experiments: AFSB RDN. Analyzed the data: AFSB PN SH. Contributed reagents/materials/analysis tools: JS GL PN SH. Wrote the paper: AFSB JM SH.

References

1. Centers for Disease Control and Prevention (2012) Prevalence of autism spectrum disorders–Autism and Developmental Disabilities Monitoring Network, 14 sites, United States, 2008. MMWR Surveill Summ 61: 1–19.
2. Splawski I, Timothy KW, Sharpe LM, Decher N, Kumar P, et al. (2004) Ca(V)1.2 calcium channel dysfunction causes a multisystem disorder including arrhythmia and autism. Cell 119: 19–31.
3. Birnbaumer L, Qin N, Olcese R, Tareilus E, Platano D, et al. (1998) Structures and functions of calcium channel beta subunits. J Bioenerg Biomembr 30: 357–375.
4. Takahashi SX, Mittman S, Colecraft HM (2003) Distinctive modulatory effects of five human auxiliary beta2 subunit splice variants on L-type calcium channel gating. Biophys J 84: 3007–3021.
5. Ludwig A, Flockerzi V, Hofmann F (1997) Regional expression and cellular localization of the alpha1 and beta subunit of high voltage-activated calcium channels in rat brain. J Neurosci 17: 1339–1349.
6. Jangsangthong W, Kuzmenkina E, Khan IF, Matthes J, Hullin R, et al. (2009) Inactivation of L-type calcium channels is determined by the length of the N terminus of mutant beta(1) subunits. Pflugers Arch 459: 399–411.
7. Cens T, Mangoni ME, Nargeot J, Charnet P (1996) Modulation of the alpha 1A Ca2+ channel by beta subunits at physiological Ca2+ concentration. FEBS Lett 391: 232–237.
8. Herzig S, Khan IF, Grundemann D, Matthes J, Ludwig A, et al. (2007) Mechanism of Ca(v)1.2 channel modulation by the amino terminus of cardiac beta2-subunits. FASEB J 21: 1527–1538.
9. Jangsangthong W, Kuzmenkina E, Khan IF, Matthes J, Hullin R, et al. (2010) Inactivation of L-type calcium channels is determined by the length of the N terminus of mutant beta(1) subunits. Pflugers Arch 459: 399–411.
10. Buraei Z, Yang J (2010) The b subunit of voltage-gated Ca2+ channels. Physiol Rev 90: 1461–1506.
11. McEnery MW, Vance CL, Begg CM, Lee WL, Choi Y, et al. (1998) Differential expression and association of calcium channel subunits in development and disease. J Bioenerg Biomembr 30: 409–418.
12. O'Roak BJ, Vives L, Girirajan S, Karakoc E, Krumm N, et al. (2012) Sporadic autism exomes reveal a highly interconnected protein network of de novo mutations. Nature 485: 246–250.
13. Hemara-Wahanui A, Berjukow S, Hope CI, Dearden PK, Wu SB, et al. (2005) A CACNA1F mutation identified in an X-linked retinal disorder shifts the voltage dependence of Cav1.4 channel activation. Proc Natl Acad Sci U S A 102: 7553–7558.
14. Strom SP, Stone JL, Ten Bosch JR, Merriman B, Cantor RM, et al. (2010) High-density SNP association study of the 17q21 chromosomal region linked to autism identifies CACNA1G as a novel candidate gene. Mol Psychiatry 15: 996–1005.
15. Splawski I, Yoo DS, Stotz SC, Cherry A, Clapham DE, et al. (2006) CACNA1H mutations in autism spectrum disorders. J Biol Chem 281: 22085–22091.
16. Limpitikul W, Johny MB, Yue DT (2013) Autism-Associated Point Mutation in CaV1.3 Calcium Channels alters their Regulation by Ca2+ [Abstract]. Biophys J 104.
17. Splawski I, Timothy KW, Decher N, Kumar P, Sachse FB, et al. (2005) Severe arrhythmia disorder caused by cardiac L-type calcium channel mutations. Proc Natl Acad Sci U S A 102: 8089–8096; discussion 8086–8088.
18. Krey JF, Pasca SP, Shcheglovitov A, Yazawa M, Schwemberger R, et al. (2013) Timothy syndrome is associated with activity-dependent dendritic retraction in rodent and human neurons. Nature Neuroscience 16: 201–209.
19. Iossifov I, Zheng T, Baron M, Gilliam TC, Rzhetsky A (2008) Genetic-linkage mapping of complex hereditary disorders to a whole-genome molecular-interaction network. Genome Res 18: 1150–1162.
20. Volsen SG, Day NC, McCormack AL, Smith W, Craig PJ, et al. (1997) The expression of voltage-dependent calcium channel beta subunits in human cerebellum. Neuroscience 80: 161–174.
21. Trikalinos TA, Karvouni A, Zintzaras E, Ylisaukko-oja T, Peltonen L, et al. (2006) A heterogeneity-based genome search meta-analysis for autism-spectrum disorders. Mol Psychiatry 11: 29–36.
22. Cross-Disorder Group of the Psychiatric Genomics Consortium (2013) Identification of risk loci with shared effects on five major psychiatric disorders: a genome-wide analysis. The Lancet 381: 1371–1379.
23. Lintas C, Altieri L, Lombardi F, Sacco R, Persico AM (2010) Association of autism with polyomavirus infection in postmortem brains. J Neurovirol 16: 141–149.
24. Geschwind DH, Sowinski J, Lord C, Iversen P, Shestack J, et al. (2001) The autism genetic resource exchange: a resource for the study of autism and related neuropsychiatric conditions. Am J Hum Genet 69: 463–466.
25. Lord C, Rutter M, Le Couteur A (1994) Autism Diagnostic Interview-Revised: a revised version of a diagnostic interview for caregivers of individuals with possible pervasive developmental disorders. J Autism Dev Disord 24: 659–685.
26. Lord C, Risi S, Lambrecht L, Cook EH, Jr., Leventhal BL, et al. (2000) The autism diagnostic observation schedule-generic: a standard measure of social and communication deficits associated with the spectrum of autism. J Autism Dev Disord 30: 205–223.
27. Glatt CE, DeYoung JA, Delgado S, Service SK, Giacomini KM, et al. (2001) Screening a large reference sample to identify very low frequency sequence variants: comparisons between two genes. Nat Genet 27: 435–438.
28. Lineweber K, Bogedain P, Wolf C, Wagner S, Weber M, et al. (2007) In patients chronically treated with metoprolol, the demand of inotropic catecholamine support after coronary artery bypass grafting is determined by the Arg389Gly-beta 1-adrenoceptor polymorphism. Naunyn Schmiedebergs Arch Pharmacol 375: 303–309.
29. Schultz D, Mikala G, Yatani A, Engle DB, Iles DE, et al. (1993) Cloning, chromosomal localization, and functional expression of the alpha 1 subunit of the L-type voltage-dependent calcium channel from normal human heart. Proc Natl Acad Sci U S A 90: 6228–6232.
30. Schleithoff L, Mehrke G, Reutlinger B, Lehmann-Horn F (1999) Genomic structure and functional expression of a human alpha(2)/delta calcium channel subunit gene (CACNA2D1). Genomics 61: 201–209.
31. Karmazinova M, Lacinova L (2010) Measurement of cellular excitability by whole cell patch clamp technique. Physiol Res 59 Suppl 1: S1–7.
32. Foell JD, Balijepalli RC, Delisle BP, Yunker AM, Robia SL, et al. (2004) Molecular heterogeneity of calcium channel beta-subunits in canine and human heart: evidence for differential subcellular localization. Physiol Genomics 17: 183–200.
33. Feinberg AP (2010) Genome-scale approaches to the epigenetics of common human disease. Virchows Arch 456: 13–21.
34. Mitchell KJ (2011) The genetics of neurodevelopmental disease. Curr Opin Neurobiol 21: 197–203.
35. Geschwind DH (2011) Genetics of autism spectrum disorders. Trends Cogn Sci 15: 409–416.
36. Colecraft HM, Alseikhan B, Takahashi SX, Chaudhuri D, Mittman S, et al. (2002) Novel functional properties of Ca(2+) channel beta subunits revealed by their expression in adult rat heart cells. J Physiol 541: 435–452.
37. Miranda-Laferte E, Schmidt S, Jara AC, Neely A, Hidalgo P (2012) A short polybasic segment between the two conserved domains of the beta2a-subunit modulates the rate of inactivation of R-type calcium channel. J Biol Chem 287: 32588–32597.
38. He LL, Zhang Y, Chen YH, Yamada Y, Yang J (2007) Functional modularity of the beta-subunit of voltage-gated Ca2+ channels. Biophys J 93: 834–845.
39. Barrett CF, Tsien RW (2008) The Timothy syndrome mutation differentially affects voltage- and calcium-dependent inactivation of CaV1.2 L-type calcium channels. Proc Natl Acad Sci U S A 105: 2157–2162.
40. Geschwind DH (2008) Autism: many genes, common pathways? Cell 135: 391–395.

41. Folstein SE, Rosen-Sheidley B (2001) Genetics of autism: complex aetiology for a heterogeneous disorder. Nat Rev Genet 2: 943–955.

42. Leblond CS, Heinrich J, Delorme R, Proepper C, Betancur C, et al. (2012) Genetic and functional analyses of SHANK2 mutations suggest a multiple hit model of autism spectrum disorders. PLoS Genet 8: e1002521.

43. Abrahams BS, Geschwind DH (2008) Advances in autism genetics: on the threshold of a new neurobiology. Nat Rev Genet 9: 341–355.

44. Ben-David E, Shifman S (2012) Networks of neuronal genes affected by common and rare variants in autism spectrum disorders. PLoS Genet 8: e1002556.

45. Skafidas E, Testa R, Zantomio D, Chana G, Everall IP, et al. (Sept 11, 2012) Predicting the diagnosis of autism spectrum disorder using gene pathway analysis. Mol Psychiatry: 10.1038/mp.2012.1126.

46. Bader PL, Faizi M, Kim LH, Owen SF, Tadross MR, et al. (2011) Mouse model of Timothy syndrome recapitulates triad of autistic traits. Proc Natl Acad Sci U S A 108: 15432–15437.

47. Liao P, Soong TW (2010) CaV1.2 channelopathies: from arrhythmias to autism, bipolar disorder, and immunodeficiency. Pflugers Arch 460: 353–359.

Brain Volumetric Correlates of Autism Spectrum Disorder Symptoms in Attention Deficit/Hyperactivity Disorder

Laurence O'Dwyer[1]*, Colby Tanner[2], Eelco V. van Dongen[1], Corina U. Greven[1,3], Janita Bralten[1,4], Marcel P. Zwiers[1], Barbara Franke[4,5], Jaap Oosterlaan[6], Dirk Heslenfeld[6,7], Pieter Hoekstra[8], Catharina A. Hartman[8], Nanda Rommelse[5,9], Jan K. Buitelaar[1,9]

1 Radboud University Medical Center, Donders Institute for Brain, Cognition and Behaviour, Department of Cognitive Neuroscience, Nijmegen, The Netherlands, 2 Department of Ecology and Evolution, University of Lausanne, Lausanne, Switzerland, 3 King's College London, Social, Genetic and Developmental Psychiatry Centre, Institute of Psychiatry, London, United Kingdom, 4 Department of Human Genetics, Radboud University Medical Center, Nijmegen, The Netherlands, 5 Radboud University Medical Center, Donders Institute for Brain, Cognition and Behaviour, Department of Psychiatry, Nijmegen, The Netherlands, 6 Department of Clinical Neuropsychology, Vrije Universiteit, Amsterdam, The Netherlands, 7 Department of Cognitive Psychology, Vrije Universiteit, Amsterdam, The Netherlands, 8 Department of Psychiatry, University Medical Center Groningen, University of Groningen, Groningen, The Netherlands, 9 Karakter Child and Adolescent Psychiatry University Center Nijmegen, Nijmegen, The Netherlands

Abstract

Autism spectrum disorder (ASD) symptoms frequently occur in subjects with attention deficit/hyperactivity disorder (ADHD). While there is evidence that both ADHD and ASD have differential structural correlates, no study to date has investigated these structural correlates within a framework that robustly accounts for the phenotypic overlap between the two disorders. The presence of ASD symptoms was measured by the parent-reported Children's Social and Behavioural Questionnaire (CSBQ) in ADHD subjects (n = 180), their unaffected siblings (n = 118) and healthy controls (n = 146). ADHD symptoms were assessed by a structured interview (K-SADS-PL) and the Conners' ADHD questionnaires. Whole brain T1-weighted MPRAGE images were acquired and the structural MRI correlates of ASD symptom scores were analysed by modelling ASD symptom scores against white matter (WM) and grey matter (GM) volumes using mixed effects models which controlled for ADHD symptom levels. ASD symptoms were significantly elevated in ADHD subjects relative to both controls and unaffected siblings. ASD scores were predicted by the interaction between WM and GM volumes. Increasing ASD score was associated with greater GM volume. Equivocal results from previous structural studies in ADHD and ASD may be due to the fact that comorbidity has not been taken into account in studies to date. The current findings stress the need to account for issues of ASD comorbidity in ADHD.

Editor: Chandan Vaidya, Georgetown University, United States of America

Funding: The NeuroIMAGE study was supported by National Institutes of Health grant R01MH62873 (to Stephen V. Faraone), NWO Large Investment Grant 1750102007010 (to Jan Buitelaar) and matching grants from Radboud University Nijmegen Medical Center, University Medical Center Groningen and Accare, and Vrije Universiteit Amsterdam. The research leading to these results also received support from the European Community's Seventh Framework Programme (FP7/2007–2013) under grant agreement number 278948 (TACTICS), and from the Innovative Medicines Initiative Joint Undertaking (IMI) under grant agreement number 115300-01 (EU-AIMS). CT was supported by a fellowship from the Irish Research Council for Science, Engineering and Technology (IRCSET). The funders had no role in study design, data collection and analysis, decision to publish, or preparation of the manuscript.

Competing Interests: Jan Buitelaar has been a consultant to/member of advisory board of and/or speaker for Janssen Cilag BV, Eli Lilly, Bristol-Myer Squibb, Organon/Shering Plough, UCB, Shire, Medice and Servier. He is not an employee of any of these companies. He is not a stock shareholder of any of these companies. He has no other financial or material support, including expert testimony, patents, royalties. There are no patents, products in development or marketed products to declare. All other authors report no biomedical financial interests or potential conflicts of interest.

* Email: larodwyer@gmail.com

Introduction

Attention-deficit/hyperactivity disorder (ADHD) and autism spectrum disorder (ASD) are both severely impairing, highly heritable neurodevelopmental disorders [1,2]. ASD is characterised by impaired social and communicative skills as well as restricted and repetitive behaviours and interests, whereas ADHD is characterised by severe inattention and/or hyperactivity and impulsivity [3]. Both disorders frequently co-occur with estimates for the presence of ADHD within ASD ranging from 30% to 80%, while the presence of ASD in ADHD is estimated at 20% to 50% [1], [2,4–6]. Deficits in executive function and motor speed have been linked to familial vulnerability for both ASD and ADHD [7–

9]. Studies have also documented an overlap of genetic factors that relate to both ASD and ADHD [4]. Overall, these findings suggest that there are shared etiological pathways for ASD and ADHD which need to be studied in more detail.

Quantitative measures that reflect the severity of ASD and ADHD symptoms may be useful to characterise both disorders in terms of a continuous distribution in which clinical disorders represent extreme variants of typical behaviour [10,11]. Studies investigating the continuous distribution of both disorders as well as their overlap, as opposed to an exclusive focus on a categorical diagnosis, may be a fruitful direction for future research [10]. Such an approach may help to better characterise the heterogeneous nature of these disorders as well as the extent to which they overlap [12]. Previously, ASD symptoms have been found to be different in various groupings of ADHD classes, with the class having the most severe ADHD symptoms also having the most severe ASD symptoms [13]. In typically developing people, recent work has found brain regions that are commonly as well as uniquely correlated with ASD and ADHD symptom severity [14]. GM volume in the left inferior frontal gyrus was found to be correlated with symptom severity in both disorders [14]. Volumetric changes in the left posterior cingulate were found to be specific to ASD, while ADHD symptom severity was found to be specifically correlated with the right parietal lobe, right temporal frontal cortex, bilateral thalamus and left hippocampus/amygdala complex [14]. The study by Geurts et al. indicates that ASD and ADHD form a continuum extending into the general population. However, the conclusions were complicated by the fact that the directions of the brain-behaviour relationships were not consistent for all regions compared to clinical studies [14].

Brain volume abnormalities are important indicators of pathophysiological processes that likely reflect disorder etiology. A number of meta-analyses have found reduced brain volume in ADHD in the majority of studies investigated (with ages ranging from ~10–37 years of age) [15], [16,17]. Regional volume reductions in ADHD subjects were robustly localised to the globus pallidus, putamen, caudate nucleus and lentiform gyrus [15], [16,17]. Total brain volume and grey matter volume have both been found to be decreased in ADHD compared with typically developing controls [15,18] [19,20]. However, both increasing age and stimulant medication were also found to be independently associated with more normal GM volumes.

It is of note that the profile of changes in brain volume in ASD is different from that of ADHD, with findings suggesting that the brain undergoes a period of accelerated growth in the first four years of life before reaching a plateau within a normal range by adolescence, which in turn is followed by volume decline in adulthood relative to typically developing controls [21], [22–27]. Importantly, in young children with autism (2–3 years old) WM enlargement has been shown to be greater than GM enlargement (18% more cerebral and 38% more cerebellar WM) [28]. This WM enlargement in young children was then found to be reversed in 12–16 year old children with autism, with WM volume reduced relative to controls [28]. In older individuals with autism, voxel-based methods have also shown less WM intensity than in age-matched controls [29,30]. However, a more recent meta-analysis has indicated consistent increases in WM volume in the right arcuate fasciculus and left inferior frontooccipital and uncinate fasciculi in adults as well as in children and adolescents with ASD [31].

For GM, several studies in adolescents and adults with ASD have reported a 6–12% increase in GM volume relative to controls [32] [31,33,34]. A meta-analysis indicated a small increase in GM volume in the left middle and inferior frontal gyri in ASD [33]. The same meta-analysis also indicated robust reductions in GM in the amgydala-hippocampus complex and medical parietal regions [33]. Overall, the GM findings were found to be more pronounced in adults, but the only statistically significant difference was a greater GM volume reduction in the precuneus in adult compared with adolescent samples [33]. However it is difficult to disentangle whether these effects are due to developmental processes or are secondary to the effects of living with cognitive differences.

Significant age-related improvements in ASD have been documented in adolescents and adults [35]. This also suggests that a selection bias exists in current studies, with older participants possibly having more severe symptoms and thus more likely to have prominent GM abnormalities.

For ADHD, the ontogenetic onset of smaller brain size is not known, but there is some evidence that smaller brain volumes in ADHD persist to the end of adolescence [18]. However, this phenomenon may attenuate in adulthood, with studies noting normal brain size in adults with ADHD [36]. In summary, the most abnormal volumes in ASD generally occur in early childhood, while the most abnormal volumes in ADHD occur in middle to late childhood [15,37,38].

Therefore, while there is evidence that both ADHD and ASD have specific and differential structural correlates, no study to date has investigated these structural correlates within a framework that robustly accounts for the phenotypic overlap between the two disorders. Only one study to date has directly compared brain volumes in ASD and ADHD [39]. The age of all subjects ranged from 10 to 16 years, and no differences were found between the two disorders in terms of total GM and WM volumes [39]. Additionally, no differences were found between either disorder and typically developing controls [39]. The relatively small size of the cohort (15 ASD subjects, 15 ADHD subjects, 15 controls) may have contributed to the negative findings.

The present study was based on the premise that the extent to which ASD symptoms occur in ADHD may have a pronounced effect on the profile of structural brain volumes in ADHD. Thus, MRI volumetric correlates of ASD symptoms in a large sample of ADHD probands, their unaffected siblings, as well as healthy controls were investigated. Mixed effects models, which controlled for ADHD symptom levels in the random effects structure of the model, were used to assess the relationship between global WM, GM and autism spectrum symptoms. As previous studies have found raised GM volume [32] in adolescent ASD subjects, we hypothesized that this profile would also be present in ADHD subjects with elevated autistic spectrum symptoms.

Methods

Participants

The study was approved by the Radboud University Medical Centre Research Ethics Committee and was in accordance with the Declaration of Helsinki. All participants over 18 years of age provided informed written consent. For participants under 18 years of age, informed written consent was obtained from the next of kin, caretakers, or guardians on behalf of the participants. This procedure was approved by the Radboud University Medical Centre Research Ethics Committee.

Participants were part of the NeuroIMAGE study. This is a prospective longitudinal MRI study (2009–2012) of the Dutch subsample of the International Multicenter ADHD Genetics (IMAGE) study performed between 2003–2006 [40–42]. All members of ADHD and control families were invited for follow-up measurement, with a mean follow-up period of 5.9 years ($SD = .72$). For the present analyses, subjects were selected from the total data set (n = 1084) when the following data was available: a high quality T1-weighted MPRAGE image, complete information from the Children's Social and Behavioural Questionnaire (that provides information on the autism spectrum symptoms), complete information from the Schedule for Affective Disorders and Schizophrenia for School-Age Children - Present and Lifetime Version (K-SADS-PL) [43] and the Conners ADHD questionnaire. IQ information and medication history were also required in order to include subjects in the current study. Subjects with a sub-threshold ADHD diagnosis (n = 75), i.e. those with significantly elevated ADHD symptoms but failed to meet the clinical criteria for a diagnosis of ADHD were excluded. Subjects were also excluded if there was inconsistency between the ADHD

Table 1. Demographic and cognitive characteristics of the sample groups.

	ADHD		Unaffected Siblings		Con		AVOVA's	P	Tukey HSD		
	Mean	SD	Mean	SD	Mean	SD			US - Con	ADHD - Con	ADHD - US
Age (years)	16.2	3.7	16.9	4.0	16.8	3.6	F(2,441) = 1.41	0.25			
IQ	98.8	14.9	101.8	14.2	106.6	13.2	F(2,441) = 12.11	<0.0001	0.017	<0.0001	0.19
Social Interest (0–24)	4.3	4.3	1.9	3.4	1.0	1.9	F(2,441) = 40.42	<0.0001	0.12	<0.0001	<0.0001
Understanding (0–14)	5.5	3.7	1.2	1.5	1.2	1.8	F(2,441) = 140.1	<0.0001	0.99	<0.0001	<0.0001
Stereotyped (0–16)	2.1	2.4	0.4	1.0	0.4	1.0	F(2,441) = 50.3	<0.0001	0.99	<0.0001	<0.0001
Resistance to Change (0–6)	1.4	1.7	0.4	0.9	0.4	0.8	F(2,441) = 33.73	<0.0001	0.96	<0.0001	<0.0001
ASD-total (0–60)	13.3	8.9	3.9	5.0	3.0	4.3	F(2,441) = 118	<0.0001	0.54	<0.0001	<0.0001
ADHD-total	13.3	2.9	1.0	1.5	0.4	0.9	F(2,441) = 2008	<0.0001	0.089	<0.0001	<0.0001
Handedness (r/l/a)	152/24/3		101/17/0		126/19/1						

Values are mean ± standard deviation. Significance was set at p<0.05. All p-values refer to ANOVAs, except for gender where the p-value refers to a chi-square test. Where ANOVA's returned a significant result, post-hoc Tukey Honest Significant Difference (Tukey HSD) tests were performed. US - Con, refers to a pairwise comparison between unaffected siblings and controls. ADHD-Con, refers to a pairwise comparison between ADHD and controls. ADHD - US, refers to a pairwise comparison between ADHD and unaffected siblings. Four subscales of the Children's Social and Behavioural Questionnaire (CSBQ) which probe ASD spectrum symptoms are shown in this table: Social Interest, Social Understanding (Understanding), Stereotypy and Resistance to Change. ASD-total is calculated as a sum of these four subscales. ADHD-total scores are calculated according to the algorithm described in detail in the supplementary information (Questionnaire Items S1).
Abbreviations: Gender (m/f), Gender (male/female); Handedness (r/l/a), Handedness (right, left, ambidextrous).

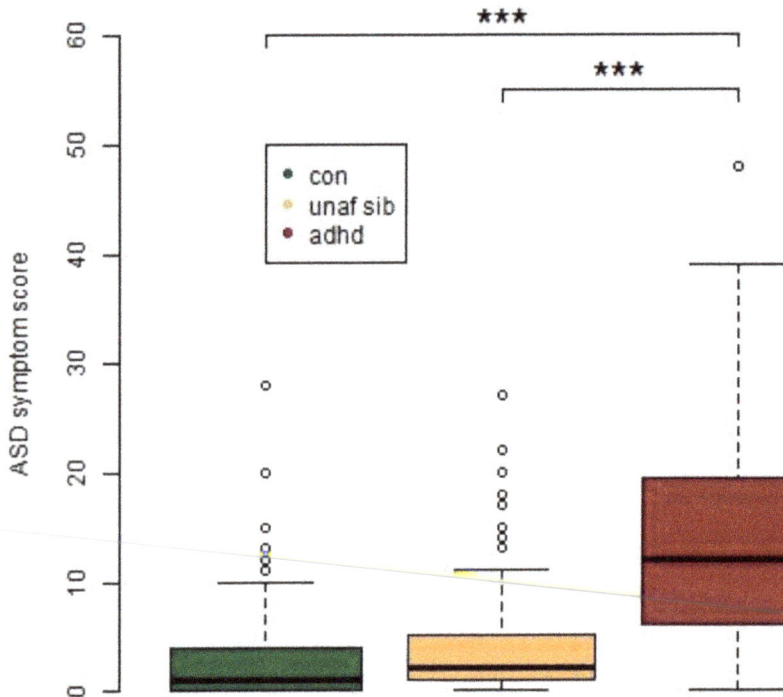

Figure 1. ASD symptoms in healthy controls, unaffected siblings and ADHD. ADHD subjects were found to have significantly higher scores relative to both unaffected siblings and healthy controls. ***$p<0.001$, with post-hoc Tukey test, following an ANOVA. ASD symptom score refers to an aggregate score from the four Children's Social and Behavioural Questionnaire (CSBQ) subscales, (1) social interest, (2) social understanding, (3) stereotypy and (4) resistance to change. Abbreviations: con, Control; unaf sib, Unaffected Siblings, adhd, Attention Deficit Hyperactivity Disorder.

Table 2. Final, generalised mixed-effect model showing fixed effects for ASD score modelled against white matter residual and grey matter volumes.

Fixed Effects	Estimate	Standard Error	t-value	p-value
WM resid	−0.485	0.206	−2.354	0.019
GM	0.013	0.013	0.994	0.321
Unaff. Sib.	−0.538	3.652	−0.147	0.883
ADHD	21.056	3.815	5.519	0.000
Age	0.071	0.177	0.398	0.691
Male	1.847	0.674	2.740	0.006
WM resid×GM	0.001	0.000	2.199	0.028
Unaff. Sib×Age	0.059	0.211	0.279	0.781
ADHD×Age	−0.675	0.207	−3.264	0.001

Formula:
$ASD\ symptoms \sim WM\ resid * GM + Diagnosis * Age + Gender +$
$\qquad (1|Total\ ADHD\ symptoms) +$
$\qquad (1|Family) +$
$\qquad (1|IQ) +$
$\qquad (1|ADHD\ medication) +$
$\qquad (1|Scanner\ type)$

"~" means modelled against, and "(1| factor)" means that a factor is included as a random effect.
A generalised mixed-effect model is run using normalised volumes of grey and white matter as explanatory variables together with age as a random effect. ASD score is set as the response variable. The final model is derived following an iterative model selection procedure that involves comparing successive models using Akaike's Information Criterion (see Methods for detailed description of model selection procedure). ASD score refers to an aggregate score from the four Children's Social and Behavioural Questionnaire (CSBQ) subscales, (1) social interest, (2) social understanding, (3) stereotypy and (4) resistance to change.
Abbreviations: WM, normalised WM volume; GM, normalised GM volume; US, unaffected siblings; WM:GM, WM by GM interaction; US: Age, unaffected sibling by Age interaction; ADHD:Age, ADHD by Age interaction.

Table 3. Final, generalised mixed-effect model showing random effects for ASD score modelled against white matter residual and grey matter volumes.

Random Effects	Variance	S.D.
Family Relatedness	8.765	2.961
IQ	1.098	1.048
Total ADHD Score	5.474	2.340
ADHD medication	0.000	0.000
Scanner Type	0.000	0.000

Formula:

$$ASD\ symptoms \sim WM\ resid * GM + Diagnosis * Age + Gender +$$
$$(1|Total\ ADHD\ symptoms) +$$
$$(1|Family) +$$
$$(1|IQ) +$$
$$(1|ADHD\ medication) +$$
$$(1|Scanner\ type)$$

"∼" means modelled against, and "(1| factor)" means that a factor is included as a random effect.

A generalised mixed-effect model is run using normalised volumes of grey and white matter as explanatory variables together with age as a random effect. ASD score is set as the response variable. The final model is derived following an iterative model selection procedure that involves comparing successive models using Akaike's Information Criterion (see Methods for detailed description of model selection procedure). ASD score refers to an aggregate score from the four Children's Social and Behavioural Questionnaire (CSBQ) subscales, (1) social interest, (2) social understanding, (3) stereotypy and (4) resistance to change.

Abbreviations: WM, normalised WM volume; GM, normalised GM volume; US, unaffected siblings; WM:GM, WM by GM interaction; US: Age, unaffected sibling by Age interaction; ADHD:Age, ADHD by Age interaction.

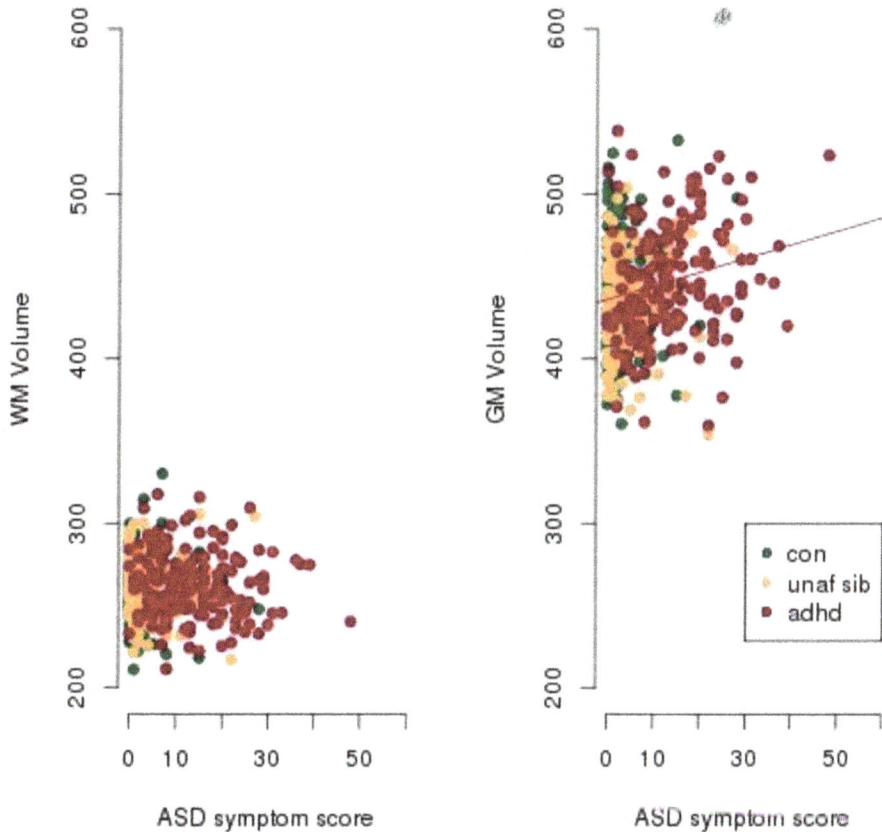

Figure 2. ASD scores are significantly positively correlated with total grey matter volume. The volumes of grey and white matter are normalised for total intracranial volume. A regression line is plotted where the Pearson's product-moment correlation is significant with p<0.05. ASD symptom score refers to an aggregate score from the four Children's Social and Behavioural Questionnaire (CSBQ) subscales, (1) social interest, (2) social understanding, (3) stereotypy and (4) resistance to change. Abbreviations: con, Control; unaf sib, Unaffected Siblings, adhd, Attention Deficit Hyperactivity Disorder; ASD, autism spectrum disorder.

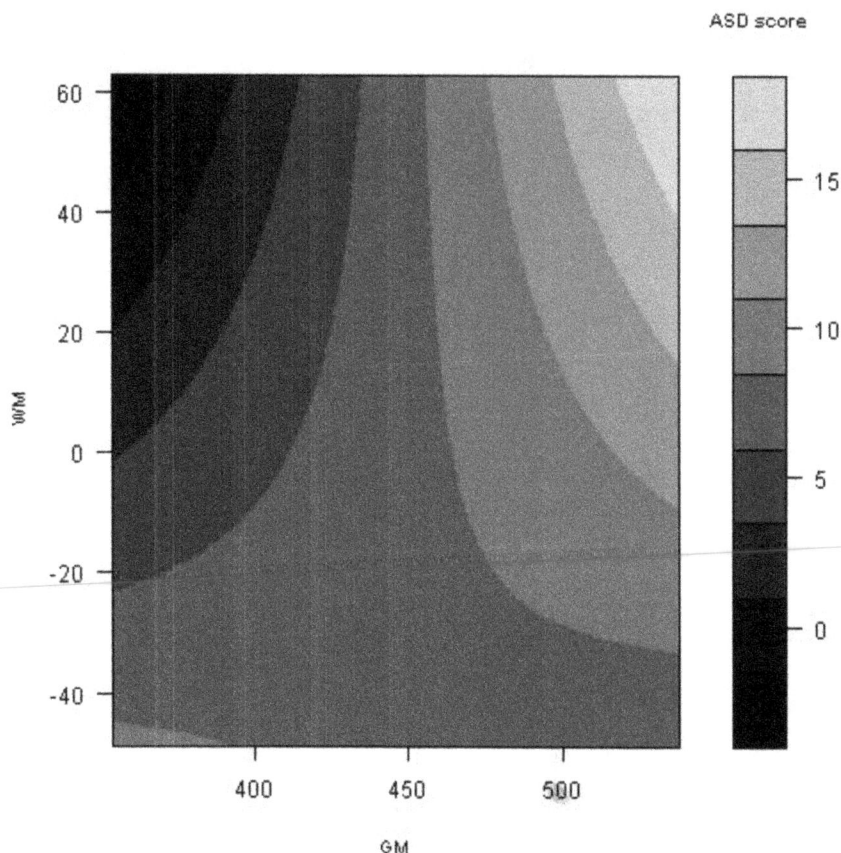

Figure 3. ASD score contour graph for the interaction between WM, GM and ASD scores. The best mixed effects model was converted into a function in R which allowed ASD scores to be extrapolated for a range of GM and WM volumes (see Methods for full description). The best mixed effects model included GM and WM residual terms (see Methods). Volumes are normalised for total intracranial volume. ASD score refers to an aggregate score from the four Children's Social and Behavioural Questionnaire (CSBQ) subscales, (1) social interest, (2) social understanding, (3) stereotypy and (4) resistance to change.

diagnosis derived from the different questionnaires employed (n = 53). The resulting data set was then age- and gender-matched; so that the current study included 90 male and 90 female ADHD subjects, 62 male and 62 female unaffected siblings of ADHD subjects and 70 male and 70 female healthy control children. The age range of participants was 7.4 to 28.5 years. All participants were of European Caucasian descent and had an IQ≥70. Demographic characteristics of each subject group are provided in Table 1. Subjects who were taking ADHD medication stopped medication (both stimulant and non-stimulant) for 48 hours prior to scanning. Regarding medication history, 71 ADHD subjects (39%) were not currently taking ADHD medication, 93 ADHD subjects (52%) were taking one ADHD medication, and 16 ADHD subjects (9%) were currently taking two ADHD medications. A complete overview of medication is provided in Table S1.

ADHD diagnosis and symptom measures

All participants were assessed using a semi-structured diagnostic interview (Dutch translation of the Schedule for Affective Disorders and Schizophrenia for School-Age Children - Present and Lifetime Version (K-SADS-PL) [43] and Conners' ADHD questionnaire to determine ADHD diagnoses. Each child was assessed with a parent-rated questionnaire (Conners' Parent Rating Scale – Revised: Long version (CPRS-R:L) combined with either a teacher-rating (Conners' Teacher Rating Scale –

Revised: Long version (CTRS-R:L) applied for children <18 years or a self-report Conners' Adult ADHD Rating Scales – Self-Report: Long version (CAARS-S:L) applied for children ≥18 years. A diagnostic algorithm was applied to combine symptom counts on the K-SADS-PL and Conners' questionnaires. A detailed description of the diagnostic algorithm is provided in the supplementary information (Diagnostic Algorithm S1). This algorithm was used to diagnose subjects and also to provide a continuous score for an overall level of ADHD symptoms that combines both inattentive and hyperactive symptoms. While ASD symptoms were present in the cohort and were significantly elevated in the ADHD group (see Results), a clinical diagnosis of autism or Asperger's syndrome had been an exclusion criterion in the original IMAGE study.

ASD measures

The Children's Social and Behavioural Questionnaire (CSBQ) [44] was used in the current study as it can measure the continuous distribution of autistic symptoms in the general population as well as in clinical groups outside of autism, including ADHD [44,45]. Most instruments for ASD are designed to assess clinical cases and are not suitable for assessing milder ASD symptoms. The CSBQ was originally developed because existing instruments did not capture more subtle social problems found in the milder end of the autism spectrum [44]. The CSBQ has previously been shown to be valuable in measuring subthreshold autistic symptoms [44–49,40]. In the current study, where clinical ASD was an exclusion criterion, but where milder autistic symptoms are expected to be elevated in the ADHD group [2,4–6,50], the CSBQ is ideally suited for the purpose of the study.

The CSBQ contains 49 items on a 3-point Likert scale. It contains items that refer directly to the DSM-IV criteria for autism, but it also captures more subtle symptoms of ASD. Therefore, it is suitable for measuring behavioural problems as seen in children with milder variants of ASD. CSBQ items are grouped into the following six subscales: (1) tuned, (2) social interest, (3) orientation, (4) social understanding, (5) resistance to change, and (6) stereotypy. It was administered in the parent-report form.

All items contained within each subscale are found in the supplemental information (Questionnaire Items S1). The CSBQ has good internal, test-retest, and inter-rater reliability, and demonstrated convergent and divergent validity [44]. The CSBQ appears to differentiate between autism and pervasive developmental disorders - not otherwise specified (PDD-NOS), and can also differentiate between PDD-NOS and ADHD [44,51]. Additionally, to assess the content validity of the CSBQ, it has previously been compared to an autism screening instrument, the Autism Behavior Checklist (ABC) [52]. A strong correlation of 0.75 was found between the total scores of both questionnaires in a large Dutch population sample [45]. The CSBQ has also been compared with the Autism Diagnostic Interview-Revised (ADI-R), Autism Diagnostic Observation Schedule (ADOS), and clinical

classification in children with mild and moderate intellectual disability [53]. In that study, the contribution of the CSBQ to a classification of ASD was most specific for the "social" and "stereotypy" subscales, with high coherence with all three classification methods [53].

An aggregate score from the four subscales, (1) social interest, (2) social understanding, (3) stereotypy and (4) resistance to change, was used in the current study to capture the core symptoms of ASD. This aggregate score has been successfully used to selectively probe ASD symptoms in previous studies [47,54]. The remaining two CSBQ subscales (tuned and orientation) probe dysfunctional social behaviours which, although characteristic for ASD, are also related to the ADHD dimensions of hyperactivity/impulsivity and attention problems, respectively [44], and were not considered in the current study for this reason.

High Resolution T1W Structural Image Acquisition and Processing

Whole brain T1 weighted MPRAGE images were acquired at 1.5T using a product 8 channel phased array headcoil on a Siemens Sonata scanner at the Free University in Amsterdam and a 1.5T Siemens Avanto MR scanner at the Donders Institute for Brain, Cognition and Behaviour in Nijmegen. A breakdown of the distribution of subjects scanned at the two sites is included in Table S2. TI/TE/TR = 1000/2.95/2730 ms, imaging matrix 256×256, 176 slices, voxel size 1×1×1 mm^3, GRAPPA acceleration 2. Brain tissue probability maps for white matter (WM), grey matter (GM) and cerebrospinal fluid (CSF) were estimated using the unified

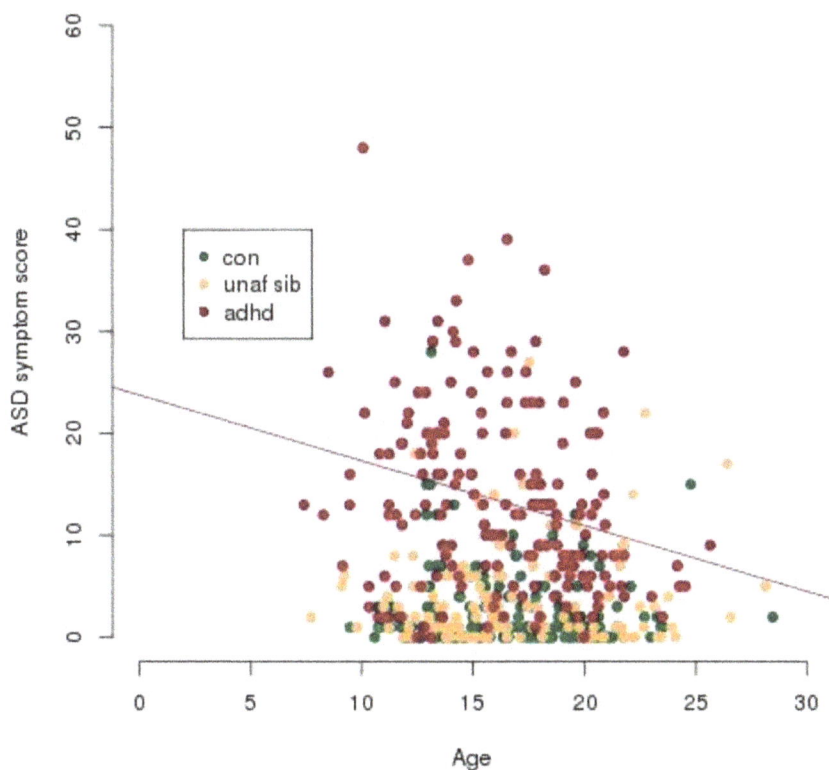

Figure 4. ASD scores decrease significantly with age within the ADHD groups. A regression line is plotted where the Pearson's product-moment correlation is significant with p<0.05. ASD score refers to an aggregate score from the four Children's Social and Behavioural Questionnaire (CSBQ) subscales, (1) social interest, (2) social understanding, (3) stereotypy and (4) resistance to change. Abbreviations: con, Control; unaf sib, Unaffected Siblings, ADHD, Attention-deficit/hyperactivity disorder; ASD, autism spectrum disorder.

segmentation algorithm as implemented in the VBM8 toolbox of SPM8 [55]. Total GM, WM and CSF volumes were computed by voxelwise summation of their probability maps. Total intracranial volume (ICV) was then computed as the sum of WM, GM and CSF volume.

The following formula was used to compute normalised volumes of global GM and WM:

total volume of GM (mm^3)/ICV (mm^3)×1000.
total volume of WM (mm^3)/ICV (mm^3)×1000.

Statistics

As ASD scores are influenced by a range of factors, mixed-effects models allow us to consider factors that potentially contribute to the understanding of the data (i.e. fixed factors), while controlling for additional factors associated with the subjects (i.e. random factors).

R statistical software (Version 2.15.1) [56], including the lme4 package [57] was used for all statistical analyses. In the current study, the "glmer" function [57] was used to fit a generalised mixed-effects model using maximum likelihood (ML). As our objective was to determine the extent to which the ASD score is influenced by the diagnosis group (i.e. control, unaffected sibling or ADHD), GM and WM, these three factors were set as fixed effects. Age was also set as a fixed factor. The total ADHD symptom score was set as a random effect, in order to control for differences in ADHD symptoms between participants, thus allowing us to focus specifically on the ASD score. IQ, ADHD medication, scanner type and family relatedness were also set as random effects. The response variable was set as ASD score, calculated as an aggregate of the four CSBQ subscales ('social interest', 'social understanding', 'stereotypy' and 'resistance to change') that probe ASD.

Models were created using normalised WM and GM volumes. Including both WM and GM variables allowed us to determine not only the extent to which GM and WM drive changes in ASD scores, but also the nature of the interactions between the explanatory variables. WM and GM volumes were co-linear (i.e. correlated with each other) and the models developed took this into account by orthogonalizing these regressors relative to each other to isolate the unique contribution of each explanatory variable independent from what is shared between them. A WM residual term was derived from the regression residuals when WM was regressed against GM. This enabled us to use GM together with a WM residual term (WM resid) in our mixed effect model. A model using WM together with a GM residual term (GM resid) was also created. Un-biased analyses and comparisons could then be carried out based on the models.

The models were fitted by maximum likelihood estimation. The starting model using GM resid and WM terms was:

ASD score ∼ GM resid * WM * Diagnosis * Age * Gender +
(1|ADHD symptoms) +
(1|Scanner type) +
(1|IQ) +
(1|Family relatedness) +
(1|ADHD medication)

where "∼" means "modelled against"; "(1| factor)" means that factor is included as a random effect, and "Diagnosis" refers to the

three diagnostic groups, i.e. control, unaffected siblings and ADHD. "*" means interacting with, and the model assesses interactions among all terms, up to a 5-way interaction among all fixed effects.

The starting model using GM and WM resid terms was:

ASD score ∼ WM resid * GM * Diagnosis * Age * Gender +
(1|ADHD symptoms) +
(1|Scanner type) +
(1|IQ) +
(1|Family relatedness) +
(1|ADHD medication)

We fit the full models as described above and then removed least significant terms in an iterative process, checking for improved fit according to Akaike's Information Criterion (AIC) [58,59] until a final model was obtained [60]. We have previously employed the AIC tool for successful model selection in an MRI and structural volume framework [61]. The models are thus primarily assessing the influence of GM and WM on the ASD scores across all healthy young controls, ADHD subjects and unaffected siblings (Sib) of ADHD subjects.

To determine if the model using GM resid or the WM resid term was a better predictor of ASD symptoms, the fits of the two final models was compared using the "anova" function in R [60].

Contour Plots

The significant interaction between GM and WM was visualized by means of a contour plot. Normalised WM and GM volumes were used for creating this contour plot. ASD scores were modelled as follows: model = lm (ASD score∼GM*WM resid); where "∼" means modelled against, "*" means interacting with, and, "lm" is used to fit a linear model in R. A matrix was created for the WM and GM volumes, and the function was run from the minimum to the maximum GM value within the matrix, and also from the minimum to the maximum WM value within the matrix. The contour plot enabled changes in ASD scores to be visualised by means of a colour key with darker colours representing lower ASD symptoms and lighter colours representing higher ASD symptoms.

Results

Demographic and Cognitive Characteristics

The demographic characteristics of the cohort are shown in Table 1. ASD scores were significantly different between groups [F(2,441) = 118, p<0.0001], with ADHD subjects having significantly raised scores relative to both controls (p<0.0001) and unaffected siblings (p<0.0001), while there was no significant difference between controls and unaffected siblings (Fig. 1; Table 1). ASD scores were found to be significantly positively correlated with ADHD scores in control group (p = 0.046, r = 0.165; Table S3) and in the ADHD group (p = 0.254, r = 0.001; Table S3).

Mixed-effects models for ASD symptoms modelled against global grey matter and white matter volumes

Following model simplification based on AIC, the optimal model for ASD symptoms is shown in Table 2 and Table 3. This model used the WM residual term together with GM (WM resid:GM model) and was found to have a lower AIC value than the alternative model that used the GM residual term together with the WM (GM resid:WM model). The alternative model is also shown in Table S4.

For the fixed effects of the WM resid:GM model, the following terms were significant: WM resid ($p = 0.019$); ADHD diagnosis ($p<0.0001$); male gender ($p = 0.006$); WM resid×GM interaction ($p = 0.028$); ADHD diagnosis×age ($p = 0.001$).

As the range of ASD scores in control and unaffected siblings is limited, a mixed effect model was also developed based on the inclusion of participants with an ASD score of 20 or higher. This model also returned a significant WM resid×GM interaction ($p = 0.0029$; Table S5).

The significant interaction between WM and GM was further visualised with a scatter plot (Fig. 2) and a contour plot (Fig. 3). A significant positive correlation was found between GM volume and ASD scores for the ADHD group ($p = 0.00025$, $r = 0.17$) (Fig. 2). No other significant correlation was found between GM volume and ASD score for control or unaffected siblings. There was also no significant correlation between WM volume and ASD score for any of the groups examined. The best mixed effects model (Table 2 and Table 3) was used to create a contour plot, which further described the interaction between GM and WM. The contour plot developed from the mixed effects model indicates that the lowest ASD scores were found in areas of low GM coupled with high WM (Fig. 3). Increasing ASD score was accompanied by greater GM volume and lower WM volume up to an ASD score on the CSBQ of ~10. For ASD scores greater than ~10, the volumetric profile indicated both raised GM and WM volume (Fig. 3).

As there was a significant interaction found between the ADHD diagnosis and age, this interaction was also visualised with a scatter plot (Fig. 4). ADHD subjects were found to have a significant negative correlation between age and ASD scores ($p<0.0005$; $r = -0.26$) while there was no correlation between age and ASD scores for unaffected siblings or controls (Fig. 4).

Total Intracranial Volume in Low and High ASD Conditions

Total intracranial volume was plotted for Control, Unaffected Sibling, ADHD with low ASD and ADHD with high ASD scores (Fig. 5). Low ASD score was defined as 20 or lower as per the CSBQ ASD score. A high ASD score was defined as greater than 20. ADHD participants with low ASD scores were found to have significantly lower total intracranial volumes than control subjects ($p<0.05$). No other significant differences were found.

Discussion

In the current study, ASD symptoms as measured by the CSBQ [44] were found to be significantly elevated in ADHD subjects relative to both controls and unaffected siblings. These findings agree with previous studies that have found elevated levels of ASD symptoms in ADHD subjects [13,62]. There was a non-significant increase in the ASD scores for unaffected siblings relative to controls, which is in line with studies showing moderate increases in ASD symptoms in unaffected siblings of ADHD subjects [40], [63]. For ADHD subjects, the co-morbid ASD symptoms were found to decrease significantly with age.

Structural MRI was used to investigate whether or not raised ASD symptoms would be accompanied by a distinct anatomical profile. When ASD scores were modelled against WM and GM volumes using mixed-effects models that controlled for ADHD symptom levels, a significant WM by GM interaction was found. Investigation of the interaction between WM, GM and ASD

scores by means of a contour graph highlighted a specific volumetric landscape with the lowest ASD scores found in areas of low GM coupled with high WM. Increasing ASD scores were accompanied by greater GM volumes and lower WM volumes. While the GM profile constantly increased with greater ASD scores, WM was found to decrease with greater ASD scores but for the highest ASD scores WM volumes were also elevated.

The profile of increased GM volume in subjects with raised ASD symptoms is in line with previous studies that have found GM volume to be significantly increased in adolescent ASD subjects [32]. Globally, decreased brain size has been the predominant finding in ADHD [15,18], while ASD is generally associated with brain overgrowth during infancy followed by a return to normal total brain size in adolescence and possible continued degeneration into middle age [64] [22–27]. Similarly, although the majority of studies have found total brain volume to be reduced in ADHD, some studies have reported no significant differences in total brain volume between ADHD subjects and typically developing controls [36,65–68]. These discrepancies may be partly accounted for by the extent to which ASD symptoms are present in the ADHD sample. The findings in the current paper that ADHD with low ASD score had significantly reduced total intracranial volume compared with control, whereas ADHD with high ASD score showed no significant difference with control, further emphasize the role that ASD symptoms may play in influencing the landscape of brain volumetrics in ADHD subjects.

Meta-analyses suggest that increasing age and medication treatment contribute to a degree of normalisation in brain volumes in ADHD [16,17]. The current findings add to these studies by indicating that ASD comorbidity may be an additional factor that plays an important role in influencing brain volume in ADHD. Decreased GM volume may be more pronounced when ASD symptoms are absent or present only to a minor degree, as was the case in the current study. Conversely, the current findings indicate that elevated ASD symptoms are accompanied by raised GM volume. The WM profile was more complex, with lower volumes found as ASD scores increase, but higher volumes found for the most extreme ASD scores. Previous studies have shown reduced WM volume in adolescent and adult ASD subjects [28], [29,30], while greater WM enlargement has been found in children with ASD [28]. A mixed effects model assessment, based on the same statistical framework as the main analysis, but including only participants with an ASD score of 20 or higher also revealed a significant GM by WM interaction. This supplementary analysis indicates that those with elevated ASD scores in the current cohort have a global volumetric profile similar to that found in ASD studies.

The volumetric landscape for different ASD scores described by the contour plot is not restricted to ADHD subjects but is also applicable to unaffected siblings and healthy controls. No significant interaction between GM, WM and ADHD was found, nor were there significant interactions between GM, WM and unaffected siblings, or between GM, WM and controls.

As ASD scores remained low in both controls and unaffected siblings, their volumetric profiles were constrained to a conjunction of low GM coupled with high WM volume. Conversely, ASD scores for ADHD subjects were more heterogeneous, with a significantly higher mean, as well as greater variance and range. Therefore, ADHD subjects exhibited a wide range of volumetric profiles that were dependent on their ASD spectrum scores.

There was a significant age-related improvement in ASD symptoms in ADHD subjects which is in agreement with previous cross-sectional and longitudinal studies that have also found age-related improvement in ASD [69,70] [71]. Neither WM nor GM volume was found to influence this age-related reduction of ASD

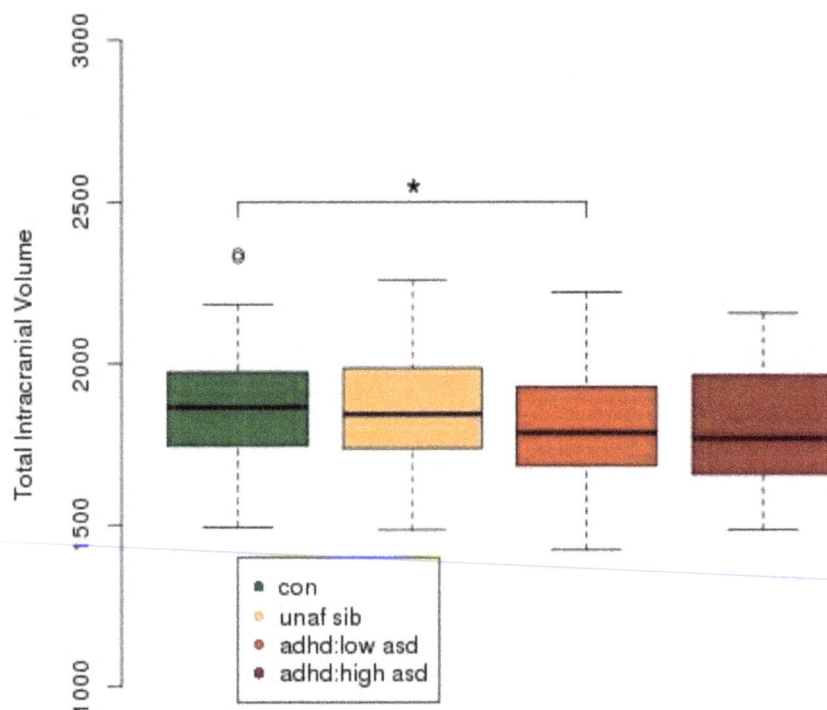

Figure 5. ADHD subjects with low ASD scores have significantly lower total intracranial volume than control subjects (p<0.05). ADHD: low ASD is defined as a participant with ADHD and an ASD score of 20 or less. ADHD: high ASD is defined as a participant with ADHD and an ASD score greater than 20.

symptoms in ADHD subjects. Therefore, the neural correlates of this finding remain unknown. Analyses of regional brain volume changes, as well as changes in WM indices of diffusion will be undertaken in a future study and may be able to shed light on this point. One possibility is that while total WM or GM volume may not have an influence on age-related changes in ASD symptoms, subtle regional changes in GM and WM structure changes may lie hidden beneath the global analysis. Structural and functional MRI studies have consistently found the caudate nucleus to be altered in ASD and to be associated with dysfunctions in multiple domains related to ASD, such as repetitive and stereotyped behaviour [72], reward processing [73–75] and executive function [73]. Caudate damage has also been related to reduced cognitive flexibility and perseverative behaviour in a range of species, including monkeys [76], birds [77], rats [78] and cats [79]. Clearly, developmental changes play a crucial role in influencing the trajectories of both disorders. Significant age-related improvements have been noted in restricted and repetitive behaviours [80] and also in overall ASD symptom counts [81]. The significant reduction of ASD scores may be related to a reduction of local short-range circuitry together with a strengthening of long-range connectivity that is seen in adolescent brain development [82]. Normal development is associated with marked changes in WM tracts, with myelination increasing throughout childhood and adolescence [83]. Increasing myelination of fronto-striatal connections during adolescence and early adulthood facilitates top-down executive control of behaviour [84]. Indices of WM integrity such as fractional anisotropy have been found to normalise in ADHD subjects as they progress to adolescence and adulthood [85]. Thus, the apparent improvements in autism symptoms with age as seen in the current study may be associated with improvements in WM integrity. Social

adaptation may contribute to a reduction of ASD symptoms with age. Initial studies have also indicated that cognitive behavioural therapy (CBT), when adapted to the special needs of patients with ASD, can offer an effective treatment modality [86], [87,88]. Although there are no pharmacological treatments that specifically target the deficits of ASD, some studies have noted improvement in behavioural symptoms with risperidone [89], while reductions in repetitive behaviours have been found following treatment with oxytocin [90]. Within the current cohort, individuals with low IQ (<70) were excluded, thus an IQ within a normal range may also facilitate compensation or adaptive mechanisms that help ADHD individuals to reduce the overt expression of ASD symptoms.

The current study should be viewed in the context of some limitations. The results are cross-sectional. Future longitudinal studies of MRI-measured developmental trajectories are needed for assessing the impact of age on developing brain structures. The results are also based on global volumetric changes and do not identify specific regional increases or decreases in WM or GM volume. Studies are underway which will assess the current data set in terms of specific regional WM and GM volumetric differences that occur with elevated ASD symptoms. The fact that clinical ASD cases were not included in the cohort is an additional limitation of the study. While the ASD score derived from the aggregate of four sub-scales of the CSBQ questionnaire (social interest, social understanding, stereotypy and resistance to change) has been successfully used to probe ASD symptoms in the past [47,54], caution is needed when interpreting this score as not all social deficits present in ADHD overlap with ASD symptoms [91]. The fact that participants were of European (Caucasian) descent is another limitation, and indicates that results may not be readily generalisable to other communities or ethnicities.

Overall, the current results highlight a specific volumetric profile that is associated with elevated ASD symptoms. This is the first study in a large cohort that robustly accounts for the phenotypic overlap between the ADHD and ASD. Equivocal findings in previous volumetric studies of ADHD and ASD may be due to the fact that issues of comorbidity have generally been ignored in studies to date. Assessing the range of volumetric profiles associated with ADHD coupled with mild ASD symptoms, through to ADHD coupled with severe ASD symptoms, will help to develop a more nuanced understanding of the pathophysiology associated with the continuous distribution and overlap of these two disorders.

Supporting Information

Table S1 Medication Information.

Table S2 Distribution of Scanning over Two Sites.

Table S3 Correlation between ASD score and ADHD symptom levels.

Table S4 Final, generalised mixed-effect model for ASD score modelled against Grey Matter Residual and White Matter Volumes.

Table S5 Final, generalised mixed-effect model for ASD score modelled against Grey Matter and White Matter Volumes using only participants with an ASD score of 20 or higher.

Diagnostic Algorithm S1 Diagnostic algorithm for ADHD in the NeuroIMAGE sample.

Questionnaire Items S1 Children's Social and Behavioural Questionnaire (CSBQ) Summary.

Author Contributions

Conceived and designed the experiments: LOD EVD JKB. Performed the experiments: LOD. Analyzed the data: LOD CT MPZ. Contributed reagents/materials/analysis tools: JKB CT MPZ. Wrote the paper: LOD. Edited the manuscript and contributed conceptual improvements: CUG JB MPZ BF JO DH PH CAH NR JKB.

References

1. Rommelse NNJ, Franke B, Geurts HM, Hartman CA, Buitelaar JK (2010) Shared heritability of attention-deficit/hyperactivity disorder and autism spectrum disorder. Eur Child Adolesc Psychiatry 19: 281–295. doi:10.1007/s00787-010-0092-x.
2. Ronald A, Simonoff E, Kuntsi J, Asherson P, Plomin R (2008) Evidence for overlapping genetic influences on autistic and ADHD behaviours in a community twin sample. J Child Psychol Psychiatry 49: 535–542. doi:10.1111/j.1469-7610.2007.01857.x.
3. Association AP (2000) Diagnostic and Statistical Manual of Mental Disorders, Fourth Edition: DSM-IV-TR. American Psychiatric Pub. 996 p.
4. Ames CS, White SJ (2011) Are ADHD traits dissociable from the autistic profile? Links between cognition and behaviour. J Autism Dev Disord 41: 357–363. doi:10.1007/s10803-010-1049-0.
5. Leyfer OT, Folstein SE, Bacalman S, Davis NO, Dinh E, et al. (2006) Comorbid psychiatric disorders in children with autism: interview development and rates of disorders. J Autism Dev Disord 36: 849–861. doi:10.1007/s10803-006-0123-0.
6. Van Steijn DJ, Richards JS, Oerlemans AM, de Ruiter SW, van Aken MAG, et al. (2012) The co-occurrence of autism spectrum disorder and attention-deficit/hyperactivity disorder symptoms in parents of children with ASD or ASD with ADHD. J Child Psychol Psychiatry 53: 954–963. doi:10.1111/j.1469-7610.2012.02556.x.
7. Corbett BA, Constantine LJ, Hendren R, Rocke D, Ozonoff S (2009) Examining executive functioning in children with autism spectrum disorder, attention deficit hyperactivity disorder and typical development. Psychiatry Res 166: 210–222. doi:10.1016/j.psychres.2008.02.005.
8. Fine JG, Semrud-Clikeman M, Butcher B, Walkowiak J (2008) Brief report: attention effect on a measure of social perception. J Autism Dev Disord 38: 1797–1802. doi:10.1007/s10803-008-0570-x.
9. Booth R, Happé F (2010) "Hunting with a knife and … fork": examining central coherence in autism, attention deficit/hyperactivity disorder, and typical development with a linguistic task. J Exp Child Psychol 107: 377–393. doi:10.1016/j.jecp.2010.06.003.
10. Chabernaud C, Mennes M, Kelly C, Nooner K, Di Martino A, et al. (2012) Dimensional brain-behavior relationships in children with attention-deficit/hyperactivity disorder. Biol Psychiatry 71: 434–442. doi:10.1016/j.biopsych.2011.08.013.
11. Shaw P, Gilliam M, Liverpool M, Weddle C, Malek M, et al. (2011) Cortical development in typically developing children with symptoms of hyperactivity and impulsivity: support for a dimensional view of attention deficit hyperactivity disorder. Am J Psychiatry 168: 143–151. doi:10.1176/appi.ajp.2010.10030385.
12. Castellanos FX, Tannock R (2002) Neuroscience of attention-deficit/hyperactivity disorder: the search for endophenotypes. Nat Rev Neurosci 3: 617–628. doi:10.1038/nrn896.
13. Reiersen AM, Constantino JN, Volk IIE, Todd RD (2007) Autistic traits in a population-based ADHD twin sample. J Child Psychol Psychiatry 48: 464–472. doi:10.1111/j.1469-7610.2006.01720.x.
14. Geurts HM, Ridderinkhof KR, Scholte HS (2013) The relationship between grey-matter and ASD and ADHD traits in typical adults. J Autism Dev Disord 43: 1630–1641. doi:10.1007/s10803-012-1708-4.
15. Valera EM, Faraone SV, Murray KE, Seidman LJ (2007) Meta-analysis of structural imaging findings in attention-deficit/hyperactivity disorder. Biol Psychiatry 61: 1361–1369. doi:10.1016/j.biopsych.2006.06.011.
16. Frodl T, Skokauskas N (2012) Meta-analysis of structural MRI studies in children and adults with attention deficit hyperactivity disorder indicates treatment effects. Acta Psychiatr Scand 125: 114–126. doi:10.1111/j.1600-0447.2011.01786.x.
17. Nakao T, Radua J, Rubia K, Mataix-Cols D (2011) Gray matter volume abnormalities in ADHD: voxel-based meta-analysis exploring the effects of age and stimulant medication. Am J Psychiatry 168: 1154–1163. doi:10.1176/appi.ajp.2011.11020281.
18. Seidman LJ, Biederman J, Liang L, Valera EM, Monuteaux MC, et al. (2011) Gray matter alterations in adults with attention-deficit/hyperactivity disorder identified by voxel based morphometry. Biol Psychiatry 69: 857–866. doi:10.1016/j.biopsych.2010.09.053.
19. Carmona S, Vilarroya O, Bielsa A, Trèmols V, Soliva JC, et al. (2005) Global and regional gray matter reductions in ADHD: a voxel-based morphometric study. Neurosci Lett 389: 88–93. doi:10.1016/j.neulet.2005.07.020.
20. Mostofsky SH, Cooper KL, Kates WR, Denckla MB, Kaufmann WE (2002) Smaller prefrontal and premotor volumes in boys with attention-deficit/hyperactivity disorder. Biol Psychiatry 52: 785–794.
21. Shaw P, Gogtay N, Rapoport J (2010) Childhood psychiatric disorders as anomalies in neurodevelopmental trajectories. Hum Brain Mapp 31: 917–925. doi:10.1002/hbm.21028.
22. Courchesne E, Carper R, Akshoomoff N (2003) Evidence of brain overgrowth in the first year of life in autism. JAMA 290: 337–344. doi:10.1001/jama.290.3.337.
23. Redcay E, Courchesne E (2005) When is the brain enlarged in autism? A meta-analysis of all brain size reports. Biol Psychiatry 58: 1–9. doi:10.1016/j.biopsych.2005.03.026.
24. Freitag CM, Luders E, Hulst HE, Narr KL, Thompson PM, et al. (2009) Total brain volume and corpus callosum size in medication-naïve adolescents and young adults with autism spectrum disorder. Biol Psychiatry 66: 316–319. doi:10.1016/j.biopsych.2009.03.011.
25. Herbert MR, Ziegler DA, Deutsch CK, O'Brien LM, Lange N, et al. (2003) Dissociations of cerebral cortex, subcortical and cerebral white matter volumes in autistic boys. Brain 126: 1182–1192.
26. Herbert MR (2005) Large brains in autism: the challenge of pervasive abnormality. Neuroscientist 11: 417–440. doi:10.1177/0091270005278866.
27. Herbert MR, Ziegler DA, Makris N, Filipek PA, Kemper TL, et al. (2004) Localization of white matter volume increase in autism and developmental language disorder. Ann Neurol 55: 530–540. doi:10.1002/ana.20032.
28. Courchesne E, Karns CM, Davis HR, Ziccardi R, Carper RA, et al. (2001) Unusual brain growth patterns in early life in patients with autistic disorder: an MRI study. Neurology 57: 245–254.
29. Chung MK, Dalton KM, Alexander AL, Davidson RJ (2004) Less white matter concentration in autism: 2D voxel-based morphometry. Neuroimage 23: 242–251. doi:10.1016/j.neuroimage.2004.04.037.
30. Waiter GD, Williams JHG, Murray AD, Gilchrist A, Perrett DI, et al. (2005) Structural white matter deficits in high-functioning individuals with autistic

spectrum disorder: a voxel-based investigation. Neuroimage 24: 455–461. doi:10.1016/j.neuroimage.2004.08.049.

31. Radua J, Via E, Catani M, Mataix-Cols D (2011) Voxel-based meta-analysis of regional white-matter volume differences in autism spectrum disorder versus healthy controls. Psychol Med 41: 1539–1550. doi:10.1017/S0033291710002187.

32. Vaccarino FM, Grigorenko EL, Smith KM, Stevens HE (2009) Regulation of cerebral cortical size and neuron number by fibroblast growth factors: implications for autism. J Autism Dev Disord 39: 511–520. doi:10.1007/s10803-008-0653-8.

33. Via E, Radua J, Cardoner N, Happé F, Mataix-Cols D (2011) Meta-analysis of gray matter abnormalities in autism spectrum disorder: should Asperger disorder be subsumed under a broader umbrella of autistic spectrum disorder? Arch Gen Psychiatry 68: 409–418. doi:10.1001/archgenpsychiatry.2011.27.

34. Nickl-Jockschat T, Habel U, Michel TM, Manning J, Laird AR, et al. (2012) Brain structure anomalies in autism spectrum disorder–a meta-analysis of VBM studies using anatomic likelihood estimation. Hum Brain Mapp 33: 1470–1489. doi:10.1002/hbm.21299.

35. Helt M, Kelley E, Kinsbourne M, Pandey J, Boorstein H, et al. (2008) Can children with autism recover? If so, how? Neuropsychol Rev 18: 339–366. doi:10.1007/s11065-008-9075-9.

36. Hesslinger B, Tebartz van Elst L, Thiel T, Haegele K, Hennig J, et al. (2002) Frontoorbital volume reductions in adult patients with attention deficit hyperactivity disorder. Neurosci Lett 328: 319–321.

37. Amaral DG, Schumann CM, Nordahl CW (2008) Neuroanatomy of autism. Trends Neurosci 31: 137–145. doi:10.1016/j.tins.2007.12.005.

38. Piven J, Arndt S, Bailey J, Andreasen N (1996) Regional brain enlargement in autism: a magnetic resonance imaging study. J Am Acad Child Adolesc Psychiatry 35: 530–536. doi:10.1097/00004583-199604000-00020.

39. Brieber S, Neufang S, Bruning N, Kamp-Becker I, Remschmidt H, et al. (2007) Structural brain abnormalities in adolescents with autism spectrum disorder and patients with attention deficit/hyperactivity disorder. J Child Psychol Psychiatry 48: 1251–1258. doi:10.1111/j.1469-7610.2007.01799.x.

40. Nijmeijer JS, Hoekstra PJ, Minderaa RB, Buitelaar JK, Altink ME, et al. (2009) PDD symptoms in ADHD, an independent familial trait? J Abnorm Child Psychol 37: 443–453. doi:10.1007/s10802-008-9282-0.

41. Müller UC, Asherson P, Banaschewski T, Buitelaar JK, Ebstein RP, et al. (2011) The impact of study design and diagnostic approach in a large multi-centre ADHD study. Part 1: ADHD symptom patterns. BMC Psychiatry 11: 54. doi:10.1186/1471-244X-11-54.

42. Müller UC, Asherson P, Banaschewski T, Buitelaar JK, Ebstein RP, et al. (2011) The impact of study design and diagnostic approach in a large multi-centre ADHD study: Part 2: Dimensional measures of psychopathology and intelligence. BMC Psychiatry 11: 55. doi:10.1186/1471-244X-11-55.

43. Kaufman J, Birmaher B, Brent D, Rao U, Flynn C, et al. (1997) Schedule for Affective Disorders and Schizophrenia for School-Age Children-Present and Lifetime Version (K-SADS-PL): initial reliability and validity data. J Am Acad Child Adolesc Psychiatry 36: 980–988. doi:10.1097/00004583-199707000-00021.

44. Hartman CA, Luteijn E, Serra M, Minderaa R (2006) Refinement of the Children's Social Behavior Questionnaire (CSBQ): an instrument that describes the diverse problems seen in milder forms of PDD. J Autism Dev Disord 36: 325–342. doi:10.1007/s10803-005-0072-z.

45. Luteijn EF, Serra M, Jackson S, Steenhuis MP, Althaus M, et al. (2000) How unspecified are disorders of children with a pervasive developmental disorder not otherwise specified? A study of social problems in children with PDD-NOS and ADHD. Eur Child Adolesc Psychiatry 9: 168–179.

46. Nijmeijer JS, Arias-Vásquez A, Rommelse NNJ, Altink ME, Buschgens CJM, et al. (2014) Quantitative Linkage for Autism Spectrum Disorders Symptoms in Attention-Deficit/Hyperactivity Disorder: Significant Locus on Chromosome 7q11. J Autism Dev Disord. doi:10.1007/s10803-014-2039-4.

47. Jaspers M, de Winter AF, Buitelaar JK, Verhulst FC, Reijneveld SA, et al. (2012) Early Childhood Assessments of Community Pediatric Professionals Predict Autism Spectrum and Attention Deficit Hyperactivity Problems. Journal of abnormal child psychology. doi:10.1007/s10802-012-9653-4.

48. Greaves-Lord K, Eussen MLJM, Verhulst FC, Minderaa RB, Mandy W, et al. (2013) Empirically based phenotypic profiles of children with pervasive developmental disorders: interpretation in the light of the DSM-5. J Autism Dev Disord 43: 1784–1797. doi:10.1007/s10803-012-1724-4.

49. Geluk CAML, Jansen LMC, Vermeiren R, Doreleijers TAH, van Domburgh L, et al. (2012) Autistic symptoms in childhood arrestees: longitudinal association with delinquent behavior. J Child Psychol Psychiatry 53: 160–167. doi:10.1111/j.1469-7610.2011.02456.x.

50. Rommelse NNJ, Geurts HM, Franke B, Buitelaar JK, Hartman CA (2011) A review on cognitive and brain endophenotypes that may be common in autism spectrum disorder and attention-deficit/hyperactivity disorder and facilitate the search for pleiotropic genes. Neurosci Biobehav Rev 35: 1363–1396. doi:10.1016/j.neubiorev.2011.02.015.

51. Geurts HM, Luman M, van Meel CS (2008) What's in a game: the effect of social motivation on interference control in boys with ADHD and autism spectrum disorders. J Child Psychol Psychiatry 49: 848–857. doi:10.1111/j.1469-7610.2008.01916.x.

52. Krug DA, Arick J, Almond P (1980) Behavior checklist for identifying severely handicapped individuals with high levels of autistic behavior. J Child Psychol Psychiatry 21: 221–229.

53. De Bildt A, Mulder EJ, Hoekstra PJ, van Lang NDJ, Minderaa RB, et al. (2009) Validity of the Children's Social Behavior Questionnaire (CSBQ) in children with intellectual disability: comparing the CSBQ with ADI-R, ADOS, and clinical DSM-IV-TR classification. J Autism Dev Disord 39: 1464–1470. doi:10.1007/s10803-009-0764-x.

54. 't Hart-Kerkhoffs LA, Jansen LM, Doreleijers TA, Vermeiren R, Minderaa RB, et al. (2009) Autism spectrum disorder symptoms in juvenile suspects of sex offenses. J Clin Psychiatry 70: 266–272.

55. Ashburner J, Friston KJ (2005) Unified segmentation. Neuroimage 26: 839–851. doi:10.1016/j.neuroimage.2005.02.018.

56. R Development Core Team (2010) R: A Language and Environment for Statistical Computing. Vienna, Austria: R Foundation for Statistical Computing. Available: http://www.R-project.org.

57. Bates D, Maechler M, Bolker B (n.d.) lme4: Linear Mixed-Effects Models Using S4 Classes. Available: http://CRAN.R-project.org/package = lme4.

58. Anderson D.R, Burnham K.P. (2002) Model selection and multimodel inference: a practical information-theoretic approach. 2nd Edition. New York, New York, USA: Springer-Verlag. 488 p.

59. Akaike H (1979) A Bayesian extension of the minimum AIC procedure of autoregressive model fitting. Biometrika 66: 237–242. doi:10.1093/biomet/66.2.237.

60. Crawley MJ (2007) The R Book. Available: http://onlinelibrary.wiley.com/book/10.1002/9780470515075. Accessed 31 August 2012.

61. O'Dwyer L, Lamberton F, Matura S, Tanner C, Scheibe M, et al. (2012) Reduced Hippocampal Volume in Healthy Young ApoE4 Carriers: An MRI Study. PLoS ONE 7: e48895. doi:10.1371/journal.pone.0048895.

62. Van der Meer JMJ, Oerlemans AM, van Steijn DJ, Lappenschaar MGA, de Sonneville LMJ, et al. (2012) Are autism spectrum disorder and attention-deficit/hyperactivity disorder different manifestations of one overarching disorder? Cognitive and symptom evidence from a clinical and population-based sample. J Am Acad Child Adolesc Psychiatry 51: 1160–1172.e3. doi:10.1016/j.jaac.2012.08.024.

63. Mulligan A, Anney RJL, O'Regan M, Chen W, Butler L, et al. (2009) Autism symptoms in Attention-Deficit/Hyperactivity Disorder: a familial trait which correlates with conduct, oppositional defiant, language and motor disorders. J Autism Dev Disord 39: 197–209. doi:10.1007/s10803-008-0621-3.

64. Courchesne E, Campbell K, Solso S (2011) Brain growth across the life span in autism: Age-specific changes in anatomical pathology. Brain Research 1380: 138–145. doi:10.1016/j.brainres.2010.09.101.

65. Hynd GW, Semrud-Clikeman M, Lorys AR, Novey ES, Eliopulos D (1990) Brain morphology in developmental dyslexia and attention deficit disorder/hyperactivity. Arch Neurol 47: 919–926.

66. Lyoo IK, Noam GG, Lee CK, Lee HK, Kennedy BP, et al. (1996) The corpus callosum and lateral ventricles in children with attention-deficit hyperactivity disorder: a brain magnetic resonance imaging study. Biol Psychiatry 40: 1060–1063.

67. Bussing R, Grudnik J, Mason D, Wasiak M, Leonard C (2002) ADHD and conduct disorder: an MRI study in a community sample. World J Biol Psychiatry 3: 216–220.

68. Durston S, Hulshoff Pol HE, Schnack HG, Buitelaar JK, Steenhuis MP, et al. (2004) Magnetic resonance imaging of boys with attention-deficit/hyperactivity disorder and their unaffected siblings. J Am Acad Child Adolesc Psychiatry 43: 332–340.

69. Happé F, Booth R, Charlton R, Hughes C (2006) Executive function deficits in autism spectrum disorders and attention-deficit/hyperactivity disorder: examining profiles across domains and ages. Brain Cogn 61: 25–39. doi:10.1016/j.bandc.2006.03.004.

70. Howlin P, Mawhood L, Rutter M (2000) Autism and developmental receptive language disorder–a follow-up comparison in early adult life. II: Social, behavioural, and psychiatric outcomes. J Child Psychol Psychiatry 41: 561–578.

71. Seltzer MM, Shattuck P, Abbeduto L, Greenberg JS (2004) Trajectory of development in adolescents and adults with autism. Mental Retardation and Developmental Disabilities Research Reviews 10: 234–247. doi:10.1002/mrdd.20038.

72. Langen M, Schnack HG, Nederveen H, Bos D, Lahuis BE, et al. (2009) Changes in the developmental trajectories of striatum in autism. Biol Psychiatry 66: 327–333. doi:10.1016/j.biopsych.2009.03.017.

73. Grahn JA, Parkinson JA, Owen AM (2009) The role of the basal ganglia in learning and memory: Neuropsychological studies. Behavioural Brain Research 199: 53–60. doi:10.1016/j.bbr.2008.11.020.

74. Schultz W, Tremblay L, Hollerman JR (2000) Reward processing in primate orbitofrontal cortex and basal ganglia. Cereb Cortex 10: 272–284.

75. Heimer L (2003) A new anatomical framework for neuropsychiatric disorders and drug abuse. Am J Psychiatry 160: 1726–1739.

76. Divac I, Rosvold HE, Szwarcbart MK (1967) Behavioral effects of selective ablation of the caudate nucleus. J Comp Physiol Psychol 63: 184–190.

77. Stettner LJ, Schultz WJ (1967) Brain lesions in birds: effects on discrimination acquisition and reversal. Science 155: 1689–1692.

78. Kirkby RJ (1969) Caudate nucleus lesions and perseverative behavior. Physiology & Behavior 4: 451–454. doi:10.1016/0031-9384(69)90135-8.

79. Thompson RL (1959) Effects of lesions in the caudate nuclei and dorsofrontal cortex on conditioned avoidance behavior in cats. J Comp Physiol Psychol 52: 650–659.

80. Esbensen AJ, Seltzer MM, Lam KSL, Bodfish JW (2009) Age-related differences in restricted repetitive behaviors in autism spectrum disorders. J Autism Dev Disord 39: 57–66. doi:10.1007/s10803-008-0599-x.

81. Taylor JL, Seltzer MM (2010) Changes in the autism behavioral phenotype during the transition to adulthood. J Autism Dev Disord 40: 1431–1446. doi:10.1007/s10803-010-1005-z.

82. Dosenbach NUF, Nardos B, Cohen AL, Fair DA, Power JD, et al. (2010) Prediction of individual brain maturity using fMRI. Science 329: 1358–1361. doi:10.1126/science.1194144.

83. Pfefferbaum A, Mathalon DH, Sullivan EV, Rawles JM, Zipursky RB, et al. (1994) A quantitative magnetic resonance imaging study of changes in brain morphology from infancy to late adulthood. Arch Neurol 51: 874–887.

84. Asato MR, Terwilliger R, Woo J, Luna B (2010) White matter development in adolescence: a DTI study. Cereb Cortex 20: 2122–2131. doi:10.1093/cercor/bhp282.

85. Kleinhans NM, Pauley G, Richards T, Neuhaus E, Martin N, et al. (2012) Age-related abnormalities in white matter microstructure in autism spectrum disorders. Brain Res 1479: 1–16. doi:10.1016/j.brainres.2012.07.056.

86. Dawson G (2008) Early behavioral intervention, brain plasticity, and the prevention of autism spectrum disorder. Development and Psychopathology 20: 775–803. doi:10.1017/S0954579408000370.

87. Scarpa A, Reyes NM (2011) Improving Emotion Regulation with CBT in Young Children with High Functioning Autism Spectrum Disorders: A Pilot Study. Behavioural and Cognitive Psychotherapy 39: 495–500. doi:10.1017/S1352465811000063.

88. Sze KM, Wood JJ (2008) Enhancing CBT for the Treatment of Autism Spectrum Disorders and Concurrent Anxiety. Behavioural and Cognitive Psychotherapy 36. Available: http://www.journals.cambridge.org/abstract_S1352465808004384. Accessed 10 March 2014.

89. Shea S, Turgay A, Carroll A, Schulz M, Orlik H, et al. (2004) Risperidone in the Treatment of Disruptive Behavioral Symptoms in Children With Autistic and Other Pervasive Developmental Disorders. Pediatrics 114: e634–e641. doi:10.1542/peds.2003-0264-F.

90. Hollander E, Novotny S, Hanratty M, Yaffe R, DeCaria CM, et al. (2003) Oxytocin infusion reduces repetitive behaviors in adults with autistic and Asperger's disorders. Neuropsychopharmacology 28: 193–198. doi:10.1038/sj.npp.1300021.

91. Matson JL, Nebel-Schwalm MS (2007) Comorbid psychopathology with autism spectrum disorder in children: an overview. Res Dev Disabil 28: 341–352. doi:10.1016/j.ridd.2005.12.004.

## 7

Violations of Personal Space by Individuals with Autism Spectrum Disorder

Daniel P. Kennedy[1,2]*, Ralph Adolphs[2,3]*

1 Department of Psychological and Brain Sciences, Indiana University, Bloomington, Indiana, United States of America, 2 Division of Humanities and Social Sciences, California Institute of Technology, Pasadena, California, United States of America, 3 Division of Biology, California Institute of Technology, Pasadena, California, United States of America

Abstract

The ability to maintain an appropriate physical distance (i.e., interpersonal distance) from others is a critical aspect of social interaction and contributes importantly to real-life social functioning. In Study 1, using parent-report data that had been acquired on a large number of individuals (ages 4–18 years) for the Autism Genetic Resource Exchange and the Simons Simplex Collection, we found that those with Autism Spectrum Disorder (ASD; n = 766) more often violated the space of others compared to their unaffected siblings (n = 766). This abnormality held equally across ASD diagnostic categories, and correlated with clinical measures of communication and social functioning. In Study 2, laboratory experiments in a sample of high-functioning adults with ASD demonstrated an altered relationship between interpersonal distance and personal space, and documented a complete absence of personal space in 3 individuals with ASD. Furthermore, anecdotal self-report from several participants confirmed that violations of social distancing conventions continue to occur in real-world interactions through adulthood. We suggest that atypical social distancing behavior offers a practical and sensitive measure of social dysfunction in ASD, and one whose psychological and neurological substrates should be further investigated.

Editor: Tiziana Zalla, Ecole Normale Supérieure, France

Funding: This work was supported by the Simons Foundation (SFARI-07-01 to R.A.), the National Institute of Mental Health (R01 MH080721 to R.A.), and the Tamagawa University global Centers of Excellence program of the Japanese Ministry of Education, Culture, Sports and Technology. The funders had no role in study design, data collection and analysis, decision to publish, or preparation of the manuscript.

Competing Interests: The authors have declared that no competing interests exist.

* Email: dpk@indiana.edu (DPK); radolphs@hss.caltech.edu (RA)

Introduction

Social dysfunction is one of the key diagnostic criteria in Autism Spectrum Disorder (ASD), and is often the single most disabling component for individuals with an ASD who otherwise might be considered high functioning. Research into the cognitive and neurobiological basis of social dysfunction has focused to a large extent on a few particular domains of social processing-most notably, face processing and mentalizing abilities [1–3]. Comparatively neglected has been research on other important aspects of social functioning, especially as they relate to real-world social interactions that can often be difficult to quantify. One such behavior is the regulation of social (i.e., interpersonal) distance, or the physical distance maintained between individuals during social interaction [4]. Though seemingly automatic and effortless, one's determination of the appropriate distance from others is a complex and dynamic social judgment that is simultaneously dependent on a number of factors, including person familiarity, cultural norms, emotional state, age, gender, and situational context, along with other variables. Social distance regulation is critical for successful social interaction, as its dysregulation can lead to personal space violations (and ensuing feelings of discomfort), as well as the inadvertent miscommunication of social intentions (e.g., aggression, defensiveness, social interest or disinterest, etc.) [4].

Anecdotally, parents, teachers, and clinicians have all described a lack of awareness of social distance norms in individuals with ASD [5], yet support for these claims is still somewhat limited.

Several studies have found abnormalities in social distancing in ASD [6–11], but these studies generally used smaller sample sizes, did not apply modern research criteria for an ASD diagnosis, and/or did not test a well-matched comparison sample, thus highlighting the need for further studies. One very recent exception to this found larger-than-normal interpersonal distance preferences in children with ASD, and that interpersonal distance failed to modulate as a function of social familiarity in this group [12]. Other studies using virtual reality have demonstrated that adolescents with an ASD seem to not respect the space of virtual characters [13], including walking directly in-between two characters seemingly engaged in a conversation with one another. However, it is currently unknown whether these types social distancing violations measured using virtual reality generalize to social distancing in the real world. In addition, these earlier studies focused solely on quantifying interpersonal distance – i.e., the readily observable physical distance between people. Less understood is whether or not individuals with ASD have an altered sense of personal space (i.e., the physical space around someone into which intrusion causes discomfort), and if so, whether this alteration relates to abnormal interpersonal distance preference.

In the current study, we took two complementary approaches to investigating the regulation of social distance in ASD – questionnaire-based data on a large number of individuals with ASD and their unaffected siblings (Study 1) and more tightly controlled laboratory experiments using the stop-distance technique [14] (Study 2). In Study 1, we analyzed phenotypic data from two large databases, the Simons Simplex Collection (SSC) and the Autism Genetic Resource Exchange (AGRE). We focused our analysis on data from the Social Responsiveness Scale (SRS), a 65-item parent- or teacher-report questionnaire designed to quantify the severity of autistic symptoms [15]. One item on the SRS explicitly assesses social distance violations at close proximity (Item 55), and we used this item as a starting point for our analyses. Our specific goals were as follows: (a) to compare probands (i.e., affected individuals; in this case, individuals with autism) and their siblings on social distance regulation, and (b) to determine the relationship between social distancing and various other parent-reported behaviors and clinical measures. In Study 2, we used controlled laboratory experiments with high-functioning adults with ASD and matched controls to complement and extend the above questionnaire-based approach. Specifically, we sought to (c) further explore whether and how such abnormalities may manifest in adulthood, and (d) attempt to gain preliminary insight into the possible psychological mechanisms underlying these social distance abnormalities. Together, such results would quantify the prevalence of social distance abnormalities in autism, identify behaviors and domains of functioning that co-segregate with this measure, and possibly suggest potential subtypes of autism (i.e., those with interpersonal distance abnormalities and those without) that may ultimately be traceable to distinct neurological and genetic profiles.

Methods

Study 1

Datasets. Phenotypic data were acquired from two publicly available databases: AGRE and SSC. The use of these de-identified data was approved by the Institutional Review Board at the California Institute of Technology. The principal difference between the two datasets was that the AGRE sample included only multiplex families (i.e., 2 or more affected individuals (in this case, children) within the family), whereas the SSC included only simplex families (i.e., only 1 affected individual). For the AGRE sample, we only included individuals that met AGRE designations of autism, which were based on fully meeting cutoff criteria on the Autism Diagnostic Interview – Revised (ADI-R) [16]. Individuals with AGRE designations of "Not Quite Autism" or "Broad Spectrum", given to those individuals that did not fully meet ADI-R cutoffs, were excluded from all analyses due to their ambiguous diagnostic status. Furthermore, since the ADI-R alone cannot differentiate between ASD subtypes, this dataset was not included in any analysis involving diagnostic subtypes. SSC diagnoses were based on the ADI-R, the Autism Diagnostic Observation Schedule (ADOS) [17], and expert clinical judgment, providing diagnoses of Autistic Disorder, Asperger's Syndrome, or PDD-NOS (Pervasive Developmental Disorder - Not Otherwise Specified).

For our analyses of both the AGRE and SSC datasets, a single ASD proband was matched with a single unaffected sibling from the same family (ASD-sib pairs). For all pairs, when multiple ASD proband or sibling options were available, individuals were chosen to best match first on gender, and then on age. Before pairs were created, specific exclusionary criteria were first applied to all cases, as detailed in Table 1 (AGRE) and Table 2 (SSC). This consisted of the following exclusionary criteria: 1) too many missing responses (greater than 6 SRS items), 2) SRS data acquired from invalid respondents (i.e., non-parent or caregiver), 3) younger than 4 years or older than 18 years, 4) evidence for non-ideopathic autism (i.e., cases with a specifically known cause, such as identified chromosomal abnormalities like Fragile X Syndrome), 5) did not meet diagnostic criteria for an ASD, 6) unaffected siblings with total SRS scores greater than T-Score cutoffs for

clinically significant social impairment (potentially indicative of an undiagnosed ASD), 7) 1 individual from monozygotic twins, or 2 individuals from monozygotic triplets, and 8) families that did not meet the multiplex designation in the AGRE sample (i.e., only 1 ASD proband) or had only 1 child in the SSC sample. The final sample consisted of 82 ASD-sib pairs (164 individuals) from the AGRE dataset (Table 1) and 684 ASD-sib pairs (1368 individuals) from the SSC dataset (Table 2). In the SSC dataset, the ASD group was comprised of 467 individuals with autism, 81 with Asperger's Syndrome, and 136 with a PDD-NOS diagnosis. Thus, after applying our exclusionary criteria, our final sample included 1532 individuals in total, consisting of 766 ASD individuals and 766 of their siblings (see **Table 3** for a detailed characterization of these groups).

Social Responsiveness Scale. The SRS is a 65-item parent- or teacher-report questionnaire that quantifies the severity of autistic impairment [15]. While designed to measure social deficits on a continuum, it has also demonstrated diagnostic utility [18]. For the present analyses, due to the larger number of parent-report compared to teacher-report data available, we restricted our analysis to parent-report data only. Individual SRS items are rated on a 4-point scale (from 0 to 3), with higher scores reflecting a higher frequency of autistic-like behaviors. Item 55 deals explicitly with social distancing (i.e., "knows when he or she is too close to someone or is invading someone's space"). Two additional items on the SRS were also of interest as they relate to the construct of social distance regulation - item 63: "Touches others in an unusual way (e.g., he or she may touch someone just to make contact and then walk away without saying anything)", and item 56: "Walks in between two people who are talking". We examined these items, as well as a third that turned out to be highly correlated with item 55 (item 52; "Knows when he or she is talking too loud or making too much noise").

Because the single item ratings are ordinal data, we used non-parametric tests for all analyses, unless stated otherwise. Furthermore, because the distributions of scores on item 55 did not differ between AGRE and SSC datasets ($U = 123535.5$, $Z = -0.42$, $p = 0.67$, $n_1 = 164$, $n_2 = 1368$, Mann-Whitney U test), these datasets were combined for all analyses, unless stated otherwise. Based on previous studies, anecdotal reports, and our own experiences, we hypothesized that individuals with an ASD would be more likely to exhibit social distancing abnormalities, compared to their unaffected siblings. All statistical tests were two-tailed. In addition, all significant correlations reported below survive Bonferroni correction for multiple comparisons.

Study 2

Participants. 18 ASD participants and 20 control participants took part in this study. Diagnosis of an ASD was confirmed using the ADOS (all module 4), ADI-R or SCQ (when a parent or guardian was available), and expert clinical judgment according to DSM-IV criteria. Groups did not differ on age, gender, or verbal, performance, or full-scale IQ (all p>0.3) (Table 4). This experiment was approved by Caltech's Institutional Review Board (IRB), and all participants gave written informed consent.

Task. In the first half of the experiment (Interpersonal Distance Condition), participants were instructed to approach the experimenter and stop at the location that felt perfectly comfortable to them. They started from approximately 3 meters away, and always approached the same experimenter, who maintained a consistent neutral expression and tried to maintain equal amounts of eye contact across participants. Once they chose the location that felt most comfortable, participants were asked to hold still while chin-to-chin distance was measured using a digital

Table 1. A list of the exclusionary criteria applied to AGRE dataset.

AGRE Subject Selection

# of Records	Exclusion Criteria
1593	Parent-Report SRS
1172	No record in pedigree
1152	Invalid respondent or missing too many responses
1097	Age less than 4 years or greater than 18 years
1065	non-ideopathic autism
825	probands did not meet ADI-R criteria for Autistic Disorder
804	unaffected siblings with total SRS scores greater than published T-score cutoffs (indicative of a potentially undiagnosed ASD)
801	duplicate entries
788	if monozygotic twins, triplets, etc., removed all except 1
623	removed simplex families
82	**Total ASD-Sib Pairs**

laser distance measurer (Bosch, model DLR165K). Distances were measured twice in immediate succession, and averaged together to account for slight variations due to body sway.

In the second half of the experiment (Personal Space Condition), the same procedures were carried out, but this time participants were asked to stop at the location that just started to feel uncomfortable to them. In addition, participants were instructed that if there was no point at which they felt uncomfortable, then they should walk as close as possible to the experimenter without physically touching them, and then to verbally tell the experimenter so. Participants completed 4 trials of each type, with the 4 Interpersonal Distance trials always preceding the 4 Personal Space trials. The order of conditions was fixed to avoid the concern that the discomfort experienced by participants during the Personal Space trials would influence their Interpersonal Distance judgments.

After all the trials were completed, participants were asked to verify that they understood the instructions by verbally explaining to the experimenter why they stopped where they did on the various trials. All participants demonstrated full understanding of the instructions (i.e., stopping at a comfortable distance for Interpersonal Distance trials, and stopping at a distance where they started to feel slightly uncomfortable for Personal Space trials), as would be expected in this group of high-functioning ASD adults and age-, gender-, and IQ-matched controls.

The relationship between mean Interpersonal Distance and mean Personal Space were examined using regression analyses, and the residuals of the regression were compared across groups.

Results

Study 1

After applying exclusionary criteria, there were no differences between groups in terms of age (proband mean ($\pm$SD) = 112.7

Table 2. A list of the exclusionary criteria applied to SSC dataset.

SSC Subject Selection

# of Records	Exclusion Criteria
1825	Parent-Report SRS
1825	No record in pedigree
1824	duplicate entries
1816	non-simplex families
1816	Invalid respondent or missing too many responses
1800	Age less than 4 years or greater than 18 years
1745	non-ideopathic autism
1745	probands did not meet best-estimate diagnosis of ASD
1713	unaffected siblings with total SRS scores greater than published T-score cutoffs (indicative of a potentially undiagnosed ASD)
1700	if monozygotic twins, triplets, etc., removed all except 1
1474	remove families with only 1 child
684	**Total ASD-Sib Pairs**

Table 3. Subject characteristics for each group.

Subject Characteristics		ASD	Siblings
Mean Age (±SD)		114.7 (±42.6) months	112.7 (±38.9) months
Male:Female ratio		5.03:1.0	0.87:1.0
Vineland		73.3 (±13.3)	104.7 (±11.6)*
Total SRS score		102.6 (±28.9)	17.5 (±11.7)
ADI-R	Social	20.7 (±5.8)	-
	Verbal Comm	16.7 (±4.2)	-
	Non-verbal Comm	9.3 (±3.5)	-
	RSB	6.4 (±2.6)	-

* = derived from the SSC dataset alone, since this information was not acquired from siblings in the AGRE dataset.
RSB = restricted, repetitive, and stereotyped patterns of behavior; SD = standard deviation.

months (±38.9); sibling = 114.7 months (±42.6); $t(1530) = 0.96$, $p = 0.34$, independent samples t-test). Not surprisingly, groups did differ in terms of total SRS scores (probands = 99.6 (±27.3); siblings = 17.8 (±11.8); $t(1530) = 76.2$, $p<0.0001$) and Vineland standard composite scores (probands = 73.3 (±13.3); siblings = 104.7 (±11.6); $t(1403) = 46.9$, $p<0.0001$) (Table 3).

Social Distancing. As hypothesized, there was a difference between probands and siblings on social distancing (item 55), with ASD probands (mean = 2.22, SD = 0.94) rated as less aware of being too close and more prone to personal space invasions than their unaffected siblings (mean = 0.70, SD = 0.95; $U = 789911.5$, $Z = -24.32$, $p<0.0001$, $n_1 = n_2 = 766$, Mann-Whitney U test; **Figure 1a**). This was true for both the AGRE dataset (ASD mean = 2.38 (0.90), sibling mean = 0.46 (0.77), $U = 9561$, $Z = -9.63$, $p<0.0001$, $n_1 = n_2 = 82$) and the SSC dataset (ASD mean = 2.20 (0.95), sibling mean = 0.73 (0.97); $U = 625713$, $Z = -22.37$, $p<0.0001$, $n_1 = n_2 = 684$), when analyzed separately. The difference in scores between ASD-sibling pairs was slightly larger in the AGRE sample compared to the SSC sample ($t(764) = 2.96$, $p = 0.003$, independent samples t-test). Furthermore, ASD and sibling groups remained different even when including those siblings with elevated total SRS scores (AGRE: ASD mean = 2.40 (0.85), sibling mean = 0.53 (0.81), $U = 11262$, $Z = -10.01$, $p<0.0001$, $n_1 = n_2 = 89$; SSC: ASD mean = 2.20

(0.76), sibling mean = 0.76 (0.98), $U = 658433.5$, $Z = -22.33$, $p<0.0001$, $n_1 = n_2 = 703$). Examination of the frequency histograms for each group reveals how well this single item (item 55) differentiates probands from their siblings (see **Figure 1b**). 78.6% of ASD-sib pairs had higher scores for probands than siblings, while the converse was true only 6.5% of the time (scores were equal for the remaining 14.9%). Relative to all other items on the SRS, this item ranks 21st out of 65 items in terms of differentiating groups (i.e., it is better than roughly two-thirds of all SRS items). There were no differences in mean ratings on this measure across the various ASD sub-categories (provided in the SSC dataset; autism mean (SD) = 2.20 (0.94); Asperger's mean = 2.22 (0.99); PDD-NOS mean = 2.17 (0.94); $H(2) = 0.47$, $p = 0.79$, $n_1 = 467$, $n_2 = 81$, $n_3 = 136$, Kruskal-Wallis test).

Ratings on item 55 correlated with total SRS scores, after removing the contribution of item 55 to the total SRS score (probands: $r = 0.29$, $p<0.0001$, siblings: $r = 0.42$, $p<0.0001$; Spearman correlation). ASD probands with higher scores on item 55 (ratings of 2 or 3) had higher total SRS scores (after removing the contribution of item 55; mean = 100.1 (25.9) out of a possible 195) compared to ASD probands with lower scores on this item (ratings of 0 or 1; mean = 86.6 (28.5); $U = 47321$, $Z = -5.21$, $p<0.0001$, $n_1 = 609$, $n_2 = 157$, Mann-Whitney U test). Given that scores on SRS items are generally positively correlated with one

Table 4. Participant characteristics for Study 2.

Subject Characteristics		ASD (n = 18)	Controls (n = 20)
Mean Age (±SD)		27.1 (±7.7) years	26.8 (±4.2) months
Males/Females		13/5	16/4
Total SRS score		98.1 (±28.2)*	-
WASI	Verbal	111.7 (±17.4)	113.7 (±8.3)
	Performance	108.2 (±9.7)	108.6 (±9.0)
	Full Scale	110.4 (±12.3)	112.6 (±8.1)
ADOS	Comm	4.5 (±1.5)	-
	Social	9.0 (±3.9)	-
	Repetitive	1.6 (±1.4)	-

* = SRS scores were not available from controls, and unavailable for 3 of the ASD participants.

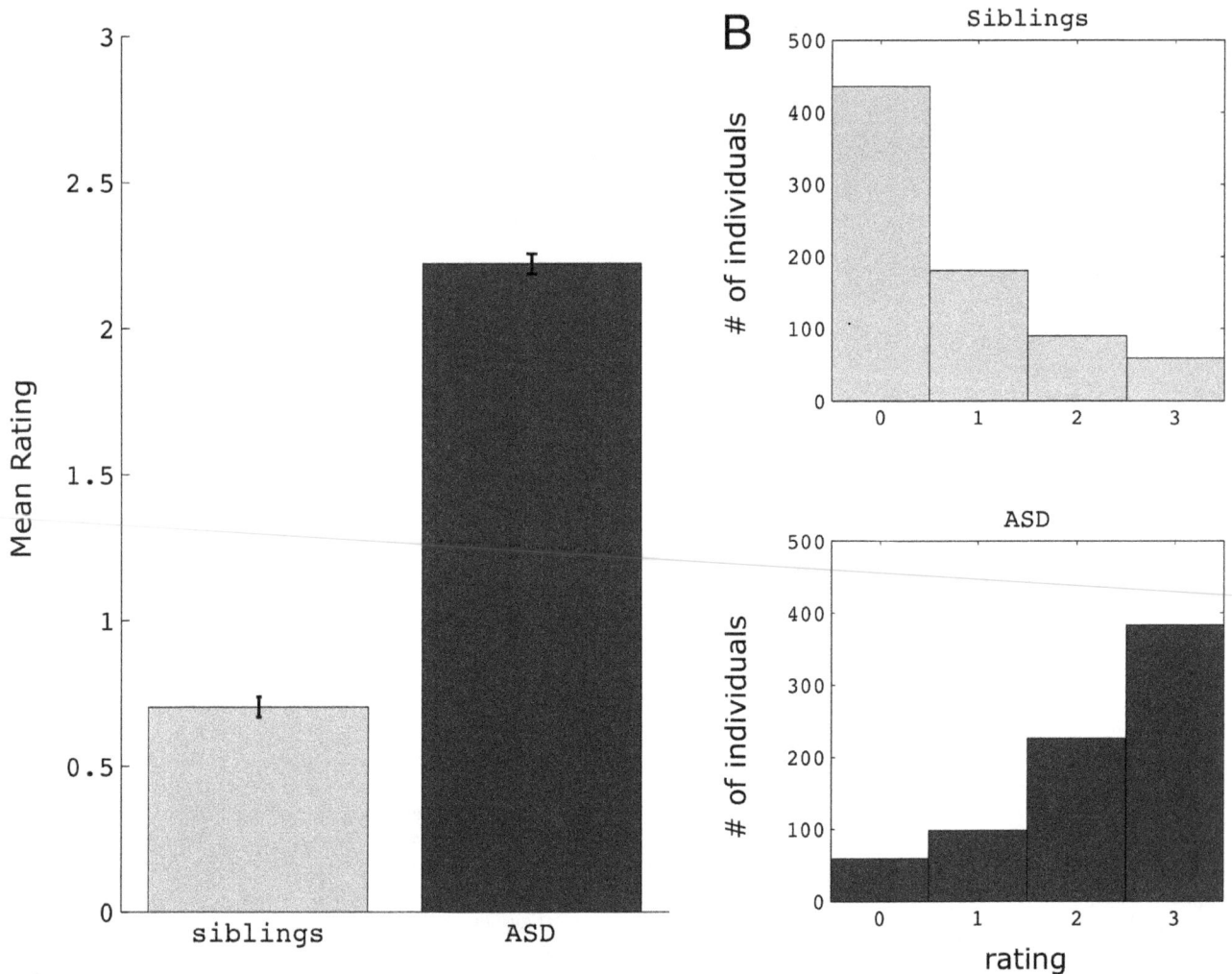

Figure 1. Ratings on item 55 (awareness of social distancing) in ASD and siblings. A) Mean ratings for each group; error bars reflect standard error of the mean (SEM). B) histograms showing the number of individuals who received each rating on item 55. Scores range from 0 to 3, with higher scores reflecting a greater frequency of social distancing abnormalities.

another [19], (in the present ASD sample, mean correlation across all pairwise item correlations, $r = 0.19$, $SD = 0.10$), it is not surprising that those with high scores on item 55 have higher overall scores. Interestingly, however, the three SRS items with the highest correlations to item 55 all seem to relate to social distancing and personal space: item 52 ($r = 0.42$, $p < 0.0001$): "Knows when he or she is talking too loud or making too much noise"; item 63 ($r = 0.31$, $p < 0.0001$): "Touches others in an unusual way (e.g., he or she may touch someone just to make contact and then walk away without saying anything)"; and item 56 ($r = 0.30$, $p < 0.0001$): "Walks in between two people who are talking" (see **Figure 2**). Correlations between item 55 and these items remained the three strongest even after accounting for age (partial correlations: $r = 0.42$, $r = 0.31$, $r = 0.30$, respectively; all $p < 0.0001$) and Vineland scores (partial correlations: $r = 0.39$, $r = 0.28$, $r = 0.27$, respectively; all $p < 0.0001$).

Correlations with ADI-R. There were positive correlations between item 55 and the ADI-R social subscale ($r = 0.13$, $p = 0.0004$) and ADI-R communication subscale (verbal: $r = 0.11$, $p = 0.006$; non-verbal: $r = 0.13$, $p = 0.0005$), but not with the ADI-R restricted and stereotyped behaviors (RSB) subscale ($r = -0.002$, $p = 0.96$). The pattern of results remained after

controlling for age (social, verbal communication, and non-verbal communication, $r = 0.16$, $r = 0.12$, $r = 0.15$, respectively, all $p < .002$; RSB, $r = 0.004$, $p = 0.90$, non-parametric partial correlation), but not after controlling for Vineland standard composite scores (all $r < 0.06$, all $p > 0.13$).

Effects of age, gender and adaptive functioning. The above described results of differences between ASD probands and siblings on item 55 cannot simply be explained by age effects. While there were slight but significant correlations between item 55 and age in both the ASD and sibling groups (probands: $r = -0.14$, $p < 0.0001$; siblings: $r = -0.30$, $p < 0.0001$; Spearman correlation), groups were well-matched with respect to age. Furthermore, group differences were found at every age from 4 years to 18 years (see **Figure 3**; for all age bins, $p < 0.005$, Mann-Whitney U test). Lastly, since the age of the control group was slightly lower than the ASD group, and since lower ages correspond to higher item 55 scores, one might, if anything, have expected to see higher scores in the sibling group compared to the ASD group if age were driving the results (i.e., an effect opposite to that observed). The results also could not be explained by differences in the number of males and females across proband and sibling groups (a consequence of the higher ratio of male:female individuals with

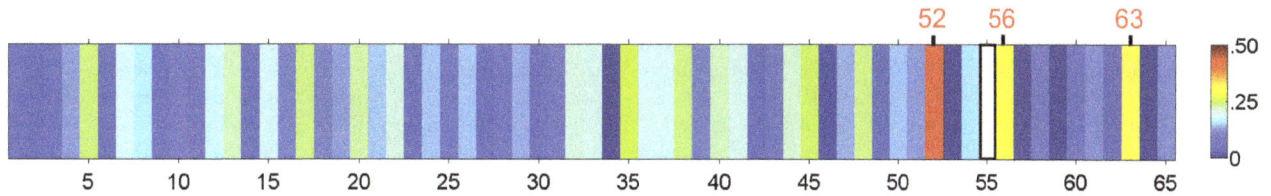

Figure 2. Correlations between ratings on item 55 (white) and all other SRS items. The three items with the highest correlations were items 52 ("Knows when he or she is talking too loud or making too much noise"), 56 ("Walks in between two people who are talking"), and 63 ("Touches others in an unusual way (e.g., he or she may touch someone just to make contact and then walk away without saying anything)"), all of which relate to the concept of social distancing.

an ASD), as there were no differences on item 55 ratings between male and female siblings (mean (SD) = 0.74 (0.98) and 0.67 (0.93), respectively; $U = 139431.5$, $Z = 1.06$, $p = 0.29$, $n_1 = 356$, $n_2 = 410$, Mann-Whitney U test), nor between male and female probands (2.24 (0.92) and 2.10 (1.04), respectively; $U = 46262$, $Z = 1.17$, $p = 0.24$, $n_1 = 639$, $n_2 = 127$, Mann-Whitney U test).

Finally, we ran an additional analysis to ensure that differences in social distancing between groups could not be accounted for by group differences in adaptive functioning, as measured with the Vineland Adaptive Behavior Scales. This was of particular concern since there were group differences in Vineland composite

scores (see above results and Table 3), and because item 55 was negatively correlated with Vineland scores in the autism group ($r = -0.19$, $p<0.0001$). Therefore, we created a subsample of the ASD and siblings groups that were well-matched on total Vineland scores, by selecting and comparing the lowest performing 20% of the sibling group and the highest performing 20% of the ASD group (ASD mean (SD) = 90.7 (5.4); Sibling mean (SD) = 90.0 (4.0); $U = 21461$, $Z = -0.30$, $p = 0.76$, $n_1 = n_2 = 147$, Mann-Whitney U test). Group differences on item 55 remained when using this subsample (ASD mean (SD) = 2.03 (0.95); Sibling mean (SD) = 0.82 (0.96); $U = 28158$, $Z = 9.18$, $p<0.0001$, $n_1 = n_2 = 147$,

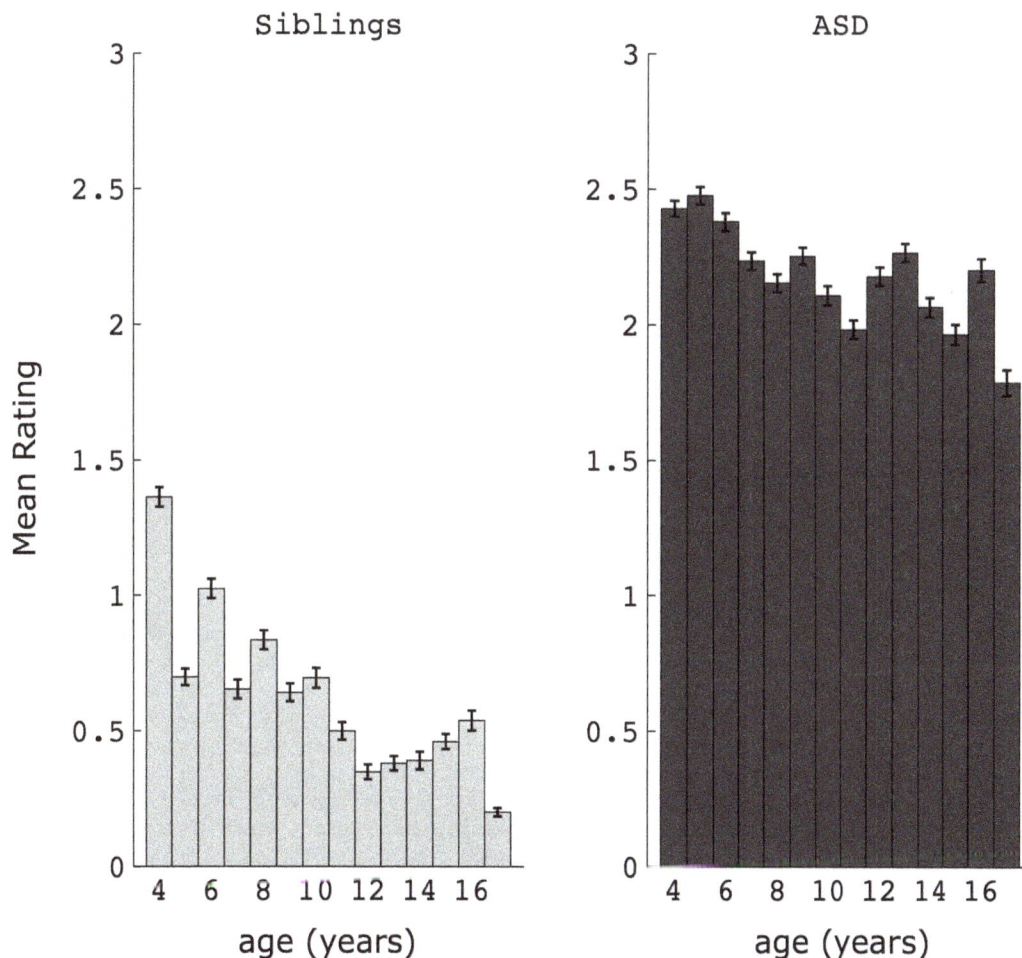

Figure 3. Ratings on item 55 (awareness of social distancing) in ASD and siblings across age bins (from 4 years to 18 years). Error bars reflect standard error of the mean (SEM). Group differences were present at every age bin (all $p<0.005$, Mann-Whitney U test).

Mann-Whitney U test). Similarly, when we restricted our analysis to groups matched on the socialization score of the Vineland (ASD mean (SD) = 89.2 (6.16), Sibling mean (SD) = 88.4, (4.50)), groups remained different on item 55 (ASD mean (SD) = 1.96 (1.03); Sibling mean (SD) = 0.81 (0.97); U = 27702, Z = 8.55, p<0.0001, $n_1 = n_2 = 147$, Mann-Whitney U test).

Study 2

Groups did not differ in terms of mean interpersonal distance (ASD = 79.9 (24.1); controls = 73.7 (17.6); [t(36) = 0.91, p = 0.37]) or mean personal space (ASD = 42.8 (29.5); controls = 42.8 (12.3); [t(36) = 0.002; p = 0.998]). Furthermore, both groups displayed a positive relationship between personal space and interpersonal distance preferences. This relationship was stronger in the control group (r = 0.881, p<0.0001) compared to the ASD group (r = 0.562, p 0.0152) (see **Figure 4a and 4b**).

To quantify the difference in the degree to which personal space predicts interpersonal distance preference in the two groups, a regression line was fit for each group separately [ASD: b = 0.46; $r^2 = 0.316$, F(1,16) = 7.4, p = 0.0151; Controls: b = 1.26; $r^2 = 0.776$, F(1,18) = 62.4, p<0.000001]. Residuals for each individual subject were then derived from their respective regression lines, and the absolute value of the residuals were compared between groups, providing a measure of how much a particular individual deviates from the regression model. We found that the groups were different from one another (t(36) = 2.95, p = 0.0055), with the ASD group having higher residuals (mean±SD = 15.3±12.2) compared to the control group (6.5±4.9) (see **Figure 4c**), indicating a less tight relationship between personal space and interpersonal distance preferences in ASD. Close examination of **Figure 4b** also reveals that 3 individuals with ASD had no sense of personal space. Importantly, these group differences were not simply driven by these individuals, since the pattern of results were unchanged if these three individuals were first excluded from the analysis (new ASD regression: ASD: b = 0.61; $r^2 = 0.325$, F(1,13) = 6.26, p = 0.026; ASD mean = 16.4±12.8; Control mean = 6.5±4.9; group difference: t(33) = 3.16, p = 0.0034). Furthermore, the results remained unchanged if a single regression line was calculated using data pooled across both groups together [b = 0.59; $r^2 = 0.38$, F(1,36) = 22.2, p<0.0001; ASD mean = 16.5±11.6; Control mean = 9.8±6.8; group difference: t(36) = 2.23, p = 0.032].

When assessing participants' understanding of the task instructions, 5 ASD participants offered additional anecdotal insight into their social distancing abnormalities, either by describing real-life events related to personal space violations (2 subjects), by providing somewhat atypical explanations for their behavior (2 subjects) or by demonstrating real-world abnormalities (1 subject). For instance, one participant described a recent event where he was explicitly told that he was standing inappropriately close to someone. Other subjects described that their discomfort was strictly due to sensory issues and restrictions (e.g., too much in my vision; can't read body language when that close). Another participant demonstrated repeated personal space violations throughout his visit to the laboratory (e.g., touching the experimenter's stomach, grabbing the experimenter's hand, touching the experimenter's face with both hands, etc.).

Discussion

In Study 1, we found that social distancing differs between individuals with an ASD and their unaffected siblings, as assessed using parent-report SRS scores in a large sample comprised of 1532 individuals. ASD individuals were rated as being less aware of their closeness to others or of invading someone's space compared to their unaffected siblings. This was true for 78.6% of ASD-sibling pairs, while the reverse was true for only 6.5% of pairs, demonstrating the robustness of this difference. Further, group differences in social distancing persisted across a wide range of ages (from 4 years to 18 years), as well as across the various ASD diagnostic sub-categories (i.e., Autistic Disorder, Asperger's, and PDD-NOS). We also found that scores on the social and communication subscales of the ADI-R correlate positively with parent ratings of social distancing abnormality. Given that social distance is a socio-communicative signal, it makes sense that a relationship would be found for both of these domains of functioning (and not with the restricted and stereotyped behaviors subscale).

In Study 2, we further explored the nature and extent of social distancing abnormalities in a sample of high-functioning adults with autism, and in a more detailed way than which was possible based on the questionnaire data. Using a controlled experimental task, we demonstrated that the tight relationship we observed in the control group between personal space and interpersonal distance was disrupted in ASD (**Figure 4**). Additional evidence for social distancing abnormality comes from anecdotal reports and direct observation of violations of social distancing conventions by our participants, and from abnormal explanations for why particular distances are preferred (i.e., sensory explanations), demonstrating that these social distancing abnormalities can persist into adulthood. Furthermore, we documented the complete absence of a sense of personal space in 3 out of 18 participants ASD participants (17%), something not seen in any of the 20 control participants.

It is particularly noteworthy that abnormalities in aspects of social distancing in ASD were detected across these two experiments (Study 1 and Study 2), since they used very different methods and 2 very different populations of participants. Given the different methodologies, a direct comparison cannot be made between children/adolescents and older adults with ASD. However, some conclusions about whether social distancing abnormalities are present and how they manifest over development can still be drawn. In Study 1, we found that abnormalities in ASD are present early in life (i.e., present at 4 years of age, which was the earliest age assessed here), and while they diminish across age (Figure 3), they continue to be present and significantly abnormal into late adolescence/young adulthood (i.e., 18 years). Study 2 demonstrated that these abnormalities are still detectable well into adulthood in some individuals. At the group level, a more subtle abnormality was detected in the relationship between personal space and interpersonal distance, suggesting either a different mechanism by which social distancing skills had been acquired over development, or a different way in which social distancing decisions are made (e.g., less reliant on personal space/feelings of discomfort). Taken together, these studies demonstrate that social distancing abnormalities are widespread in childhood and adolescence, and may be a persistent, life-long feature of ASD, especially apparent in some individuals with an ASD.

In Study 1, scores on the parent-report measure of social distancing competency were most strongly correlated with several other items that also relate to social distancing. Two of these items were *a priori* items of interest ("Touches others in an unusual way…" and "walks in between two people who are talking") since they explicitly assess violations of two aspects of social distancing - namely, personal space and social space. A third item, which actually had the highest correlation with item 55, is less obviously related to social distancing ("Knows when he or she is talking too loud or making too much noise"). However, one's sense of space is

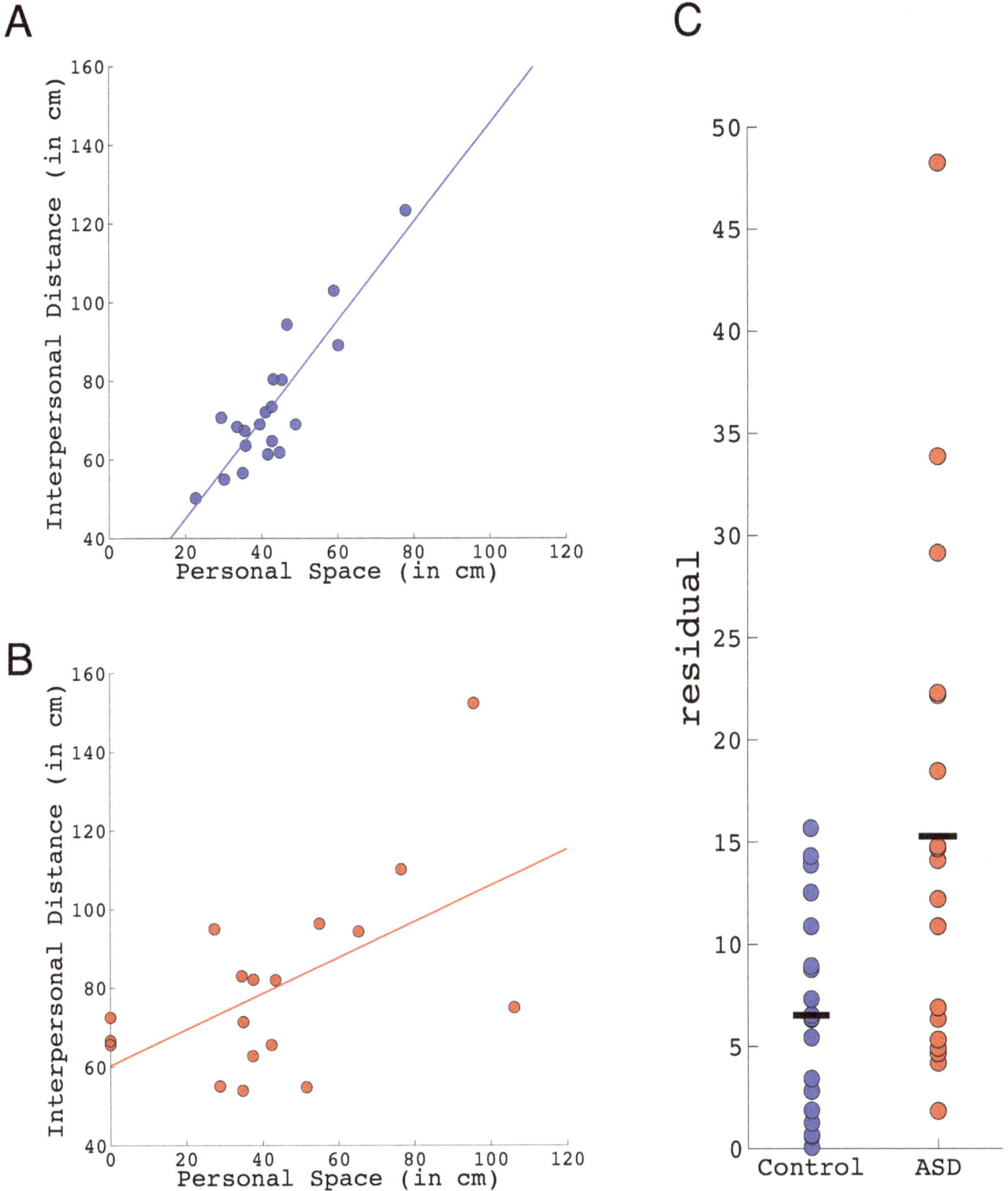

Figure 4. Relationship between personal space and interpersonal distance preferences in ASD and control adults. The correlation between these two measures is stronger in the control group (Panel A; r = 0.881, p<0.000001) than in the ASD group (Panel B; r = 0.562, p = 0.0151). Residuals were derived from regression lines fit to each group separately. Absolute values of the residuals are plotted for control and ASD groups (Panel C). Groups were different on this measure (t(36) = 2.95, p = 0.0055), with the ASD group displaying greater residuals, indicating a less tight relationship between personal space and interpersonal distance preferences.

a multimodal construct and can be violated by a number of sensory modalities [4,20], including audition (e.g., talking too loud in a public area). Thus, it is not surprising that an individual that violates the space of another person tends to do so through more than one sensory modality.

In regard to the finding of a group difference in social distancing competency between individuals with an ASD and their unaffected siblings in Study 1, one potential concern is that families were preselected according to specific criteria that could have biased the results toward finding such a difference. For instance, inclusion of a family into the SSC dataset requires that there be only 1 affected individual, and that siblings are not diagnosed with or referred for possible ASD, along with additional exclusionary criteria applied to siblings (adaptive functioning levels below 70, identified as having a developmental delay other than Down Syndrome, diagnosed with schizophrenia or psychiatric disorders requiring treatment with more than 1 psychotropic medication, or having an Individualized Education Plan). The criteria for inclusion into the AGRE dataset, however, are less restrictive with regard to siblings, and allowed for inclusion of siblings that might have been referred for a possible ASD. Even within this AGRE sample, the group difference was still significant, the magnitude of this difference was larger compared to the SSC sample, and it remained significant even when we included those siblings that had elevated total SRS scores (indicative of clinically significant social impairment and a possible undiagnosed ASD). It is also worth pointing out that this concern regarding sibling selection would not influence the description of the social distancing phenotype within the ASD group (e.g., clinical correlates).

One particularly interesting finding, underscored by the integration of Study 1 and Study 2, is that social distancing abnormalities in ASD cannot be entirely explained by adaptive functioning (as measured with the Vineland) or intelligence. In Study 1, although there was a relationship between composite Vineland scores and social distancing in ASD (r = −0.19), this relationship alone could not account for the group difference in social distancing, since this difference persisted even when groups were carefully matched on composite Vineland scores (or specifically matched on the Vineland socialization domain). Similarly, in Study 2, an altered relationship between interpersonal distance preference and personal space was found in Study 2, where full-scale IQ scores were in the average to above average range (93–133). In fact, the three ASD participants without a sense of personal space had full-scale IQ scores of 100, 106 and 108. These findings together suggest that social distancing is a social competency that is at least partly separable from more general impairments in social, communicative, and daily living abilities as well as intelligence. We suggest that social distancing should be thought of as one specific facet of the composite set of abilities that constitute social functioning in real life; future studies should investigate the possibility that it may depend on partly dissociable underlying neurobiological mechanisms and/or genetic causes that could provide a window into subtypes of ASD.

Preliminary evidence regarding the neural systems underlying social distance regulation comes from a recent study that identified a critical role for the amygdala [21], a brain region with known anatomical and functional abnormalities in autism [22]. By studying a patient with complete bilateral lesions of the amygdala, Kennedy et al. [21] found that an intact amygdala is necessary for feelings of discomfort following personal space violations, thus helping to automatically regulate interpersonal distance. Furthermore, this prior study found that in neurotypical individuals, the amygdala exhibits greater activity when another person is standing close-by compared to when that person is far away. Given findings of anatomical abnormality [23–25] and functional abnormality [26] of the amygdala in individuals with ASD, it is possible that dysregulation of the relationship between personal space and interpersonal distance relates directly to amygdala dysfunction. The future demonstration of such a relationship could provide evidence that social distance regulation serves as an endophenotype for amygdala dysfunction in ASD.

Some limitations of the current studies should be noted. First, because the datasets analyzed in Study 1 were based on already acquired SRS data, our analysis was necessarily restricted to and limited by the specific items that comprise the SRS (and other phenotypic data). Given that these measures were not designed specifically to assess social distancing, we lacked the richness of measurement that one might obtain in an observational or experimental study. Another limitation is that, given the wording of item 55, we were only able to assess social distance violations arising from abnormally close proximity, and not social distance violations arising from abnormally far proximity. While our data clearly show that people with ASD generally are abnormal with respect to being too close, it remains an open question whether a subset of individuals with ASD might also sometimes be abnormally too far away from others. The wording of item 55 also inquires specifically about the child's *knowledge* about social distancing, rather than the child's behavior. Had the questionnaire explicitly assessed behavior, one might expect an even greater group difference, since rating a behavior is more objective and less open to interpretation and justification. The present study was unable to determine which specific factors may (or may not) influence social distancing in ASD. Past research in children with an ASD has shown that social distance is dependent on several factors, including the age and familiarity of the other person [8], opening the possibility that social distancing abnormalities in ASD may be highly context dependent, and that there may be at least some preserved aspects of social distance regulation, depending on the circumstances. Therefore, it should be emphasized that this study does not replace the need for observational and experimental research. Study 2 helped to address some of the above concerns by carrying out experimental laboratory tasks aimed at investigating the nature of social distancing abnormalities in more detail. However, this experiment also had limitations, especially given that the task was somewhat unnatural, especially in terms of the explicit nature of the task. It was made clear to participants that social distancing was being measured (both through instructions and also because of repeated measurements of distances), which is very different than typical social interactions where social distancing judgments are generally made in a more automatic and spontaneous manner. Thus, it is possible the explicit nature of the task may have masked real-world impairment that may still be present in some adults with ASD. This may be an additional factor underlying why our finding of a lack of an overall group difference in interpersonal distance preference in Study 2 was different from some previous reports (e.g., [13]). Other factors, including heterogeneity in symptom expression across individuals or social learning and adaptation over a protracted developmental timecourse may have also accounted for our lack of group-level differences in personal space and interpersonal distance measures.

From the current data, we are unable to determine the precise psychological mechanisms underlying social distancing abnormality in ASD. It is presently unclear whether abnormality in some individuals arises specifically from a lack of one's own sense of personal space (which is observed in several participants in Study 2), from a lack of awareness of others' personal space, a combination of the two, or abnormality in the mapping between one's sense of personal space and interpersonal distance preference. This information would be crucial to know in order to develop strategic interventions [5], as each mechanism would dictate a different interventional emphasis (e.g., a focus on one's own space, or a focus on other people's personal space). However, the results from Study 2 might provide initial clues regarding one possible mechanism underlying social distancing abnormalities in ASD. Given the tight relationship between personal space and interpersonal distance in our control group, we suggest that decisions regarding interpersonal distance may normally be related to the feelings of discomfort – in other words, the larger one's requirement for personal space, the proportionally greater interpersonal distance required by that individual. If feelings of discomfort were lacking or abnormal in individuals with ASD, then establishing a proper interpersonal distance would need to rely on other, non-visceral cues. While very preliminary, this hypothesis is supported by reports from two of our ASD participants, who described using sensory feedback, rather than visceral feelings of discomfort, to regulate their distance. Subsequent studies using a larger sample size, more sensitive and naturalistic measures of personal space and interpersonal distancing, and further probing how social distancing decisions are made by individuals with an ASD might help to provide further insight into these issues. In addition, further research aimed at understanding how personal space and interpersonal distance relate to and influence each other in both neurotypical subjects and those with ASD would be useful in this regard.

In sum, we have shown that social distance abnormalities are remarkably prevalent in ASD, and have detailed the relationships between social distancing and age, diagnosis, and clinical measures of social, communicative, and adaptive functioning. Using parent questionnaire data, in addition to interactive laboratory experiments and anecdotal report and observation, we have demonstrated that social distancing abnormalities persist over a wide range of ages and levels of functioning, and are still present in at least some cognitively-able high functioning adults with ASD. What we have not quantified here, however, is how abnormal

regulation of social distance might negatively impact an individual's real-world functioning in terms of the potentially serious consequences that might ensue. We have heard reports by parents of significant social and legal problems arising from personal space violations. Given the present findings, we suspect that this might be a widespread problem for individuals with an ASD and their families, and one that deserves careful consideration. Further understanding of this important aspect of social behavior, along with the psychological and neural mechanisms underlying its regulation and dysregulation, will be important in developing effective interventions aimed at ameliorating social distancing abnormalities, and potentially for improving social functioning in ASD more generally.

Acknowledgments

We are grateful to all of the families at the participating SFARI Simplex Collection (SSC) sites, as well as the principal investigators (A. Beaudet, R. Bernier, J. Constantino, E. Cook, E. Fombonne, D. Geschwind, D. Grice, A. Klin, D. Ledbetter, C. Lord, C. Martin, D. Martin, R. Maxim, J. Miles, O. Ousley, B. Peterson, J. Piggot, C. Saulnier, M. State, W. Stone, J. Sutcliffe, C. Walsh, E. Wijsman). We appreciate obtaining access to phenotypic data on SFARI Base. Approved researchers can obtain the SSC population dataset described in this study by applying at https://base.sfari.org. We also gratefully acknowledge the resources provided by the Autism Genetic Resource Exchange (AGRE) Consortium and the participating AGRE families. The Autism Genetic Resource Exchange is a program of Autism Speaks and is supported, in part, by grant 1U24MH081810 from the National Institute of Mental Health to Clara M. Lajonchere (PI). We also thank John Constantino (Washington University) for helpful discussions at all stages of this project. Portions of this work have been presented at the 2010 International Meeting For Autism Research in Philadelphia.

Author Contributions

Conceived and designed the experiments: DPK RA. Performed the experiments: DPK. Analyzed the data: DPK. Wrote the paper: DPK RA.

References

1. Dawson G, Webb SJ, McPartland J (2005) Understanding the nature of face processing impairment in autism: insights from behavioral and electrophysiological studies. Dev Neuropsychol 27: 403–424.
2. Schultz RT (2005) Developmental deficits in social perception in autism: the role of the amygdala and fusiform face area. Int J Dev Neurosci 23: 125–141.
3. Frith U (2001) Mind blindness and the brain in autism. Neuron 32: 969–979.
4. Hall E (1966) The Hidden Dimension. Garden City, New York: Doubleday.
5. Garfin DG, Lord C (1986) Communication as a social problem in autism. In: Schopler E, Mesibov GB, editors. Social Behavior in Autism. New York: Plenum Press.
6. Donnellan AM, Anderson JL, Mesaros RA (1984) An observational study of stereotypic behavior and proximity related to the occurrence of autistic child-family member interactions. J Autism Dev Disord 14: 205–210.
7. van Engeland H, Bodnar FA, Bolhuis G (1985) Some qualitative aspects of the social behaviour of autistic children: an ethological approach. J Child Psychol Psychiatry 26: 879–893.
8. Lord C, Hopkins JM (1986) The social behavior of autistic children with younger and same-age nonhandicapped peers. J Autism Dev Disord 16: 249–262.
9. McGee GG, Feldman RS, Morrier MJ (1997) Benchmarks of social treatment for children with autism. J Autism Dev Disord 27: 353–364.
10. Pedersen J, Livoir-Petersen MF, Schelde JT (1989) An ethological approach to autism: an analysis of visual behaviour and interpersonal contact in a child versus adult interaction. Acta Psychiatr Scand 80: 346–355.
11. Howlin P (1986) An overview of social behavior in autism. In: Schopler E, Mesibov GB, editors. Social Behavior in Autism. New York: Plenum Press.
12. Gessaroli E, Santelli E, di Pellegrino G, Frassinetti F (2013) Personal space regulation in childhood autism spectrum disorders. PLoS One 8: e74959.
13. Parsons S, Mitchell P, Leonard A (2004) The use and understanding of virtual environments by adolescents with autistic spectrum disorders. J Autism Dev Disord 34: 449–466.
14. Hayduk LA (1978) Personal-Space - Evaluative and Orienting Overview. Psychological Bulletin 85: 117–134.
15. Constantino JN, Gruber CP (2005) The social responsiveness scale: Western Psychological Services.
16. Le Couteur A, Rutter M, Lord C, Rios P, Robertson S, et al. (1989) Autism diagnostic interview: a standardized investigator-based instrument. J Autism Dev Disord 19: 363–387.
17. Lord C, Rutter M, Goode S, Heemsbergen J, Jordan H, et al. (1989) Autism diagnostic observation schedule: a standardized observation of communicative and social behavior. J Autism Dev Disord 19: 185–212.
18. Constantino JN, Davis SA, Todd RD, Schindler MK, Gross MM, et al. (2003) Validation of a brief quantitative measure of autistic traits: comparison of the social responsiveness scale with the autism diagnostic interview-revised. J Autism Dev Disord 33: 427–433.
19. Constantino JN, Gruber CP, Davis S, Hayes S, Passanante N, et al. (2004) The factor structure of autistic traits. J Child Psychol Psychiatry 45: 719–726.
20. Nesbitt PD, Steven G (1974) Personal space and stimulus intensity at a Southern California amusement park. Sociometry 37: 105–115.
21. Kennedy DP, Glascher J, Tyszka JM, Adolphs R (2009) Personal space regulation by the human amygdala. Nat Neurosci 12: 1226–1227.
22. Pelphrey K, Adolphs R, Morris JP (2004) Neuroanatomical substrates of social cognition dysfunction in autism. Ment Retard Dev Disabil Res Rev 10: 259–271.
23. Bauman M, Kemper TL (1985) Histoanatomic observations of the brain in early infantile autism. Neurology 35: 866–874.
24. Schumann CM, Amaral DG (2006) Stereological analysis of amygdala neuron number in autism. J Neurosci 26: 7674–7679.
25. Schumann CM, Hamstra J, Goodlin-Jones BL, Lotspeich LJ, Kwon H, et al. (2004) The amygdala is enlarged in children but not adolescents with autism; the hippocampus is enlarged at all ages. J Neurosci 24: 6392–6401.
26. Dalton KM, Nacewicz BM, Johnstone T, Schaefer HS, Gernsbacher MA, et al. (2005) Gaze fixation and the neural circuitry of face processing in autism. Nat Neurosci 8: 519–526.

## 8

Altered Network Topologies and Hub Organization in Adults with Autism: A Resting-State fMRI Study

Takashi Itahashi[1], Takashi Yamada[2], Hiromi Watanabe[2], Motoaki Nakamura[2,3], Daiki Jimbo[4], Seiji Shioda[4], Kazuo Toriizuka[1], Nobumasa Kato[2], Ryuichiro Hashimoto[2,5]*

1 Department of Pharmacognosy and Phytochemistry, Showa University School of Pharmacy, Tokyo, Japan, 2 Department of Psychiatry, Showa University School of Medicine, Tokyo, Japan, 3 Kinko Hospital, Kanagawa Psychiatric Center, Kanagawa, Japan, 4 Department of Anatomy, Showa University School of Medicine, Tokyo, Japan, 5 Department of Language Sciences, Graduate School of Humanities, Tokyo Metropolitan University, Tokyo, Japan

Abstract

Recent functional magnetic resonance imaging (fMRI) studies on autism spectrum condition (ASC) have identified dysfunctions in specific brain networks involved in social and non-social cognition that persist into adulthood. Although increasing numbers of fMRI studies have revealed atypical functional connectivity in the adult ASC brain, such functional alterations at the network level have not yet been fully characterized within the recently developed graph-theoretical framework. Here, we applied a graph-theoretical analysis to resting-state fMRI data acquired from 46 adults with ASC and 46 age- and gender-matched controls, to investigate the topological properties and organization of autistic brain network. Analyses of global metrics revealed that, relative to the controls, participants with ASC exhibited significant decreases in clustering coefficient and characteristic path length, indicating a shift towards randomized organization. Furthermore, analyses of local metrics revealed a significantly altered organization of the hub nodes in ASC, as shown by analyses of hub disruption indices using multiple local metrics and by a loss of "hubness" in several nodes (e.g., the bilateral superior temporal sulcus, right dorsolateral prefrontal cortex, and precuneus) that are critical for social and non-social cognitive functions. In particular, local metrics of the anterior cingulate cortex consistently showed significant negative correlations with the Autism-Spectrum Quotient score. Our results demonstrate altered patterns of global and local topological properties that may underlie impaired social and non-social cognition in ASC.

Editor: Satoru Hayasaka, Wake Forest School of Medicine, United States of America

Funding: A part of this study is the result of "Development of BMI Technologies for Clinical Application" carried out under the Strategic Research Program for Brain Sciences by the Ministry of Education, Culture, Sports, Science and Technology of Japan. This work was also supported by the Japan Society for the Promotion of Science (JSPS) Grant-in-Aid for Young Scientists (B) (25870738 to T.I.) and by a Grant-in-Aid for Scientific Research on Innovative Areas (23118003; Adolescent Mind & Self-Regulation to R.H.) from the Ministry of Education, Culture, Sports, Science, and Technology of Japan. The funders had no role in study design, data collection and analysis, decision to publish, or preparation of the manuscript.

Competing Interests: The authors have declared that no competing interests exist.

* E-mail: dbridges50@gmail.com

Introduction

Autism spectrum condition (ASC) has been characterized by impairments in social and communication skills, combined with repetitive and restricted behavior. However, this spectrum comprises a range of heterogeneous populations with varying degrees of severity. The debates surrounding the precise definition of its core symptoms, as well as the choice of the term for characterizing this spectrum (i.e., "disorder" or "condition"), have not been settled even in the latest version of the American Psychiatry Association's Diagnostic and Statistical Manual of Mental Disorders-Fifth Edition (DSM-V) has been published [1]. In an effort to reveal functional brain alterations underlying the clinical symptoms of ASC, an increasing number of functional magnetic resonance imaging (fMRI) studies have recently examined intrinsic activity in the absence of externally imposed tasks. Such resting-state fMRI (rs-fMRI) studies have found atypical intrinsic connectivity in ASC (for overview, see [2]): for instance, under-connectivity within a default mode network [3,4], and over- and under-connectivity between many pairs of brain regions [5,6]. These abnormal functional interactions between distributed brain areas lend support to the hypothesis that brain abnormalities in ASC can best be understood as a network disorder [7].

In neuroscience research, network studies (connectomics) of the human brain are becoming the key to understanding brain functions and mechanisms of neuropathological disorders [8]. In particular, advances in graph-theoretical analysis of rs-fMRI data have provided a new perspective on the functional organization of the human brain. This approach enables the representation of the whole brain as a large-scale network composed of nodes (brain regions) and edges (connections between nodes), and allows the examination of the topological properties of the network [9]. At the network level, for example, a small-world network is characterized by high clustering and short characteristic path length [10], which is a hallmark of the human brain network [11,12]. At the nodal level, the degree of a node quantifies the connectedness of the node with the rest of nodes in a network and therefore is useful in identifying highly connected nodes (i.e., hubs) that may play critical roles in information integration [13]. Several studies have identified functional hubs, particularly along the midline cortical regions (e.g., the supplementary motor area and precuneus) in neurotypical individuals [14–17]. While network structure and topological metrics change during the normal course of development [18–21], hub organization is stable from adolescence to young adulthood in neurotypical individuals [17], providing the notion that hub organization may serve as a functional backbone of the human brain. On the other hand, there is evidence for atypical neurodevelopment during adolescence in individuals with ASC [22], which raises the possibility that significant changes in hub organization occur between adolescence and adulthood.

A number of studies have applied graph-theoretical analysis to clinical populations, including patients with schizophrenia [23–27], major depressive disorder [28], and other disorders [29,30]. Although the graph-theoretical approaches are now being applied to studies on different aspects of the ASC brain (e.g., white matter connectivity and electrophysiological connectivity) [31–35], only a few have applied graph-theoretical analysis to rs-fMRI data of this disorder [36–39]. Rudie et al. [39] recently described disrupted local segregation and enhanced global integration in adolescents with ASC compared to neurotypical counterparts, while Barttfeld et al. [36] have reported that changes in the small-worldness measure occurring at shifts between different cognitive states show opposite patterns in patients with ASC and controls. However, basic questions regarding global network organization and possible alterations of "hubness" in adults with ASC have not been fully addressed.

Growing evidence suggests that people with ASC exhibit atypical neurodevelopmental process at least persisting immediately before adulthood [22,40–42]. For instance, individuals with ASC show brain over-growth in early childhood, followed by a period with an accelerated rate of decline in brain size from adolescence to middle age [42]. In addition, the developmental trajectories of subcortical regions (e.g., putamen and caudate) are known to be different in individuals with ASC relative to normal controls [43]. Furthermore, functional abnormalities of ASC vary with age [44], as corroborated by a meta-analysis revealing that the neural anomalies in adults with ASC differed significantly from those in children [45]. Therefore, in addition to the previous pediatric data, it is important to investigate the topological properties of the brain network in adults with ASC to complement the time-course of changes in topological properties from adolescence to adulthood.

The present study applied a graph-theoretical analysis to rs-fMRI data and compared the local and global topological properties of the brain network of adults with ASC to those of age- and gender-matched controls. In particular, we focused on the analysis of hub organization using local metrics and examined whether the order of node importance is altered in the autistic brain network. Since previous findings suggested that adults with ASC showed under-connectivity when compared to normal controls [2], we hypothesized that: 1) adults with ASC would show aberrant network organization as quantified by several global metrics, such as decreases in clustering coefficient and characteristic path length; 2) local network metrics would be altered in several regions for which activation and/or connectivity have been shown to be abnormal in ASC (e.g., the anterior cingulate cortex); 3) several topological properties altered in ASC would be linked with the autistic trait as assessed by the Autism Spectrum Quotient (AQ) test [46]; and 4) given the altered pattern of behavioral strengths and weaknesses in ASC, participants with ASC would exhibit significantly altered hub organization and alterations of "hubness" in nodes (e.g., superior temporal sulcus) responsible for a broad range of dysfunctions in ASC.

Materials and Methods

1. Participants

Forty-six adults with ASC were recruited from outpatient units of the Karasuyama Hospital, Tokyo, Japan. The inclusion criteria were: (1) age between 18 and 55 years and (2) a formal diagnosis of pervasive developmental disorder (PDD) based on the Diagnostic and Statistical Manual of Mental Disorders, Fourth Edition (DSM-IV). Exclusion criteria included a history of electroconvulsive therapy, alcohol or other drug abuse or dependence, or any neurological illness affecting the central nervous system. PDD was diagnosed by a team of three experienced psychiatrists and one clinical psychologist, based on two detailed interviews with the patients regarding their development and behavior from infancy through adolescence and family history. The interviews were conducted independently by one of the psychiatrists and the clinical psychologist in the team. The patients were also asked to bring along suitable informants who had known them in early childhood. The psychiatrist gave the final diagnosis, after consultation with the other psychiatrist and the clinical psychologist, a process requiring approximately three hours. This team confirmed that none of the participants met the DSM-IV criteria for any other psychiatric disorder. Although there were some individuals with ASC who showed some levels of anxiety, mood, or attention deficit and hyperactivity disorders, the severity of the problems did not meet the diagnostic criteria for other mental disorders.

A total of 46 normal controls (NCs) were recruited by advertisements and acquaintances. None of the NCs reported any severe medical problem or history of any neurological or psychiatric problems. Moreover, the Mini-International Neuropsychiatric Interview was used to confirm that none of the NCs met the diagnostic criteria for any psychiatric disorder.

The intelligence quotient (IQ) scores of participants with ASC were evaluated using either the Wechsler Adult Intelligence Scale-Third Edition (WAIS-III) or the WAIS-Revised (WAIS-R), while those of NCs were estimated using a Japanese version of the National Adult Reading Test (JART) [47]. Based on the National Adult Reading Test (NART) for English-speaking population [48], the JART has been developed to estimate the IQ of a Japanese subject by scoring his or her reading ability of 25 words printed in Kanji (adopted logographic Chinese characters). It has been widely used in Japanese clinical studies both for normal and patient groups [49,50]. Every participant with ASC was considered as being high-functioning, because his or her full-scale IQ score was higher than 80. Although the IQ score was missing for one male participant with ASC, he was also regarded as being high-functioning, because his predicted IQ was 114 based on the JART. Handedness was assessed using the Edinburgh Handedness Inventory [51]. Furthermore, participants completed the Japanese version of the Autism-Spectrum Quotient (AQ) test [46,52]. All of the participants of this study had normal or corrected-to-normal vision. Within the ASC group, 14 of the 46 participants were using either one or more of the following medications: antidepressants (9 patients), hypnotic drugs (9 patients), anti-anxiety drugs (8 patients), antipsychotic drugs (6 patients), and antiepileptic drugs (3 patients). The summary of participant demographic information can be found in Table 1.

The Ethics Committee of the Faculty of Medicine of Showa University approved all of the procedures used in this study, including the method of obtaining consent, in accordance with the Declaration of Helsinki. Written informed consent was obtained from participants after fully explaining the purpose of this study. Since all participants were high-functioning (IQ>80) adults

Table 1. Demographics and rating scale of the participants.

	NC			ASC			Statistics	
	Mean ± s.d.	Range	N	Mean ± s.d.	Range	N	df	p-value
Sample size			46 (7 female)			46 (7 female)		
Age (years)	32.02±7.94	19–50	46	31.11±8.14	19–51	46	90	0.68
Handedness	80.68±49.40	-100–100	41	69.49±63.59	-130–100	45	84	0.37
Estimated IQ	107.59±8.64	87.46–119.8	44	105.8±14.12	83–134	45	87	0.47
AQ score	15.08±5.27	8–30	38	36.20±5.63	24–47	46	82	<0.001

NC: normal control, ASC: autism spectrum condition, s.d.: standard deviation, N: the sample size for each of demographic information, AQ: Autism Spectrum Quotient.

without any other comorbidities, they were able to fully understand the content and nature of this study. Guardians' verbal consent was neither documented nor recorded because every patient was judged to possess the full ability to give consent on his or her own by his or her primary doctor (TY, WH, MN, or NK). Any concern regarding the possibility of reduced capacity to consent on his or her own was not voiced by either the ethics committee or patients' primary doctors. Every participant was assigned an arbitrary identification number for this study, so that all the data, including imaging and demographic data, could be analyzed anonymously. The data were stored locally, at a single location in the Department of Psychiatry, Showa University. In accordance with the obtained written informed consent, the data were only available for use by our research group.

2. MRI Data Acquisition

All MRI data were acquired using a 1.5-Tesla GE Signa system (General Electric, Milwaukee, WI, USA) with a phased-array whole-head coil. The functional images were acquired using a gradient echo-planar imaging sequence (in-plane resolution: 3.4375×3.4375 mm, echo time (TE): 40 ms, repetition time (TR): 2000 ms, flip angle: 90°, slice thickness: 4 mm with a 1-mm slice gap [11,53], matrix size: 64×64, 27 axial slices). Two hundred and eight volumes were acquired in a single run. The first four volumes were discarded to allow for T1 equilibration. In addition, a high-resolution T1-weighted spoiled gradient recalled (SPGR) 3D MRI image was collected (in-plane resolution: 0.9375×0.9375 mm, 1.4 mm slice thickness, TR: 25 ms, TE: 9.2 ms, matrix size: 256×256, 128 sagittal slices). Each participant was instructed to lie relaxed in the scanner and to remain as still as possible with his or her eyes closed, yet to stay awake in the dim scanner room.

3. Data Preprocessing

SPM8 software (http://www.fil.ion.ucl.ac.uk/spm/software/spm8/) was used to perform fMRI data preprocessing. First, slice timing and head motion were corrected. No participant was excluded due to excessive motion (>±2 mm translation and > ±2° rotation from the first volume in any axis). We also evaluated the amount of translation and rotation of the head during the scanning of each subject according to the following equation [54]:

$$\text{Translation/Rotation} = \frac{1}{T}\sum_{t=2}^{T}\sqrt{\Delta x_t^2 + \Delta y_t^2 + \Delta z_t^2},$$

where T is the number of volumes (i.e., $T = 204$ in this study); variables x, y, and z stand for translation or rotation values in each of the three axes; and Δx_i is the difference between x_i and x_{i-1} in the x-axis. The amount of head motion was comparable between the two groups in both translation (NC: 0.049±0.026 (mean ± standard deviation); ASC: 0.043±0.024; t-test: $t = 1.140, p = 0.257$) and rotation (NC: 0.037±0.014; ASC: 0.034±0.014; t-test: $t = 1.016, p = 0.312$). For each participant, a T1-weighted SPGR image was realigned along the mid-sagittal anterior-posterior commissure line, and then the realigned T1-weighted image was segmented and reconstructed in order to generate a skull-tripped T1-weighted image. The realigned fMRI images were co-registered to the skull-stripped T1-weighted image; the fMRI images were then spatially normalized to the standard Montreal Neurological Institute (MNI) template, and were resampled to a resolution of 3×3×3 mm. Finally, the images were spatially smoothed using a 6-mm full-width half-maximum Gaussian kernel.

4. Network Construction

4.1. Definitions of nodes and edges. Functional brain networks consist of nodes and edges. In this study, nodes and edges corresponded to regions of interest (ROIs) and functional connectivity between all possible pairs of the ROIs, respectively. We used the MNI coordinates of 160 brain regions provided by a previous meta-analytic study [55], and constructed a ROI consisting of voxels within a 5-mm radius sphere around the coordinate for each node. The mean time-series was extracted from each ROI, and then artifactual components were removed from the mean time-series using the CompCor method [56] implemented in the Functional Connectivity Toolbox (http://www.nitrc.org/projects/conn/). Briefly, this method first identifies five principal components associated with physiological signals from the segmented white matter and cerebrospinal fluid regions in each participant, and then regresses out those time-series, together with those associated with six head motion parameters and their temporal derivatives from the extracted mean time-series in each ROI. In this study, no global signal regression was performed to avoid the risk of yielding spurious negative correlations [57].

To reduce systematic biases in functional connectivity induced by sub-millimeter head motions during the scan [58,59], we adopted the "scrubbing" method together with a frame-wise displacement (FD) threshold of 0.5 mm and a band-pass filter (0.009–0.08 Hz) [58] (see Text S1 and Figure S1 for details and the effect of scrubbing). We confirmed that the mean FD was comparable between the two groups (NC: 0.1153±0.0423; ASC: 0.1034±0.0466; $t = 1.28$, $p = 0.201$). After these scrubbing steps, the number of retained volumes was comparable between the groups (NC: 203.17±1.51 volumes; ASC: 202.93±2.51 volumes; t-test: $t = 0.554$, $p = 0.581$), and each group retained approximately 99.5% of their original volumes. For measuring functional connectivity, correlation coefficients between all possible pairs of the ROIs were then calculated, which resulted in a 160×160 correlation matrix for each participant. Finally, each correlation matrix was transformed into an adjacency matrix by applying a predefined threshold (see next section), where the i-th and the j-th nodes were connected if the (i,j)-th element of the adjacency matrix is equal to one. See Text S2 for functional connectivity analysis.

4.2. Threshold selection. A binary undirected graph was constructed by applying a correlation threshold, ranging from zero to one, to each element of the correlation matrix; however, applying a single common threshold across all participants yields a different number of edges and nodes, which in turn may induce spurious between-group differences in network topology [60]. To avoid this problem, the sparsity-based threshold, S, the ratio of the number of existing edges to the maximum possible number of edges in a graph ($= 12720$), was employed [26,28].

The range of sparsity-based thresholds S was determined using the following procedures. First, we identified the minimum number of positive elements in the correlation matrix to determine the maximum sparsity (i.e., higher limit) for each participant, and then identified the minimum sparsity (i.e., lower limit), in which there was no fragmentation of the graph into several components for each participant. All graphs satisfied the property of the small-world network (i.e., the small-worldness scalar σ is greater than one). See the following section for a description of the small-worldness scalar. The range of sparsity was determined as 19.50% $\leq S \leq 48.43\%$. Over this range, we repeatedly calculated the global and local network metrics of interest (see next section) with an interval of 0.63% (47 steps).

5. Network Metrics

To assess topological properties of graphs, local and global metrics were calculated on a graph at each of the 47 sparsity levels. Brief descriptions of the metrics used in this study are listed in Table S1. More detailed definitions and descriptions of the metrics can be found in a recent review [61]. For each node, we calculated the three local metrics: degree k, betweenness b, and nodal efficiency e. For global metrics, we calculated global efficiency E_{glob}, local efficiency E_{loc}, and assortativity r. In addition to those global metrics, we computed the small-world parameters [10], including clustering coefficient C, characteristic path length L, normalized clustering coefficient γ, normalized characteristic path length λ, and small-worldness scalar σ. Small-world network should satisfy the conditions of $\gamma > 1$ and $\lambda \approx 1$ (i.e., $\sigma > 1$). Although we calculated all the above-mentioned global metrics, we reported mainly on r, C, L, and σ because some metrics bore a certain relationship (i.e., proportional or inverse) to other metrics. For example, clustering coefficient C bears a proportional relationship to local efficiency E_{loc}, while characteristic path length L is inversely proportional to global efficiency E_{glob} [62]. All metrics were calculated using the Brain Connectivity Toolbox (http://www.brain-connectivity-toolbox.net/).

While each of the metrics is highly dependent upon the threshold, there is no standard threshold currently accepted for the network construction. To avoid arbitrariness in network thresholding, we calculated the area under the curve (AUC) of each metric. The AUC provides an integrated scalar value representing the metric under investigation across the examined range of sparsity. The robustness of the AUC analysis for metrics has been demonstrated in previous studies [28,63].

6. Hubness

Hubs are often identified using degree k, betweenness b, and nodal efficiency e. High-degree nodes can be considered as centers for information integration; those with high betweenness may serve as way stations for network traffic, and those with high nodal efficiency have superior information propagation ability and hence contribute to efficient information flow [13,64]. In this study, hubs were defined as nodes with a k, b, or e value more than one standard deviation above the mean of all the nodes in the network [15].

7. Hub Disruption Index

Differences in local metrics are usually evaluated at each nodal level rather than at the network level. The hub disruption index is a useful metric for summarizing and visualizing the pattern of nodal abnormalities in a clinical group compared to a neurotypical group [65].

We calculated the hub disruption index, κ, in order to evaluate alteration in network topology in each individual brain, with reference to the normative network topology of the NC group. For each node in the network, we first subtracted the mean local metric (e.g., degree) in the NC group from the normalized degree in a participant, and then plotted the value against the mean of the NC group. We estimated slope using linear regression analysis, and defined the obtained slope as κ. When the resulting data are scattered along a horizontal line ($\kappa = 0$), there is no disruption in that participant. In contrast, data scattered along a negatively sloping line ($\kappa < 0$) indicates some disruption in that participant. For instance, in comatose patients, high-degree nodes in the NC group showed a significant reduction of degree in the patients, while some low-degree nodes in the NC group showed a significant increase of degree in the patients, resulting in a significant negative slope for the patient group [65]. We expected that the ASC group would show some altered patterns in their local metrics. The hub disruption index was calculated separately for the three local metrics of degree κ_D, betweenness κ_B, and nodal efficiency κ_E. Of note, the calculation of the hub disruption index was performed on the normalized AUC metric of each local metric.

8. Statistical Analysis

8.1. Differences in network metrics. For between-group comparison of each of the metrics described above, permutation-based nonparametric tests with 5000 permutations were performed on the AUC of that metric, including age and gender as nuisance covariates. For each measure over the range of thresholds, two-sample two-tailed t-tests were performed in order to evaluate between-group differences, and a false discovery rate (FDR) correction was used for multiple comparisons [66].

8.2. Reproducibility of hubs. As described previously, hubs were identified using a predefined threshold for degree k, betweenness b, or nodal efficiency e. Although several studies have identified functional hubs according to this manner, it is difficult to confirm whether or not those hubs are reproducible. In this study, we evaluated reproducibility using the bootstrapping method [67]. Within each group, each of the local metrics was resampled, and then hubs were identified using the resampled data and a predefined threshold. This procedure was repeated 10,000 times, and then we counted the occurrence frequency of hubness at each node. Finally, we computed the summation of the frequencies across all the three metrics at each node as a score of hubness of the node. We regarded a node as a functional hub if its score was higher than 2.1 (i.e., the frequency at each local metric was greater than 0.7 on average).

8.3. Relationship between network metrics and AQ score. If a between-group difference in any of the global metrics or hub disruption indices was observed, we further investigated the relationship between the metric and the AQ score using a partial correlation analysis, with age and gender as controlling variables. For the local metrics, we repeated the partial correlation analysis only on nodes where significant group difference was found on all the three local metrics without correction for multiple comparisons, to minimize the problem of multiple comparisons.

Results

1. Global Network Metrics

The global metrics of assortativity r, clustering coefficient C, characteristic path length L, and small-worldness σ in each group are depicted in Figure 1. Figures 1A to D represent the mean and standard error of these metrics, calculated at each sparsity level. For other global metrics (i.e., global efficiency E_{glob}, local efficiency E_{loc}, normalized clustering coefficient γ, and normalized characteristic path length λ), see Figures S2 and S3. As shown in Figure 1D and Figures S2C and S2D, the networks of both the NC and ASC groups exhibited the small-world properties ($\gamma > 1$, $\lambda \approx 1$, and $\sigma > 1$) over the entire range of thresholds. The AUC analyses revealed that, while σ was comparable between the groups, r, C, and L were significantly lower in participants with ASC than in NCs (r: $p = 0.013$; C: $p = 0.014$; L: $p = 0.002$) (Figure 2).

2. Local Network Metrics

Group comparisons of the local metrics are shown in Figure 3 and Table S2. In total, we identified 28 nodes showing a significant group difference ($p<0.05$) in at least 1 metric: 5 in the fronto-parietal (FP) network, 6 in the cingulo-opercular (CO) network, 4 in the default-mode (DEF) network, 5 in the occipital

(OC) network, 5 in the sensorimotor (SE) network, and 3 in the cerebellar (CER) network. While increased local metrics in the ASC group were mainly observed in the OC network, reductions were found in the FP and CO networks (Table 2). Notably, all three local metrics were significantly decreased at the left anterior cingulate cortex (ACC) [−2, 30, 27] and right superior temporal sulcus (STS) [52, −15, −13] and increased at the supplementary motor area (SMA) [0, −1, 52] in the ASC group.

3. Hubness

Hubs were identified using each of the normalized local metrics and the bootstrapping method described previously. For the sake of simplicity, a node is referred to as a *common* hub if that node was identified as a hub in both groups, and a node is referred to as a *group-specific* hub if that node was identified as a hub in only one group.

In total, we identified 15 nodes that showed *common* or *group-specific* hub properties in the whole brain (Figure 4 and Table 3). Among those nodes, we found that five NC-specific hubs were in the right hemisphere (e.g., the bilateral STS, right dorsolateral prefrontal cortex (dlPFC), and precuneus), six ASC-specific hubs located bilaterally in the brain (e.g., the bilateral Heschl's gyri and bilateral precentral gyri), and four common hubs located mainly in the frontal and parietal regions (the bilateral temporoparietal junction (TPJ), right inferior frontal gyrus (IFG) pars opercularis, and precentral/IFG). For functional hubs identified based on each local metric, see Figures S4, S5, and S6. The existence of group-specific hubs indicates an alteration of hub organization in the ASC group.

4. Hub Disruption Indices

Consistent with the possibility of altered hub organization in ASC, the hub disruption index κ exhibited significant negative values for the ASC group in all three metrics (κ_D: $p = 0.007$; κ_B: $p < 0.001$; κ_E: $p = 0.006$) (Figures 5A to C). For instance, the right STS consistently held hub properties across all three local metrics in the NC group, and its averaged network topology in the ASC group was smaller than the normative network topology of the NC group; on the other hand, the right ventrolateral PFC (vlPFC) [46, 39, −15] consistently held hub properties across all three local metrics in the ASC group, and its averaged network topology in the ASC group was greater than the reference calculated from the NC group (Figures 5D to F).

5. Relationship between Altered Network Topology and the AQ Score

No significant correlation was found between the AQ score and any of the global metrics or any of the hub disruption indices. For the local metrics, we only focused on nodes that showed significant alterations in all three local metrics. Thus, the left ACC, SMA, and right STS were selected as candidates for further partial correlation analyses. As shown in Figure 6, we found significant correlations between the AQ score and two of the local metrics of the ACC (k: $r = -0.291$, $p = 0.049$; e: $r = -0.298$, $p = 0.044$), suggesting that the severity of autistic traits may be reflected in the alterations of nodal metrics.

Discussion

This study examined the topological properties of the resting-state functional brain network in participants with ASC using a graph-theoretical analysis. Participants with ASC showed significant decreases in clustering coefficient C and characteristic path length L, which is consistent with previous findings in adolescents

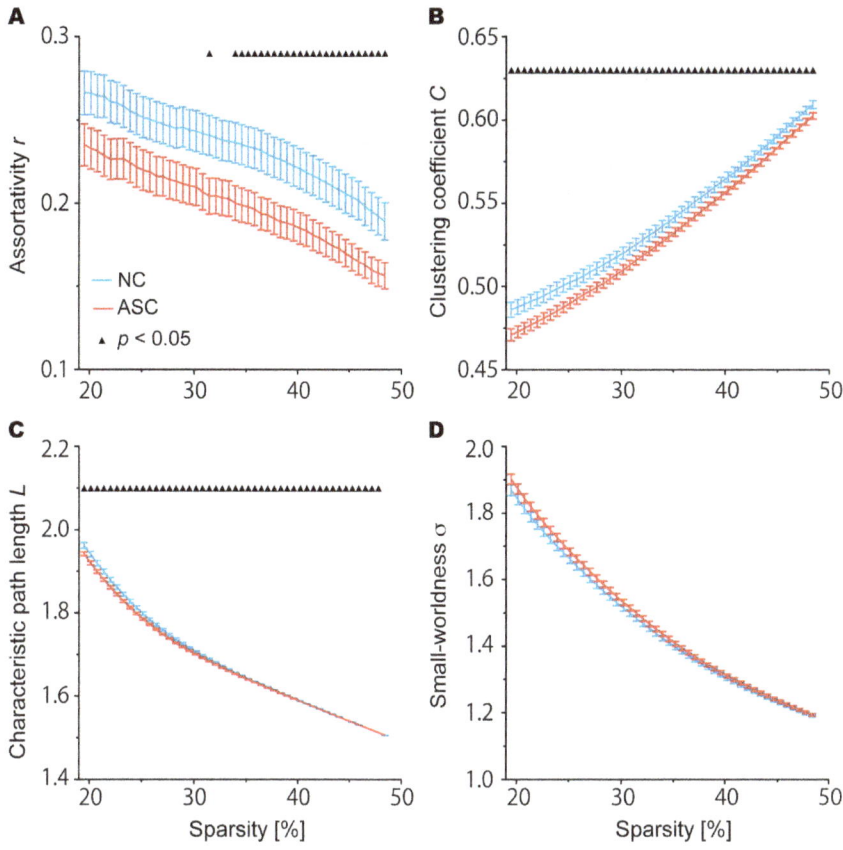

Figure 1. Global metrics of the assortativity, r; clustering coefficient, C; characteristic path length, L; and small-worldness scalar, σ as functions of the sparsity threshold. The ASC group (red line) exhibited lower C (B) and L (C) than the NC group (blue) over the range of sparsity thresholds ($p<0.05$, FDR corrected), while σ was comparable between groups (D). In addition, r was significantly lower in participants with ASC than in NCs over 33.9% of sparsity threshold values (A). The error bar indicates the standard error of the mean (SEM).

with ASC [39]. Furthermore, reduced assortativity was found in ASC, implying that high-degree nodes tended to connect with low-degree nodes to a greater degree in the ASC brain than in the neurotypical brain. These findings are consistent with the view

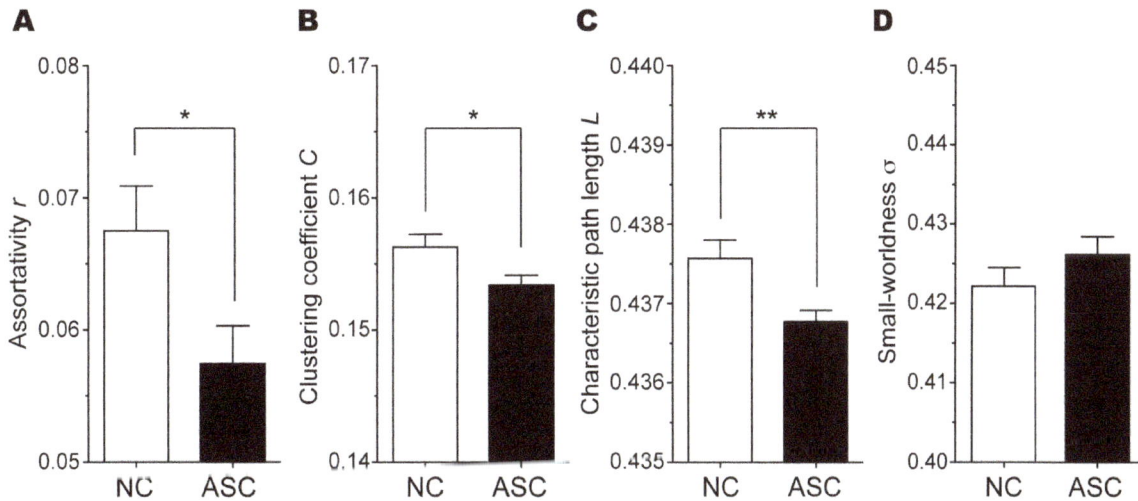

Figure 2. Between-group differences in the AUC values of assortativity, r; clustering coefficient, C; characteristic path length, L; and small-worldness scalar, σ. In the AUC analyses, participants in the ASC group (black) also showed significantly lower r ($p = 0.013$) (A), C ($p = 0.014$) (B), and L ($p = 0.002$) (C) than those in the NC group (white), whereas there were no significant differences in the small-worldness scalar σ (D) between the groups. The error bar indicates the standard error of the mean (SEM). Significance levels are represented by *$p<0.05$ and **$p<0.01$, respectively.

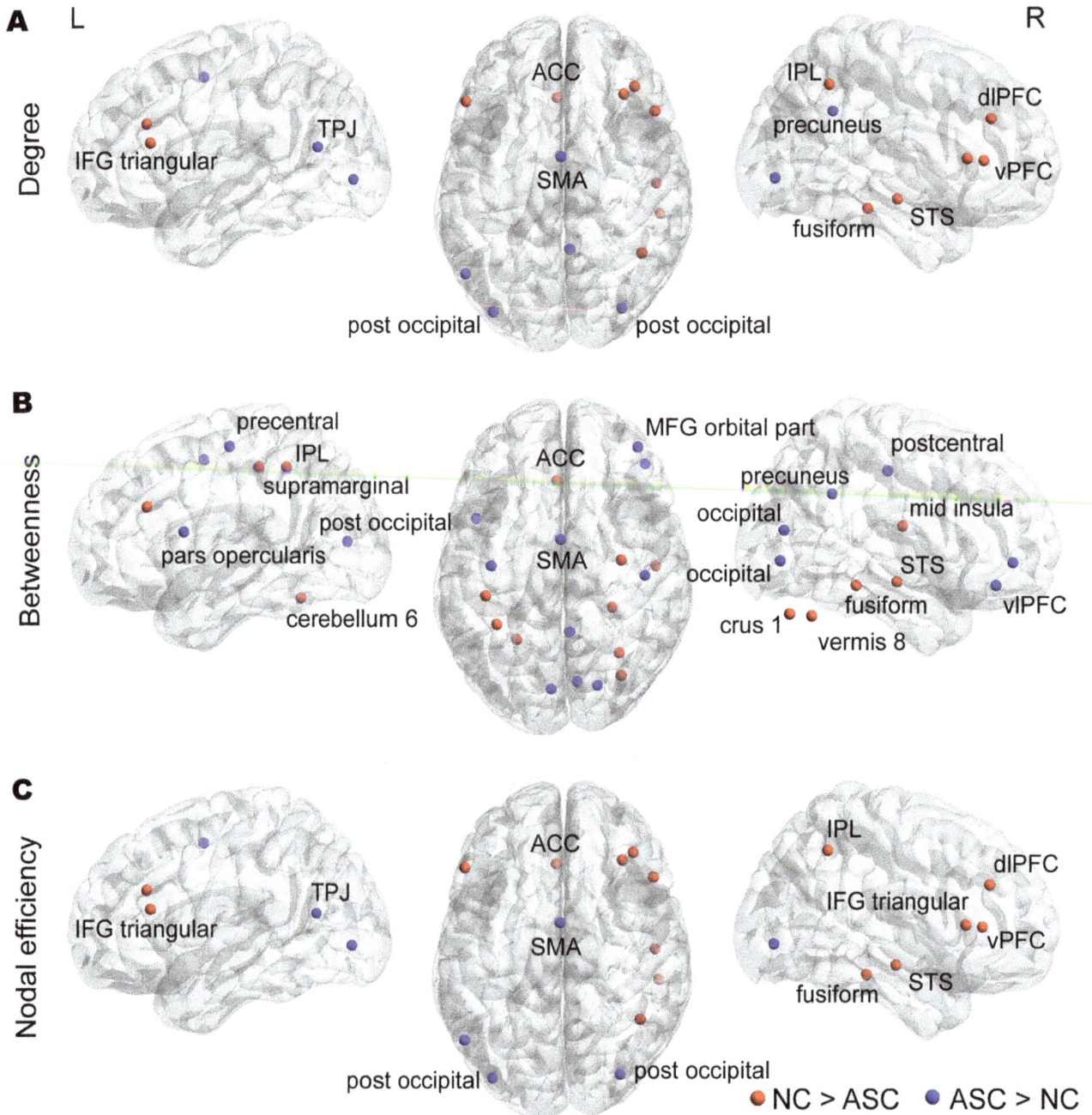

Figure 3. Altered local metrics of degree; betweenness; and nodal efficiency. Alterations in each of local metrics, including degree (A), betweenness (B), and nodal efficiency (C), were observed. The red sphere indicates NC>ASC, while the blue sphere denotes ASC>NC. Of note, in this study, the right inferior temporal [52, −15, −13] was regarded as the right superior temporal sulcus (STS), because this node was anatomically located on the STS rather than the inferior temporal. See Table S3 for other nodes re-labeled in this study. The distributions of nodes showing altered local metrics were visualized with the Brain Net Viewer (http://www.nitrc.org/projects/bnv/).

that network organization in the ASC brain shifts toward randomization compared to that in the NC brain [39,68]. In analyses of the local metrics, increases were observed primarily in the occipital (OC) and sensorimotor (SE) networks, while reductions were found in the fronto-parietal (FP) and cingulo-opercular (CO) networks in participants with ASC, compared with NCs. We also observed that, while both groups shared some nodes as common hubs, each group had several group-specific hubs, indicating changes in hub organization in ASC. Indeed, such changes were confirmed by analyses of all the three hub disruption indices. Subsequent partial correlation analyses demonstrated significant associations between the total AQ score and two local metrics (degree k and nodal efficiency e) of the left ACC. These findings indicate that the influence of nodes is significantly altered in the ASC brain and such alteration is particularly characterized by changes of "hubness" in several nodes critical for social and non-social cognition, both of which are profoundly impaired in people with ASC.

Table 2. The number of affected nodes (NC>ASC or ASC>NC) and non-affected nodes.

Type[†]	Affected nodes[††]		Non-affected nodes[††]
	NC>ASC	ASC>NC	
FP (21)	4 (19%)	1 (4.8%)	16 (76.2%)
CO (32)	4 (12.5%)	2 (6.3%)	26 (81.3%)
DEF (34)	2 (5.9%)	2 (5.9%)	30 (88.2%)
OC (22)	0 (0%)	5 (22.7%)	17 (77.3%)
SE (33)	2 (6.1%)	3 (9.1%)	28 (84.9%)
CER (18)	3 (16.7%)	0 (0%)	15 (83.3%)

[†]The numbers in parentheses indicate the number of nodes in each sub-network.
[††]The percentages in parentheses indicate the proportion of affected (or non-affected) nodes to the total number of nodes in each sub-network.
FP: fronto-parietal, CO: cingulo-opercular, DEF: default-mode, OC: occipital, SE: sensorimotor, CER: cerebellar.

1. Altered Global Network Organization in ASC

A recent study demonstrated that adolescents with ASC exhibited enhanced global integration (decreased characteristic path length L) and disrupted local segregation (decreased clustering coefficient C) compared with neurotypical counterparts [39]. Although almost all of the examined global metrics in adults with ASC were consistent with those previously reported for adolescents with ASC [39], only normalized clustering coefficient γ showed a discrepancy between adolescents and adults with ASC; while adolescents with ASC showed a significant reduction in this metric, it was comparable in adults (see Figure S2C). This discrepancy may reflect a normalization process from puberty to adulthood in ASC, which has been often observed for other structural measures (e.g., fractional anisotropy [69]). To investigate this possibility, future investigations need to directly compare data from the two developmental stages obtained in the same experimental setting.

In addition to C and L, we examined the assortativity r of the network; r quantifies whether nodes preferentially connect to nodes with similar degrees. A network is assortative if $r>0$ and random if $r = 0$ [70]. Compared with neurotypical brain networks, autistic brain networks were less assortative but not disassortative (i.e., $r>0$), providing further evidence of increased randomness in the network [39,68]. Given that functional connectivity used for constructing a network in this study could be considered as an indirect measure of anatomical connectivity, disruptions of anatomical brain network may possibly induce atypical organization of functional brain network in ASC. Indeed, several diffusion tensor imaging (DTI) studies have demonstrated that people with ASC show alterations in local anatomical pathways, such as the inferior longitudinal fasciculus and uncinate fasciculus [71]. Although no DTI data are available to confirm the link between anatomical and functional brain networks of ASC on a topological space, our findings on global metrics indicate that the tendency of increased randomness in functional network may reflect disrupted anatomical network organization in the ASC brain.

2. Alterations of Local Metrics in ASC

At the nodal level, increased local metrics of degree k, betweenness b, and nodal efficiency e, were primarily observed within the occipital (OC) and sensorimotor (SE) networks, while reductions were mainly observed in the fronto-parietal (FP) and cingulo-opercular (CO) networks in ASC. The FP and CO networks are thought to be critical for adaptive control and stable set maintenance, respectively [72,73]. Previous fMRI studies have

revealed that individuals with ASC often show abnormal activation or atypical connections within the FP network during cognitive control and executive function tasks [74–76]. Furthermore, a recent fMRI study using pattern classification analysis demonstrated that the degree of nodes within the CO network contributed to improved classification of the diagnostic status between neurotypical and ASC individuals [36], indicating significant functional alterations in the CO network that may be characteristic to ASC.

Within the CO network, the left ACC exhibited significant reductions in all three local metrics, together with significant negative correlations between the AQ score and k and e. Previous studies on ASC have reported reduced brain activation in the ACC during a number of different cognitive tasks [77,78], as well as during rest [3]. This region is thought to be important for various cognitive and affective functions, including emotional processing [79], conflict monitoring [80], and the learning and selection of high-level behavioral plans [81]. Together with these previous findings, our results suggest that malfunction of the ACC may contribute to impairments in these diverse cognitive and affective functions in ASC.

Notably, significant increases in all three local metrics were observed in the SMA, which is implicated in multiple roles mainly related to movement (e.g., memory-guided movement sequencing) [82]. Although motor dysfunctions may not be always included in the core clinical symptoms of ASC [83,84], clinical observations related to abnormal motions are frequently reported in people with ASC, raising the possibility that people with ASC may have motor network dysfunctions. Indeed, several neuroimaging studies have reported that people with ASC exhibit altered brain activity or functional connectivity in the SMA during motor tasks [85–88]. For example, Takarae et al. demonstrated reduced brain activation in the portion of the SMA (supplementary eye field) during visually guided saccades [87]. Taken together, increased local metrics in this node may reflect such atypical brain activation or connectivity that underlies motor dysfunctions in ASC.

3. Loss of Hubs in the Social-Communication Network of Autism

Several studies have identified functional hubs using several topological metrics (e.g., degree, betweenness, and nodal efficiency) [13–17,89]. In this study, most of the previously reported hubs were replicated using at least one of the three local metrics (e.g., the right precuneus, anterior insula, left inferior parietal lobule) (see Figures S4, S5, and S6), except in a few nodes (e.g., the SMA).

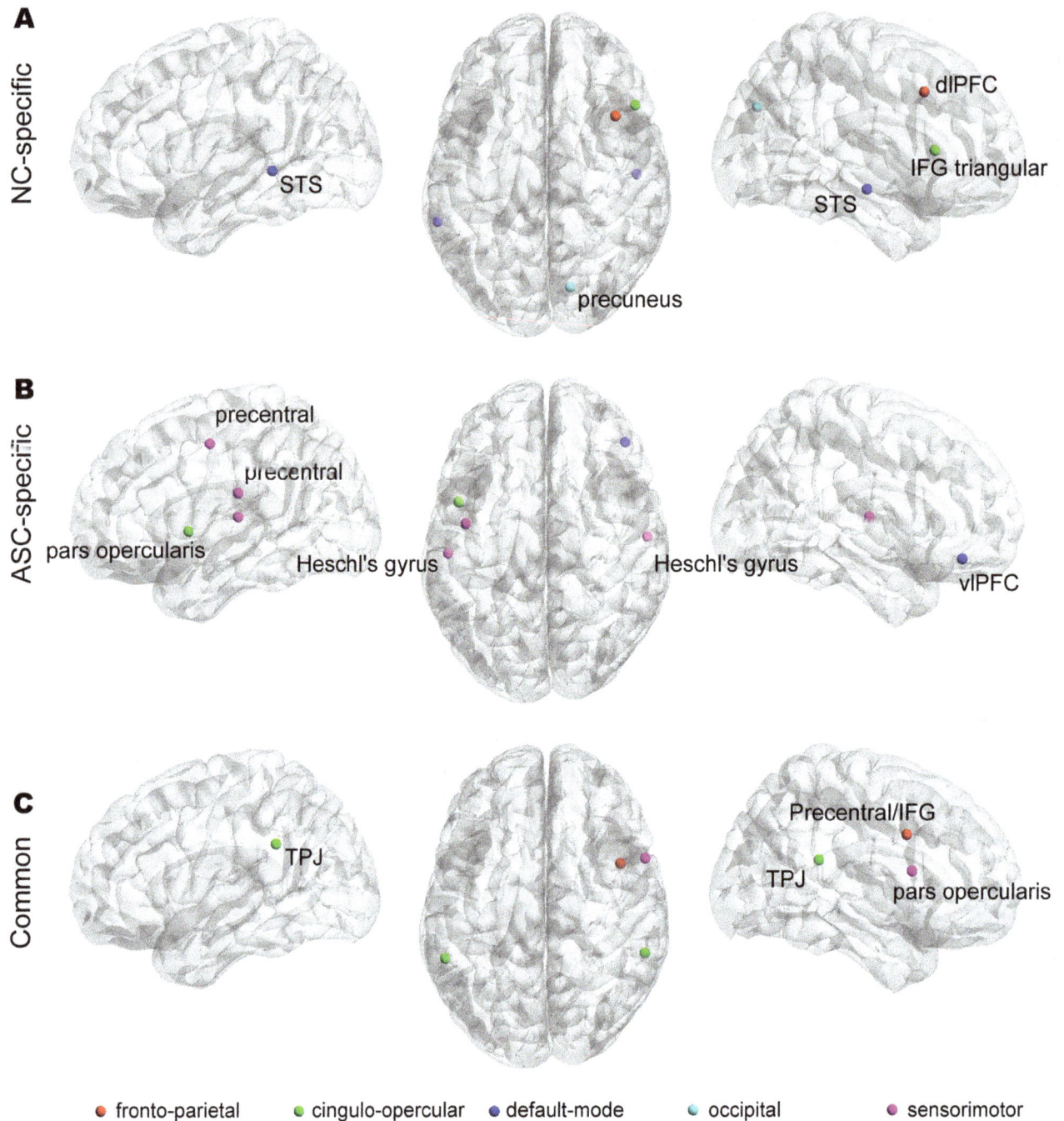

Figure 4. Hub nodes identified using the bootstrap method. The first row shows five NC-specific hubs (A), the second row shows six ASC-specific hubs (B), and the last row shows four common hubs (C). Hub distribution was visualized with the BrainNet Viewer (http://www.nitrc.org/projects/bnv/). Correspondences between colors and networks are as follows: fronto-parietal = red; cingulo-opercular = green; default mode = blue; occipital = cyan; sensorimotor = magenta.

Notably, four nodes (the right precentral/IFG, bilateral TPJ, and right IFG pars opercularis) were identified as common hubs, while five nodes (the bilateral STS, right dlPFC, and right precuneus) and six nodes (the right vlPFC, left IFG pars opercularis, bilateral precentral gyri, and bilateral Heschl's gyri) were identified as NC-specific and ASC-specific hubs, respectively.

Several lines of evidence suggest that dysfunction of the mirror neuron system (MNS) may account for a socio-communicative deficit, which is one of the core clinical symptoms in people with

ASC [90,91]. This system involves the right IFG and STS [92] and is thought to represent the actions of others and intentions associated with those actions. The right IFG is one of the central nodes in the MNS and is involved in directing social interaction [93]. Several studies have reported morphological and functional abnormalities in ASC, including reduced gray matter volume [94,95] and reduced neural activity during social tasks [96]. In this study, the right IFG pars opercularis was determined to be a hub in both NC and ASC networks, whereas functional connections

Table 3. A list of hub nodes identified using the Bootstrapping method.

Label	Coordinate	Type	Hub score[†]	
			NC	ASC
NC-specific hubs				
dlPFC R	40, 17, 40	FP	**2.48**	1.61
IFG triangular R	51, 23, 8	CO	**2.95**	1.10
STS R	52, −15, −13	DEF	**2.15**	0.38
STS L	−61, −41, −2	DEF	**2.43**	1.19
Precuneus R	15, −77, 32	OC	**2.31**	1.08
ASC-specific hubs				
IFG pars opercularis L	−48, 6, 1	CO	1.86	**2.85**
vlPFC R	46, 39, −15	DEF	0.45	**2.76**
Precentral L	−44, −6, 49	SE	1.75	**2.82**
Precentral L	−54, −22, 22	SE	1.12	**2.66**
Heschl's gyrus R	59, −13, 8	SE	1.93	**2.69**
Heschl's gyrus L	−54, −22, 9	SE	1.16	**2.32**
Common hubs				
Precentral/IFG R	44, 8, 34	FP	**2.71**	**2.28**
TPJ R	58, −41, 20	CO	**2.42**	**2.12**
TPJ L	−55, −44, 30	CO	**2.35**	**2.55**
IFG pars opercularis R	58, 11, 14	SE	**2.88**	**2.99**

[†]Hub score was calculated as the summation of frequencies across all the three local metrics, and then a node with high hub score ($\geq$2.1) was considered as a hub in this study.
FP: fronto-parietal, CO: cingulo-opercular, DEF: default-mode, OC: occipital, SE: sensorimotor.

between this node and several nodes (e.g., the right anterior insula and left ACC) were decreased for ASC, as indicated by functional connectivity analysis (see Figure S7 and Table S4). Although no over-connections with this node were observed in this study, a recent fMRI study reported over-connectivity between this region and others, involving the bilateral OFC, right putamen, and accumbens [97]. Therefore, the observation that the right IFG retained hubness in ASC in the presence of several reduced functional connections may be suggestive of the existence of complementary over-connection with other nodes, possibly at sub-threshold levels.

The right STS was the only NC-specific hub and showed significant reductions across all three local metrics in the ASC group. This region has been demonstrated to play key roles in several social perceptions, such as the perception of eye gaze and biological motion [93]. This node, particularly the posterior part of the STS, has been proposed as one of the core regions responsible for social perceptual impairments in ASC [98]. Consistent with this view, a number of previous studies on ASC have reported abnormalities in this area, such as cortical thinning [99], volumetric reductions [100], under-connectivity between this node and other regions (e.g., amygdala) [101], and atypical functional segregation of the posterior STS [102]. In this study, no under-connections with this node were observed, and no significant associations between any of the local metrics of this node and the AQ score were found. However, in support of the view of mirror neuron dysfunction, the loss of hubness in the right STS together with significant reductions in all three local metrics may underlie socio-cognitive deficits in ASC.

It is noteworthy that six ASC-specific hubs, including the right vlPFC, bilateral precentral gyri, bilateral primary auditory cortices

(Heschl's gyri), and left pars opercularis, were identified in this study. As shown in some behavioral studies [103,104], people with ASC have difficulties in the inhibition of inappropriate behaviors. A recent fMRI study demonstrated that, while neurotypical adults showed no recruitment of the right vlPFC, adults with ASC showed atypical hyper-recruitment of the right vlPFC during inhibition control to socially relevant stimuli [74]. Therefore, the hubness in this node may reflect the atypical functional circuitry in the ASC brain. In addition to deficits in social and communicative functions, people with ASC often show impairments in sensory processing. In particular, auditory hypersensitivity is one of the common sensory impairments in ASC, and several behavioral studies have reported deficits in auditory filtering [105–107]. A recent magnetoencephalographic study reported that children with ASC showed longer M50 and M100 peak latencies compared to neurotypical children and that those long latencies were negatively correlated with the severity of auditory hypersensitivity [108]. Furthermore, Hyde et al. recently reported increased cortical thickness in the bilateral primary auditory cortices in the ASC brain [109]. Although no clinical and behavioral data regarding altered sensations are available in this study, our findings on the primary auditory cortex may reflect abnormalities in auditory processing in ASC.

The altered hub organization revealed in this study was also summarized as a disruption of hub rank order. Even though declines in the hub disruption indices were moderate compared to those in comatose patients (ASC: $\kappa_D = -0.22$; comatose [65]: $\kappa_D = -0.82$), the ASC group still showed clear significant reductions of the indices in all three local metrics such that some hubs in the normal brain network (e.g., the right STS) were non-hubs in the ASC brain. Although no significant correlations

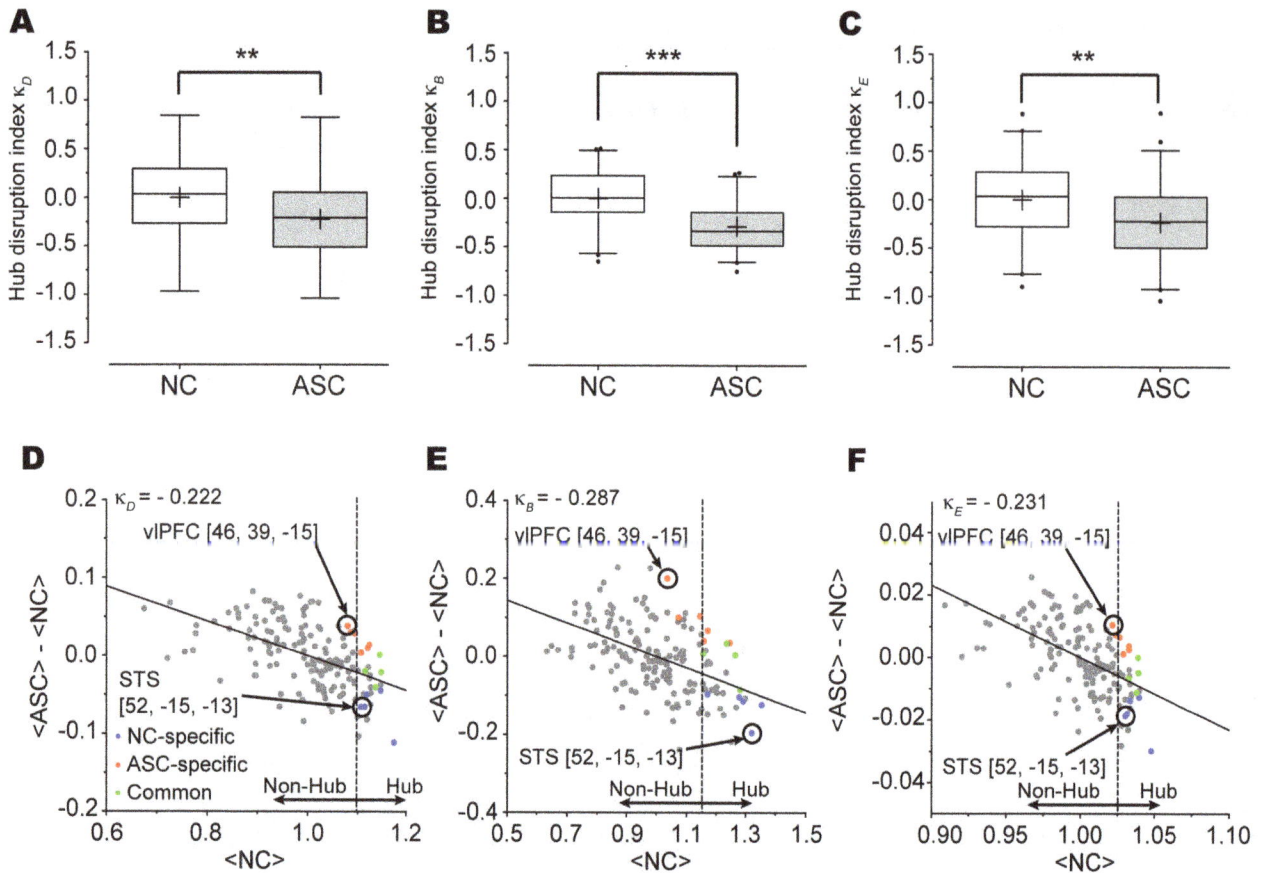

Figure 5. Hub disruption index for each of the three normalized local network metrics of degree; betweenness; and nodal efficiency. The ASC group (gray) exhibited significant reductions in all the three hub disruption indices (κ_D: $p = 0.007$; κ_B: $p < 0.001$; κ_E: $p = 0.006$) (A, B, and C). For illustrative purposes, each of the local metrics was averaged, and then the hub disruption index was calculated at the group level (D, E, and F). Each of hub disruption indices showed significantly negative values in the ASC group, indicating the disruption of hub organization. The colors represent the following groups: NC-specific hub: blue, ASC-specific hub: red, common hub: green. Of note, nodes with high hub scores (≥ 2.1) were considered as hubs in this study. Significance levels are denoted by **$p < 0.01$ and ***$p < 0.001$, respectively.

between hub disruption indices and the AQ score were found in this study, future studies are needed to address the possibility that a range of dysfunctions involving socio-communicative deficits, dyspraxia, auditory hypersensitivity in ASC might arise from changes in the order of node importance in functional brain network.

Consistent with our results regarding hubness and hub disruption indices, functional connectivity analyses revealed weakened functional connections between nodes in the large-scale system composed of the MNS, limbic system, and insula (see Text S2 and Table S4). The insula is anatomically connected with brain regions within the MNS and limbic system, and this system as a whole has been proposed to facilitate the understanding of other people's emotions through action representation [110]. Therefore, our results suggest that poor communication between the MNS and limbic system through the anterior insula may contribute to social cognitive and affective dysfunctions in ASC. In addition, reduced functional connections were also found in the motor network involving the precentral gyrus, cerebellum, and putamen, which may potentially explain ASC-associated motor deficits [86,87,111,112]. Taken together, our findings on functional connectivity are in line with the view that ASC is characterized by an array of dysfunctions including the hallmark deficits in social and communicative functions.

It would also be important in future studies to link the observed pattern of altered functional networks with molecular and genetic findings to advance our understanding of the pathological mechanisms of ASC. Molecular basis of ASC is associated with many of the synaptic cell-adhesion molecules, including neurexins, neuroligins, and cadherins [113–116], all of which play important roles in determining aspects of neural connections including synaptic formation and axonal guidance. Altered expressions of genes encoding these molecules might lead to the development of altered functional network for ASC that displays the characteristics of brain connectivity revealed by the present study.

4. Limitations

There are several limitations in the present study. Firstly, functional brain networks were constructed using the 160 functional ROIs defined by Dosenbach et al. [55], while previous studies have often employed anatomical ROIs (e.g., an automated anatomical labeling atlas). There is evidence that differences in node definition can affect the resulting topological architecture [117–119]. In addition, the set of nodes used in this study does not include certain limbic regions (e.g., amygdala) that are important in clinical populations. However, the set of nodes used here exhibited better reliability than the anatomical scheme for calculating the network topology [120], and the same node

A

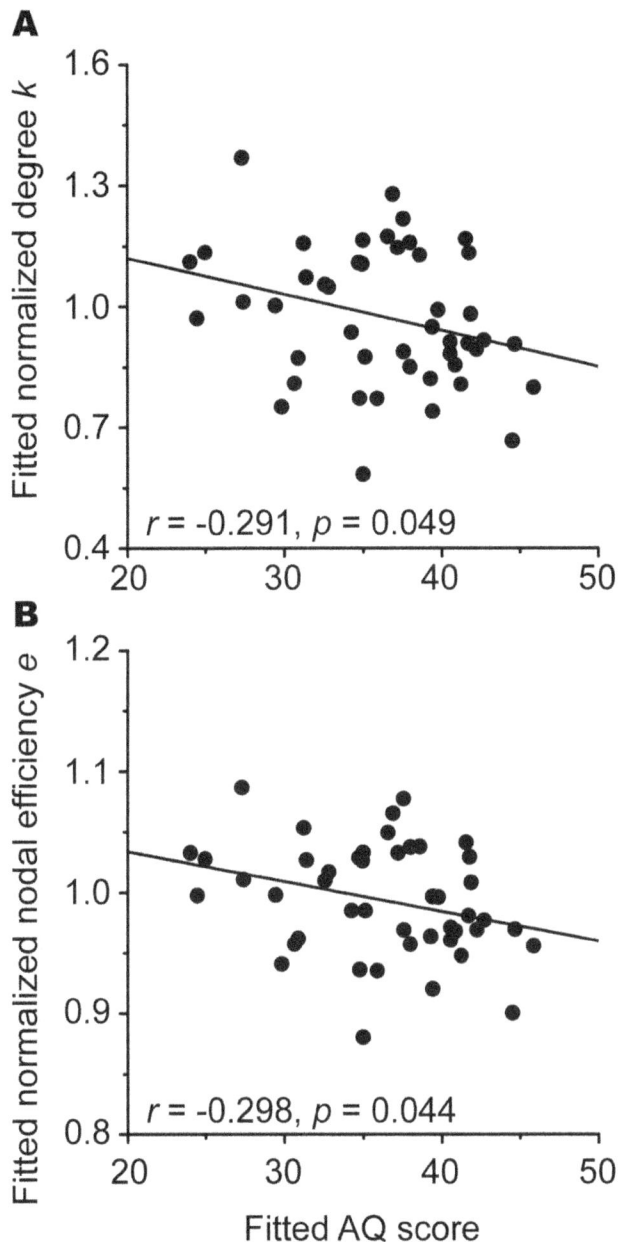

$r = -0.291, p = 0.049$

B

$r = -0.298, p = 0.044$

Fitted AQ score

Figure 6. Scatter plots of degree and nodal efficiency of the left ACC against AQ score. Partial correlation analyses revealed that there were the significant negative correlations between the AQ score and two of the local metrics of the ACC (k: $r = -0.291$, $p = 0.049$; e: $r = -0.298$, $p = 0.044$).

activities in different frequency bands have been reported in people with ASC based on electroencephalography (EEG) data [31,34]. In future studies, it will be important to examine the topological properties of the functional brain network in individuals with ASC using both electrophysiologically and hemodynamically derived signals.

Thirdly, some demographic information (IQ and handedness) was missing in this study. To validate our main findings, we repeated the second-level analyses of all the 8 global metrics on 39 NCs and 45 participants with ASC, and confirmed that, in spite of reduced statistical power, statistical conclusions were preserved for all the 8 measures (see Figure S8). Although gender differences might be one of the confounding factors, the small number of female participants ($n = 7$ in each group) did not allow us to draw statistically rigorous conclusions regarding possible gender effects on the network measures. Further investigations will be needed to examine the gender effects on the topological metrics.

Lastly, we examined the topological properties of the resting-state functional brain network, while state-dependent topological changes have been reported in ASC [36] and schizophrenia [25]. Hence, exploring network topologies during tasks would also be important for developing a complete understanding of the ASC brain.

Conclusions

Our findings revealed significant alterations in global network topologies, as well as changes in the order of node importance and the loss of hubness associated with social and non-social functions in ASC. Consistent with previous findings [39,68], our results suggest that the autistic brain network is likely to be randomized compared to the neurotypical one. At the nodal level, the left ACC and right STS might contribute to socio-communicative deficiencies in ASC. Advances in the modeling of functional brain networks have provided powerful methodological frameworks to reveal the neuronal alterations underlying atypical behaviors in ASC.

Supporting Information

Figure S1 Effects of the scrubbing method. Using the frame-wise displacement metric with a 0.5 mm threshold, the motion-contaminated volumes were detected in 16 NCs and 12 participants with ASC, respectively. The first row shows the effects of the scrubbing method for the average of 16 NCs (A to C), and the second row shows the effects for the average of 12 participants with ASC (D to F). The first column shows the correlation matrices for both groups, calculated without applying the scrubbing method (for simplicity, we will refer these as "standard") (A and D); the second column shows the correlation matrices calculated with the scrubbing method (henceforth, we will refer these as "scrubbed") (B and E); the last column shows the difference between the standard and scrubbed matrices (C and F). We observed slightly decreased correlation values in the short-range, and increased correlation values in the long-range after adopting the scrubbing method. For example, the correlation between the right vPFC [34,32,7] and right vlPFC [39,42,16] was decreased after the removal of motion contaminated volumes ($D = 14.25$ mm; $\Delta r = -0.01$), while the correlation between the right vmPFC [6,64,3] and left post occipital [$-37, -83, -2$] was increased after scrubbing ($D = 153.24$ mm; $\Delta r = 0.016$). FP: fronto-parietal, CO: cingulo-opercular, DEF: default mode, OC: occipital, SE: sensorimotor, CER: cerebellar, D: the Euclidean distance between node A and node B.

definition was used in several network studies [17,36]. Moreover, the fact that our findings on global metrics were consistent with the results of a previous study of adolescents with ASC [39] further supports the validity of our analyses.

Secondly, the frequency band of the analyzed resting-state brain activity was restricted to the low frequency range due to limitations in the temporal resolution of fMRI, and the relatively sluggish nature of the hemodynamic response. In this study, we applied a band-pass filter (0.009–0.08 Hz) to remove artifacts, because low-frequency spontaneous fluctuations of rs-fMRI signals within this range are thought to reflect neurophysiological processes of the human brain [121,122]. On the other hand, abnormal brain

Figure S2　Global metrics of global efficiency, E_{glob}, local efficiency, E_{loc}, normalized clustering coefficient, γ, and normalized characteristic path length, λ, as functions of the sparsity threshold. The error bar indicates the standard error of the mean (SEM). Compared with the NC group (blue line), the ASC group (red line) showed significantly higher E_{glob} and lower E_{loc} and λ ($p<0.05$, FDR corrected) over the range of sparsity thresholds (A, B, and D), whereas γ was comparable between the groups (C).

Figure S3　Between-group differences in the AUC values of global efficiency, E_{glob}, local efficiency, E_{loc}, normalized clustering coefficient, γ, and normalized characteristic path length, λ. In the AUC analyses, participants with ASC (black) exhibited significantly higher E_{glob} ($p = 0.02$) (A), and significantly lower E_{loc} ($p = 0.011$) (B) and λ ($p = 0.001$) (D), while γ was comparable between the groups (D). Significance levels are represented by *$p<0.05$ and **$p<0.01$, respectively.

Figure S4　Functional hubs were identified using degree and bootstrapping method. The first row shows ten "NC-specific" hubs, involving the bilateral anterior insula, left STS, the bilateral dlPFC, and right IFG triangular; the second row shows six "ASC-specific" hubs, including the right vlPFC, left precentral gyrus, and left Heschl's gyrus; and the last row shows five "common" hubs (the right dlPFC, left IPL, TPJ, and left IFG pars opercularis). Correspondences between colors and networks are as follows: fronto-parietal = red; cingulo-opercular = green; default mode = blue; sensorimotor = magenta. Hubs were visualized with the BrainNet Viewer (http://www.nitrc.org/projects/bnv/).

Figure S5　Functional hubs were identified using betweenness and bootstrapping method. The first row shows eight "NC-specific" hubs, involving the bilateral STS, left precuneus, the bilateral crus 1, and right IFG triangular; the second row shows 11 "ASC-specific" hubs, including the SMA, the right vlPFC, left TPJ, and right Heschl's gyrus; and the last row shows seven "common" hub, encompassing the bilateral precuneus, the right TPJ, the right IFG pars opercularis, and left precentral. Correspondences between colors and networks are as follows: fronto-parietal = red; cingulo-opercular = green; default mode = blue; occipital = cyan; sensorimotor = magenta; cerebellar = yellow. Hubs were visualized with the BrainNet Viewer (http://www.nitrc.org/projects/bnv/).

Figure S6　Functional hubs were identified using nodal efficiency and bootstrapping method. The first row shows nine "NC-specific" hubs, involving the bilateral anterior insula, the left STS, the left ACC, the right dlPFC, and right IFG triangular; the second row shows five "ASC-specific" hubs, including the right vlPFC, left precentral, left angular gyrus, and left Heschl's gyrus; and the last row shows seven "common" hub, encompassing the bilateral IFG pars opercularis, and right dlPFC.

References

1. American Psychiatric Association (2013) Diagnostic and statistical manual of mental disorders: DSM-5. Arlington, VA: American Psychiatric Publishing.
2. Uddin LQ, Supekar K, Menon V (2013) Reconceptualizing functional brain connectivity in autism from a developmental perspective. Front Hum Neurosci 7: 458.
3. Assaf M, Jagannathan K, Calhoun VD, Miller L, Stevens MC, et al. (2010) Abnormal functional connectivity of default mode sub-networks in autism spectrum disorder patients. Neuroimage 53: 247–256.

Correspondences between colors and networks are as follows: fronto-parietal = red; cingulo-opercular = green; default mode = blue; sensorimotor = magenta. Hubs were visualized with the BrainNet Viewer (http://www.nitrc.org/projects/bnv/).

Figure S7　Reduced functional connectivity in participants with ASC identified using the network-based statistic approach. The reduced connections were found mainly within the cingulo-opercular network rather than within the default mode network. Correspondences between colors and networks are as follows: fronto-parietal = red; cingulo-opercular = green; default mode = blue; sensorimotor = magenta; cerebellar = yellow. These reduced connections were visualized with the BrainNet Viewer (http://www.nitrc.org/projects/bnv/).

Figure S8　Between group differences in the AUC values of all the global measures performed on 39 NCs and 45 participants with ASC. The second-level analyses were reconducted on 39 NCs and 45 ASC participants to ensure that between-group differences were not due to differences in handedness. Statistical conclusions were preserved for all the global metrics (clustering coefficient: $p = 0.048$, characteristic path length: $p = 0.012$; assortativity: $p = 0.032$; small-worldness: $p = 0.083$; global efficiency: $p = 0.018$; local efficiency: $p = 0.044$; normalized clustering coefficient: $p = 0.170$; normalized characteristic path length: $p = 0.013$). Significance levels are represented by *$p<0.05$ and **$p<0.01$, respectively.

Table S1　Brief description of network metrics used in this study.

Table S2　Altered local network metrics (degree k, betweenness b, and nodal efficiency e) in the ASC group compared to the NC group.

Table S3　A list of re-labeled nodes in this study.

Table S4　Reduced functional connectivity in participants with ASC compared to NCs.

Text S1　The details of scrubbing method used in this study.

Text S2　Functional connectivity analysis.

Author Contributions

Conceived and designed the experiments: RH. Performed the experiments: TY HW MN RH. Analyzed the data: TI RH. Contributed reagents/materials/analysis tools: TI RH. Wrote the paper: TI RH. Supervision: NK KT DJ SS.

4. von dem Hagen EA, Stoyanova RS, Baron-Cohen S, Calder AJ (2013) Reduced functional connectivity within and between 'social' resting state networks in autism spectrum conditions. Soc Cogn Affect Neurosci 8: 694–701.
5. Di Martino A, Yan CG, Li Q, Denio E, Castellanos FX, et al. (2013) The autism brain imaging data exchange: towards a large-scale evaluation of the intrinsic brain architecture in autism. Mol Psychiatry.
6. Supekar K, Uddin LQ, Khouzam A, Phillips J, Gaillard WD, et al. (2013) Brain hyperconnectivity in children with autism and its links to social deficits. Cell Rep 5: 738–747.

7. Muller RA (2007) The study of autism as a distributed disorder. Ment Retard Dev Disabil Res Rev 13: 85–95.

8. Bullmore ET, Bassett DS (2011) Brain graphs: graphical models of the human brain connectome. Annu Rev Clin Psychol 7: 113–140.

9. Bullmore E, Sporns O (2009) Complex brain networks: graph theoretical analysis of structural and functional systems. Nat Rev Neurosci 10: 186–198.

10. Watts DJ, Strogatz SH (1998) Collective dynamics of 'small-world' networks. Nature 393: 440–442.

11. Achard S, Salvador R, Whitcher B, Suckling J, Bullmore E (2006) A resilient, low-frequency, small-world human brain functional network with highly connected association cortical hubs. J Neurosci 26: 63–72.

12. Bassett DS, Bullmore E (2006) Small-world brain networks. Neuroscientist 12: 512–523.

13. Tian L, Wang J, Yan C, He Y (2011) Hemisphere- and gender-related differences in small-world brain networks: a resting-state functional MRI study. Neuroimage 54: 191–202.

14. Fransson P, Aden U, Blennow M, Lagercrantz H (2011) The functional architecture of the infant brain as revealed by resting-state fMRI. Cereb Cortex 21: 145–154.

15. He Y, Wang J, Wang L, Chen ZJ, Yan C, et al. (2009) Uncovering intrinsic modular organization of spontaneous brain activity in humans. PLoS One 4: e5226.

16. Buckner RL, Sepulcre J, Talukdar T, Krienen FM, Liu H, et al. (2009) Cortical hubs revealed by intrinsic functional connectivity: mapping, assessment of stability, and relation to Alzheimer's disease. J Neurosci 29: 1860–1873.

17. Hwang K, Hallquist MN, Luna B (2013) The development of hub architecture in the human functional brain network. Cereb Cortex 23: 2380–2393.

18. Fair DA, Cohen AL, Power JD, Dosenbach NU, Church JA, et al. (2009) Functional brain networks develop from a "local to distributed" organization. PLoS Comput Biol 5: e1000381.

19. Fan Y, Shi F, Smith JK, Lin W, Gilmore JH, et al. (2011) Brain anatomical networks in early human brain development. Neuroimage 54: 1862–1871.

20. Meunier D, Achard S, Morcom A, Bullmore E (2009) Age-related changes in modular organization of human brain functional networks. Neuroimage 44: 715–723.

21. Menon V (2013) Developmental pathways to functional brain networks: emerging principles. Trends Cogn Sci 17: 627–640.

22. Kleinhans NM, Pauley G, Richards T, Neuhaus E, Martin N, et al. (2012) Age-related abnormalities in white matter microstructure in autism spectrum disorders. Brain Res 1479: 1–16.

23. Alexander-Bloch AF, Gogtay N, Meunier D, Birn R, Clasen L, et al. (2010) Disrupted modularity and local connectivity of brain functional networks in childhood-onset schizophrenia. Front Syst Neurosci 4: 147.

24. Bassett DS, Nelson BG, Mueller BA, Camchong J, Lim KO (2012) Altered resting state complexity in schizophrenia. Neuroimage 59: 2196–2207.

25. Fornito A, Zalesky A, Pantelis C, Bullmore ET (2012) Schizophrenia, neuroimaging and connectomics. Neuroimage 62: 2296–2314.

26. Liu Y, Liang M, Zhou Y, He Y, Hao Y, et al. (2008) Disrupted small-world networks in schizophrenia. Brain 131: 945–961.

27. Lynall ME, Bassett DS, Kerwin R, McKenna PJ, Kitzbichler M, et al. (2010) Functional connectivity and brain networks in schizophrenia. J Neurosci 30: 9477–9487.

28. Zhang J, Wang J, Wu Q, Kuang W, Huang X, et al. (2011) Disrupted brain connectivity networks in drug-naive, first-episode major depressive disorder. Biol Psychiatry 70: 334–342.

29. Bruno J, Hosseini SM, Kesler S (2012) Altered resting state functional brain network topology in chemotherapy-treated breast cancer survivors. Neurobiol Dis 48: 329–338.

30. Sanz-Arigita EJ, Schoonheim MM, Damoiseaux JS, Rombouts SA, Maris E, et al. (2010) Loss of 'small-world' networks in Alzheimer's disease: graph analysis of FMRI resting-state functional connectivity. PLoS One 5: e13788.

31. Barttfeld P, Wicker B, Cukier S, Navarta S, Lew S, et al. (2011) A big-world network in ASD: dynamical connectivity analysis reflects a deficit in long-range connections and an excess of short-range connections. Neuropsychologia 49: 254–263.

32. Tsiaras V, Simos PG, Rezaie R, Sheth BR, Garyfallidis E, et al. (2011) Extracting biomarkers of autism from MEG resting-state functional connectivity networks. Comput Biol Med 41: 1166–1177.

33. Li H, Xue Z, Ellmore TM, Frye RE, Wong ST (2012) Network-based analysis reveals stronger local diffusion-based connectivity and different correlations with oral language skills in brains of children with high functioning autism spectrum disorders. Hum Brain Mapp.

34. Peters JM, Taquet M, Vega C, Jeste SS, Fernandez IS, et al. (2013) Brain functional networks in syndromic and non-syndromic autism: a graph theoretical study of EEG connectivity. BMC Med 11: 54.

35. Jakab A, Emri M, Spisak T, Szeman-Nagy A, Beres M, et al. (2013) Autistic traits in neurotypical adults: correlates of graph theoretical functional network topology and white matter anisotropy patterns. PLoS One 8: e60982.

36. Barttfeld P, Wicker B, Cukier S, Navarta S, Lew S, et al. (2012) State-dependent changes of connectivity patterns and functional brain network topology in autism spectrum disorder. Neuropsychologia 50: 3653–3662.

37. Redcay E, Moran JM, Mavros PL, Tager-Flusberg H, Gabrieli JD, et al. (2013) Intrinsic functional network organization in high-functioning adolescents with autism spectrum disorder. Front Hum Neurosci 7: 573.

38. Di Martino A, Zuo XN, Kelly C, Grzadzinski R, Mennes M, et al. (2013) Shared and distinct intrinsic functional network centrality in autism and attention-deficit/hyperactivity disorder. Biol Psychiatry 74: 623–632.

39. Rudie JD, Brown JA, Beck-Pancer D, Hernandez LM, Dennis EL, et al. (2012) Altered functional and structural brain network organization in autism. Neuroimage Clin 2: 79–94.

40. Hua X, Thompson PM, Leow AD, Madsen SK, Caplan R, et al. (2013) Brain growth rate abnormalities visualized in adolescents with autism. Hum Brain Mapp 34: 425–436.

41. Amaral DG, Schumann CM, Nordahl CW (2008) Neuroanatomy of autism. Trends Neurosci 31: 137–145.

42. Courchesne E, Campbell K, Solso S (2011) Brain growth across the life span in autism: age-specific changes in anatomical pathology. Brain Res 1380: 138–145.

43. Langen M, Schnack HG, Nederveen H, Bos D, Lahuis BE, et al. (2009) Changes in the developmental trajectories of striatum in autism. Biol Psychiatry 66: 327–333.

44. Williams DL, Cherkassky VL, Mason RA, Keller TA, Minshew NJ, et al. (2013) Brain function differences in language processing in children and adults with autism. Autism Res 6: 288–302.

45. Dickstein DP, Pescosolido MF, Reidy BL, Galvan T, Kim KL, et al. (2013) Developmental meta-analysis of the functional neural correlates of autism spectrum disorders. J Am Acad Child Adolesc Psychiatry 52: 279–289 e216.

46. Baron-Cohen S, Wheelwright S, Skinner R, Martin J, Clubley E (2001) The autism-spectrum quotient (AQ): evidence from Asperger syndrome/high-functioning autism, males and females, scientists and mathematicians. J Autism Dev Disord 31: 5–17.

47. Matsuoka K (2006) Estimation of premorbid IQ in individuals with Alzheimer's disease using Japanese ideographic script (Kanji) compound words: Japanese version of National Adult Reading Test. Psychiatry Clin Neurosci 60: 332–339.

48. Nelson HE (1982) National Adult Reading Test (NART): For the Assessment of Premorbid Intelligence in Patients with Dementia: Test Manual. NFER-Nelson, Windsor, UK.

49. Nakano M, Matsuo K, Nakashima M, Matsubara T, Harada K, et al. (2014) Gray matter volume and rapid decision-making in major depressive disorder. Prog Neuropsychopharmacol Biol Psychiatry 48: 51–56.

50. Watanabe T, Yahata N, Abe O, Kuwabara H, Inoue H, et al. (2012) Diminished medial prefrontal activity behind autistic social judgments of incongruent information. PLoS One 7: e39561.

51. Oldfield RC (1971) The assessment and analysis of handedness: The Edinburgh inventory. Neuropsychologia 9: 97–113.

52. Wakabayashi A, Baron-Cohen S, Wheelwright S, Tojo Y (2006) The Autism-Spectrum Quotient (AQ) in Japan: A cross-cultural comparison. J Autism Dev Disord 36: 263–270.

53. Cao H, Plichta MM, Schafer A, Haddad L, Grimm O, et al. (2014) Test-retest reliability of fMRI-based graph theoretical properties during working memory, emotion processing, and resting state. Neuroimage 84: 888–900.

54. Liu Y, Liang M, Zhou Y, He Y, Hao Y, et al. (2008) Disrupted small-world networks in schizophrenia. Brain 131: 945–961.

55. Dosenbach NU, Nardos B, Cohen AL, Fair DA, Power JD, et al. (2010) Prediction of individual brain maturity using fMRI. Science 329: 1358–1361.

56. Behzadi Y, Restom K, Liau J, Liu TT (2007) A component based noise correction method (CompCor) for BOLD and perfusion based fMRI. Neuroimage 37: 90–101.

57. Murphy K, Birn RM, Handwerker DA, Jones TB, Bandettini PA (2009) The impact of global signal regression on resting state correlations: are anti-correlated networks introduced? Neuroimage 44: 893–905.

58. Power JD, Barnes KA, Snyder AZ, Schlaggar BL, Petersen SE (2012) Spurious but systematic correlations in functional connectivity MRI networks arise from subject motion. Neuroimage 59: 2142–2154.

59. Van Dijk KR, Sabuncu MR, Buckner RL (2012) The influence of head motion on intrinsic functional connectivity MRI. Neuroimage 59: 431–438.

60. van Wijk BC, Stam CJ, Daffertshofer A (2010) Comparing brain networks of different size and connectivity density using graph theory. PLoS One 5: e13701.

61. Rubinov M, Sporns O (2010) Complex network measures of brain connectivity: uses and interpretations. Neuroimage 52: 1059–1069.

62. Newman M (2003) The Structure and Function of Complex Networks. SIAM Review 45: 167–256.

63. Achard S, Bullmore E (2007) Efficiency and cost of economical brain functional networks. PLoS Comput Biol 3: e17.

64. Zhang Z, Liao W, Chen H, Mantini D, Ding JR, et al. (2011) Altered functional-structural coupling of large-scale brain networks in idiopathic generalized epilepsy. Brain 134: 2912–2928.

65. Achard S, Delon-Martin C, Vértes PE, Renard F, Schenck M, et al. (2012) Hubs of brain functional networks are radically reorganized in comatose patients. Proceedings of the National Academy of Sciences 109: 20608–20613.

66. Benjamini Y, Hochberg Y (1995) Controlling the False Discovery Rate: A Practical and Powerful Approach to Multiple Testing. Journal of the Royal Statistical Society Series B (Methodological) 57: 289–300.

67. Efron B (1979) Bootstrap Methods: Another Look at the Jackknife. The Annals of Statistics 7: 1–26.

68. Lai MC, Lombardo MV, Chakrabarti B, Sadek SA, Pasco G, et al. (2010) A shift to randomness of brain oscillations in people with autism. Biol Psychiatry 68: 1092–1099.

69. Bakhtiari R, Zurcher NR, Rogier O, Russo B, Hippolyte L, et al. (2012) Differences in white matter reflect atypical developmental trajectory in autism: A Tract-based Spatial Statistics study. Neuroimage Clin 1: 48–56.

70. Newman MEJ (2002) Assortative Mixing in Networks. Physical Review Letters 89: 208701.

71. Aoki Y, Abe O, Nippashi Y, Yamasue H (2013) Comparison of white matter integrity between autism spectrum disorder subjects and typically developing individuals: a meta-analysis of diffusion tensor imaging tractography studies. Mol Autism 4: 25.

72. Dosenbach NU, Fair DA, Miezin FM, Cohen AL, Wenger KK, et al. (2007) Distinct brain networks for adaptive and stable task control in humans. Proc Natl Acad Sci U S A 104: 11073–11078.

73. Dosenbach NU, Visscher KM, Palmer ED, Miezin FM, Wenger KK, et al. (2006) A core system for the implementation of task sets. Neuron 50: 799–812.

74. Duerden EG, Taylor MJ, Soorya LV, Wang T, Fan J, et al. (2013) Neural correlates of inhibition of socially relevant stimuli in adults with autism spectrum disorder. Brain Research 1533: 80–90.

75. Greimel E, Nehrkorn B, Fink GR, Kukolja J, Kohls G, et al. (2012) Neural mechanisms of encoding social and non-social context information in autism spectrum disorder. Neuropsychologia 50: 3440–3449.

76. Just MA, Cherkassky VL, Keller TA, Kana RK, Minshew NJ (2007) Functional and anatomical cortical underconnectivity in autism: evidence from an FMRI study of an executive function task and corpus callosum morphometry. Cereb Cortex 17: 951–961.

77. Kana RK, Keller TA, Minshew NJ, Just MA (2007) Inhibitory control in high-functioning autism: decreased activation and underconnectivity in inhibition networks. Biol Psychiatry 62: 198–206.

78. Solomon M, Ozonoff SJ, Ursu S, Ravizza S, Cummings N, et al. (2009) The neural substrates of cognitive control deficits in autism spectrum disorders. Neuropsychologia 47: 2515–2526.

79. Etkin A, Egner T, Kalisch R (2011) Emotional processing in anterior cingulate and medial prefrontal cortex. Trends Cogn Sci 15: 85–93.

80. Botvinick MM, Cohen JD, Carter CS (2004) Conflict monitoring and anterior cingulate cortex: an update. Trends Cogn Sci 8: 539–546.

81. Holroyd CB, Yeung N (2012) Motivation of extended behaviors by anterior cingulate cortex. Trends Cogn Sci 16: 122–128.

82. Gaymard B, Rivaud S, Pierrot-Deseilligny C (1993) Role of the left and right supplementary motor areas in memory-guided saccade sequences. Ann Neurol 34: 404–406.

83. Dowell LR, Mahone EM, Mostofsky SH (2009) Associations of postural knowledge and basic motor skill with dyspraxia in autism: implication for abnormalities in distributed connectivity and motor learning. Neuropsychology 23: 563–570.

84. Dziuk MA, Gidley Larson JC, Apostu A, Mahone EM, Denckla MB, et al. (2007) Dyspraxia in autism: association with motor, social, and communicative deficits. Dev Med Child Neurol 49: 734–739.

85. Di Martino A, Ross K, Uddin LQ, Sklar AB, Castellanos FX, et al. (2009) Functional brain correlates of social and nonsocial processes in autism spectrum disorders: an activation likelihood estimation meta-analysis. Biol Psychiatry 65: 63–74.

86. Mostofsky SH, Powell SK, Simmonds DJ, Goldberg MC, Caffo B, et al. (2009) Decreased connectivity and cerebellar activity in autism during motor task performance. Brain 132: 2413–2425.

87. Takarae Y, Minshew NJ, Luna B, Sweeney JA (2007) Atypical involvement of frontostriatal systems during sensorimotor control in autism. Psychiatry Res 156: 117–127.

88. Muller RA, Cauich C, Rubio MA, Mizuno A, Courchesne E (2004) Abnormal activity patterns in premotor cortex during sequence learning in autistic patients. Biol Psychiatry 56: 323–332.

89. Power JD, Schlaggar BL, Lessov-Schlaggar CN, Petersen SE (2013) Evidence for hubs in human functional brain networks. Neuron 79: 798–813.

90. Iacoboni M, Dapretto M (2006) The mirror neuron system and the consequences of its dysfunction. Nat Rev Neurosci 7: 942–951.

91. Rizzolatti G, Fabbri-Destro M, Cattaneo L (2009) Mirror neurons and their clinical relevance. Nat Clin Pract Neurol 5: 24–34.

92. Rizzolatti G, Fabbri-Destro M (2008) The mirror system and its role in social cognition. Curr Opin Neurobiol 18: 179–184.

93. Blakemore SJ (2008) The social brain in adolescence. Nat Rev Neurosci 9: 267–277.

94. Kosaka H, Omori M, Munesue T, Ishitobi M, Matsumura Y, et al. (2010) Smaller insula and inferior frontal volumes in young adults with pervasive developmental disorders. Neuroimage 50: 1357–1363.

95. Yamasaki S, Yamasue H, Abe O, Suga M, Yamada H, et al. (2010) Reduced gray matter volume of pars opercularis is associated with impaired social communication in high-functioning autism spectrum disorders. Biol Psychiatry 68: 1141–1147.

96. Kana RK, Libero LE, Hu CP, Deshpande HD, Colburn JS (2012) Functional Brain Networks and White Matter Underlying Theory-of-Mind in Autism. Social Cognitive and Affective Neuroscience.

97. Rudie JD, Shehzad Z, Hernandez LM, Colich NL, Bookheimer SY, et al. (2012) Reduced functional integration and segregation of distributed neural systems underlying social and emotional information processing in autism spectrum disorders. Cereb Cortex 22: 1025–1037.

98. Pelphrey KA, Carter EJ (2008) Brain mechanisms for social perception: lessons from autism and typical development. Ann N Y Acad Sci 1145: 283–299.

99. Hadjikhani N, Joseph RM, Snyder J, Tager-Flusberg H (2006) Anatomical differences in the mirror neuron system and social cognition network in autism. Cereb Cortex 16: 1276–1282.

100. Boddaert N, Chabane N, Gervais H, Good CD, Bourgeois M, et al. (2004) Superior temporal sulcus anatomical abnormalities in childhood autism: a voxel-based morphometry MRI study. Neuroimage 23: 364–369.

101. Abrams DA, Lynch CJ, Cheng KM, Phillips J, Supekar K, et al. (2013) Underconnectivity between voice-selective cortex and reward circuitry in children with autism. Proceedings of the National Academy of Sciences 110: 12060–12065.

102. Shih P, Keehn B, Oram JK, Leyden KM, Keown CL, et al. (2011) Functional differentiation of posterior superior temporal sulcus in autism: a functional connectivity magnetic resonance imaging study. Biol Psychiatry 70: 270–277.

103. Christ SE, Holt DD, White DA, Green L (2007) Inhibitory control in children with autism spectrum disorder. J Autism Dev Disord 37: 1155–1165.

104. Mosconi MW, Kay M, D'Cruz AM, Seidenfeld A, Guter S, et al. (2009) Impaired inhibitory control is associated with higher-order repetitive behaviors in autism spectrum disorders. Psychol Med 39: 1559–1566.

105. Ashburner J, Ziviani J, Rodger S (2008) Sensory processing and classroom emotional, behavioral, and educational outcomes in children with autism spectrum disorder. Am J Occup Ther 62: 564–573.

106. Dunn MA, Gomes H, Gravel J (2008) Mismatch negativity in children with autism and typical development. J Autism Dev Disord 38: 52–71.

107. Lane A, Young R, Baker AZ, Angley M (2010) Sensory Processing Subtypes in Autism: Association with Adaptive Behavior. Journal of Autism and Developmental Disorders 40: 112–122.

108. Matsuzaki J, Kagitani-Shimono K, Goto T, Sanefuji W, Yamamoto T, et al. (2012) Differential responses of primary auditory cortex in autistic spectrum disorder with auditory hypersensitivity. Neuroreport 23: 113–118.

109. Hyde KL, Samson F, Evans AC, Mottron L (2010) Neuroanatomical differences in brain areas implicated in perceptual and other core features of autism revealed by cortical thickness analysis and voxel-based morphometry. Hum Brain Mapp 31: 556–566.

110. Carr L, Iacoboni M, Dubeau MC, Mazziotta JC, Lenzi GL (2003) Neural mechanisms of empathy in humans: a relay from neural systems for imitation to limbic areas. Proc Natl Acad Sci U S A 100: 5497–5502.

111. Allen G, Muller RA, Courchesne E (2004) Cerebellar function in autism: functional magnetic resonance image activation during a simple motor task. Biol Psychiatry 56: 269–278.

112. Nebel MB, Joel SE, Muschelli J, Barber AD, Caffo BS, et al. (2012) Disruption of functional organization within the primary motor cortex in children with autism. Hum Brain Mapp.

113. Arons MH, Thynne CJ, Grabrucker AM, Li D, Schoen M, et al. (2012) Autism-associated mutations in ProSAP2/Shank3 impair synaptic transmission and neurexin-neuroligin-mediated transsynaptic signaling. J Neurosci 32: 14966–14978.

114. Foldy C, Malenka RC, Sudhof TC (2013) Autism-associated neuroligin-3 mutations commonly disrupt tonic endocannabinoid signaling. Neuron 78: 498–509.

115. Redies C, Hertel N, Hubner CA (2012) Cadherins and neuropsychiatric disorders. Brain Res 1470: 130–144.

116. Jamain S, Quach H, Betancur C, Rastam M, Colineaux C, et al. (2003) Mutations of the X-linked genes encoding neuroligins NLGN3 and NLGN4 are associated with autism. Nat Genet 34: 27–29.

117. Hayasaka S, Laurienti PJ (2010) Comparison of characteristics between region- and voxel-based network analyses in resting-state fMRI data. Neuroimage 50: 499–508.

118. Wang J, Wang L, Zang Y, Yang H, Tang H, et al. (2009) Parcellation-dependent small-world brain functional networks: a resting-state fMRI study. Hum Brain Mapp 30: 1511–1523.

119. Zalesky A, Fornito A, Harding IH, Cocchi L, Yucel M, et al. (2010) Whole-brain anatomical networks: does the choice of nodes matter? Neuroimage 50: 970–983.

120. Wang JH, Zuo XN, Gohel S, Milham MP, Biswal BB, et al. (2011) Graph theoretical analysis of functional brain networks: test-retest evaluation on short- and long-term resting-state functional MRI data. PLoS One 6: e21976.

121. Fox MD, Raichle ME (2007) Spontaneous fluctuations in brain activity observed with functional magnetic resonance imaging. Nat Rev Neurosci 8: 700–711.

122. Raichle ME, MacLeod AM, Snyder AZ, Powers WJ, Gusnard DA, et al. (2001) A default mode of brain function. Proc Natl Acad Sci U S A 98: 676–682.

## 9

Autism-Specific Covariation in Perceptual Performances: "*g*" or "*p*" Factor?

Andrée-Anne S. Meilleur[1], Claude Berthiaume[1], Armando Bertone[1,2], Laurent Mottron[1]*

1 The University of Montreal Center of Excellence for Pervasive Developmental Disorders (CETEDUM), Hôpital Rivière-des-Prairies, Montreal, Quebec, Canada, **2** School/ Applied Child Psychology, Department of Education and Counselling Psychology, McGill University, Montreal, Quebec, Canada

Abstract

Background: Autistic perception is characterized by atypical and sometimes exceptional performance in several low- (e.g., discrimination) and mid-level (e.g., pattern matching) tasks in both visual and auditory domains. A factor that specifically affects perceptive abilities in autistic individuals should manifest as an autism-specific association between perceptual tasks. The first purpose of this study was to explore how perceptual performances are associated within or across processing levels and/or modalities. The second purpose was to determine if general intelligence, the major factor that accounts for covariation in task performances in non-autistic individuals, equally controls perceptual abilities in autistic individuals.

Methods: We asked 46 autistic individuals and 46 typically developing controls to perform four tasks measuring low- or mid-level visual or auditory processing. Intelligence was measured with the Wechsler's Intelligence Scale (FSIQ) and Raven Progressive Matrices (RPM). We conducted linear regression models to compare task performances between groups and patterns of covariation between tasks. The addition of either Wechsler's FSIQ or RPM in the regression models controlled for the effects of intelligence.

Results: In typically developing individuals, most perceptual tasks were associated with intelligence measured either by RPM or Wechsler FSIQ. The residual covariation between unimodal tasks, i.e. covariation not explained by intelligence, could be explained by a modality-specific factor. In the autistic group, residual covariation revealed the presence of a plurimodal factor specific to autism.

Conclusions: Autistic individuals show exceptional performance in some perceptual tasks. Here, we demonstrate the existence of specific, plurimodal covariation that does not dependent on general intelligence (or "g" factor). Instead, this residual covariation is accounted for by a common perceptual process (or "p" factor), which may drive perceptual abilities differently in autistic and non-autistic individuals.

Editor: Leonardo Chelazzi, University of Verona, Italy

Funding: This work was supported by grants from CIHR (171795); Autism Speaks Foundation (2706) and the Frederick Banting and Charles Best Canada Graduate Scholarships Doctoral Award (CGS-D) (AASM). The funders had no role in study design, data collection and analysis, decision to publish, or preparation of the manuscript.

Competing Interests: The authors have declared that no competing interests exist.

* Email: laurent.mottron@gmail.com

Introduction

In addition to socio-communicative alterations, autistic individuals present lifelong behavioural characteristics related to visual and auditory perception [1]. These include hypersensitivity to noise [2], prolonged visual exploration of objects [3], early preference for geometric figures over social information [4], and early detection of cross-modal synchrony [5]. The prominence of these behaviours has led to the inclusion of sensory atypicalities and behaviours among the diagnostic criteria for the Autism Spectrum Disorder in the latest version of the Diagnostic and Statistical Manual of Mental Disorders (DSM-5) [6]. Note that, in keeping with the current consensus on language in autism research, the term "autistic" rather than "person with autism" is employed in a respectful way [7] [8].

Atypical perceptual abilities have also been demonstrated in experimental settings with tasks that assess low- and mid-level information processing. Low-level refers to the early stages of information processing upon entry into the perceptual system. This is mediated by primary cortical areas (e.g., visual area V1) that extract elementary perceptual dimensions (e.g., luminance-contrast, spatial frequency, pitch.) and send feedforward signals to mid-level cortical systems for further processing. Autistic atypical ities are mostly characterized by exceptionable extraction of low-level physical dimensions of auditory [9–12] (see Bhatara et al. 2013 [13]) and visual [14–18] (see Schwarzkopf et al. 2014 [19]) information. As a result, autistic individuals perform better in discrimination tasks than age- and intelligence-matched typically developing participants.

Mid-level perceptual mechanisms involve later stages of perceptual processing (i.e., extra striate, associative cortical areas, etc.) and the integration of low-level signals and grouping processes (e.g., pattern recognition and manipulation). Mid-level information processing is more susceptible than low-level systems to the influences of expectations and semantic knowledge. In autism, high performance in mid-level tasks is primarily the result of a non-mandatory influence of global/gestalt effects. High performances are consistently demonstrated during visuospatial tasks requiring pattern extraction, detection, matching and/or manipulation [20,21], but have also been documented in the auditory domain during musical tasks [22–24]. Some of these perceptual capabilities are evident as early as three years of age [25], indicating that high perception in autistic individuals manifests at various steps of processing in different modalities and relatively early in development.

Knowledge of how perceptual performances are associated within or across levels of processing and/or modalities is crucial to determine whether altered autistic perception results from the effect of a factor, or atypical process, specific to autism. Although high perceptual processing in both auditory and visual modalities has been associated with autism, most studies demonstrating autistic perceptual alterations have examined one modality or level in isolation. Therefore, it remains unknown whether high processing in a particular domain of perception is related to performance in other perceptual functions, levels and modalities, despite the frequent assumption that this is the case [26,27].

There is a correlation between perceptual and other cognitive abilities in typically developing individuals. Spearman used factorial analyses to suggest that correlation between diverse cognitive abilities may be explained by a general intelligence factor, which he labelled the "g-factor" [28]. In autism, recent data suggest that perception makes a strong contribution to intelligence and that its high autonomy involves the optional use of higher cortical areas (e.g., low functional activation of prefrontal areas) during the processing of perceptual and non-perceptual information [29]. The identification of a relationship between perceptual abilities, besides general intelligence in autistic individuals but not in typically developing individuals would provide evidence for a perceptual factor specific to autism. The existence of a general perceptual factor would be consistent with the Enhanced Perceptual Functioning (EPF) model of autistic cognition [30,31]. According to the EPF model, autistic cognition is characterized by a bottom-up processing style dominated by the strong activation of early neural mechanisms across perceptual modalities [32] and autonomy of perceptual processes toward top-down influences (i.e., a weak effect of expectations on percepts such as visual illusions [33]).

Research on autistic perceptual strengths and weaknesses has been largely conducted with control groups most frequently matched to the autism group with the Wechsler scale (i.e, FSIQ), and, to a lesser extent, Raven's Progressive Matrices (RPM) as a measure of intelligence [34]. The RPM assesses fluid intelligence, which is strongly associated with general intelligence in typical development. It is administered as a series of multiple-choice questions, requiring no verbal instructions. In contrast, the Wechsler Intelligence Scale, which is based on a multidimensional theory of intelligence, assesses different cognitive abilities to measure overall intellectual performance. Several of its subtests assess comprehension and verbal expression skills. Although the Wechsler Intelligence Scale is the most commonly used tool for cognitive assessment, RPM may be more suitable to measure intelligence in some people with a handicap that alters the encoding of information. For instance, children with a hearing impairment perform in the average range on the RPM, whereas they perform in the range for intellectual disability on the Wechsler verbal IQ scale [35]. This result supports the importance of using a measure of general intelligence tailored to the population being tested to obtain an adequate estimate of overall intellectual capacity without bias from secondary factors.

Although matching autistic and non-autistic groups with an intelligence measure is necessary to control for general cognitive ability between groups, the method used to match intelligence may also significantly affect the results and their interpretation. In some cases, significant differences in the performance of perceptual tasks between groups matched on Wechsler Full Scale IQ disappear when the same groups are matched on Raven Progressive Matrices [36], a measure that is considered by some as a more accurate reflection of autistic intelligence [37,38]. This lack of equivalence between measures of intelligence that are strongly correlated in typical development further suggests that the components of general intelligence in autism may differ from those in non-autistic individuals.

The main purpose of this study was therefore to determine how perceptual performances are associated within or across processing levels (low- and mid-level) and/or modalities (visual and auditory) in autism. We sought to examine the effect of intelligence on perceptual performances, and whether patterns of covariation differ between autistic and non-autistic individuals. Based on studies of intelligence, we expect that covariation between perceptual abilities are explained by general intelligence in typically developing individuals. In contrast, in autistic individuals, we expect to find residual covariation between perceptual abilities that is explained by another factor besides general intelligence. This residual covariation would be indicative of a hidden factor, which exerts a common influence on perceptual tasks, irrespective of intelligence (Figure 1a).

We chose a luminance-contrast discrimination task [39] and a modified block design task [40] to examine low- and mid-level visual processes, respectively. For auditory perception, we used a low-level pitch discrimination task and a mid-level melody discrimination task [41]. Tasks were chosen on the basis of evidence suggesting that they are able to detect high performances associated with autism. These tasks were selected to examine both the relationship between modalities and between different levels of processing. Figure 2 provides a schematic representation of the study's factorial design.

Methods

Participants

The target clinical population was comprised of adolescents and adults on the Autism Spectrum (AS). Forty-six autistic individuals and 46 typically developing (TD) participants completed the study. Most autistic individuals had delayed or abnormal language development, because this particular subgroup has been shown to have superior perceptual performance more consistently than AS individuals without developmental language abnormalities [10]. All but three autistic participants presented either a delay in speech onset (30/46) defined according to the ADI-R (first word onset after 24 months or first phrase onset after 33 months) or a score >1 on any of the following ADI items: immediate echolalia, stereotyped speech/delayed echolalia or pronoun reversal suggesting atypical language development (11/46). Standardized information on language development was not available for two participants without language delay or atypicalities in language development. These individuals were diagnosed with autism on the basis of expert clinical judgment and DSM-IV criteria only.

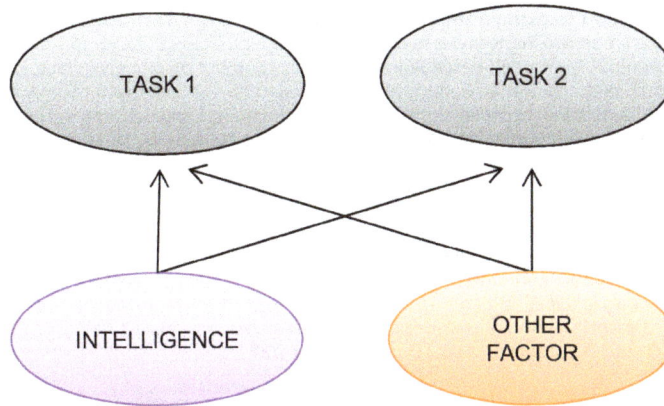

A. Generic Model

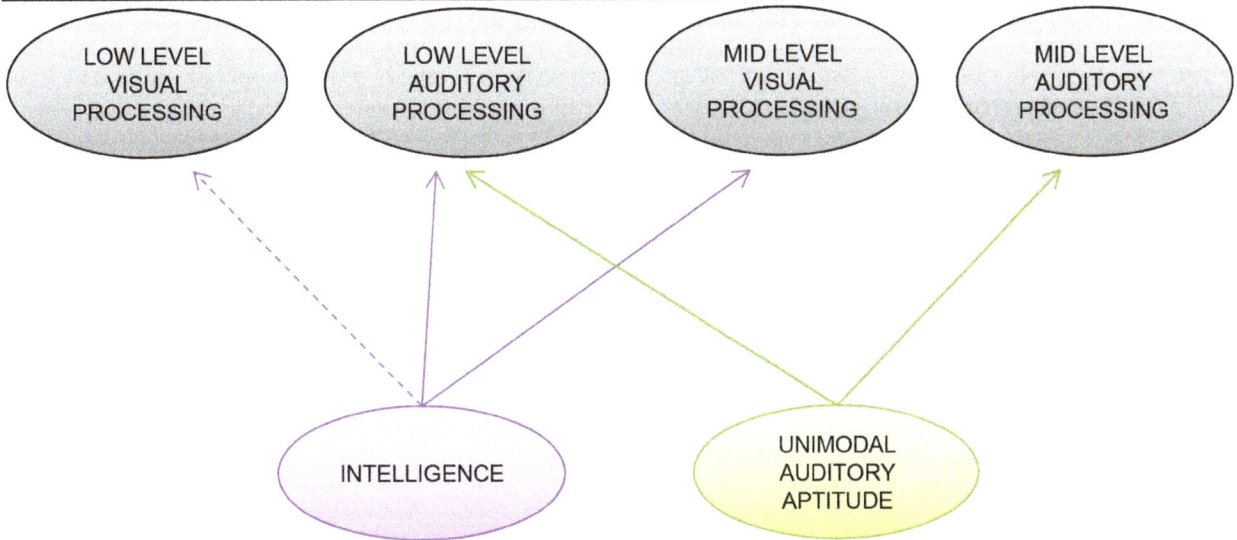

B. TD Controls

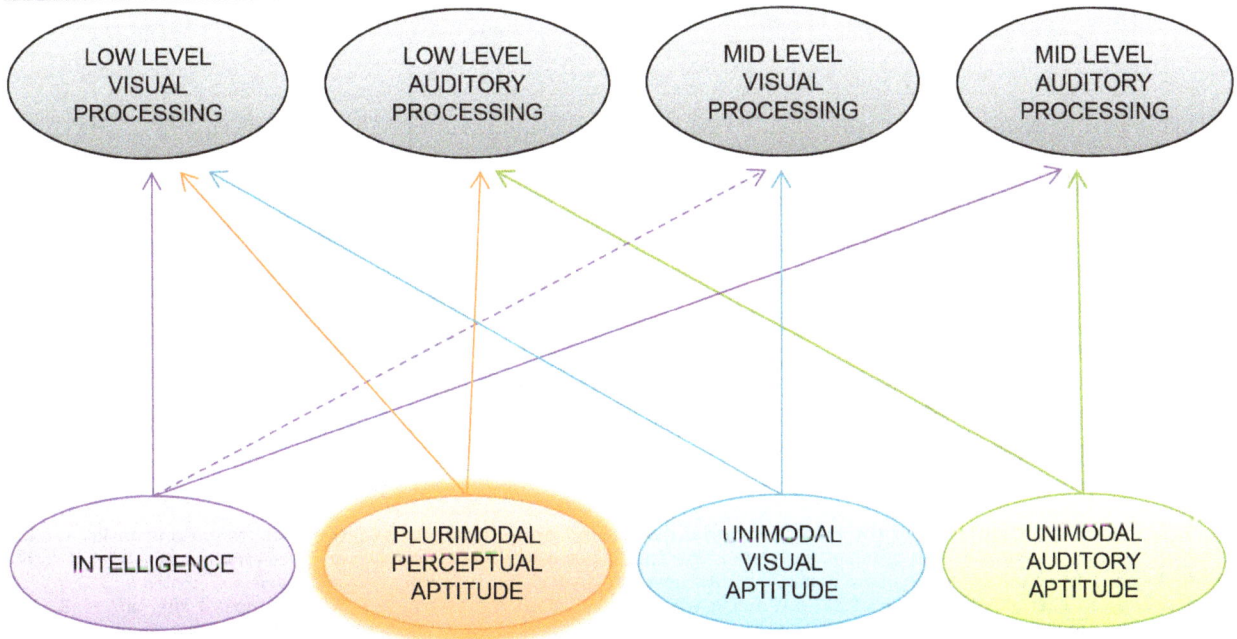

C. Autistic Individuals

Figure 1. Illustration of theoretical models to explain the pattern of covariation between tasks. Across all figures, experimental tasks are presented in the top row, in grey. Factors are shown in the lower row, in colour. The "Intelligence" factor (purple) includes the effect of RPM, FSIQ or both, depending on the variable and group. These models describe the significant contribution of a given factor (i.e., intelligence or other factor) to the variance of any given perceptual task performance. **A.** Generic model. Arrows from the same factor (here, intelligence) pointing towards two tasks (here, 1 and 2) indicate that the correlation between these two tasks can be explained by their common relationship with the factor, represented here as intelligence. In the example presented, the intelligence factor does not fully explain the variance of tasks 1 and 2, and a residual covariation attributed to "another factor" (orange), not dependent on intelligence, explains this residual correlation. **B.** (TD controls) and **C.** (Autistic individuals). Models that fit the observed patterns of covariation in this study for each group separately (statistics available in Table 2 and 4). The factors not dependent on intelligence, that contribute to residual covariations include: the "Unimodal Auditory Aptitude" factor (green), the "Unimodal Visual Aptitude" factor (blue) and the "Plurimodal Perceptual Aptitude" factor (orange). The "Unimodal Auditory Aptitude" factor is a common factor found in both autistic individuals and in the general TD population and explains the relationship between levels of processing within a single perceptual modality. The "Unimodal Visual Aptitude" factor is an analogue to the "Unimodal Auditory Aptitude" factor, but within the visual modality. This factor reaches significance only in the autistics group in the current study. The "Plurimodal Perceptual Aptitude" factor is different from the unimodal aptitude factors and is present only in autistic individuals. This factor is the main finding of the current study and is given the abbreviated "p-factor" label in the discussion. Full Lines: $p<0.05$; Dotted lines: $p<0.1$.

Participants were recruited from the «Centre d'Excellence des Troubles Envahissants du Développement de l'Université de Montréal» (CETEDUM) database. No Research Resource Identifier (RRID) can be provided for this population database because it is not publically available. Nonetheless, additional information regarding population characteristics can be requested within the limits of confidentiality. Forty-three autistic participants were diagnosed with the Autism Diagnostic Interview (ADI-R) [42] and/or the Autism Diagnostic Observation Schedule (ADOS-G) [43] (ADI only: three; ADOS only: two; ADI+ADOS: 38). Trained clinical professionals working at the specialized clinic at the Rivière-des-Prairies Hospital carried out both diagnostic tests.

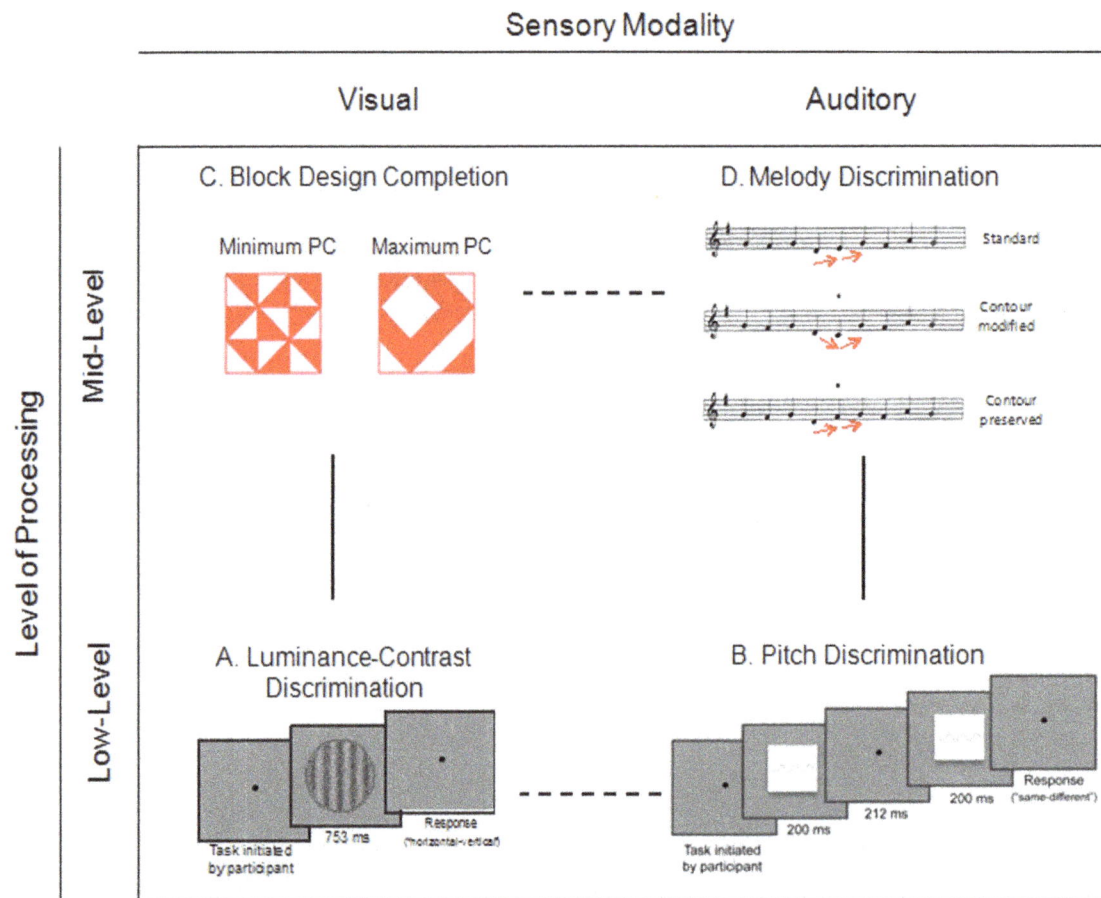

Figure 2. Schematic representation of the study's factorial design and presentation of experimental stimuli and tasks. The four experimental tasks are presented in each quadrant. Each task is characterized by a sensory modality (visual or auditory) and by a level of cortical processing engaged during task completion (low- or mid-level). **A.** Luminance-contrast (LC) discrimination: gratings were presented for 753 ms each and separated by an inter-stimulus interval of 271 ms, during which a noise mask was presented to minimize spatial after effects. **B.** Pitch discrimination: pure tones were presented for 200 ms each and separated by an inter-stimulus interval of 212 ms. **C.** Block design completion: examples of minimum and maximum perceptual cohesiveness (PC) models. **D.** Melody discrimination: examples of a standard melody compared to contour modified and contour preserved conditions. Red arrows represent contour direction. Lines represent relationships of interest in the current study. Full lines: unimodal relationships, between levels of processing; Dotted lines: plurimodal relationships, within levels of processing.

Three autistic participants were diagnosed based on DSM-IV criteria and expert (LM) clinical judgment. Neither TD participants nor their first-degree relatives had any history of AS, or other neurodevelopmental or neurological conditions. All participants completed the Autism Quotient (AQ) questionnaire [44]. One control participant reached a score of 30, which is above the recommended cut-off score of 26 [44]. This participant was excluded from the analysis of auditory tasks due to formal musical training; however, the participant was included in the analysis of visual tasks because his performance was comparable to that of other TD controls. All of the participants had a full scale IQ score above the range of intellectual disability (FSIQ greater than 70). Participants who could not complete practice trials (conducted a maximum of 3 times) and those who scored minimally in the first test items or did not complete enough trials to obtain a valid threshold measure, were excluded. The number of excluded participants by analysis is available as supporting information (Table S1). In addition, eight controls and three autistic participants with more than five years of formal music education, as measured with an in-house 20-item questionnaire, were excluded from the auditory task analyses [45,46]. Table 1 shows the descriptive statistics for age, AQ, intelligence, and baseline motor speed. Participants and their caregiver, for those under the legal age, gave informed, written consent. The research ethics committee (CER) of the Riviere-des-Prairies Hospital approved the study.

Stimuli and Procedure

All participants underwent preliminary visual and auditory acuity testing with standard tests [Runge test and Snellen chart for vision and a pure-tone audiogram (250–8000 Hz) for audition] and had normal to correct-to-normal vision; none of the participants had hearing aids or hearing loss. Testing was conducted in the auditory testing room of the Perceptual Neurosciences Laboratory (PNLab) for Autism and Development, located at Rivière-des-Prairies Hospital. This room is designed to minimize external noise and light sources. Auditory and visual stimuli were produced and presented via the DataPixx graphics and data acquisition toolbox and run on an Apple Macintosh G4 platform with an 18-inch Viewsonic E90FB .25 CRT (1280×1024 pixels) monitor refreshed at a rate of 75 Hz. The background of

the display was kept as a grey colour ($x = 0.2783 | y = 0.321$) with an average intensity of 40 cd/m^2, with a minimum (L_{min}) luminance value of 0.50 cd/m^2 and a maximum (L_{max}) luminance value of 89.50 cd/m^2. Auditory stimuli were presented to both ears simultaneously with Sennheiser HD280 earphones at an intensity of 65 db SPL. The stability of parameters defining the auditory and visual stimuli was assessed with a Quest 1100 sonometer and Minolta CS-100 colorimeter, respectively. All participants underwent preliminary visual and auditory acuity testing with standard tests [Runge test and Snellen chart for vision and a pure-tone audiogram (250–8000 Hz) for audition] and had normal to correct-to-normal vision; none of the participants had hearing aids or hearing loss. The auditory and visual tasks were carried out in a semi-randomized order to counterbalance for crossover, learning, and/or fatigue effects. Tasks involving the same modality were never presented in succession.

Low-level Visual Task. Luminance-contrast (LC) discrimination was examined with a task from a study by Bertone et al. (2005) [39]. In this task, participants are asked to fixate a dot on a screen and identify the spatial orientation of sine-wave static gratings by pressing the "right" or "up" arrow of a standard computer keyboard to indicate horizontal or vertical orientation, respectively. Gratings are a regularly spaced collection of identical, parallel, elongated elements. A sine-wave grating is a repeated number of fuzzy dark and light bars, or cycles defined by its level of luminance. An example of a vertically oriented sine-wave grating is shown in Figure 2a. Gratings were presented alone on the screen and the participant initiated each subsequent trial by pressing the spacebar of the keyboard; no time limit was imposed. The task started with five practice trials in which the participant needed to reach a minimum score of 80% correct before continuing to the experimental task. The task used a constant stimuli procedure to determine the identification threshold. Stimuli were presented 10 times for each level of luminance modulation (10%, 5%, 3.5%, 2%, 1.25%, and 0.625%) and for each orientation for a total of 120 trials. Spatial frequency was kept constant at 1 cpd. A Weibull psychometric function [47] was then applied to the set of responses to determine the discrimination threshold for a performance level of 75% correct. This measure of LC discrimination threshold served as the variable of interest (the lower the threshold score, the better the performance). Given that

Table 1. Descriptive statistics for all participants including age and Wechsler's Intelligence Scale IQ (FSIQ, VIQ, NVIQ) and Raven Progressive Matrices (RPM) scores: mean (standard deviation); range.

	TD Controls	Autistic Individuals	Statistics	p
n (males: females)	46 (38M: 8F)	46 (38M: 8F)	-	-
Age in years	20.20 (3.74); 18–28	20.57 (5.83); 14–36	t(76.669) = −.362	.718
Autism Quotient	13.74 (4.55); 7–30	25.93 (8.22); 9–45	t(70.177) = −8.802	<.001***
Wechsler FSIQ[a]	108.65 (12.59); 80–131	94.70 (15.41); 71–130	t(90) = 4.757	<.001***
VIQ	108.89 (12.23); 78–128	92.86 (19.64); 47–128	t(67.765) = 4.534	<.001***
NVIQ	107.33 (13.64); 79–133	99.70 (13.54); 71–131	t(88) = 2.659	.009**
RPM[b]	67.13 (23.00); 23–99	71.30 (22.10); 10–99	U = 927	.306
Motor speed in seconds	12.63 (3.63); 8.28–22.54	13.40 (3.42); 7.60–21,69	t(82) = .990	.325

[a]Standard scores on the Wechsler's Intelligence Scales;
[b]Percentile on the Raven Progressive Matrices; TD: Typically Developing, FSIQ: Full Scale IQ (n total = 92), VIQ: Verbal IQ (n total = 87), NVIQ: Non-verbal IQ (n total = 90), RPM: Raven Progressive Matrices (n total = 92); Significance levels:
*p<0.05,
**p<0.01,
***p<0.005.

values were very small, LC discrimination threshold scores multiplied by 100 were used in the analyses. This linear transformation had no effect on statistical significance.

Low-level Auditory Task. Pitch discrimination was used to investigate low-level auditory processing. Participants listened to a standard pure-tone of fixed value (500, 1000, or 1500 Hz), followed or preceded by a comparison pure-tone, and were asked to indicate whether the two stimuli perceived were the same or different (Figure 2b). Participants held a VPixx response box in each hand and pressed the top button of the box in the left hand if they thought that the pitch was the same and the top button of the box in the right hand if they thought that it was different. Subsequent trials were initiated 750 ms after the participant pressed the bottom button with either hand; no time limit was imposed. Thresholds for the three standard stimuli were obtained within a single adaptive staircase procedure, Harvey's ML-PEST [48]. Thresholds were measured 3 times and averaged to obtain an accurate threshold estimation for each standard stimulus. Before the experimental trials, each participant completed 10 practice trials and had to reach a minimum score of 80% correct responses before continuing the experimental task. The average pitch discrimination threshold served as the variable of interest (the lower the threshold score, the better the performance). The discrimination threshold is expressed as a Weber fraction (w): the fractional change in frequency required to discriminate each standard condition ($\Delta f/f$), where Δf is the minimum difference in frequency required to discriminate accurately between standard and comparison stimuli, and f is the reference standard frequency.

Mid-Level Visual Task. Hierarchical local-global processing of visual information was investigated with a modified version of the Block Design subtest of Wechsler's Intelligence Scale from Caron et al. (2006) [21]. This block design task incorporates a large range of difficulty and target figures that vary in their level of perceptual cohesiveness (PC). The PC level is manipulated by changing the number of opposite-coloured edges, or *edge cues*. The higher the number of edge cues, the lower the PC and the faster the task is completed. There were three PC levels: minimum, intermediate and maximum (Figure 2c), corresponding to easy, moderate and hard levels of difficulty, respectively. Task difficulty also increased with the number of blocks included in the model (4, 9, or 16). Participants were encouraged to work as quickly and precisely as possible. A time limit of 120, 180, and 240 seconds was established for the 4, 9 and 16 block models, respectively. A measure of baseline motor speed was obtained by administering a control condition consisting of a plain red target figure for each model size. Completion time for construction of the target figure was recorded, in seconds, with a standard stopwatch. Timing began upon presentation of the model and ended once the figure was completed or the time limit was reached. The variable of interest was the average completion time of the most difficult maximum PC condition in the six different trials (the faster completion time, i.e. the lower the score, the better the performance). Performance in the maximum PC condition was chosen as the variable of interest because it detects differences between groups with the highest level of sensitivity.

Mid-Level Auditory Task. Hierarchical local-global processing of auditory information was investigated with a melody discrimination task inspired by an earlier study by Peretz (1987) [49]. The melodies were made up of nine notes each lasting 350 ms except for the last note which lasted twice as long (700 ms). In the "contour-modified condition", a change in the frequency of one note resulted in a change in the interval direction, whereas in the "contour-preserved condition" a change in frequency did not alter the interval direction (Figure 2d). The modified note was either at the beginning, middle or end of the melody, but never the first or last note. There were a total of 48 trials, including 12 identical melodies presented twice, 12 contour-modified melodies and 12 contour-preserved melodies. Participants had to determine whether the two melodies presented were the same or different. Similar to the pitch discrimination task, participants held a VPixx response box in each hand and pressed the top button of the box in the left hand if they thought that the two melodies were the same and top button of the box in the right hand if they thought that they were different. The task started after two successful practice trials. Sensitivity d-prime values were calculated for each condition, which included 12 "different" and 24 "same" trials. The variable of interest was the level of sensitivity to changes in the most difficult contour-preserved condition, regardless of when the note change was made (beginning, middle or end). Performance in this condition was chosen as the variable of interest because it reflects sensitivity to local changes within a non-automatic situation that generally promotes global processing. For consistency with the other measures, mean d' scores are presented as inverted values, such that the lower the score, the better the performance. All values were converted to positive values by subtracting d' scores from a constant: inverted melody discrimination score $= 4 - d'$. This linear transformation had no effect on statistical significance.

Statistical Analyses

Experiments were designed and the results were interpreted to answer four questions, using two regression models. *Model 1:* 1) For each perceptual task, is the association between intelligence and performance the same for autistic and control groups? 2) Does the relationship between intelligence and performance depend on the measure of intelligence used (FSIQ or RPM)? 3) Does controlling for intelligence with FSIQ or RPM affect differences in performance between groups? *Model 2:* 4) Do patterns of covariation in task performances differ between groups?

Model 1: Effect of intelligence on performance and between group-differences in performances. Regression analyses conducted separately for each task and each measure of intelligence examined the effect of intelligence on performance and differences between groups in performance, with the following multiple linear regression model:

$$PERF = B_0 + B_1 * INTEL + B_2 * GR$$
$$+ B_3 * INTELXGR + residual$$

where PERF = task performance, INTEL: intelligence measure, RPM or Wechsler's FSIQ (z-scores), GR: group variable (0 if TD control, 1 if AS)

According to the coding scheme of the independent variables, B_1 indicates the expected linear increase in mean performance for a one SD increase along the intelligence scale, for the control group. B_3 indicates the expected between groups difference in linear increase in mean performance for a one SD increase along the intelligence scale. That is, $B_1 + B_3$ indicates the expected linear increase in mean performance for a one SD increase along the intelligence scale, for the AS group. B_2 indicates the expected between groups difference in mean performance, for groups with average intelligence (z-score = 0). When B_3 is not statistically significant and its estimate near 0, B_2 indicates the expected between groups difference in mean performance, in this case, constant all along the intelligence scale. When B_3 is statistically significant or its estimate not close to 0, the expected between groups difference in mean performance vary along the intelligence scale and could be estimated by $B_2 + B_3 *$INTEL.

Model 2: Between group differences in residual covariation in task performance. The following multiple linear regression model was used to analyse how covariation in performances differed between groups, taking into consideration the effect of intelligence (or *residual* covariation):

$$PERF1 = B'_0 + B'_1 * INTEL + B'_2 * GR + B'_3 * INTELXGR + B'_4 * PERF2 + B'_5 * PERF2XGR + residual$$

where PERF1 = performance in task 1, PERF2 = performance in task 2 INTEL = intelligence measure (Wechsler's FSIQ or RPM, z-score), GR = group (0 if TD control, 1 if AS).

According to the coding scheme of the independent variables, B_4 indicates the expected linear increase in mean performance at task 1 for a one unit increase in the performance at task 2 for the control group, while controlling for the effect of intelligence. In other words, B_4 is the expected residual covariation between tasks for the control group. Similarly, B_5 indicates the expected difference in residual covariation between groups. Thus, $B_4 + B_5$ indicates the expected residual covariation between tasks for the AS group.

Statistical significance was set at $p < 0.05$. For each model, assumptions (normality, linearity, homoscedasticity) were checked from residual analysis. Standardised residuals greater than 3 were considered as outliers and were excluded from the analysis. Baseline motor speed was added as an additional covariate if block task performance was part of the regression model (dependent or independent variable).

Results

Effect of intelligence on performance

Table 2 shows the main results from model 1. There was a statistically significant FSIQ X Group interaction for pitch and block, but not for the LC and melody discrimination tasks. However, when we controlled for intelligence with RPM, we found a RPM X Group interaction for LC and melody discrimination, but not for the pitch and block tasks. This finding provides a clear yes-answer to our first question, demonstrating that the effect of intelligence on performance is not the same for autistic and controls individuals. Consequently, between group difference in performance vary along the intelligence scale (graphs illustrating these differences are available as Figure S1).

Qualitative inspection of simple effects (Table 2) revealed that for TD controls, the association between intelligence and tasks (LC, pitch, and block) was stronger when FSIQ was used as an intelligence measure than when RPM was used. However, for autistic individuals, performance in tasks (LC and melody) was more strongly associated with RPM than with FSIQ. These observations provide a clear yes-answer to our second question, showing that the effect of intelligence on performance differs according to the measure of intelligence used.

It has been proposed that RPM is a better measure of general intelligence than FSIQ in autism; therefore, we carried out a complementary stepwise regression analysis to test the effect of FSIQ over that of RPM among controls, and the effect of RPM over that of FSIQ among autistic individuals. We began the analyses by including the least accurate intelligence measure in the model, and then added the most accurate measure. In controls, FSIQ contributed significantly to the regression model, in addition to the contribution made by RPM, for LC ($p = .077$), pitch ($p = .005$), and block ($p = .001$) tasks. However, in autistic individuals, RPM contributed significantly to the regression model, in addition to the contribution made by FSIQ, for LC ($p = .002$) and melody ($p = .003$) tasks. This finding will be considered during the interpretation of results of residual covariation, because inaccurate measures of intelligence can produce false positive conclusions.

Between group differences in task performance

Table 3 shows the expected group means, according to model 1, at average intelligence and at one standard deviation above average intelligence. When we controlled for intelligence with FSIQ, autistic individuals performed better in pitch discrimination and block tasks than controls, although there were no significant differences in performance in LC and melody tasks between groups. When we controlled for intelligence with RPM, autistic individuals performed better in the pitch discrimination task, whereas controls performed better in LC and melody discrimination tasks. Performance in the block task was not statistically different between groups. These findings provide a yes answer to our third question, because they show that between group differences in performance depend on the measure used to control for general intelligence (FSIQ or RPM). Interestingly, the difference in performance between groups with average intelligence was larger than between groups with an intelligence level one standard deviation above average, regardless of the measure of intelligence used.

Between group difference in residual co-variation in task performances

Table 4 shows the main results from model 2. In line with the yes answer to our first question (Is the association between intelligence and performance the same for autistic and control groups?), intelligence X group interaction was included in the 16 multiple linear regression models.

Plurimodal co-variation. The upper parts of Table 4 (a and b) show the residual covariation of performances between low- and mid-level tasks. When intelligence was measured by FSIQ (Table 4a), we found significant residual covariation for low-level tasks in autistic individuals. This residual covariation was significantly different from that of the TD control group. However, there was only a trend in covariation for low-level tasks in autistic individuals ($p < 0.10$) when intelligence was measured by RPM (Table 4b).

Unimodal co-variation. The lower parts of Table 4 (a and b) show results of the residual covariation of performances between visual tasks and auditory tasks. There was significant residual covariation for auditory tasks in both groups when intelligence was measured by FSIQ (4a). In addition, there was significant residual covariation for visual tasks in the autistic group. This residual covariation was significantly different from that of the TD control group. When intelligence was measured by RPM (4b), we found significant residual covariation for auditory tasks in the control group and significant residual covariation for visual tasks in both groups. We found no significant differences between groups, although trends ($p < 0.10$) were observed. These findings provide a yes answer to our fourth, and main question, showing a different pattern of residual covariation in task performance between groups.

Discussion

Summary of findings

In this study, we report the first systematic assessment of the association of autistic perceptual performance across processing

Table 2. Model 1 (Effect of intelligence on performance and between group differences in performances) main results: a. Wechsler's Full Scale IQ (FSIQ) or b. Raven Progressive Matrices (RPM).

a.

	FSIQ X Group	FSIQ Simple Effects				Group Effects[a]	
		TD Controls		Autistic Individuals		TD Controls vs AS	
	B3	B1		B1+B3		B2	
	p	estimate	p	estimate	p	estimate	p
LC	.267	-.082	.063	-.145	<.001***	-.050	.396
Pitch	.005**	-.795	<.001***	.006	.976	-1.329	<.001***
Music	.140	-.035	.807	-.311	.011***	-.142	.453
Block[b]	.034 *	-10.233	.001***	-3.348	.149	-15.909	<.001***

b.

	RPM X Group	RPM Simple Effects				Group Effects[a]	
		TD Controls		Autistic Individuals		TD Controls vs AS	
	B3	B1		B1+B3		B2	
	p	estimate	p	estimate	p	estimate	p
LC	.007**	-.045	.329	-.223	<.001***	.278	<.001***
Pitch	.270	-.715	.005**	-.310	.253	-.950	.012*
Music	.020*	-.055	.720	-.551	<.001***	.402	.046*
Block[b]	.760	-6.106	.013*	-4.995	.075	-5.444	.167

For a graphic representation, see Figure S1.

[a]AS: Autism Spectrum (Autistic) Individuals; TD: Typically Developing; B: Unstandardized regression coefficient. Negative B values indicate that autistic individuals perform better (i.e. lower score) than controls, and vice versa for positive B values;

[b]Baseline motor speed is added to the model; Significance levels:

*$p<.05$,

**$p<.01$,

***$p<.005$.

Table 3. Expected mean performance according to Model 1 at average intelligence and one SD above average intelligence a. Wechsler's Full Scale IQ (FSIQ) or b. Raven Progressive Matrices (RPM).

a.

| | Expected Means at FSIQ=0 SD | | | | | | Expected Means at FSIQ=+1 SD | | | | | |
| | TD Controls | | Autistic Individuals | | | | TD Controls | | Autistic Individuals | | | |
	Mean	SE	Mean	SE	p		Mean	SE	Mean	SE	p	
LC	0.832	0.044	0.882	0.039	.396		0.750	0.040	0.737	0.060	.859	
Pitch	3.022	0.202	1.692	0.183	<.001***		2.227	0.201	1.698	0.293	.142	
Music	2.719	0.140	2.577	0.125	.453		2.684	0.142	2.266	0.201	.093	
Block[a]	51.707	2.552	35.798	2.106	<.001***		41.474	2.323	32.450	3.416	.024*	

b.

| | Expected Means at RPM=0 SD | | | | | | Expected Means at RPM=+1 SD | | | | | |
| | TD Controls | | Autistic Individuals | | | | TD Controls | | Autistic Individuals | | | |
	Mean	SE	Mean	SE	p		Mean	SE	Mean	SE	p	
LC	0.809	0.042	1.087	0.051	<.001***		0.765	0.039	0.864	0.036	.066	
Pitch	2.920	0.208	1.970	0.303	.012*		2.204	0.231	1.660	0.185	.071	
Music	2.783	0.125	3.185	0.154	.046*		2.729	0.139	2.634	0.106	.590	
Block[a]	46.147	2.281	40.703	3.145	.167		40.040	2.023	35.707	1.803	.116	

[a]Baseline motor speed is added to the model. For FSIQ: predicted mean for motor speed = 12.875, For RPM: predicted mean for motor speed = 12.998; TD: Typically Developing; SE: Standard Error; Significance levels:
*p<.05,
**p<.01,
***p<.005.

Table 4. Model 2 (Between group differences in residual covariation) main results: a. Wechsler's Full Scale IQ (FSIQ), or b. Raven Progressive Matrices (RPM).

a.		Covariation	Covariation by Group			
Independent Variable →		X Group	TD Controls		Autistic Individuals	
Dependent Variable		B_5	B_4		B_4+B_5	
		p	estimate	p	estimate	p
Low-Level Tasks	Pitch→LC	.011*	−.002	.951	.134	.003***
	LC→Pitch	.179	.042	.964	1.691	.032*
Mid-Level Tasks[a]	Music→Block	.291	4.253	.220	−.438	.876
	Block→Music	.583	.006	.417	−.003	.841
Visual Modality[a]	LC→Block	.921	10.494	.386	9.076	.240
	Block→LC	.025*	.001	.558	.012	.008**
Auditory Modality	Pitch→Music	.452	.263	.005**	.392	.009**
	Music→Pitch	.111	1.003	<.001***	.441	.058

b.		Covariation	Covariation by Group			
Independent Variable →		X Group	TD Controls		Autistic Individuals	
Dependent Variable		B_5	B_4		B_4+B_5	
		p	estimate	p	estimate	p
Low-Level Tasks	Pitch→LC	.086	.019	.484	.113	.086
	LC→Pitch	.740	1.010	.273	1.423	.094
Mid-Level Tasks[a]	Music→Block	.312	3.524	.308	−.939	.737
	Block→Music	.815	.002	.819	−.002	.893
Visual Modality[a]	LC→Block	.190	24.509	.022*	8.261	.236
	Block→LC	.058	.002	.310	.010	.019*
Auditory Modality	Pitch→Music	.668	.211	.010**	.281	.077
	Music→Pitch	.092	.948	.002***	.296	.240

[a]Motor speed was also statistically controlled for; TD: Typically Developing, LC: Luminance-Contrast Discrimination Task; SE: Standard Error, B: Unstandardized regression coefficient; Significance levels:
*$p<.05$,
**$p<.01$,
***$p<.005$.

levels (low- vs. mid-) and modalities (auditory vs. visual), and we examine the role of intelligence in this covariation. Our main finding is that perceptual performances in auditory and visual tasks are associated in autistic individuals, and this association cannot be explained by intelligence alone. In the following discussion, we will propose a plausible interpretation of this finding and its relation with intelligence, in the context of the current literature.

Comparison of task performances between groups. The autism group outperformed the TD control group in the pitch discrimination (low-level, auditory) and modified block design tasks (mid-level, visual). These findings are consistent with previous studies demonstrating that autistic individuals perform better than non-autistic individuals in similar pitch discrimination tasks, which is now considered to be the most replicated low-level perceptual strength in autism (for a review, see Mottron et al. 2013 [31]). Autistic individuals showed a higher performance in pitch discrimination tasks than non-autistic individuals regardless of whether intelligence was controlled for with Wechsler's FSIQ or RPM. This suggests that such superior low-level auditory performance is not a by-product of a more (RPM) or less (Wechsler's Intelligence Scales) conservative IQ matching strategy. This supports the hypothesis that a fundamental difference in the

neural encoding of pitch underlies this autistic perceptual superiority.

In accordance with previous studies, we found that autistic individuals performed better than non-autistic individuals in the modified block design task; however, this was only true when the Wechsler's FSIQ was used as a covariate (see also Stevenson and Gernsbacher, 2013 [50]). Indeed, group differences were no longer observed when we controlled for intelligence with the RPM. This result is consistent with the findings of Dawson et al. (2007) [37]. They demonstrated that autistic individuals who performed on average within the 60th percentile in the block design subtest, versus the 25th percentile for TD controls with the same FSIQ level, had a mean RPM intelligence score also in the 60th percentile. This study demonstrated that particular perceptual performances in autism depend on the matching variable, with some peaks of ability disappearing when groups are matched with IQ measures that do not underestimate intelligence (i.e., RPM). In addition to the mid-level, block design task, a similar matching effect has also been found for other low-level visual tasks, such as inspection time [36].

In contrast, we found no differences between groups for performances in low-level visual and mid-level auditory tasks included in our design. Therefore, our analysis did not replicate previous studies controlling for Wechsler's FSIQ, in which autistic individuals [14] and children at risk of autism [15] were shown to be more sensitive to luminance-defined information than control individuals. Moreover, we found that the TD control group performed better in this task than the autistic group when we controlled for intelligence with RPM. In addition, our results do not replicate previous findings that autism is associated with a local processing advantage for melody processing, because TD controls of average RPM intelligence were more sensitive than autistic individuals to local changes in simple melodies. This discrepancy may be due to differences in task sensitivity between studies. Indeed, Bouvet et al. (2014) [24] showed that autistic individuals were more adept at detecting local elements within musical stimuli than RPM and Wechsler's performance IQ-matched controls; however, global to local interference was poorer in autistic individuals than in controls.

Overall, these findings suggest that although high performance in perceptual tasks is a defining indicator of atypical perception in autism, perceptual particularities cannot be simply interpreted as "stronger than typical" perception. For instance, autism-associated proficiency in the block design test results from autonomy from the top down influence of perceptual cohesiveness, which may or not result in exceptional performance according to the difficulty of the task [21].

Explaining the residual covariation between tasks beyond the g-factor: the *p*-factor

Figure 1 shows a plausible model that may account for the different pattern of covariation between tasks, and the relationship between tasks and intelligence observed among autistic and non-autistic groups. As indicated in the theoretical model accounting for our results, a significant part of the covariance in task performance could not be explained by intelligence both in the autistic and the TD control group, although different factors may account for this trend in autistic and non-autistic individuals (Table 4). Figure 1b and c shows a plausible model that may account for the different pattern of covariation between tasks, and the relationship between tasks and intelligence observed among autistic and non-autistic groups. For non-autistic participants, all observed covariation could either be explained by a common relationship with intelligence, or with a unimodal, auditory aptitude factor. A residual covariation between visual tasks is found in non-autistics when statistical control is made with RPM, but it vanished when the statistical control is made with FSIQ. Since the FSIQ is considered a more accurate measure than RPM in this group, the unimodal visual aptitude factor is not included in the model. However, in the autistic group, a different pattern of covariation emerges in which covariation across visual tasks and between plurimodal tasks requires additional, explanatory factors.

General intelligence (i.e., the g-factor) accounts for around one fifth of the variance in perceptual tasks in the typically developing population. Intelligence is typically related to performance in perceptual tasks such as inspection time [51], motion perception [52] or pitch discrimination [53] in typically developing individuals. According to the Cattell-Horn-Carroll theory [54], several broad abilities are responsible for the variance that cannot be explained by fluid and crystallized intelligence, or by their combination [55]. The proportion of variance that cannot be explained by intelligence increases with IQ, and has been attributed to the differentiation of specific abilities [55]. This explanation may also account for covariation in the autistic group that cannot be explained by the g-factor. Current data suggest *the differentiation of perception at large*, in addition to covariation

explained by the broad, modality-specific abilities in typical individuals. Accordingly, covariation of performance in low-level tasks involving *two different modalities* (thereby involving anatomically independent processing systems), as well as *two different levels of perceptual integration* (low- and mid-level), indicates that several perceptual abilities may be influenced by a specific plurimodal perceptual aptitude factor in autism. We propose to label this factor the *p*-factor, to distinguish it from the g-factor. Such an altered perceptual factor in autism is likely to underlie and generate cascade effects on several cognitive and adaptive mechanisms [56,57], including, but not limited to, various perceptual abilities across modalities.

Reports of these alterations suggest a model in which several genetic mutations promote the construction of local neural networks [58], which would plausibly have a greater effect on low-level coding mechanisms than subsequent, more complex stages of processing. According to several, recent systematic analyses and reviews, most mutations involved in autism converge toward enhanced plasticity mechanisms [59]. One hypothesis therefore is that the *p*-factor represents the interface between the final common genetic pathway of mutation involved in autism, and neurocognitive cascade effects. Both early visual and auditory sensory systems are selectively responsive to frequency-defined perceptual attributes (spectral or spatial frequency); therefore, we propose that atypical, probably overstimulated, tuning of frequency-selective mechanisms is a type of local alteration common to both perceptual modalities in autism. Frequency-selective mechanisms are modulated by the balance of excitatory/inhibitory activity which encodes elementary information [60]. Both animal and human studies have shown that GABA mediates this balance in both visual and auditory modalities [61–63]. The implication of altered lateral GABAergic inhibition in perceptual anomalies in autism is consistent with behavioural, physiological and genetic demonstrations of altered lateral inhibition within early visual areas in autism [56,64,65]. There is also evidence that high concentrations of GABA in humans are related to enhanced line orientation [61] and tactile discrimination thresholds [66], supporting the hypothesis that GABAergic mechanisms play an important role in cross-modal alteration of perception in autism.

Limitations and Conclusions

Our findings may have been influenced by the choice of task. Indeed, the identity of the *p*-factor that is responsible for perceptual covariation is unknown, and some tasks may be more dependent than others on this mechanism. This is the first study of its kind; therefore, the analyses were mostly exploratory and not corrected for multiple analyses. Statistical adjustments (Bonferonni type) became overly conservative when analyses involved correlated independent variables, or when analyses were repeated on multiple correlated dependent variables. Moreover, our analytic strategy was limited by samples size and the number of tasks. We recommend that large scale studies should be carried out in the future. Such studies should include several tasks within and between levels and modalities and use statistical methods such as factor analysis and structural equation modelling to identify the precise components of the perceptual *p*-factor. A similar study involving tasks associated with exceptional performance in autism (e.g. for mid-level auditory level [24] and for low-level visual level [67]) may also unravel strong effects.

The results of multiple linear regression analyses should be considered as underestimates of the link between observable performances and the unobservable *p*-factor. Furthermore, previous studies have assumed equal regression slopes when applying standard methods to control for intelligence (e.g., matching participants within groups). However, as demonstrated in this study, unequal regression slopes can indicate varying group differences along the intelligence scale and/or inaccuracy of the measure of intelligence used. This highlights the importance of testing this assumption whenever sample size and available data make it possible, regardless of the method of control (matching or statistical) and the measure of intelligence (e.g., RPM or Wechsler) chosen. Only then can we make accurate interpretations about the generalization of findings.

Supporting Information

Figure S1 Task performance – Intelligence relationships: groups differences. Raw performance for each experimental task (y axes) plotted on intelligence level (x axes). Autistic individuals are in green, TD controls are in blue. These graphs represent the statistics found in Table 2. The statistics presented in Table 3 can also be visualized on this figure by looking at differential group performances for intelligence levels at 0SD and +1SD. Note that the graph for the block design task does not exactly illustrate the statistics from Table 2 and 3 since a 2D

representation of the data could not include motor speed as a covariate.

Table S1 Number of participants excluded a. in each task, because of failure to complete task. Numbers in Table S1.a. also include the 3 autistic and 8 control participants with musical experience who are excluded solely from auditory task (i.e., Pitch and Music), and b. within regression analysis because of residuals >3 standard deviations.

Acknowledgments

We thank Dr. Kate Plaisted and HRDP autism research team members for comments on the manuscript, as well as our research assistant Chloé Paquin-Hodge for testing the participants.

Author Contributions

Conceived and designed the experiments: AASM LM AB CB. Performed the experiments: AASM. Analyzed the data: AASM CB. Contributed reagents/materials/analysis tools: LM AB CB. Contributed to the writing of the manuscript: AASM LM AB CB.

References

1. Mottron L, Dawson M, Soulieres I, Hubert B, Burack J (2006) Enhanced perceptual functioning in autism: an update, and eight principles of autistic perception. J Autism Dev Disord 36: 27–43.
2. Gomes E, Pedroso FS, Wagner MB (2008) Auditory hypersensitivity in the autistic spectrum disorder. Pro Fono 20: 279–284.
3. Zwaigenbaum L (2010) Advances in the early detection of autism. Curr Opin Neurol 23: 97–102.
4. Pierce K, Conant D, Hazin R, Stoner R, Desmond J (2011) Preference for geometric patterns early in life as a risk factor for autism. Arch Gen Psychiatry 68: 101–109.
5. Klin A, Lin DJ, Gorrindo P, Ramsay G, Jones W (2009) Two-year-olds with autism orient to non-social contingencies rather than biological motion. Nature 459: 257–261.
6. American Psychiatric Association (2013) Diagnostic and Statistical Manual of Mental Disorders, Fifth Edition. Arlington, VA, American Psychiatric Association. pp. 50–59.
7. Pellicano E, Stears M (2011) Bridging autism, science and society: moving toward an ethically informed approach to autism research. Autism Res 4: 271–281.
8. Sinclair J (1999) Why I dislike "person first" language. http://www.jimsinclair.org/person_first.htm. Accessed 2014 Jul 10.
9. Bonnel A, Mottron L, Peretz I, Trudel M, Gallun E, et al. (2003) Enhanced pitch sensitivity in individuals with autism: a signal detection analysis. J Cogn Neurosci 15: 226–235.
10. Bonnel A, McAdams S, Smith B, Berthiaume C, Bertone A, et al. (2010) Enhanced pure-tone pitch discrimination among persons with autism but not Asperger syndrome. Neuropsychologia 48: 2465–2475.
11. Jones CR, Happe F, Baird G, Simonoff E, Marsden AJ, et al. (2009) Auditory discrimination and auditory sensory behaviours in autism spectrum disorders. Neuropsychologia 47: 2850–2858.
12. Heaton P, Williams K, Cummins O, Happe F (2008) Autism and pitch processing splinter skills: a group and subgroup analysis. Autism 12: 203–219.
13. Bhatara A, Babikian T, Laugeson E, Tachdjian R, Sininger YS (2013) Impaired timing and frequency discrimination in high-functioning autism spectrum disorders. J Autism Dev Disord 43: 2312–2328.
14. Bertone A, Mottron L, Jelenic P, Faubert J, Bertone A, et al. (2005) Enhanced and diminished visuo-spatial information processing in autism depends on stimulus complexity. Brain 128: 2430–2441.
15. McCleery JP, Allman E, Carver LJ, Dobkins KR (2007) Abnormal magnocellular pathway visual processing in infants at risk for autism. Biol Psychiatry 62: 1007–1014.
16. Jemel B, Mimeault D, Saint-Amour D, Hosein A, Mottron L (2010) VEP contrast sensitivity responses reveal reduced functional segregation of mid and high filters of visual channels in autism. J Vis 10:13.
17. Falter CM, Braeutigam S, Nathan R, Carrington S, Bailey AJ (2012) Enhanced Access to Early Visual Processing of Perceptual Simultaneity in Autism Spectrum Disorders. J Autism Dev Disord 43:1857–1866.
18. Remington AM, Swettenham JG, Lavie N (2012) Lightening the load: perceptual load impairs visual detection in typical adults but not in autism. J Abnorm Psychol 121: 544–551.

19. Schwarzkopf DS, Anderson EJ, de Haas B, White SJ, Rees G (2014) Larger extrastriate population receptive fields in autism spectrum disorders. J Neurosci 34: 2713–2724.
20. Perreault A, Gurnsey R, Dawson M, Mottron L, Bertone A (2011) Increased sensitivity to mirror symmetry in autism. PLoS One 6: e19519.
21. Caron MJ, Mottron L, Berthiaume C, Dawson M (2006) Cognitive mechanisms, specificity and neural underpinnings of visuospatial peaks in autism. Brain 129: 1789–1802.
22. Heaton P, Hudry K, Ludlow A, Hill E (2008) Superior discrimination of speech pitch and its relationship to verbal ability in autism spectrum disorders. Cogn Neuropsychol 25: 771–782.
23. Mottron L, Peretz I, Menard E (2000) Local and global processing of music in high-functioning persons with autism: beyond central coherence? J Child Psychol Psychiatry 41: 1057–1065.
24. Bouvet L, Simard-Meilleur AA, Paignon A, Mottron L, Donnadieu S (2014) Auditory local bias and reduced global interference in autism. Cognition 131: 367–372.
25. Kaldy Z, Kraper C, Carter AS, Blaser E (2011) Toddlers with Autism Spectrum Disorder are more successful at visual search than typically developing toddlers. Dev Sci 14: 980–988.
26. Jarvinen-Pasley A, Wallace GL, Ramus F, Happe F, Heaton P, et al. (2008) Enhanced perceptual processing of speech in autism. Developmental Science 11: 109–121.
27. Vlamings PH, Jonkman LM, van Daalen E, van der Gaag RJ, Kemner C (2010) Basic abnormalities in visual processing affect face processing at an early age in autism spectrum disorder. Biol Psychiatry 68: 1107–1113.
28. Spearman C (1904) General Intelligence, Objectively Determined and Measured. The American Journal of Psychology 12: 201–292.
29. Soulières I, Dawson M, Samson F, Barbeau EB, Sahyoun CP, et al. (2009) Enhanced visual processing contributes to matrix reasoning in autism. Hum Brain Mapp 30: 4082–4107.
30. Mottron L, Dawson M, Soulieres I, Hubert B, Burack J (2006) Enhanced Perceptual Functioning in Autism: An Update, and Eight Principles of Autistic Perception. Journal of Autism & Developmental Disorders 36: 27–43.
31. Mottron L, Bouvet L, Bonnel A, Samson F, Burack JA, et al. (2013) Veridical mapping in the development of exceptional autistic abilities. Neurosci Biobehav Rev 37: 209–228.
32. Samson F, Mottron L, Soulieres I, Zeffiro TA (2012) Enhanced visual functioning in autism: an ALE meta-analysis. Hum Brain Mapp 33: 1553–1581.
33. Mitchell P, Mottron L, Soulieres I, Ropar D (2010) Susceptibility to the Shepard illusion in participants with autism: reduced top-down influences within perception? Autism Res 3: 113–119.
34. Mottron L (2004) Matching strategies in cognitive research with individuals with high-functioning autism: current practices, instrument biases, and recommendations. J Autism Dev Disord 34: 19–27.
35. Conrad R (1979) The deaf schoolchild: Language and cognitive function: Harper Collins Publishers.
36. Barbeau EB, Soulieres I, Dawson M, Zeffiro TA, Mottron L (2013) The level and nature of autistic intelligence III: Inspection time. J Abnorm Psychol 122: 295–301.
37. Dawson M, Soulieres I, Gernsbacher MA, Mottron L (2007) The level and nature of autistic intelligence. Psychol Sci 18: 657–662.

38. Hayashi M, Kato M, Igarashi K, Kashima H (2007) Superior fluid intelligence in children with Asperger's disorder. Brain and Cognition 66: 306–310.

39. Bertone A, Mottron L, Jelenic P, Faubert J (2005) Enhanced and diminished visuo-spatial information processing in autism depends on stimulus complexity. Brain 128: 2430–2441.

40. Caron MJ, Mottron L, Berthiaume C, Dawson M (2006) Cognitive mechanisms, specificity and neural underpinnings of visuospatial peaks in autism. Brain 129: 1789–1802.

41. Mottron L, Peretz I, Menard E (2000) Local and global processing of music in high-functioning persons with autism: beyond central coherence? Journal of Child Psychology & Psychiatry & Allied Disciplines 41: 1057–1065.

42. Lord C, Rutter M, Le Couteur A (1994) Autism Diagnostic Interview-Revised: a revised version of a diagnostic interview for caregivers of individuals with possible pervasive developmental disorders. J Autism Dev Disord 24: 659–685.

43. Lord C, Rutter M, DiLavore PC, Risi S (1999) Autism Diagnostic Observation Schedule-WPS (ADOS-WPS).Los Angeles. CA: Western Psychological Services.

44. Woodbury-Smith MR, Robinson J, Wheelwright S, Baron-Cohen S (2005) Screening adults for Asperger Syndrome using the AQ: a preliminary study of its diagnostic validity in clinical practice. J Autism Dev Disord 35: 331–335.

45. Micheyl C, Delhommeau K, Perrot X, Oxenham AJ (2006) Influence of musical and psychoacoustical training on pitch discrimination. Hear Res 219: 36–47.

46. Tervaniemi M, Kruck S, De Baene W, Schroger E, Alter K, et al. (2009) Top-down modulation of auditory processing: effects of sound context, musical expertise and attentional focus. Eur J Neurosci 30: 1636–1642.

47. Weibull W (1951) A statistical distribution function of wide applicability. Journal of Applied Mechanics 18: 293–297.

48. Harvey LO, Jr. (1997) Efficient estimation of sensory thresholds with ML-PEST. Spat Vis 11: 121–128.

49. Peretz I (1987) Shifting ear differences in melody comparison through transposition. Cortex 23: 317–323.

50. Stevenson JL, Gernsbacher MA (2013) Abstract spatial reasoning as an autistic strength. PLoS One 8: e59329.

51. Grudnik JL, Kranzler JH (2001) Meta-analysis of the relationship between intelligence and inspection time. Intelligence 29: 523–535.

52. Melnick MD, Harrison BR, Park S, Bennetto L, Tadin D (2013) A Strong Interactive Link between Sensory Discriminations and Intelligence. Current biology: CB 23: 1013–1017.

53. Acton GS, Schroeder DH (2001) Sensory discrimination as related to general intelligence. Intelligence 29: 263–271.

54. McGrew KS (2005) The Cattell-Horn-Carroll theory of cognitive abilities: Past, present, and future. In: Flanagan DP, Genshaft JL, Harrison PL, editors. Contemporary intellectual assessment: Theories, tests, and issues New York: Guilford. pp. 136–182.

55. Mackintosh N (2011) IQ and Human Intelligence. United States: Oxford university Press.

56. Bertone A, Hanck J, Kogan C, Chaudhuri A, Cornish K (2010) Associating neural alterations and genotype in autism and fragile x syndrome: incorporating perceptual phenotypes in causal modeling. J Autism Dev Disord 40: 1541–1548.

57. Vattikuti S, Chow CC (2010) A computational model for cerebral cortical dysfunction in autism spectrum disorders. Biol Psychiatry 67: 672–678.

58. Ben-David E, Shifman S (2012) Networks of neuronal genes affected by common and rare variants in autism spectrum disorders. PLoS Genet 8: e1002556.

59. Poulin-Lord MP, Barbeau E, Soulières I, Monchi O, Doyon J, et al. (2014) Increased Topographical Variability of Task-related Activation in Perceptive and Motor Associative Regions in Adult Autistics. Neuroimage: Clinical 4:444–453.

60. Ferster D, Miller KD (2000) Neural mechanisms of orientation selectivity in the visual cortex. Annu Rev Neurosci 23: 441–471.

61. Edden RA, Muthukumaraswamy SD, Freeman TC, Singh KD (2009) Orientation discrimination performance is predicted by GABA concentration and gamma oscillation frequency in human primary visual cortex. J Neurosci 29: 15721–15726.

62. Razak KA, Fuzessery ZM (2010) GABA shapes a systematic map of binaural sensitivity in the auditory cortex. J Neurophysiol 104: 517–528.

63. Razak KA, Fuzessery ZM (2009) GABA shapes selectivity for the rate and direction of frequency-modulated sweeps in the auditory cortex. J Neurophysiol 102: 1366–1378.

64. Fatemi SH, Folsom TD, Reutiman TJ, Thuras PD (2009) Expression of GABA(B) receptors is altered in brains of subjects with autism. Cerebellum 8: 64–69.

65. Fatemi SH, Reutiman TJ, Folsom TD, Thuras PD (2009) GABA(A) receptor downregulation in brains of subjects with autism. J Autism Dev Disord 39: 223–230.

66. Puts NA, Edden RA, Evans CJ, McGlone F, McGonigle DJ (2011) Regionally specific human GABA concentration correlates with tactile discrimination thresholds. J Neurosci 31: 16556–16560.

67. Keïta L, Guy J, Berthiaume C, Mottron L, Bertone A (2014) An early origin for detailed perception in autism: biased sensitivity for high-spatial frequency information. Nature Science Reports 4: 5475.

## 10

Neural Correlates of Own Name and Own Face Detection in Autism Spectrum Disorder

Hanna B. Cygan[1], Pawel Tacikowski[1,2], Pawel Ostaszewski[3], Izabela Chojnicka[4], Anna Nowicka[1]*

1 Nencki Institute of Experimental Biology, Department of Neurophysiology, Laboratory of Psychophysiology, Warsaw, Poland, **2** Karolinska Institute, Department of Neuroscience, Brain, Body and Self Laboratory, Stockholm, Sweden, **3** University of Social Sciences and Humanities, Department of Psychology, Warsaw, Poland, **4** Medical University of Warsaw, Department of Medical Genetics, Warsaw, Poland

Abstract

Autism spectrum disorder (ASD) is a heterogeneous neurodevelopmental condition clinically characterized by social interaction and communication difficulties. To date, the majority of research efforts have focused on brain mechanisms underlying the deficits in interpersonal social cognition associated with ASD. Recent empirical and theoretical work has begun to reveal evidence for a reduced or even absent self-preference effect in patients with ASD. One may hypothesize that this is related to the impaired attentional processing of self-referential stimuli. The aim of our study was to test this hypothesis. We investigated the neural correlates of face and name detection in ASD. Four categories of face/name stimuli were used: own, close-other, famous, and unknown. Event-related potentials were recorded from 62 electrodes in 23 subjects with ASD and 23 matched control subjects. P100, N170, and P300 components were analyzed. The control group clearly showed a significant self-preference effect: higher P300 amplitude to the presentation of own face and own name than to the close-other, famous, and unknown categories, indicating preferential attentional engagement in processing of self-related information. In contrast, detection of both own and close-other's face and name in the ASD group was associated with enhanced P300, suggesting similar attention allocation for self and close-other related information. These findings suggest that attention allocation in the ASD group is modulated by the personal significance factor, and that the self-preference effect is absent if self is compared to close-other. These effects are similar for physical and non-physical aspects of the autistic self. In addition, lateralization of face and name processing is attenuated in ASD, suggesting atypical brain organization.

Editor: Karen Lidzba, University Children's Hospital Tuebingen, Germany

Funding: This work was supported by the National Science Centre, Warsaw, Poland (grant 2011/01/B/HS6/00683). The funders had no role in study design, data collection and analysis, decision to publish, or preparation of the manuscript.

Competing Interests: The authors have declared that no competing interests exist.

* E-mail: a.nowicka@nencki.gov.pl

Introduction

Autism spectrum disorder (ASD) is a heterogeneous neurodevelopmental disorder which affects, according to various sources, from 1 in 160 children (WHO: www.who.int) to 1 in 88 (CDC: www.cdc.gov). The main clinical hallmarks of ASD include impairments in social functioning and communication, existence of stereotyped repetitive behaviors, and a highly restricted scope of interests. The precise neuropathophysiology of ASD is still unclear [1], [2].

While previous research has been largely focused on deficits in interpersonal (social) interaction in ASD [3–6], the current approach emphasizes the need for also understanding alterations in intrapersonal (self-referential) cognition [7], [8]. This need seems to be fully justified, as the term 'autism' (derived from the Greek word 'autos', meaning 'self') was first applied by Kanner to describe young patients from his clinic who were extremely self-focused [9]. Recently, Lombardo and Baron-Cohen [10] proposed that individuals with ASD can be both egocentric and impaired in self-referential cognition. The authors also pointed to the atypical neural circuitry underlying the processing of self-relevant information in ASD. In addition, Rogers and Pennington [11] suggested that a disturbed process of forming and coordinating representations of the self and the other may be linked to specific deficits observed in ASD.

Despite distinct methodological approaches and operationalizations of self-concept, many studies on autistic self consistently point to a lack of differences between representations of self and other [8], [12–14]. For example, in Gunji's event-related potentials (ERP) study [12], children with pervasive developmental disorder (PDD; PDD includes ASD) were passively viewing their own, familiar, and unfamiliar faces. Their ERP response to own face did not differ from ERP responses to familiar and unfamiliar faces, whereas in typically developing participants ERPs were enhanced in the self face condition in comparison to the familiar face condition. Parallel effects were found by Lombardo et al. [8] in a study using functional magnetic resonance imaging (fMRI). They asked individuals with ASD and control participants to make reflective mentalizing or physical judgments about themselves and an "other" (the British Queen). In ASD participants, the self and other conditions resulted in similar ventromedial prefrontal cortex activations, and the middle cingulate cortex responded even stronger to other-mentalizing than self-mentalizing. In contrast, neurotypical individuals preferentially recruited those regions in response to self when compared to other referential processing. Reduced or even absent self-preference effects in ASD participants

Table 1. Participants' characteristics in the ASD group (age, handedness, IQ, ADOS, and ADI-R scores) and in the control group (age, handedness, and IQ scores).

subject	group	age	handedness	IQ			ADI-R			ADOS		
				verbal	performance	full scale	social (cutoff = 10)	communication (cutoff = 8)	repetitive behavior (cutoff = 3)	social (cutoff = 4)	communication (cutoff = 2)	repetitive behavior
A1	ASD	18	L	113	112	113	25	20	6	11	4	2
A2	ASD	23	R	100	69	86	25	23	7	3	3	1
A3	ASD	23	R	108	122	114	30	26	12	9	6	0
A4	ASD	19	R	96	90	93	26	18	8	8	5	0
A5	ASD	19	R	109	103	106	27	26	12	6	3	0
A6	ASD	18	R	116	93	106	27	21	11	8	3	2
A7	ASD	17	R	104	118	112	26	14	5	11	6	2
A8	ASD	17	L	119	121	122	27	21	8	5	3	3
A9	ASD	22	R	119	122	121	25	17	5	9	3	3
A10	ASD	18	R	96	109	102	25	23	8	8	5	2
A11	ASD	19	R	108	83	97	21	22	8	6	6	7
A12	ASD	18	R	125	107	117	25	22	10	7	3	3
A13	ASD	19	R	114	123	118	24	17	9	12	4	1
A14	ASD	24	R	124	93	111	16	21	7	5	2	4
A15	ASD	19	R	85	95	89	30	20	12	13	4	1
A16	ASD	22	R	97	121	108	24	17	2	4	2	0
A17	ASD	27	R	98	121	108	23	42	11	3	3	0
A18	ASD	21	R	99	104	101	26	22	9	8	3	2
A19	ASD	24	R	143	107	128	8	20	5	5	5	2
A20	ASD	21	R	114	118	116	14	8	8	3	3	0
A21	ASD	18	R	123	110	118	14	16	11	10	4	0
A22	ASD	21	R	119	99	110	12	15	1	4	2	0
A23	ASD	23	R	112	101	108	24	18	4	8	4	2
mean		20,4		109	104	107,13						
(s.d.)		2,76		11,3	16,43	11,51						
C1	Control	18	L	110	110	110						
C2	Control	17	L	122	92	109						
C3	Control	19	R	130	97	116						
C4	Control	19	R	86	99	91						
C5	Control	18	R	120	112	117						
C6	Control	19	R	111	108	110						
C7	Control	22	R	116	126	121						

Table 1. Cont.

subject	group	age	handedness	IQ			ADI-R			ADOS		
				verbal	performance	full scale	social (cutoff=10)	communication (cutoff=8)	repetetive behavior (cutoff=3)	social (cutoff=4)	communication (cutoff=2)	repetitive behavior
C8	Control	23	R	107	114	110						
C9	Control	18	R	130	123	128						
C10	Control	23	R	139	122	132						
C11	Control	18	R	86	93	89						
C12	Control	22	R	120	125	123						
C13	Control	23	R	99	93	97						
C14	Control	17	R	116	117	117						
C15	Control	19	R	114	112	113						
C16	Control	22	R	120	125	123						
C17	Control	27	R	113	113	113						
C18	Control	21	R	111	118	114						
C19	Control	24	R	117	116	117						
C20	Control	21	R	119	103	112						
C21	Control	24	R	113	101	108						
C22	Control	21	R	119	118	119						
C23	Control	23	R	120	121	121						
mean	Control	20,8		114	109,53	112,20						
(s.d.)	Control	2,66		15	12,13	12,36						

All subjects were male.

were also reported in studies on the self-reference effect in memory (i.e. enhanced memory for stimuli encoded in reference to oneself). In Henderson's et al. [13] study, participants read a list of words and decided whether the word described something about themselves, something about Harry Potter, or contained a certain number of letters. In the following session, subjects were asked to recognize previously presented words on a long list. Consistent with previous studies [7], [14], ASD subjects showed a reduced or absent self-reference effect.

The aforementioned studies revealed some significant alterations in self-related information processing in ASD individuals and in the associated neuronal circuitry. These alterations may be viewed in the light of the absent-self hypothesis [15–21] and the impaired I-concept hypothesis [22]. The absent-self hypothesis proposes that a specific kind of higher order self-awareness, possibly involved in top-down control, may be missing in autism. The second hypothesis posits that development of I-concept in patients with autism is disturbed or even absent. Specifically, Glezerman [22] pointed to the impairment of the 'symbolic' self that is developed in the neurotypical population through lifetime experience and enables the perception of self as unique and separate from others.

One may hypothesize, however, that explanations referring to attentional processes seem to be reasonable. The impaired self-preference observed in many ASD studies may be related to weaker engagement of attentional resources in processing of self-related information. It is well-documented that in a typically developing population, stimuli referring to one's own person attract attention automatically [23] and are selectively detected among other stimuli in the environment. A good example is the so called 'cocktail party' effect. Even when engaged in another cognitive task, a person can still detect own name in the unattended ear or visual field [24–27]. Moreover, one's own name is particularly resistant to attentional blink [28], and is preferentially processed even without reaching conscious awareness [29]. Studies on the neural processing of self-related cues (one's own name or face) generally support this notion of preferential attention allocation [30–36].

Thus the question arises whether attention allocation for self-related stimuli is also disturbed in ASD patients. In order to answer this question, the present study investigated detection of one's own face and one's own name in ASD participants and matching control subjects. We decided to use a simple detection task because such tasks do not require any intentional discrimination between presented stimuli, engage attention automatically, and require the same motor reaction (i.e., pressing the same button) for all stimuli. As a result we can imply that any plausible differences between stimuli, conditions, or groups can be related to different activation of attentional processes. It is important to note that detection is an obligatory initial stage in the processing of any incoming stimulus. One may suppose that any impairment present at this stage of information processing determines alterations at later stages.

Up to now, no studies have compared the processing of own face and own name in the same group of ASD participants while using the same experimental paradigm. Such a comparison would enable us to relate to Uddin's hypothesis [37], stating that 'physical' aspects of the autistic self are less disturbed than 'psychological' (i.e. non-physical) aspects. Whereas self-face directly refers to the 'physical self', self-name refers rather to the 'non-physical self'. If there is an atypical pattern of attention allocation for all self-related stimuli in ASD, similar results for names and faces should be observed; otherwise, some alterations might be observed for one type of stimulus only.

It is noteworthy that little is known about neural processing of one's own name in ASD. This is quite surprising given that names are highly relevant stimuli in the context of communication, i.e., the domain which is clearly impaired in this clinical group. To the best of our knowledge, there is only one published study on the neural basis of the own name processing in ASD. Carmody et al. [38] compared neural correlates of processing of one's own name, numbers, and the word 'Hello' in one ASD patient. Own name was associated with activations in the right frontal medial and middle gyri. Interestingly, self-name processing typically results in increased medial prefrontal cortex activation in normal populations [39–42]. However, because it was a single case study and because the subject was sedated during scanning, the results need to be treated with caution. Thus the investigation of own-name processing in ASD is of interest *per se* and may be viewed as a novel contribution to the field of ASD research.

In our study, control conditions consisted of names and faces belonging to three categories: unfamiliar, famous, and related to significant other. The latter category was introduced because 'me' vs. 'not-me' distinction may be modulated by the level of familiarity of the person used in the self-other comparison; it might be stronger for distant (not personally known and significant) other and weaker for close-other. Such modulation was reported in our previous studies of the neurotypical populations [42], [43]. The name and face of the close-other share many features with own name and face: their emotional load is very high, they are very familiar, and they are encountered extremely often in every-day life. Thus attention allocation for self and close-other related information may be similar, and processing of information related to close-other may resemble processing of self-related information.

The goal of this ERP study is to investigate the neural correlates of name and face detection in ASD. Specifically, we aim to verify our hypothesis stating that attention allocation for self-related stimuli is disturbed in ASD patients. This hypothesis would be confirmed if the self-preference effect expected in the control group is absent in the ASD group. Moreover, we are interested in whether the attentional involvement in detection of stimuli related to the 'physical' self (i.e., the own face) differs from attentional engagement in detection of stimuli related to the 'non-physical' self (i.e., the own name). Showing that the processing of own face is less disturbed than processing of own name would be supportive of Uddin's hypothesis [37].

The ERP method was chosen because it provides insights into the neural mechanisms that underlie covert cognitive processing that may not be evident in overt behaviors. Therefore, this method is particularly helpful when there might be no difference in a measured behavior between groups despite the supposition that the underlying neural substrate of that behavior may be different [44]. Amplitudes and latencies of the following ERP components were analyzed: P100 (a positive component peaking approximately 100 ms after the stimulus onset), N170 (a negative deflection reaching its maximum 170 ms after the stimulus onset), and P300 (an ERP component starting around 300 ms after the stimulus onset).

P100 and N170 components reflect exogenous processes modulated by the physical attributes of stimuli but not by cognitive processes [45]. Herrmann and Knight [46] proposed that these components are related to attention processes, operating at the early stage and influencing stimulus processing at the later stage. Many studies have shown that P100 reflects a facilitation of early sensory processing of attended stimuli [47], [48] and it may serve as a marker of early stimulus-driven attention allocation [49], [50]. In addition, it has been also proposed that P100 component

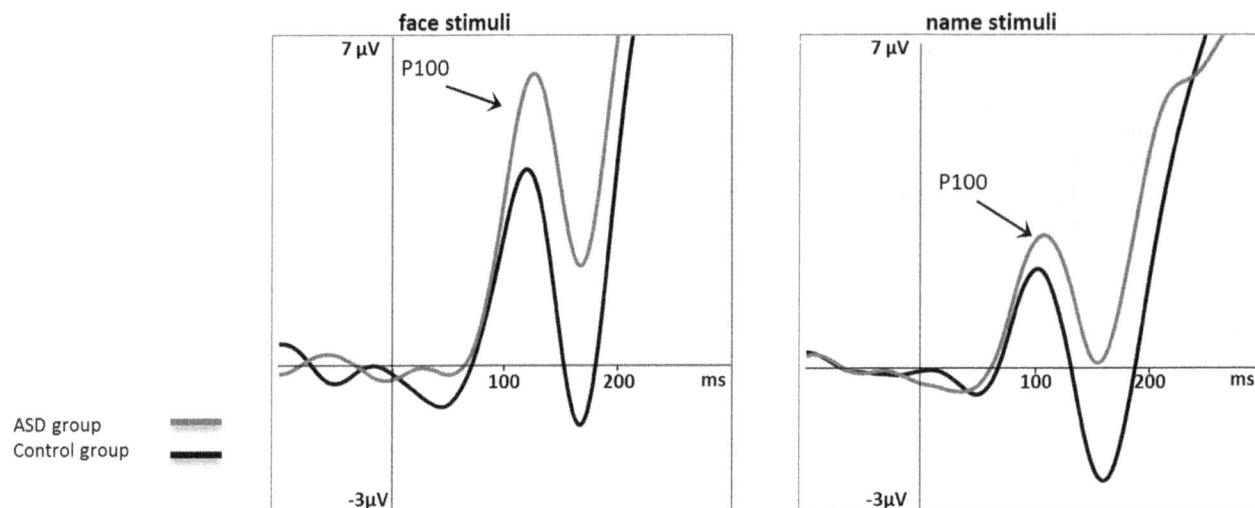

Figure 1. Grand average event-related potentials (ERP) in the P100 time window in the ASD group vs. the control group, pooled for PO7 and PO8 electrodes. left panel presents response to face stimuli, right panel presents response to name stimuli, with all categories taken together.

may serve as a sign of processing effort [51]. In other words, the higher P100 amplitude (and/or the longer latency) the stronger need for engagement of brain resources.

In typical adults, the N170 component is related to early stage encoding of faces [52], [53]. The N170 is maximal over posterior areas and is faster and larger in response to face stimuli compared to non-face stimuli [53]. N170 was shown to be sensitive to face inversion [52]. Some studies revealed that it is affected by face familiarity whereas other did not find such effect [52–55]. It is now generally acknowledged that N170 represents the analysis of structural information of faces [53], [56–59]. Importantly, N170 is also specific to other stimuli processing that required expertise and was associated with word form analysis in case of names [43], [60].

The P300 component, in turn, has been mainly associated with the processes of attention and is often treated as an index of ability to sustain attention on targets [61]. Attention allocation reflected in P300 is independent of stimulus modality and is influenced by the familiarity factor [34], [36], [43]. The P300 also seems to vary with the emotional value of the stimulus - emotionally charged stimuli (regardless of their valence) produced larger P300 then neutral ones [62], [63]. There is still much debate on the underlying generator(s) but the prevailing opinion is that multiple neural sources contribute to the P300 [64].

These ERP components (i.e., P100, N170, P300) were observed and analyzed in previous studies on processing of faces and names in typically developing population [31], [32], [36], [65–74]. However, in the case of adult individuals with ASD, studies on face processing (there is no ERP study on name processing in the ASD) reported findings mainly related to P100 and N170 components. It has been demonstrated that adults with autism had delayed P100 and N170 latencies and lower N170 amplitudes for faces [75]. Other studies confirmed longer N170 latency in response to face stimuli in individuals with ASD but no significant effects for P100 and N170 amplitude and P100 latency were identified [76], [77]. In the recent Webb et al. study [78] no group differences in early ERP correlates of attention (P100) and structural face processing (N170) were found, suggesting that the P100 and N170 responses to upright faces in adults with ASD can resemble those seen in controls.

The majority of ERP studies on the topic of own name and own face processing report the self-preference effect in amplitudes of P300 in typically developing population [31], [32], [36], [72–74] (but see [79]). While P100 and P300 are the main candidates to differentiate attentional processes involved in detection of names and faces in the ASD group and the control group, only the latter component is associated both with the self-preference effect and attention allocation. Therefore, we expect that amplitudes of P300 in the ASD group will reflect plausible impairment of attentional processes involved in the processing of self-related stimuli. Such impairment should be manifested as a lack of differences between P300 amplitudes in the self vs. other condition and may be influenced by the personal relevance of 'the other'.

Methods

Ethics statement

The experimental protocol was approved by the Bioethics Committee of Warsaw Medical University (Warsaw, Poland). Informed written consent was obtained prior to the study from all participants and their legal caregivers.

Participants

Twenty three adolescents and young adults with ASD and 23 control subjects participated in this study (age range 17–27 years). ASD subjects were recruited from the SYNAPSIS Foundation which provides diagnosis and therapy for people with ASD. The subjects' IQs were evaluated on the basis of the Wechsler Intelligence Scale for Adults - Revised (WAIS-R) Polish adaptation [80]. The control group was matched in terms of age, handedness, and IQ-score (see Table 1). ASD subjects were clinically diagnosed by psychiatrists prior to the experiment and the clinical diagnosis was confirmed using standardized tests: the Autism Diagnostic Observation Schedule (ADOS) and Autism Diagnostic Interview-Revised (ADI-R) (see Table 1). Handedness was confirmed with the Edinburgh Inventory [81]. Subjects had normal or corrected-to-normal vision. All subjects were financially compensated for their participation in the experiment.

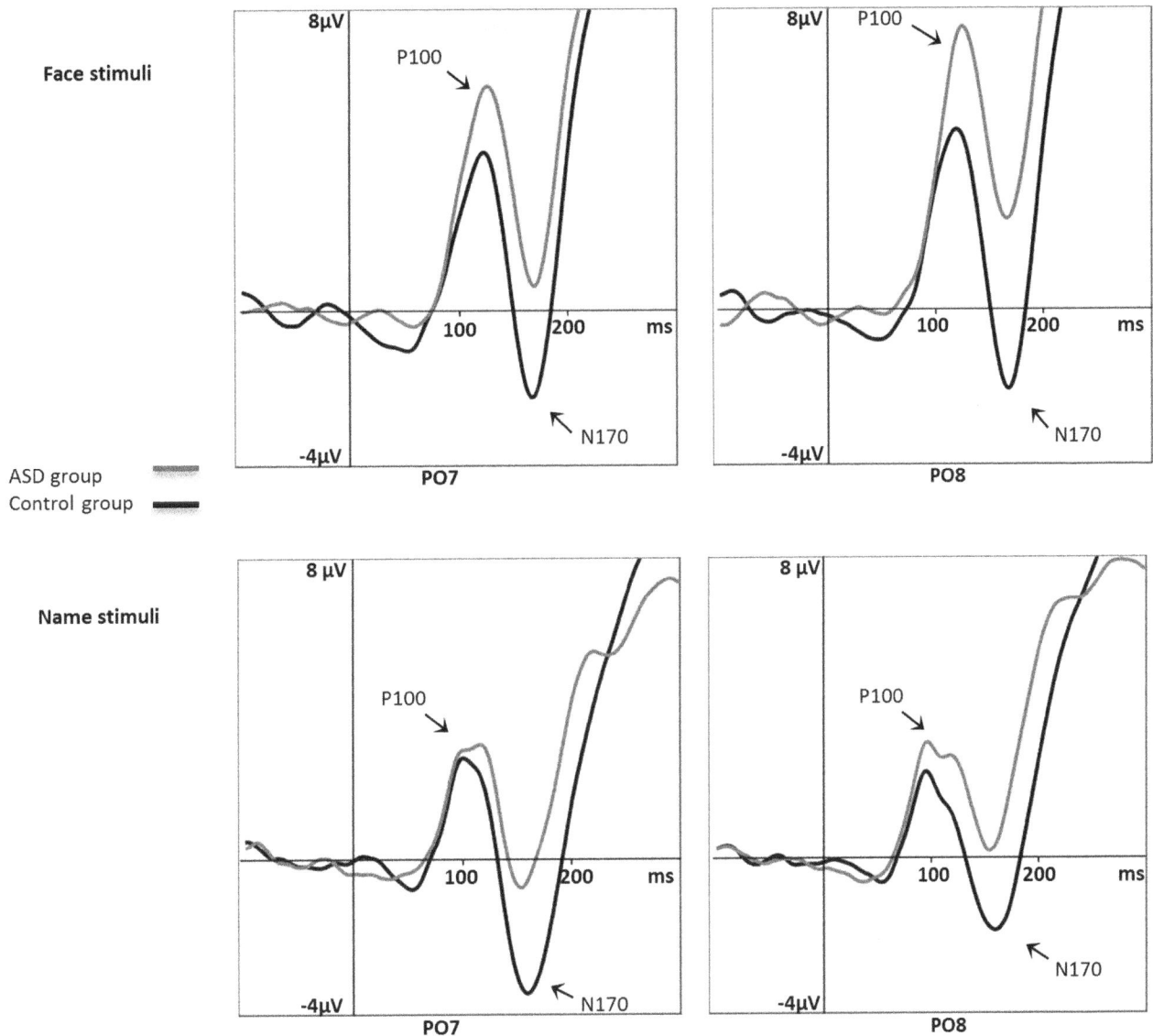

Figure 2. Grand average event-related potentials (ERP) in the N170 time window in the ASD group vs. the control group, separately for each analyzed scalp position (PO7, PO8). upper panels present response to face stimuli, bottom panels present response to name stimuli, with all categories taken together. For faces, amplitudes of N170 (peak-to-peak vs. P100) were higher on PO8 than on PO7 and for names amplitudes were higher on PO7 than on PO8.

Stimuli

Faces and names (first and last names) were presented visually on a computer screen in two separate sessions. The sequence of the two sessions was randomized between subjects: half started with the name-detection task, while the other half with the face-detection task.

In the face-detection session, grey-scaled images of faces were presented against a black background. All photos were extracted from the original background using Adobe Photoshop CS5® software (Adobe Systems Incorporated), so that only the face, ears, and hair were visible. Faces belonged to four categories: (1) subjects own, (2) close-other's, (3) famous person (e.g., actor), and (4) unknown face. A face from each category was presented 32 times. The photos of famous and unknown people were downloaded from the internet. The luminance of pictures was matched to color statistics of one image, eliminating possible differences between stimuli. The size of the face stimuli ranged from $6° × 6°$ to $6° × 5°$, and did not differ between categories or groups.

Names were written in white, capital letters and presented against a black background. Categories of names were analogous to categories of faces: (1) subjects own, (2) close-other's, (3) famous person (e.g., actor), and (4) unknown name. A name from each category was presented 32 times. The size of the name stimuli ranged from $3° × 6°$ to $3° × 9°$ and did not differ between categories or groups. Stimuli in both series were presented in pseudo-random order, so that no more than three stimuli of the same category or type were presented consecutively.

The set of all stimuli was individually tailored. Different famous and unknown faces/names were chosen for each subject to match gender of faces and length of the own and close-other's names. Names and faces of analogous categories referred to the same person. Before the experiment each participant was asked to

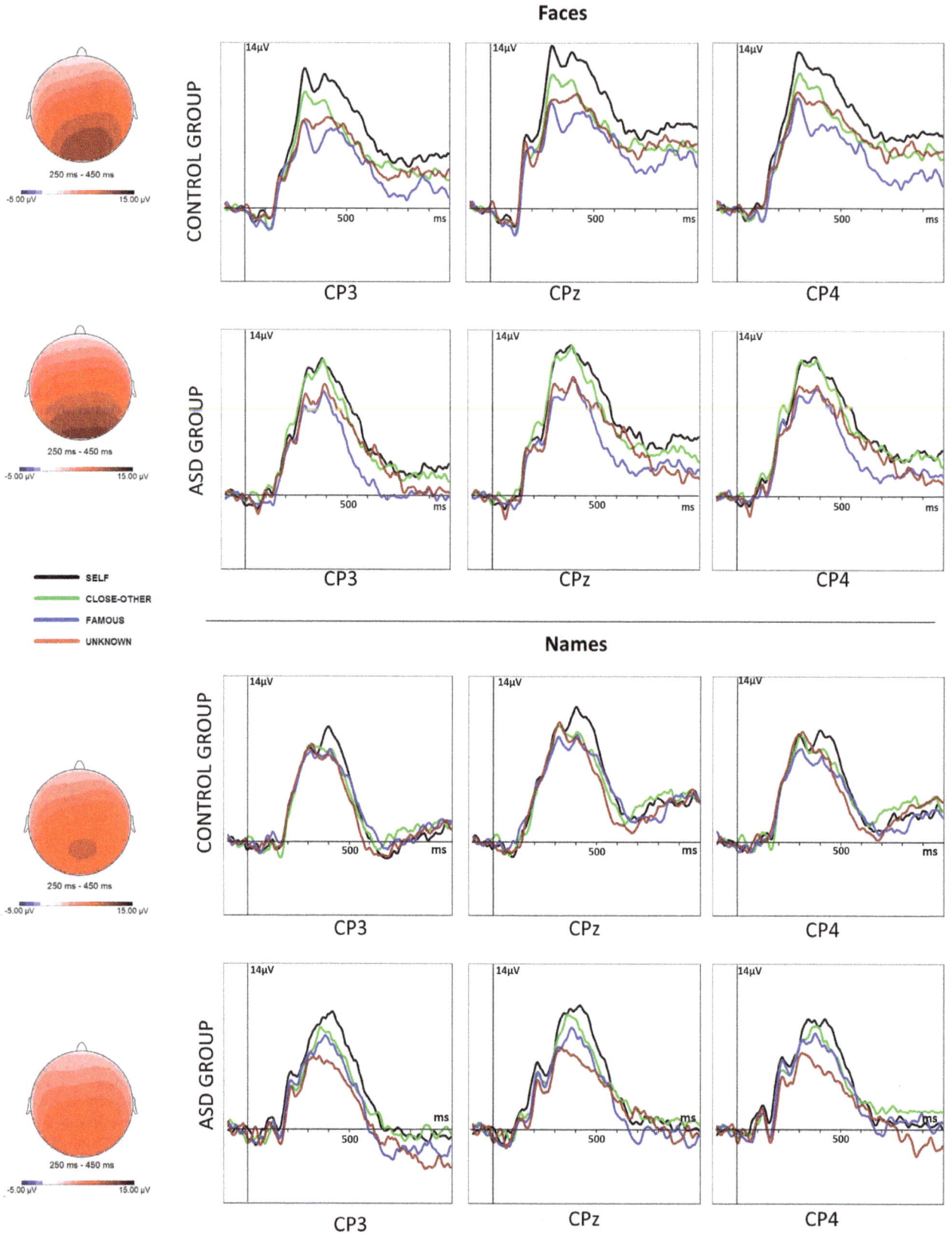

Figure 3. Grand average event-related potentials (ERP) in the ASD group vs. the control group, presented separately for each category of stimuli (own, close-other, famous, unknown), each analyzed centro-parietal scalp position (CP3, CPz, CP4), and each type of stimuli (face, name).

confirm that he knows the famous person and does not know the unknown names. No restriction was put on the subjects choice of the close-other because we wanted to avoid a situation where predefined the 'close-other' is not really close to the subject. In the ASD group 16 participants chose their parent, three their sibling, three their grandmother, and one their best friend. In the control group, seven participants chose their parent, four their sibling, three their best friend, and nine their girlfriend.

Experimental procedure

Stimuli were displayed in central vision on a 19-inch NEC MultiSync LCD 1990Fx monitor. Presentation® software (Neurobehavioral Systems, Albany, CA, USA) was used for stimuli presentation and measurement of the subject responses. The participants were seated in an acoustically and electrically shielded dark room at a distance of 60 cm from the computer monitor. The subjects performed a simple detection task: they were to respond to each stimulus as quickly as possible by pressing the same button with their index finger on a Cedrus response pad (RB-830, San Pedro, USA).

After reading instructions displayed on the computer screen, each session began with the participant completing a trial session in which feedback information was displayed (i.e., "correct", "response too slow"). During this session stimuli from each category were presented twice. After succesful completion, subjects began the actual study.

The sequence of events in each trial was as follows: presentation of a fixation point (a white "+" against a black background) for 100 ms, a blank screen for 300 to 1200 ms, and a target item displayed for 500 ms. Onset of the consecutive trial was driven by the subjects response and appeared 2000 ms after pressing the response button. Following the first session, the second one (preceded by the training session) was initiated by the subject by pressing a response button. Each session lasted about 7 minutes.

EEG recordings

EEG was continuously recorded from 62 scalp sites using a 136-channel amplifier (QuickAmp, Brain Products, Enschede, the Netherlands) and BrainVisionRecorder® software (Brain Products, Munich, Germany). Ag-AgCl electrodes were mounted on an elastic cap (ActiCAP, Munich, Germany) and positioned according to the extended 10–20 system. Electrode impedance was kept below 5 kΩ. The EEG signal was recorded against an average of all channels calculated by the amplifier hardware. The sampling rate was 500 Hz.

Behavioral data analysis

Responses were scored as correct if the button was pressed within 150–1000 ms after the stimulus onset. Response times (RTs) were analyzed using mixed-model ANOVA, with the following factors: group (ASD, control), type (face, name), and category (own, close-other, famous, and unknown). RTs were averaged across correct trials only.

ERP analysis

Off-line analysis of the EEG signal was performed using BrainVisionAnalyzer® software (Brain Products, Gilching, Germany). The first step was the implementation of butterworth zero phase filters: high-pass – 0.1 Hz, 12 dB/oct; low-pass – 30 Hz, 12 dB/oct; and notch filter – 50 Hz. Next, we corrected ocular artifacts using Independent Component Analysis [82]. After the decomposition of each data set into maximally statistically independent components based on visual inspection of the component map [83], components representing eye blinks were rejected. Ocular-artifact-free EEG data were obtained by multiplying the remaining ICA components using the reduced component-mixing matrix. Then, the EEG signal was segmented to obtain epochs extending from 100 ms before to 1000 ms after the stimulus onset (baseline correction from -100 to 0 ms). In the automatic artifact rejection, the maximum permitted voltage step per sampling point was 50 μV. The maximum permitted absolute difference between two values in the segment was 200 μV. The minimum and maximum permitted amplitudes were -200 μV and 200 μV respectively, and the lowest permitted activity in the 100 ms interval was 0.5 μV. Finally, the data were re-referenced to the mean from both earlobes and averaged for each stimuli category.

The ERPs for own, close-other's, famous, and unknown faces/ names were computed for correct trials only. The mean number of segments used to compute ERPs in the ASD group was 29 for names and 30 for faces. In the control group, 31 for names and 31 for faces. We did not find significant differences in the number of epochs used to compute ERPs between types and categories of stimuli or between groups.

In the statistical analysis, peak latencies and amplitudes were used. We analyzed amplitudes and latencies of P100, N170, and P300 previously reported in studies with visual presentation of faces and names, at previously reported locations [31], [32], [36], [65], [71–74], [79]. Based on the visual inspection of grand-average ERPs and on the existing literature, the peak detection was performed for the following time-windows: P100 (50–150 ms after the stimulus onset), N170 (150–220 ms), and P300 (250–450 ms). We focused on scalp regions in which those ERP components had their maximum amplitudes. P100 and N170 were analyzed in the left and right occipital regions (PO7 and PO8). P300 was analyzed in the central-parietal region (CPz, CP3 and CP4). Including two lateral electrodes (i.e., CP3, CP4) into the subset of centro-parietal electrodes enabled us to relate to the issue of plausible differences in the left and right hemisphere involvement in processing of names and faces in the ASD group. Our choice of electrodes was confirmed by the topography of brain activity in the time windows corresponding to P100, N170, and P300.

Taking into account that P100 and N170 were analyzed at the same electrode sites, amplitude of the second component was analyzed as a peak-to-peak against P100. Visual analysis of the P300 revealed double maxima within chosen time window. Thus peak detection was performed in two time windows: early P300 (250–350 ms) and late P300 (350–450 ms). Epochs were visually inspected to ensure that for each participant ERP components reached their maximum/minimum within the selected time window.

We performed mixed-model ANOVA on amplitudes and latencies of each component with the following factors: group (a between-subject factor at two levels: ASD, control), type (a within-subject factor at two levels: face, name), category (a within-subject factor at four levels: own, close-other, famous and unknown), and location. This within-subject factor was at two levels (left, right) in the case of P100 and N170 and at three levels (left, central, right) in the case of P300. All effects with more than one degree of freedom in the numerator were adjusted for violations of sphericity according to the Greenhouse and Geisser formula [84]. T-tests with Bonferroni correction for multiple comparisons were applied to post-hoc analyses. Only interactions involving the between-subjects factor of group that were necessary to address the main aims of the present study were further analyzed.

Results

Behavioral data

No significant main effects or interaction were found.

Electrophysiological data

P100. Statistical analysis on P100 amplitudes revealed a significant main effect of the type of stimulus ($F_{1,44} = 20.968$; p< .0001; $\eta^2 = .323$) and two interactions: type × location ($F_{3,90} = 4.971$; p = .031; $\eta^2 = .102$) and type × group ($F_{1,44} = 3.916$; p = .05; $\eta^2 = .820$). All other main factors and interactions were insignificant. Faces, in general, were associated with higher P100 amplitudes than names. Post hoc tests showed that only face amplitudes were significantly higher in the right than in the left hemisphere (p = .019). Between-group differences referring to the type of stimulus showed that face amplitudes of P100 were higher in ASD than in the control group (p = .036) (see Figure 1). Analysis of the P100 latencies revealed a main effect of the type factor ($F_{1,44} = 67.581$; p<.0001; $\eta^2 = .606$). Latencies for faces were significantly longer than for names.

N170. Statistical analysis of N170 amplitudes revealed a main effect of category ($F_{1,44} = 2.837$; p = .04; $\eta^2 = .061$) and a significant 3-way interaction: group × type × location ($F_{1,44} = 5.138$; p = .028; $\eta^2 = .105$). Post hoc analysis showed that in the control group N170 amplitudes for names were higher in the left hemisphere than in the right (p = .014), and N170 amplitudes for faces were marginally higher in the right hemisphere than in the left (p = .085). Moreover, N170 amplitudes in the left hemisphere were higher in the control than in the ASD group (p = .004). Analysis of N170 latencies revealed a main effect of the type of stimuli ($F_{1,44} = 12.954$; p = .001; $\eta^2 = .227$). N170 latency for faces was significantly longer than for names (see Figure 2).

P300. ANOVA for early P300 (see Figure 3) amplitudes revealed a main effect of the type of stimuli ($F_{1,44} = 9.558$; p = .003; $\eta^2 = 0.178$), category of stimuli ($F_{3,42} = 9.741$; p<.001; $\eta^2 = .181$), electrode location ($F_{2,43} = 12.099$; p<.001; $\eta^2 = .216$), and interactions: type × category ($F_{3,42} = 4.621$; p = .004; $\eta^2 = .095$), group × type × category ($F_{3,42} = 3.997$; p = .013; $\eta^2 = .083$), group × type × location ($F_{2,43} = 5.013$; p = .009; $\eta^2 = .102$), and group × category × location ($F_{6,39} = 3.451$; p = .005; $\eta^2 = .073$). All other effects were insignificant. Post hoc tests of 'group × type × category' interaction showed that in both groups there were no differences in early P300 between categories of names. However, significant differences appeared in response to faces. In the ASD group, response to own face did not differ from the response to close-other's face and unknown face. However, amplitudes to own and close-other's face were higher than for famous face (p = .005 and p = .001, respectively). In the control group, response to own face was significantly higher than to the close-other's (p = .001), famous (p<.001), and unknown face (p = .001).

Post hoc tests of 'group × type × location' interaction showed that in the ASD group amplitudes for faces were higher than for names at each investigated location: left (p = .008), right (p = .007), and central (p = .002). In the control group, this effect appeared only on the right side of the scalp (p = .041). Post hoc analyses of the 'group × category × location' interaction revealed that in typically developing participants, amplitudes of early P300 to all categories of faces and names were higher at the right (CP4) and central (CPz) electrode sites in comparison to the left (CP3). In contrast, this effect (CPz, CP4>CP3) was observed in ASD subjects only for the close-other category.

Analysis of early P300 latencies revealed a main effect of the group ($F_{1,44} = 4.776$; p = .034; $\eta^2 = .970$). Longer latencies of early P300 latencies were observed in the ASD group than in the control.

ANOVA on late P300 peak amplitudes (see Figure 3) revealed a main effects of the type of stimuli ($F_{1,44} = 4.904$; p = .032; $\eta^2 = .100$), category of stimuli ($F_{3,42} = 19.522$; p<.001; $\eta^2 = .307$), location ($F_{2,43} = 8.978$; p<.001; $\eta^2 = .169$), and statistical significance of interactions: group × category ($F_{3,42} = 3.243$; p = .024; $\eta^2 = .068$), category × location ($F_{6,39} = 3.022$; p = .013; $\eta^2 = .064$), type × location ($F_{2,43} = 3.168$; p = .047; $\eta^2 = .067$), and group × category × location ($F_{6,39} = 3.699$; p = .004; $\eta^2 = .078$). All other main factors and interactions were insignificant. Post hoc tests of 'group × category' interaction indicated that in the ASD group, regardless of the type of stimuli, late P300 response to own face/name was higher than for famous (p = .002) and unknown face/name (p<.001). Peak amplitude for the close-other category was higher than for famous (p = .023) and unknown (p = .008). No differences between the self and close-other category were found. In the control group, response for the own face/name was higher than for the close-other's (p = .001), famous (p<.001), and unknown face/name (p = .001). In this group, peak amplitude for close-other's face/name was higher than for famous face/name (p = .014). Post hoc tests for the 'group × category × location' interaction showed that the described effects in each group were significant at each investigated electrode location. However, they were the strongest at the central site. No significant differences regarding P300 peak latencies were observed in the late time window.

Discussion

The goal of this ERP study was to investigate the neural correlates of name and face detection in ASD. Names and faces differed in respect to their personal significance (own, close-other's, famous, unknown). Specifically, we were interested whether preferential attention allocation for self-related stimuli was impaired in ASD participants, and whether the same effects could be observed for the 'physical self' (one's own face) and the 'non-physical self' (one's own name).

On the behavioral level, we did not find differences in RTs between groups and experimental conditions. It should be stressed, however, that the task we used was very simple and did not require discriminating between stimuli. No in-depth processing of incoming information was required to successfully accomplish the task, and only high-functioning ASD participants were tested.

On the neural level, several significant effects were observed. In general, faces were associated with higher P100 amplitudes than names in both groups. It has been well documented that the amplitude of P100 is sensitive to perceptual features of visual stimuli, such as brightness, contrast, visual acuity, and size [85], [86]. Interestingly, some studies report face-sensitive effects at the level of P100 [73], [87]. It has been argued, however, that this may just result from perceptual differences between faces and visual stimuli used for comparison [88]. Thus increased P100 to faces in both our groups is possibly a consequence of the size and complexity of these stimuli. We observed no self-preference effect in this early ERP component for both the ASD and control group.

Besides the effects common for the two groups, some between-group differences appeared about 100 ms after the stimulus onset: P100 amplitudes in response to all categories of faces were higher in the ASD group than in the control group. This effect may reflect the enhanced visual processing often reported in ASD [89]. Alternatively, it could be also attributed to early stimulus-driven attention allocation [49], [50], i.e., enhanced P100 to faces in the ASD group may reflect increased orienting/attention to these stimuli. However, increased attention operating at the early stage of face processing did not exert influence on the later stages, related to face recognition (see discussion referring to the P300 findings below). Actually, one may speculate that this enhanced P100 indicates the higher processing effort present at earliest stage of face perception in this clinical group [51]. However, none of previously published studies on face processing reported P100 amplitudes to faces higher in individuals with ASD than in control individuals [75–78]. This discrepancy between our P100 results and findings of previously published studies may result from crucial differences in experimental paradigms, i.e. different attentional requirements, different stimuli and different subject's tasks. Specifically, in Webb et al. [78] and MacPartland et al. [77] studies, presentation of faces was task-irrelevant, thus faces were out of focus of attention: subjects were supposed to detect (i.e., press a button) houses [78] or butterflies [77]. In two other studies, emotional faces were presented [75], [76] and subjects were asked either to indicate whether the face was neutral or sad [76] or to verbalize the word which described how the person in the photograph was feeling [75].

Subsequently, amplitudes of N170 differentiated the two groups: N170 recorded in the left hemisphere to names was higher in the control group than in the ASD group. In addition, lateral effects related to the type of presented information were present only in the control group. Specifically, N170 amplitude to names was higher in the left hemisphere than in the right one and to faces higher in right than in the left one, however the second effect was only marginally significant. Although general enhancement of N170 amplitudes to faces is typically observed when faces are compared to other visual objects [90], some studies revealed higher amplitudes of N170 component in the right hemisphere only [43], [52], [91]. Increased N170 for names in the left hemisphere, in turn, was also previously reported in healthy subjects [73], [86], [92] and seems to be in line with typical dominance of the left side of the human brain in language processing.

While in the control group on the early stage of information processing, left hemisphere dominance appeared for visually presented names and right hemisphere dominance – for faces, such effects were absent in the ASD group. In the case of names, the lack of lateral effects is generally in line with the previously found dysfunction of the left hemisphere in the ASD [93], [94] (but see [95]) and atypical patterns of lateralization of language processing in this clinical group [96], [97]. In the case of faces, presence of the right hemispheric dominance in ASD groups is still unclear. For example lack of lateral differences in ASD was previously reported in N170 component by [98] while other studies report such lateralization for both control and ASD subjects [75], [76], [78].

With regard to the main aim of our study, the most important findings were between-group differences found in the 250–350 ms and 350–450 ms time windows. In both groups, P300 amplitudes in the early time window were significantly modulated by categories of faces, not names. In the control group, the own face was associated with higher P300 amplitudes than all other faces, whereas in the ASD group the own and close-other's face did not differ. Both resulted in enhanced P300 in comparison to the famous but not unknown face. The latter is in line with findings of a study reporting that children with autism fail to show differential late positive ERP component to their mother's face versus an unfamiliar face [99]. These higher amplitudes of early P300 to own and the close-other's face but not to the famous face

seem to reflect the personal relevance of those stimuli. The lack of significant differences between personally relevant faces (i.e., own and close-other faces) and unknown faces possibly results from equivalent attention allocation for those stimuli. A similar effect in ASD children was found by Gunji et al. [12]. In this study, no significant differences in P300 components were observed among the own, familiar, and unfamiliar face conditions. We argue that this elevated level of attention may be due to an elementary adaptive mechanism that guarantees that events/information with a potentially high survival value would not be missed [100]. It might be the case that novel objects (unknown faces) attracted ASD participants' attention to the same extent as personally relevant but not famous faces. Latency of early P300 also differentiated the two groups. It was significantly longer in the ASD group than in the control group for all names and faces, indicating some delay in processing of these socially-relevant stimuli.

Importantly, in the late time window we observed common patterns of P300 amplitudes for both types of stimuli, indicating the self-preference effect in the control group and the personal relevance effect in the ASD group. Specifically, in the control group own name/face processing resulted in the highest amplitudes of P300 in comparison to all other names/faces (i.e., close-other's, famous, unknown name/face). In the ASD group, P300 for own name/face did not differ from P300 for close-other name/face. However, P300 to own and close-other's name/face was significantly higher than P300 to other (famous and unknown) name/face.

Our P300 results showing preferential processing of the self-related stimuli in the control group are in line with previous ERP studies in healthy subjects [32], [34], [36], [68], [72], [73]. The novel finding in the control group is that amplitudes of P300 to own name and face were also higher than P300 to close-other's name and face. To our knowledge, none of the previous ERP studies used such stimuli together with self, famous, and unknown names and faces. Enhanced P300 in a own face condition in comparison to a friend's face condition was reported in one study only [12].

In contrast to the control group, late P300 findings in the ASD group revealed that the self-preference effect was present only when own name/face was compared to distant others' names/faces and absent when close-other's name/face was used as a reference to the self-related stimuli. The latter suggests equivalent attention allocation for own and close-other's faces and names in the ASD group. Thus, at the level of detection, the self-related stimuli are not differentiated from the close-other related stimuli, but they are differentiated from stimuli related to the more distant other (i.e. a famous person and the unknown person). It seems that in the case of ASD individuals, preferential processing was not restricted only to the self-related stimuli but to all personally relevant stimuli. Enhanced P300 to both own and close-other's name and face in the ASD group may reflect not only similar attentional characteristics [61] of these stimuli but also emotional ones [63]. Attention and emotion may complement each other as the model of motivated attention [101] states that emotional cues prompt motivational regulation and draw attentional resources. This is supported by findings of behavioral [100] and electrophysiological studies [102]. Although lower impact of emotion in guiding attention to socially-relevant stimuli might be expected in ASD [103], it is plausible that higher P300 amplitudes to the self and close-other related stimuli in the ASD group reflect similar emotionally motivated attentional load of these stimuli. One may speculate that in the case of ASD participants, motivated attention allocation to those stimuli might be associated with a kind of behavioral learning. This supposition is supported by the fact that most participants from our ASD group (22 out of 23) chose a family member as the 'close other'. Taking into account that they spent most of the time at home, extensive contact with that person and his/her significance in fulfilling daily needs may result in intensive stimulus- reward learning [104].

Alternative interpretations of P300 findings, not referring to the attentional processes, are also plausible. For example, our P300 findings may be interpreted in the context of the person recognition model [105–108] and its ERP adaptations [73], [92], [109], [110]. P300 is considered to reflect activation of semantic knowledge about a person [110]. Thus, P300 findings in the ASD group may suggest similar levels of person-specific semantic knowledge, referring to the self and the significant other. In contrast, the control group mainly displayed activation of self-knowledge. This result may support the theoretical view of a poorly developed or even absent 'I-concept' [22]. This is related to a distorted perception of oneself as unique and distinct from others. As a result, we can observe insufficient elaboration of the self-concept and impaired differentiation of the self from the significant other in autistic individuals [10], [22].

The P300 findings in the ASD group may also be viewed in the light of Uddin's [37] hypothesis, stating that psychological but not physical aspects of the self are altered in ASD. In other words, it might be expected that processing of 'symbolic' self-related stimuli (e.g. own name) is more impaired in ASD patients than processing of 'physical' self-related stimuli (e.g. own face). However, investigating these two types of stimuli at the same time, using the same experimental procedure, the same modality of stimuli, and with the same participants, we observed an analogous pattern of late P300 amplitudes for own name and own face. Thus our P300 results indicate that the 'physical self' and 'non-physical self' are processed in a similar way not only in the control group but also in the ASD group. Although our findings seems to disprove Uddin's hypothesis one may speculate that some in-depth processing, absent in our detection task, would be required to reveal disturbances in the 'psychological self'. The only difference between detection of names and faces (including one's own name and one's own face) observed in both groups was related to the temporal delay of the former in comparison to the later. P300 amplitude differentiated categories of faces in the early time window and categories of names in the late time window. This may be linked to the time consuming semantic processing of name stimuli.

ERP findings of this study also reveal attenuated lateralization of face and name processing in ASD. In the control group only, name detection in general was associated with higher activity in the left hemisphere whereas face detection was associated with enhanced activity in the right hemisphere, as revealed by N170 and P300 amplitudes, respectively. In contrast, lateral differences were absent in the ASD group. All of these effects support the notion of atypical functional brain organization [111], [112] in ASD participants during social stimuli processing.

Finally, one may hypothesize that aurally presented names should bring more ecologically valid findings. The auditory version of a name is more adequate in the context of communication and social interactions. However, we used the visual version of names in order to investigate self-related stimuli that differed only in respect to their domain ('physical', i.e., face vs. 'non-physical', i.e. name), but not their modality. Results from our own neuroimaging study [42] on healthy participants suggest that the involvement of the medial prefrontal cortex, is largely independent from the modality of one's own name. However, in some other brain regions (e.g. inferior frontal gyri) the preference in processing of one's own name vs. the close-other's name was present only for the auditory modality [42]. Therefore, it cannot be ruled out that using auditory presentations of the names would reveal a different pattern of results.

In conclusion, the present study provides evidence indicating equivalent engagement of attentional resources in detection of visually presented stimuli related to the self and to the close-other in adolescent and young adults with ASD. Similar effects were observed for names and for faces. In contrast, preferential attention allocation for the self-face and self-name was observed in typically developing individuals. Further research with different tasks and stimuli is needed to fully explain the impaired 'me' vs. 'not-me' distinction in autism.

Acknowledgments

We would like to thank all participants and their families, as well as Michał Wroniszewski, Joanna Grochowska, and Urszula Wójcik from the SYNAPSIS Foundation for their help in selecting the groups of participants.

Author Contributions

Conceived and designed the experiments: HBC PT PO IC AN. Performed the experiments: HBC PT IC PO AN. Analyzed the data: HBC AN. Wrote the paper: HBC PT PO IC AN.

References

1. Amaral DG, Schumann CM, Nordahl CW (2008) Neuroanatomy of autism. Trends in Neurosciences 31: 137–145. doi: 10.1016/j.tins.2007.12.005.

2. Williams DL, Minshew NJ (2007) Understanding autism and related disorders: what has imaging taught us. Neuroimaging Clinics of North America 17: 495–509. doi: 10.1016/j.nic.2007.07.007.

3. Hadjikhani N, Joseph RM, Snyder J, Tager-Flusberg H (2006) Anatomical differences in the mirror neuron system and social cognition network in autism. Cerebral Cortex 16: 1276–1282. doi: 10.1093/cercor/bhj069.

4. Baron-Cohen S, Baldwin DA, Crowson M (1997) Do children with autism use the speaker's direction of gaze strategy to crack the code of language? Child Development 681: 48–57. doi: 10.1111/j.1467-8624.1997.tb01924.x.

5. DePape AMR, Chen A, Hall GBC, Trainor LJ (2012) Use of prosody and information structure in high functioning adults with autism in relation to language ability. Frontiers in Psychology 3: 72. doi: 10.3389/fpsyg.2012.00072.

6. Wang AT, Lee SS, Sigman M, Dapretto M (2006) Neural basis of irony comprehension in children with autism: the role of prosody and context. Brain 129: 932–943. doi: 10. 1093/brain/awl032.

7. Lombardo MV, Barnes JL, Wheelwright SJ, Baron-Cohen S (2007) Self-referential cognition and empathy in autism. PLoS ONE 2: e883. doi: 10.1371/journal.pone.0000883.

8. Lombardo MV, Chakrabarti B, Bullmore ET, Sadek SA, Pasco G, et al. (2010) Atypical neural self-representation in autism. Brain 133: 611–624. doi: 10.1093/brain/awp306.

9. Kanner L (1943) Autistic disturbances of affective contact. Nervous Child 2: 217–250.

10. Lombardo MV, Baron-Cohen S (2010) Unraveling the paradox of the autistic self. Wiley Interdisciplinary Reviews: Cognitive Science 1: 393–403. doi: 10.1002/wcs.45.

11. Rogers SJ, Pennington BF (1991) A theoretical approach to the deficits in infantile autism. Development and Psychopathology 3: 137–162. doi: 10.1017/S0954579400000043.

12. Gunji A, Inagaki M, Inoue Y, Takeshima Y, Kaga M (2009) Event-related potentials of self-face recognition in children with pervasive developmental disorders. Brain and Development 31:139–147. doi: 10.1016/j.braindev.2008.04.011.

13. Henderson HA, Zahka NE, Kojkowski NM, Inge AP, Schwartz CB, et al. (2009) Self-Referenced Memory, Social Cognition, and Symptom Presentation in Autism. Journal of Child Psychology and Psychiatry 50: 853–861. doi: 10.1111/j.1469-7610.2008.02059.x.

14. Toichi M, Kamio Y, Okada T, Sakihama M, Youngstrom EA, et al. (2002) A lack of self-consciousness in autism. American Journal of Psychiatry 159: 1422–1424. doi: 10.1176/appi.ajp.159.8.1422.

15. Hurlburt RT, Happe F, Frith U (1994) Sampling the form of inner experience in three adults with Asperger syndrome. Psychological Medicine 24: 385–395. doi: 10.1017/S0033291700027367.

16. Frith U, Happe F (1999). Theory of mind and self-consciousness: what it is like to be autistic. Mind and Language 14:1–22. doi: 10.1111/1468-0017.00100.

17. Frith U (2003) Autism: explaining the enigma. 2nd. Malden, MA: Blackwell.

18. Happe F (2003) Theory of mind and the self. Annals of the New York Academy of Sciences 1001: 134–144. doi: 10.1196/annals.1279.008.

19. Baron-Cohen S (2005) Autism – 'autos': Literally, a total focus on the self? In: Feinberg TE, Keenan JP, editors. The lost self: pathologies of the brain and identity. Oxford: Oxford University Press.

20. Frith U, de Vignemont F (2005). Egocentrism, allocentrism, and Asperger syndrome. Consciousness and Cognition 14: 719–738. doi: 10.1016/j.concog.2005.04.006.

21. Hobson PR, Chidambi G, Lee A, Meyer J (2006) Foundations for self-awareness: an exploration through autism. Monographs of the Society for Research in Child Development 71: vii–166. doi: 10.1111/j.1540-5834.2006.00387.x

22. Glezerman T (2013) Autistic person's sense of self. Autism and the brain. New York: Springer. p. 194.

23. Alexopoulos T, Muller D, Ric F, Marendaz C (2012) I, me, mine: Automatic attentional capture by self-related stimuli. European Journal of Social Psychology, 42: 770–779. doi: 10.1002/ejsp.1882.

24. Cherry EC (1953) Some experiments on the recognition of speech, with one and with two ears. Journal of the Acoustical Society of America, 25: 975–979.doi: 10.1121/1.1907229.

25. Moray N (1959) Attention in dichotic listening: Affective cues and the influence of instructions. Quarterly Journal of Experimental Psychology 11: 56–60. doi: 10.1080/17470215908416289.

26. Wolford G, Morrison F (1980) Processing of unattended visual information. Memory and Cognition 8: 521–527. doi: 10.3758/BF03213771.

27. Wood N, Cowan N (1995) The cocktail party phenomenon revisited: how frequent are attention shifts to one's name in an irrelevant auditory channel? Journal of Experimental Psychology: Learning, Memory and Cognition 21: 255–260. doi: 10.1037/0278-7393.21.1. 255.

28. Shapiro KL, Caldwell J, Sorensen RE (1997) Personal names and the attentional blink: A visual "cocktail party" effect. Journal of Experimental Psychology-Human Perception and Performance 23: 504–514. doi: 10.1037/0096-1523.23.2.504.

29. Pfister R, Pohl C, Kiesel A, Kunde W (2012) Your unconscious knows your name. PLoS One 7: e32402. doi: 10.1371/journal.pone.0032402.

30. Berlad I, Pratt H (1995) P300 in response to the subject's own name. Electroencephalography and Clinical Neurophysiology 96, 472–474. doi: 10.1016/0168-5597(95)00116-A.

31. Müller HM, Kutas M (1996) What's in a name? Electrophysiological differences between spoken nouns, proper names. NeuroReport 8: 221–225. doi: 10.1097/00001756-199612200-00045.

32. Folmer RL, Yingling CD (1997) Auditory P3 responses to name stimuli. Brain and Language 56: 306–311. doi: 10.1006/brln.1997.1828.

33. Gray HM, Ambady N, Lowenthal WT, Deldin P (2004) P300 as an index of attention to self-relevant stimuli. Journal of Experimental and Social Psychology, 40: 216–224. doi: 10.1016/S0022-1031(03)00092-1

34. Sui J, Zhu Y, Han S (2006) Self-face recognition in attended and unattended conditions: an event-related brain potential study. NeuroReport 17: 423–427. doi: 10.1097/01.wnr. 0000203357.65190.6161.

35. Scott LS, Luciana M, Wewerka S, Nelson CA (2005) Electrophysiological correlates of facial self-recognition in adults and children. Cognitie, Creier, Comportament (Romanian Journal-Translation: Cognition, Brain, Behavior) 9: 211–238.

36. Tacikowski P, Nowicka A (2010) Allocation of attention to self-name and self-face: An ERP study. Biological Psychology 84: 318–324. doi: 10.1016/j.biopsycho.2010.03.009.

37. Uddin LQ (2011) The self in autism: An emerging view from neuroimaging. Neurocase 17: 201–208. doi: 10.1080/13554794.2010.509320.

38. Carmody DP, Moreno R, Mars AE, Seshadri K, Lambert GH, et al. (2007) Brief report: brain activation to social words in a sedated child with autism. Journal of Autism and Developmental Disorders 37: 1381–1385. doi: 10.1007/s10803-006-0270-3.

39. Carmody DP, Lewis M (2006) Brain activation when hearing one's own and others' names. Brain Research 1116: 153–158. doi: 10.1016/j.brainres.2006.07.121.

40. Holeckova I, Fischer C, Morlet D, Delpuech C, Costes N, et al. (2008) Subject's own name as a novel in a MMN design: a combined ERP and PET study. Brain Research 1189: 152–165. doi: 10.1016/j.brainres.2007.10.091.

41. Kampe KK, Frith CD, Frith U (2003) Hey John: Signals conveying communicative intention toward the self active brain regions associated with mentalizing, regardless of modality. Journal of Neuroscience 23: 5258–5263.

42. Tacikowski P, Brechmann A, Nowicka A (2013) Cross-modal pattern of brain activations associated with the processing of self- and significant other's name. Human Brain Mapping 34: 2069–2077. doi: 10.1002/hbm.22048.

43. Tacikowski P, Brechmann A, Marchewka A, Jednoróg K, Dobrowolny M, et al. (2011) Is it about the self or the significance? An fMRI study of self-name recognition. Social Neuroscience 6: 98–107. doi: 10.1080/17470919.2010.490665.

44. Jeste SS, Nelson CA 3rd (2009) Event related potentials in the understanding of Autism Spectrum Disorders: An analytical review. Journal of Autism and Developmental Disorders 39: 495–510. doi: 10.1007/s10803-008-0652-9.

45. Coles MGH, Rugg MD (1995) Event-related brain potentials: An introduction. In: Rugg MD, Coles MGH, editors. Electrophysiology of mind. Event-related brain potentials and cognition. Oxford: Oxford University Press, pp. 40–85.

46. Herrmann CS, Knight RT (2001) Mechanisms of human attention: Event related potentials and oscillations. Neuroscience and Biobehavioral Reviews 25: 465–476. doi:10.1016/S0149-7634(01)00027-6.

47. Hillyard SA, Anllo-Vento L (1998) Event-related brain potentials in the study of visual selective attention. Proceedings of the National Academy of Sciences of the United States of America 95: 781–787. doi:10.1073/pnas.95.3.781.

48. Luck SJ, Heinze H, Mangun GR, Hillyard SA (1990) Visual event-related potentials index focused attention within bilateral stimulus arrays. II. Functional dissociation of P1 and N1 components. Electroencephalography and Clinical Neurophysiology 75: 528–542. doi:10. 1016/0013-4694(90)90139-B.

49. Luck SJ, Woodman GE, Vogel EK (2000) Event-related potential studies of attention. Trends in Cognitive Sciences 4: 432–440. doi: 10.1016/S1364-6613(00)01545-X.

50. Mangun GR (1995) Neural mechanisms of visual selective attention. Psychophysiology 32: 4–18. doi: 10.1111/j.1469-8986.1995.tb03400.x.

51. Hileman CM, Henderson H, Mundy P, Newell L, Jaime M (2011) Developmental and individual differences on the P1 and N170 ERP components in children with and without autism. Developmental Neuropsychology 36: 214–236. doi: 10.1080/87565641.2010.549870.

52. Bentin S, Allison T, Puce A, Perez E, McCarthy G (1996) Electrophysiological studies of face perception in humans. Journal of Cognitive Neuroscience 8: 551–565. doi: 10.1162/jocn. 1996.8.6.551.

53. Eimer M (2000) Event-related brain potentials distinguish processing stages involved in face perception and recognition. Clinical Neurophysiology 111: 694–705. doi: 10.1016/S1388-2457(99)00285-0.

54. Rossion B, Gauthier I, Tarr MJ, Despland P, Bruyer R, et al. (2000) The N170 occipito-temporal component is delayed and enhanced to inverted faces but not to inverted objects: an electrophysiological account of face-specific processes in the human brain. Neuroreport 11: 69–74. doi: 10.1097/00001756-200001170-00014.

55. Caharel S, Poiroux S, Bernard C, Thibaut F, Lalonde R, et al. (2002) ERPs associated with familiarity and degree of familiarity during face recognition. International Journal of Neuroscience 112: Pages 1499–1512. doi: 10.1080/00207450290158368

56. Carbon CC, Schweinberger SR, Kaufmann JM, Leder H (2005) The Thatcher illusion seen by the brain: an event-related brain potentials study. Cognitive Brain Research 24: 544–555. doi: 10.1016/j.cogbrainres.2005.03.008.

57. Herzmann G, Schweinberger SR, Sommer W, Jentzsch I (2004) What's special about personally familiar faces? A multimodal approach. Psychophysiology 41: 688–701. doi: 10. 1111/j.1469-8986.2004.00196.x.

58. Schweinberger SR, Pickering EC, Jentzsch I, Burton M, Kaufmann JM (2002) Event-related brain potential evidence for a response of inferior temporal cortex to familiar face repetitions. Cognitive Brain Research 14: 398–409. doi: 10.1016/S0926-6410(02)00142-8.

59. Bentin S, Deouell LY (2000) Structural encoding and identification in face processing; ERP evidence for separate mechanisms. Cognitive Neuropsychology 17: 35–54. doi:10.1080/026432900380472.

60. Bentin S, Mouchetant-Rostaing Y, Giard MH, Echallier JF, Pernier J (1999) ERP manifestations of processing printed words at different psycholinguistic levels: time course and scalp distribution. Journal of Cognitive Neuroscience 11: 235–260. doi: 10.1162/089892 999563373

61. Polich J (2007) Updating P300: An integrative theory of P3a and P3b. Clinical Neurophysiology 118: 2128–2148. doi: 10.1016/j.clinph.2007.04.019.

62. Johnston VS, Miller DR, Burleson MH (1986) Multiple P3s to emotional stimuli and their theoretical significance. Psychophysiology, 23: 684–694. doi: 10.1111/j.1469-8986.1986.tb0 0694.x.

63. Dietrich DE, Waller C, Johannes S, Wieringa BM, Emrich HM, et al. (2001) Differential effects of emotional content on event-related potentials in word recognition memory. Neuropsychobiology 43: 96–101. doi:10.1159/000054874.

64. Polich J, Kok A (1995) Cognitive and biological determinants of P300: An integrative review. Biological Psychology 41: 103–146. doi: 10.1016/0301-0511(95)05130-9.

65. Dering B, Martin CD, Moro S, Pegna AJ, Thierry G (2011) Face-sensitive processes one hundred milliseconds after picture onset. Frontiers in Human Neuroscience 5: 93. doi: 10. 3389/fnhum.2011.00093.

66. Rossion B, Caharel S (2011) ERP evidence for the speed of face categorization in the human brain. Disentangling the contribution of low-level visual cues from face perception. Vision Research 51: 1297–1311. doi: 10.1016/j.visres.2011.04.003.

67. Mitsudo T, Kamio Y, Goto Y, Nakashima T, Tobimatsu S (2011) Neural responses in the occipital cortex to unrecognizable faces. Clinical Neurophysiology 122: 708–718. doi: 10.1016/j.clinph.2010.10.004.

68. Dawson G, Webb SJ, McPartland J (2005) Understanding the nature of face processing impairment in autism: Insights from behavioral and electrophysiological studies. Developmental Neuropsychology 27: 403–424. doi: 10.1207/s15326942dn2703_6.

69. Herrmann MJ, Ehlis AC, Ellgring H, Fallgatter AJ (2005) Early stages (P100) of face perception in humans as measured with event-related potentials (ERPs). Journal of Neural Transmission 112: 1073–1081. doi: 10.1007/s00702-004-0250-8.

70. Caharel S, Courtay N, Bernard C, Lalonde R, Rebai M (2005) Familiarity and emotional expression influence an early stage of face processing: An electrophysiological study. Brain and Cognition 59: 96–100. doi: 10.1016/j.bandc.2005.05.0.

71. Caharel S, Poiroux S, Bernard C, Thibaut F, Lalonde R, et al. (2002) ERPs associated with familiarity and degree of familiarity during face recognition. International Journal of Neuroscience 112: 1499–512. doi: 10.1080/00207450290158368.

72. Perrin F, Maquet P, Peigneux P, Ruby P, Degueldre C, et al. (2005) Neural mechanisms involved in the detection of our first name: a combined ERPs and PET study. Neuropsychologia 43: 12–19. doi: 10.1016/j. neuropsychologia.2004.07.0.

73. Tacikowski P, Jednorog K, Marchewka A, Nowicka A (2011) How multiple repetitions influence the processing of self-, famous and unknown names and faces: an ERP study. International Journal of Psychophysiology 79: 219–230. doi: 10.1016/j.ijpsycho.2010.10.010.

74. Zhao K, Yuan J, Zhong Y, Peng Y, Chen J, et al. (2009) Event-related potential correlates of the collective self-relevant effect. Neuroscience Letters 464: 57–61. doi: 10.1016/j.neulet.2009.07.017.

75. O'Connor K, Hamm JP, Kirk IJ (2005) The neurophysiological correlates of face processing in adults and children with Asperger's syndrom. Brain and Cognition 59; 82–95. doi: 10.1016/j.bandc.2005.05.004.

76. O'Connor K, Hamm JP, Kirk IJ (2007). Neurophysiological responses to face, facial regions and objects in adults with Asperger's syndrome: An ERP investigation. International Journal of Psychophysiology 63: 283–293. doi: 10.1016/j.ijpsycho.2006.12.001.

77. McPartland J, Dawson G, Webb SJ, Panagiotides H, Carver LJ (2004) Event-related brain potentials reveal anomalies in temporal processing of faces in autism spectrum disorder. Journal of Child Psychology and Psychiatry 45: 1235–1245. doi: 10.1111/j.1469-7610. 2004.00318.x.

78. Webb SJ, Jones E, Merkle K, Murias M, Greenson J, et al. (2010). Response to familiar faces, newly familiar faces, and novel faces as submitted by ERPs is intact in adults with autism spectrum disorders. International Journal of Psychophysiology 77: 106–117. doi: 10.1016/j.ijpsycho.2010.04.011.

79. Höller Y, Kronbichler M, Bergmann J, Crone JS, Ladurner G, et al. (2011) EEG frequency analysis of responses to the own-name stimulus. Clinical Neurophysiology 122: 99–106. doi: 10.1016/j.clinph.2010.05.029.

80. Brzeziński J, Gaul M, Hornowska E, Jaworowska A, Machowski A, et al. (2004) WAIS-R(PL) – Skala inteligencji Wechslera dla dorosłych – wersja zrewidowana. [Wechsler Adult Intelligence Scale - revised] Warsaw: Pracownia Testów Psychologicznych Polskiego Towarzystwa Psychologicznego.

81. Oldfield RC (1971) The assessment and analysis of handedness: the Edinburgh inventory. Neuropsychologia 9: 97–113. doi: 10.1016/0028-3932(71)90067-4.

82. Bell AJ, Sejnowski TJ (1995) An information-maximization approach to blind separation and blind deconvolution. Neural Computation 7: 1129–1159. doi: 10.1162/neco.1995.7.6. 1129.

83. Jung TP, Makeig S, Westerfield M, Townsend J, Courchesne E, et al. (2001) Analysis and visualization of single-trial event-related potentials. Human Brain Mapping 14: 166–185. doi: 10.1002/hbm.1050.

84. Greenhouse SW, Geisser S (1959) On Methods in the Analysis of Profile Data. Psychometrika 24: 95–112. doi: 10.1007/BF02289823.

85. Allison T, Puce A, Spencer DD, McCarthy G (1999) Electrophysiological studies of human face ferception. I: Potentials generated in occipitotemporal cortex by face and non-face stimuli. Cerebral Cortex 9: 415–430. doi:10.1093/cercor/9.5.415.

86. Pfütze EM, Sommer W, Schweinberger SR (2002) Age-related slowing in face and name recognition: Evidence from event-related brain potentials. Psychology and Aging 17: 140–160. doi: 10.1037/0882-7974.17.1.140.

87. Itier RJ, Taylor MJ (2004) Effects of repetition learning on upright, inverted and contrast-reversed face processing using ERPs. Neuroimage 21: 1518–1532. doi: 10.1016/j. neuroimage.2003.12.016.

88. Rossion B, Jacques C (2008) Does physical interstimulus variance account for early electrophysiological face sensitive responses in the human brain? Ten lessons on the N170. NeuroImage 39: 1959–1979. doi: 10.1016/j.neuroimage. 2007.10.

89. Samson F, Mottron L, Soulières I, Zeffiro TA (2012) Enhanced visual functioning in autism: an ALE meta-analysis. Human Brain Mapping 33: 1553–1581. doi: 10.1002/hbm. 21307.

90. Eimer M (2011) The face sensitivity in the N170 components. Frontiers in Human Neuroscience 5: 119. doi: 10.3389/fnhum.2011.00119.

91. Sadeh B, Zhdanov A, Podlipsky I, Hendler T, Yovel G (2008) The validity of the face-selective ERP N170 component during simultaneous recording with functional MRI. Neuroimage 42: 778–786. doi: 10.1016/j.neuroimage.2008.04.168.

92. Schweinberger SR, Ramsay LA, Kaufmann JM (2006) Hemispheric asymmetries in font-specific and abstractive priming of written personal names: Evidence from event-related brain potentials. Brain Research 1117: 195–205. doi: 10.1016/j.brainres.2006.08.070.

93. Chiron C, Leboyer M, Leon F, Jambaqué I, Nuttin C, et al. (1995) SPECT of the brain in childhood autism: evidence for a lack of normal hemispheric asymmetry. Developmental Medicine and Child Neurology 37: 849–860. doi: 10.1111/j.1469-8749.1995.tb11938.x.

94. Eyler LT, Pierce K, Courchesne E (2012) A failure of left temporal cortex to specialize for language is an early emerging and fundamental property of autism. Brain 135: 949–960. doi: 10.1093/brain/awr364.

95. Floris DL, Chura LR, J. Holt RJ, Suckling J, Bullmore ET, et al. (2013) Psychological correlates of handedness and corpus callosum asymmetry in autism: The left hemisphere dysfunction theory revisited. Journal of Autism and Developmental Disorders 43: 1758–1772. doi: 10.1007/s10803-012-1720-8.

96. Kleinhans NM, Muller RA, Cohen DN, Courchesne E (2008) Atypical functional lateralization of language in autism spectrum disorders. Brain Research 1221: 115–125. doi: 10.1016/j.brainres.2008.04.080.

97. Knaus TA, Silver AM, Kennedy M, Lindgren KA, Dominick KC, et al. (2010) Language laterality in autism spectrum disorder and typical controls: a functional, volumetric, and diffusion tensor MRI study. Brain and Language 112: 113–120. doi: 10. 1016/j.bandl.2009.11.005.

98. McPartland JC, Wu J, Bailey CA, Mayes LC, Schultz RT, et al. (2011) Atypical neural specialization for social percepts in autism spectrum disorder. Social Neuroscience 6: 436–451. doi: 10.1080/17470919.2011.586880.

99. Dawson G, Carver L, Meltzoff AN, Panagiotides H, McPartland J, et al. (2002) Neural correlates of face and object recognition in young children with autism spectrum disorder, developmental delay, and typical development. Child Development 73: 700–717. doi: 10. 1111/1467-8624.00433.

100. Öhman A, Flykt A, Esteves F (2001) Emotion drives attention: detecting the snake in the grass. Journal of Experimental Psychology: General 130:466–478. doi: 10.1037/0096-3445.130.3.466.

101. Lang PJ, Bradley MM, Cuthbert BN (1997) Motivated attention: Affect, activation and action. In: Lang PJ, Simons RF, Balaban MT, editors. Attention and Orienting: Sensory and Motivational Processes. Manhwah, New Jersey: Lawrence Erlbaum Associates Publishers, pp. 97–135.

102. Briggs KE, Martin FH (2009) Affective picture processing and motivational relevance: arousal and valence effects on ERPs in an oddball task. International Journal of Psychophysiology 72: 299–306. doi: 10.1016/j.ijpsycho. 2009.01.009.

103. Nuske HJ, Vivanti G, Dissanayake C (2013) Are emotion impairments unique to, universal, or specific in autism spectrum disorder? A comprehensive review. Cognition & Emotion 27: 1042–1061. doi: 10.1080/02699931.2012.762900.

104. Pierce K, Heist F, Sedaghat F, Courchesne E (2004) The brain response to personally familiar faces in autism: findings of fusiform activity and beyond. Brain 127: 2703–2716. doi: 10.1093/brain/awh289.

105. Bruce V, Young A (1986) Understanding face recognition. British Journal of Psychology 77: 305–327. doi: 10.1111/j.2044-8295.1986.tb02199.

106. Morton J (1969) Interaction of information in word recognition. Psychological Review 76: 165–178. doi: 10.1037/h0027366.

107. Morton J (1979) Facilitation in word recognition: experiments causing change in the logogen model. In: Kolers PA, Wrolstal M, Bouma H, editors. Processing of Visible Language. New York: Plenum Press, pp. 259–268.

108. Valentine T, Moore V, Brédart S (1995) Priming production of people's names. The Quarterly Journal of Experimental Psychology Section A: Human Experimental Psychology 48: 513–535. doi: 10.1080/14640749508401404.

109. Herzmann G, Sommer W (2007) Memory-related ERP components for experimentally learned faces and names: characteristics and parallel-test reliabilities. Psychophysiology 44: 262–276. doi: 10.1111/j.1469-8986.2007.00505.x.

110. Paller KA, Gonsalves B, Grabowecky M, Bozic VS, Yamada S (2000) Electrophysiological correlates of recollecting faces of known and unknown individuals. NeuroImage 11: 98–110.doi: 10.1006/nimg/1999.0521.

111. Escalante-Mead PR, Minshew NJ, Sweeney JA (2003) Abnormal brain lateralization in high-functioning autism. Journal of Autism and Developmental Disorders 33: 539–543. doi: 10.1023/A:1025887713788.

112. D'Cruz AM, Mosconi MW, Steele S, Rubin LH, Luna B, et al. (2009) Lateralized response timing deficits in autism. Biological Psychiatry 66: 393–397. doi: 10. 1016/j.biopsych.2009.01.008.

Screening for Autism Spectrum Disorders with the Brief Infant-Toddler Social and Emotional Assessment

Ingrid Kruizinga[1], Janne C. Visser[2], Tamara van Batenburg-Eddes[3], Alice S. Carter[4], Wilma Jansen[5], Hein Raat[1]*

1 Department of Public Health, Erasmus University Medical Center, Rotterdam, the Netherlands, 2 Karakter University Center Nijmegen, Nijmegen, the Netherlands, 3 Department of Psychology and Education, VU University, Amsterdam, the Netherlands, 4 Department of Psychology, University of Massachusetts Boston, Boston, Massachusetts, United States of America, 5 Department of Youth Policy, Rotterdam Municipal Health Service (GGD Rotterdam-Rijnmond), Rotterdam, the Netherlands

Abstract

Objective: Using parent-completed questionnaires in (preventive) child health care can facilitate the early detection of psychosocial problems and psychopathology, including autism spectrum disorders (ASD). A promising questionnaire for this purpose is the Brief Infant-Toddler Social and Emotional Assessment (BITSEA). The screening accuracy with regard to ASD of the BITSEA Problem and Competence scales and a newly calculated Autism score were evaluated.

Method: Data, that was collected between April 2010 and April 2011, from a community sample of 2-year-olds (N = 3127), was combined with a sample of preschool children diagnosed with ASD (N = 159). For the total population and for subgroups by child's gender, area under the Receiver Operating Characteristic (ROC) curve was examined, and across a range of BITSEA Problem, Competence and Autism scores, sensitivity, specificity, positive and negative likelihood ratio's, diagnostic odds ratio and Youden's index were reported.

Results: The area under the ROC curve (95% confidence interval, [95%CI]) of the Problem scale was 0.90(0.87–0.92), of the Competence scale 0.93(0.91–0.95), and of the Autism score 0.95(0.93–0.97). For the total population, the screening accuracy of the Autism score was significantly better, compared to the Problem scale. The screening accuracy of the Competence scale was significantly better for girls (AUC = 0.97; 95%CI = 0.95–0.98) than for boys (AUC = 0.91; 95%CI = 0.88–0.94).

Conclusion: The results indicate that the BITSEA scales and newly calculated Autism score have good discriminative power to differentiate children with and without ASD. Therefore, the BITSEA may be helpful in the early detection of ASD, which could have beneficial effects on the child's development.

Editor: Gabriel S. Dichter, UNC Chapel Hill, United States of America

Funding: This study is funded by a grant from the funding body ZonMw, The Netherlands Organization for Health Research and Development (www.zonmw.nl), project number: 80-82435-98-8058. The funders had no role in study design, data collection and analysis, decision to publish, or preparation of the manuscript.

Competing Interests: Alice S. Carter gets royalties on the sale of the BITSEA from Pearson Assessment (not in the context of this study). The other authors have no conflicts of interest relevant to this article to disclose.

* E-mail: h.raat@erasmusmc.nl

Introduction

Preventive child health care offers a systematic opportunity for the early detection of psychosocial problems and psychopathology, such as autism spectrum disorders (ASD), among toddlers. In the Netherlands, preventive child health care for children of ages 0–4 years is delivered through community well-child clinics that provide routine developmental assessment and vaccinations (i.e. well-child visits) and that are free of charge [1].

ASD represents a set of neurodevelopmental disorders that are characterized by impairments in the domains of reciprocal social interactions and communication and by restrictive, stereotyped patterns of behavior [2]. In the current Diagnostic and Statistical Manual of Mental disorders, 5th edition, ASD's are part of the pervasive developmental disorders and classified into three main categories, namely: autistic disorder, Asperger's disorder and pervasive developmental disorder-not otherwise specified [2]. Studies report ASD prevalence rates of about 1.0% [3,4].

Abnormal functioning that is indicative of ASD starts before 3 years of age [2]. On average, the first symptoms to arouse parental concerns about children eventually diagnosed with ASD occur before the second birthday. However, the average age of ASD diagnosis is approximately three years of age and often occurs later [5]. These findings suggest that it should be possible to detect and diagnose ASD earlier. Early detection of ASD is important because early access to interventions may improve children's outcomes, [6,7] and diagnosis may enhance parent's understanding and coping with the impairments of their child [8].

One approach for facilitating early identification of ASD is the population-based screening of children as part of well-child visits using parent-completed questionnaires [9,10] Several instruments are developed for the early detection of ASD, of which the use of the Checklist for Autism in Toddlers (CHAT) [11] and the Modified Checklist for Autism in Toddlers (M-CHAT) [12] is advocated by autism support organizations [13]. However, early detection instruments that are used in a preventive health care setting should cover a broad range of psychosocial problems, since limited time and capacity in the preventive child health care make it undesirable to screen for each psychosocial problem separately. Also, it has been shown that psychosocial problems tend to co-occur, [14,15] and that individual problems may apply to more than one disorder [16]. In addition to measuring problem domains, it is crucial to also measure competence domains. Delays in the acquisition of competencies are strongly related to a wide range of psychosocial problems later in life [17] and are often the prodromal signs of developmental disorders, such as ASD [18].

The Brief Infant-Toddler Social and Emotional Assessment (BITSEA) [19] is a promising and short (42 items) questionnaire, that measures both problems (Problem scale) and delays in the acquisition of competencies (Competence scale) in 1–3 year olds, and also consists of items designed to measure ASD symptoms. The BITSEA is not designed to diagnose ASD, but it may be useful as a screener for identifying children with this disorder [20]. Previous studies have shown that the BITSEA Problem and Competence scale has adequate reliability for the Problem scale and validity for the Problem and Competence scale [19,21–23]. The study performed in the Netherlands [23] evaluated among others the internal consistency, test-retest reliability, concurrent validity and discriminant validity. An adequate Cronbach's alpha (i.e. >0.70[24]) was found for the Problem scale (0.76) and marginal for the Competence scale (0.63). Test-retest reliability was adequate (>0.70 [25]) for the Problem scale (0.75) and marginal for the Competence scale (0.61). The BITSEA Problem scale was positively correlated with the CBCL, Pearson coefficients of 0.66 (Internalizing), 0.65 (Externalizing) and 0.75 (Total Problem). The BITSEA Competence score was negatively correlated with the CBCL, Pearson coefficients of −0.26 (Internalizing), −0.23 (Externalizing) and −0.26 (Total Problem). All correlations were significant (p<0.01). The mean BITSEA score was compared between a group of parents that worried about the development of their child and a group that did not worry. The Problem and Competence score were significantly less favourable in the group of parents that worried, compared to the group of parents that did not worry (effect sizes were respectively 0.93 and 0.52)."

Also the sensitivity and specificity of the BITSEA has been evaluated in several studies [19,26,27] One study, conducted in the United States [19], examined its sensitivity and specificity in a community sample of 1280 children. In this study, children with scores in the clinical range on the Child Behavioral Checklist (CBCL1.5-5) [28] and Infant-Toddler Social and Emotional Assessment (ITSEA) [29,30] were used as reference groups for the evaluation of the Problem scale. A sensitivity of respectively 93.2% and 78.1% and a specificity of respectively 78.0% and 88.8% were found. The Competence scale was evaluated against a group of children with a score in the clinical range on the ITSEA and had a sensitivity of 68.9% and a specificity of 95.1%. Problem scale cutpoints were chosen at scores of $\geq 75^{th}$ percentile and Competence scale cutpoints were chosen at scores of $<15^{th}$ percentile [31]. In a Turkish study [26], in a community sample of 462 children, sensitivity and specificity of only the Competence scale was examined relative to children treated in a child psychiatry outpatient clinic with an autism diagnosis (n = 35). In this study, the sensitivity was 72%–93% and specificity was 76%–85%, depending on the cutpoint chosen. A Dutch study [27] evaluated the screening accuracy of the BITSEA Problem scale more extensively than prior studies. The screening accuracy was evaluated with multiple indices (i.e. area under the curve, sensitivity, specificity, likelihood ratio's, diagnostic odds ratios and Youden's index) by calculating receiver operating character-

istic (ROC) curves of the BITSEA Problem scale relative to the CBCL Total Problem scale. Indices of screening accuracy for a range of BITSEA Problem scores were presented, because different cutpoints might be chosen in different settings (e.g. clinical application versus epidemiological research). In that study, the screening accuracy of the BITSEA Competence scale was not evaluated with a reference group of children with a CBCL Total Problem score in the clinical range, since the CBCL Total Problem score does not measure competencies.

In the present study we aim to evaluate the screening accuracy of both the BITSEA Problem and Competence scales with regard to an ASD diagnosis. Additionally, we will evaluate the screening accuracy of the BITSEA items that are specifically intended to signal ASD, since little is known about the performance of these items in the detection of ASD. Previous studies showed differences in mean BITSEA scores between boys and girls (with boys scoring less favourably) [19,22,23], therefore the screening accuracy is also evaluated in subgroups by child gender.

Method

Ethics Statement

Regarding the data collection of the community sample; only anonymous data were used and the questionnaires were completed on a voluntary basis by the parents. Parents received written information on these questionnaires and were free to refuse to participation. Observational research with data does not fall within the ambit of the Dutch Act on research involving human subjects [32] and does not require the approval of an ethics review board. The Medical Ethics Committee of the Erasmus Medical Centre Rotterdam declared to have no objection ('formal waiver') regarding the study protocol and consent procedures. The Medical Ethical Committee of the University Medical Centre St. Radboud Nijmegen approved the study protocol regarding the ASD-study. We are prepared to make the data available upon request.

Design and participants

For the present study, data from two separate samples were combined. First, data from a community sample of 2-year old children was used. These data were gathered between April 2010 and April 2011 by child health care organizations in the context of routine health examinations in the Rotterdam area, the Netherlands. Parents of 3170 children that attended the well-child visit handed in the questionnaire (95.5% of all parents that attended the well-child visit). Children were excluded from the analyses if there were too many missing items on both BITSEA scales [20] (n = 43), leaving a study population of 3127 (94.2%) children. No children in the community sample were under treatment of a mental health professional at the time of inclusion. Details on the design and participants of the community sample are described elsewhere [23].

Second, data from a sample of children diagnosed with ASD were used (i.e. ASD-sample). Children between the ages of 12–40 months were recruited in the DIANE-study (Diagnosis and Intervention of Autism in the Netherlands) [33] at Karakter Child and Adolescent Psychiatry University Center Nijmegen, the Netherlands. Children with a positive score on the Early Screening of Autistic Traits Questionnaire [34] and/or for whom there were major concerns regarding social and communicative development entered the study between spring 2004 and spring 2007. Parents of the ASD-sample completed the ITSEA (i.e. a more comprehensive measure that includes the BITSEA items) at home before their first visit for diagnostic assessments and all children underwent an extensive psychiatric assessment (i.e. administration of the Autism

Diagnostic Observation Schedule and Autism Diagnostic Interview-Revised) observations of standardised parent-child play and standardised assessment of cognitive and language skills). Details on the design and participants of the ASD-sample are described elsewhere [35]. For the purpose of this study, answers on BITSEA items were extracted from the larger pool of ITSEA items. Children were excluded from the analyses if they did not receive a diagnosis (n = 29), if they received a diagnosis other than ASD (n = 69) (i.e. false positives), if there were too many missing items on the BITSEA scales [20] (n = 19), or if they were younger than 12 months (n = 2) leaving a study population of 159 (57%) children.

Measures

The BITSEA, designed for 1-to-3-year old children, consists of 42 items with three response options ('not true/rarely'(0), 'somewhat true/sometimes'(1), 'very true/often'(2)) and comprises two multi-item scales; a Problem scale (31 items) and a Competence scale (11 items). The Problem scale assesses social-emotional/behavioral problems such as aggression, defiance, overactivity, negative emotionality, anxiety, and withdrawal. The Competence scale assesses social-emotional abilities such as empathy, prosocial behaviors, and compliance [31]. Responses can be summed for each scale: a high score on the Problem scale and/or a low score on the Competence scale is less favourable [20]. The BITSEA also consists of 17 items that are specifically included for the early detection of ASD belonging to either the Problem scale (9 items) or the Competence scale (8 items). The autism items reflect problems behaviors that are typical of children with ASD (e.g. *put things in a special order over and over*) and competencies in which deficits are often present in children with ASD (e.g. *points to show you something far away*) [20]. Although these items formally do not represent a separate scale, we calculated the Autism score analogous to the Problem scale score, yielding a good internal consistency (Cronbach's alpha = 0.77). Answers on the autism items belonging to the Competence scale were first reversed before all autism items were summed, so a higher Autism score would represent more problems and fewer competencies. Children with more than 3 missing items were excluded for analyses (n = 48). Excluded children were all part of the community sample.

Items on standard socio-demographic variables were included: child age and gender.

Analyses

Demographic characteristics and mean BITSEA scores. Differences in mean BITSEA scores and child age between the community sample and the ASD-sample were tested with independent sample t-tests. Differences in gender composition of the community sample and ASD-sample were tested with Chi-square tests.

Screening accuracy. Screening accuracy was evaluated by calculating receiver operating characteristic (ROC) curves, with a reference group that consists of children with a diagnosis of ASD. The area under the ROC curve was examined, along with, for a range of Problem and Competence scale scores and the Autism score; sensitivity, specificity, positive test likelihood ratio (LHR$^+$) and negative test likelihood ratio (LHR$^-$), diagnostic odds ratio (OR) and Youden's index. All indices for screening accuracy were evaluated for the total sample as well as for boys and girls separately.

The ROC curve is a plot of sensitivity as a function of 1-specificity for all possible cutpoints of the BITSEA. The greater the area under the curve (AUC), the more discriminative power

the BITSEA has in differentiating children with and without ASD. An AUC>0.90 indicates high accuracy; 0.70≤AUC<0.90 indicates moderate accuracy; 0.50≤AUC<0.70 indicates low accuracy; and AUC = 0.50 is chance level accuracy [36]. We examined the 95% confidence intervals of the AUCs to evaluate whether the screening accuracy differed significantly between subgroups.

To determine the optimal cutpoint, the Youden index was used, which is defined as the maximum vertical distance between the ROC curve and the diagonal or chance line and is calculated as *Youden's index = sensitivity+specificity-1* [37].

Sensitivity is the proportion of true positives that are correctly identified by the test; specificity is the proportion of true negatives that are correctly identified by the test. To further investigate the correctness of classification, likelihood ratios were calculated. *LHR$^+$ = sensitvitiy/(1-specificity)* is the ratio of the probability of a positive test result if the outcome is positive (true positive) to the probability of a positive test result if the outcome is negative (false positive); *LHR$^-$ = (1-sensitivity)/specificity* is the ratio of the probability of a negative test result if the outcome is positive (false negative) to the probability of a negative test result if the outcome is negative (true negative). LHR$^+$>7.00 and LHR$^-$<0.30 indicate high screening accuracy [38].

The *OR = sensitivity*specificity/((1-sensitivity)*(1-specificity)) = LHR$^+$/LHR$^-$* of a test is the ratio of the odds of a positive test result when having the 'disorder' relative to the odds of a positive test result when not having the 'disorder'. The values of OR ranges from zero to infinity, with higher values indicating better discriminatory test performance. OR>20.00 indicate high screening accuracy [38].

The AUC, Youden's index, sensitivity, specificity, LHR$^+$, LHR$^-$ and OR are independent of prevalence of the 'disorder', as opposed to the positive predictive value and negative predictive value, therefore the latter were not evaluated in this study. [38].

All analyses were performed in SPSS 20.0 (SPSS Inc. 2011).

Results

The demographic characteristics of the multiethnic community sample and ASD-sample are presented in Table 1. In comparison to the community sample, the ASD-sample consisted of older children (t = 58.3, p<0.001) and more boys (X^2 = 50.2, p<0.001).

Mean BITSEA scores

The mean Problem and Competence scale scores and the Autism score are presented in Table 1. In comparison to children in the community sample, children in the ASD-sample scored less favourably on the Problem scale (t = 28.1, p<0.001), the Competence scale (t = 29.9, p<0.001) and Autism score (t = 37.3, p< 0.001).

Screening accuracy

ROC curves of the Problem and Competence scale scores and Autism score are presented in Figure 1. In Table 2, the AUC and sensitivity, specificity, LHR$^+$, LHR$^-$, OR and Youden's index are presented for a range of BITSEA scale, for the total population and for subgroups by child gender.

The AUC's (95% confidence interval [CI]) of the Problem scale was 0.90(0.87–0.92), and of the Competence scale 0.93(0.91–0.95). The screening accuracy of the Problem scale was equal for girls (AUC = 0.93; 95%CI = 0.89–0.97) and boys (AUC = 0.88; 95%CI = 0.85–0.91). The screening accuracy of the Competence scale was better for girls (AUC = 0.97; 95%CI = 0.95–0.98) than for boys (AUC = 0.91; 95%CI = 0.88–0.94). The Youden index

Table 1. Child characteristics of the autism spectrum disorder (ASD) sample and community sample.

	ASD-sample N = 159	Community sample N = 3127
	Percentage (N)	Percentage (N)
Gender[a]*		
boys	79.2 (126)	50.0 (1564)
girls	20.8 (33)	49.1 (1535)
	Mean (SD)	Mean (SD)
Age (months)*	31.8 (6.4)	23.7 (0.7)
BITSEA Problem scale score*	20.5 (8.7)	7.8 (5.3)
BITSEA Competence scale score*	10.0 (4.0)	17.5 (3.0)
BITSEA Autism score*	14.6 (5.2)	4.1 (3.3)

a. Percentages do not sum to 100% due to missing values.
* Significant differences in composition between ASD-sample and community sample with regard to gender, and age and mean Problem scale score, Competence scale score, and Autism score, $p < 0.001$.

indicated the same optimal cutpoint for the total population and for boys and girls for the Problem scale (score 13) and for the Competence scale (score 15).

In Table 3 AUCs and sensitivity, specificity, LHR⁺, LHR⁻, OR and Youden's index are presented for a range of Autism scores for the total population and for subgroups by child gender. The AUC was 0.95(0.93–0.97) and the screening accuracy was equal for girls (AUC = 0.97; 95%CI = 0.95–0.99) and boys (AUC = 0.93; 95%CI = 0.91–0.96). The Youden index indicated different optimal cutpoint for the total population (score 10) and for boys (score 9) and girls (score 8).

The scores in the general population with the highest Youden index as cutpoints for the Problem and Competence scale and Autism score yielded concern level of ASD of respectively 16.1%, 10.1% and 6.9% children.

Discussion

The present study evaluated the screening accuracy of the Problem and Competence scales and the newly calculated Autism score for a community sample in comparison to a sample that consists of children with an ASD diagnosis. Our results indicate that the Problem and Competence scales and the Autism score have high screening accuracy to detect ASD (i.e. AUC>0.90).

In our study we present the sensitivity and specificity for a range of BITSEA scores, because different cutpoints might be chosen in different settings (e.g. clinical application versus epidemiological research). For the comparison of the sensitivity and specificity with results of other studies we chose to discuss the sensitivity and specificity for the optimal cutpoint as indicated by the Youden index. In comparison with the prior Dutch study [27] on the screening accuracy of the BITSEA Problem scale with regard a CBCL Total Problem score in the clinical range, we found similar

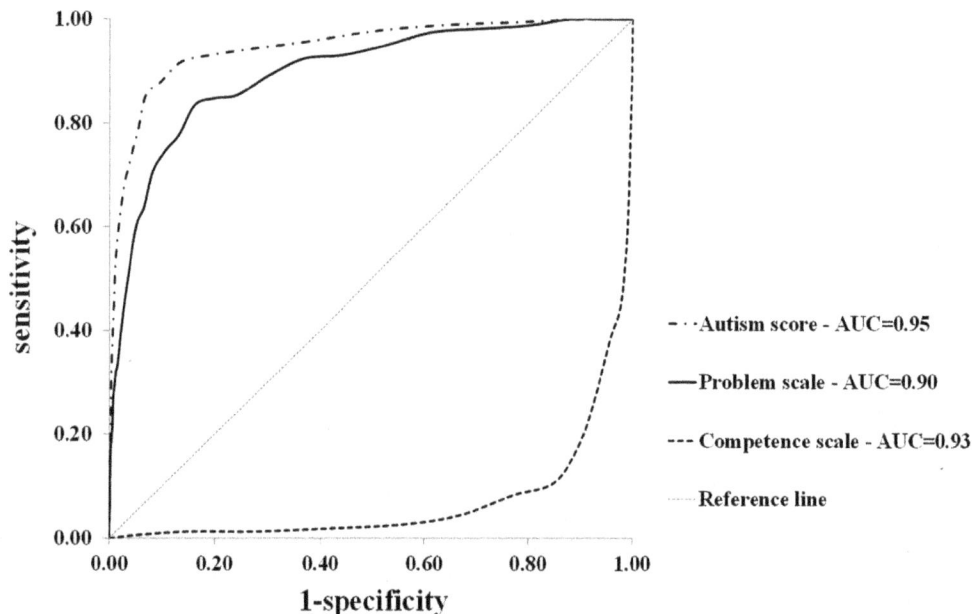

Figure 1. ROC curves and AUC of the BITSEA Problem and Competence scale and BITSEA Autism score relative to a sample of children with a diagnosis of autism spectrum disorder.

Table 2. The screening accuracy of the BITSEA scales with regard to autism spectrum disorders: Area Under the Curve and sensitivity, specificity, liklihood ratio's, diagnostic odd ratio and Youden's index for a range of Problem and Competence scores, for the total sample and for subgroups by gender.

Scale	BITSEA Problem							BITSEA Competence						
Total	AUC = 0.90 (95% CI = 0.87–0.92)							AUC = 0.93 (95% CI = 0.91–0.95)						
N = 3286	score	sens	spec	LHR⁺	LHR⁻	OR	J	score	sens	spec	LHR⁺	LHR⁻	OR	J
	9	0.92	0.63	2.51	0.12	20.73	0.56	11	0.98	0.56	2.20	0.04	52.97	0.53
	10	0.89	0.70	2.94	0.16	18.92	0.59	12	0.96	0.61	2.48	0.07	37.00	0.57
	11	0.85	0.76	3.53	0.19	18.24	0.61	13	0.93	0.72	3.34	0.10	35.01	0.65
	12	0.85	0.80	4.22	0.19	22.05	0.65	14	0.90	0.82	4.91	0.12	40.41	0.72
	13	**0.83**	**0.84**	**5.18**	**0.20**	**26.22**	**0.67**	**15**	**0.85**	**0.89**	**7.92**	**0.17**	**47.95**	**0.74**
	14	0.78	0.87	5.92	0.26	23.06	0.65	16	0.77	0.92	9.38	0.25	37.71	0.69
	15	0.75	0.89	7.08	0.28	24.85	0.64	17	0.67	0.96	15.19	0.34	44.37	0.63
	16	0.71	0.92	8.60	0.32	26.93	0.62	18	0.56	0.97	21.95	0.46	48.15	0.53
	17	0.64	0.93	9.75	0.39	25.10	0.57	19	0.43	0.98	22.48	0.58	38.49	0.41
Boys	AUC = 0.88 (95% CI = 0.85–0.91)							AUC = 0.91 (95% CI = 0.88–0.94)*						
N = 1690	9	0.92	0.60	2.31	0.13	17.48	0.52	11	0.97	0.53	2.08	0.05	42.04	0.51
	10	0.88	0.67	2.64	0.18	14.80	0.55	12	0.95	0.60	2.34	0.09	27.19	0.54
	11	0.85	0.73	3.19	0.21	15.50	0.58	13	0.92	0.71	3.12	0.12	26.66	0.62
	12	0.84	0.78	3.88	0.20	19.17	0.62	14	0.88	0.82	4.84	0.14	33.88	0.70
	13	**0.83**	**0.82**	**4.61**	**0.20**	**22.63**	**0.65**	**15**	**0.82**	**0.88**	**6.92**	**0.20**	**34.70**	**0.71**
	14	0.77	0.85	5.18	0.27	19.18	0.62	16	0.73	0.90	7.65	0.30	25.51	0.63
	15	0.74	0.88	6.02	0.30	20.17	0.62	17	0.62	0.94	11.23	0.40	28.23	0.57
	16	0.70	0.90	7.28	0.33	21.81	0.60	18	0.50	0.97	15.66	0.52	30.15	0.47
	17	0.63	0.92	8.06	0.40	19.92	0.55	19	0.37	0.98	15.54	0.65	24.09	0.35
Girls	AUC = 0.93 (95% CI = 0.89–0.97)							AUC = 0.97 (95% CI = 0.95–0.98)*						
N = 1568	9	0.94	0.66	2.79	0.10	28.74	0.60	11	0.98	0.66	2.85	0.03	91.70	0.64
	10	0.94	0.73	3.46	0.09	39.10	0.66	12	0.97	0.69	3.11	0.04	72.11	0.66
	11	0.87	0.79	4.05	0.16	24.65	0.66	13	0.95	0.78	4.32	0.07	62.63	0.73
	12	0.87	0.82	4.79	0.16	30.36	0.69	14	0.92	0.81	4.90	0.10	49.22	0.73
	13	**0.84**	**0.86**	**6.04**	**0.19**	**32.24**	**0.70**	**15**	**0.88**	**0.94**	**14.14**	**0.12**	**113.81**	**0.82**
	14	0.81	0.89	7.22	0.22	33.11	0.69	16	0.82	0.97	26.15	0.19	138.50	0.79
	15	0.77	0.91	8.94	0.25	36.14	0.69	17	0.73	1.00	x	0.27	x	0.73
	16	0.74	0.93	10.89	0.28	39.33	0.67	18	0.62	1.00	x	0.38	x	0.62
	17	0.68	0.95	12.97	0.34	38.09	0.63	19	0.49	1.00	x	0.51	x	0.49

* The Competence scale AUCs differ significantly between boys and girls (i.e. the 95% confidence intervals do not overlap)
Note: AUC = area under the curve; 95%CI = 95% confidence interval; sens = sensitivity; spec = specificity; LHR⁺ = likelihood ratio positive test; LHR⁻ = likelihood ratio negative test; OR = diagnostic odds ratio; J = Youden's index.
All AUC's were significant (p<0.001). Scores with the highest unrounded Youden's index are indicated in bold.

results; also a AUC>0.90 and no differences between subgroups. Multiple values for sensitivity and specificity of the BITSEA are reported in the study conducted in the US, because different indicators were used to classify a 'clinical group', and also in the Turkish study, because in their study a range of BITSEA cutpoints was applied. The US-study [19] found comparable mean sensitivity and specificity for the Problem scale as in our study. However, for the Competence scale in the US-study, a lower sensitivity and slightly higher specificity were found, compared to our study. The Turkish study [26] found slightly higher mean sensitivity and lower mean specificity for the Competence scale, compared to our study. However, the different methods to determine sensitivity and specificity (i.e. different indicators of a

'clinical group' and different methods to determine cutpoints), make it difficult to compare results across these studies.

The Youden index yielded the same cutpoints for boys and girls on the Problem and Competence scales. These results differ from what was found in the US-study [19], where the cutpoints on the Problem scale in children aged 24–29 months differed between boys (score 14) and girls (score 13) and also differed on the Competence scale (girls, score 15; boys, score 14). The Turkish study [26] found the same cutpoint (score 12) on the Competence scale in children aged 24–35 months, for both boys and girls. These differences between studies might be attributed to different characteristics of the study populations. Also, in the Turkish study, the ASD sample size (n = 35) was much smaller compared to our ASD sample size (n = 159).

Table 3. The screening accuracy of the BITSEA Autism score: Area Under the Curve and sensitivity, specificity, liklihood ratio's, diagnostic odds ratio and Youden's index for a range of Autism scores, for the total sample and for subgroups by gender.

	BITSEA Autism score						
Total	**AUC = 0.95 (95% CI = 0.93–0.97)**						
N = 3236	score	sens	spec	LHR⁺	LHR⁻	OR	J
	6	0.94	0.72	3.43	0.08	43.33	0.67
	7	0.93	0.81	4.86	0.09	56.11	0.74
	8	0.92	0.86	6.77	0.10	70.71	0.78
	9	0.88	0.90	9.05	0.13	67.53	0.78
	10	**0.85**	**0.93**	**12.40**	**0.16**	**78.79**	**0.78**
	11	0.79	0.95	14.39	0.22	64.70	0.73
	12	0.72	0.96	19.44	0.29	66.80	0.68
	13	0.68	0.97	25.35	0.33	75.96	0.65
	14	0.59	0.98	37.59	0.42	89.38	0.57
Boys	AUC = 0.93 (95% CI = 0.91–0.96)						
N = 1671	5	0.94	0.59	2.29	0.09	24.30	0.53
	6	0.94	0.70	3.08	0.09	33.74	0.63
	7	0.92	0.78	4.10	0.10	40.05	0.70
	8	0.90	0.84	5.66	0.11	49.92	0.74
	9	**0.88**	**0.89**	**7.73**	**0.13**	**57.56**	**0.77**
	10	0.85	0.91	9.94	0.16	60.28	0.76
	11	0.79	0.93	11.79	0.23	51.33	0.72
	12	0.70	0.95	14.20	0.32	44.76	0.65
	13	0.65	0.97	18.97	0.36	52.46	0.62
Girls	AUC = 0.97 (95% CI = 0.95–0.99)						
N = 1543	4	1.00	0.57	2.33	0.00	x	0.57
	5	1.00	0.67	3.07	0.00	x	0.67
	6	0.97	0.76	4.00	0.04	93.93	0.73
	7	0.97	0.84	6.23	0.04	163.02	0.81
	8	**0.97**	**0.89**	**8.76**	**0.04**	**241.62**	**0.86**
	9	0.87	0.92	10.79	0.14	76.91	0.79
	10	0.87	0.95	16.46	0.14	120.83	0.82
	11	0.81	0.96	18.48	0.20	91.29	0.76
	12	0.81	0.97	32.09	0.20	161.62	0.78

Note: AUC = area under the curve; 95%CI = 95% confidence interval; sens = sensitivity; spec = specificity; LHR⁺ = likelihood ratio positive test; LHR⁻ = likelihood ratio negative test; OR = diagnostic odds ratio; J = Youden's index. All AUC's were significant (p<0.001). Scores with the highest unrounded Youden's index are indicated in bold.

The screening accuracy of the newly calculated Autism score was equal for boys and girls, however, the scores with the highest Youden's index differed between boys (score 9) and girls (score 8). Even though the Autism score consists of less items (17 items), its screening accuracy for ASD was better for the total population than the Problem scale (31 items), but not better than the Competence scale (11 items). The Autism score is formally not a separate BITSEA scale and the findings of the present study imply that calculation of the Autism score is unnecessary when the Competence score is known. It was to be expected that the screening accuracy of the Autism score would be at least equally well as the screening accuracy of the Competence scale, since the Autism score consists of 8 of the 11 Competence items. However, the addition of the items from the Problem scale does not further improve the screening accuracy of the Autism score.

Limitations and strengths

Our study has some limitations. First, the BITSEA scores for the ASD-sample are based on BITSEA items that were extracted from the larger pool of ITSEA items, since parents of children in the ASD-sample completed the ITSEA.

Second, as it is expected that children with *typical* development acquire more competencies with age, previous studies have found higher Competence scores in older children, compared to younger children.[19,22]. Our community sample consisted of a homogeneous sample with regard to age ($M = 23.7$, $SD = 0.7$). Therefore, it may not be appropriate to generalise our findings on screening accuracy of the Competence scale to children of other ages.

Third, the ASD-sample differed significantly from the community sample with regard to child's gender (more boys), and age (older children). It is likely that these characteristics might have influenced mean BITSEA scale scores; previous studies have found

Screening for Autism Spectrum Disorders with the Brief Infant-Toddler Social and Emotional Assessment

that mean BITSEA scores for boys are less favourable [19,22,23] and that mean Competence scores increase with age [19,22]. Therefore, differences in mean BITSEA scores between the community and ASD-sample might not solely be attributed to the ASD, but also to the demographic characteristics of the samples. To compensate for these differences between conditions, we applied propensity score matching post-hoc. This yielded a sample of 900 matched cases: 750 children in the community sample en 150 in the ASD-sample, with a statistically equal boy/girl ratio (community sample: 74.5% boys, ASD-sample: 80,0% boys). There was still a significant (p<0.001) difference between matched cases regarding age (community sample: M = 28.9; SD = 7.5, ASD-sample: M = 31.8; SD = 6.4), however the effect size, Cohen's d, was small; 0.38 [39]. We calculated the AUC for the ROC-curves again for the matched sample, and no significant differences (i.e. no overlapping confidence intervals) were found compared to our prior results (data not shown). ·

Fourth, we do not have follow-up data on the community sample with regard to an ASD diagnosis. However, since the estimated prevalence of ASD is 1% [3,4], we may assume that 31 children out of 3127 children will receive a diagnosis of ASD. It is difficult to estimate exactly what the effect is on our results. However, if the effect would be significant (i.e. a community sample with definitely no children with ASD would lead to other results), the mean BITSEA scores of that community sample would be more favourable than in the present study. This would mean an even larger difference in BITSEA scores, compared to the ASD sample, possibly leading to larger AUC and better sensitivity and specificity than we have found in the present study. So, due to this limitation we rather underestimate than overestimate the 'true' results.

A strength of our study is that the analyses were performed on a large community sample and ASD-sample which adds to the power of the study. Moreover, children in the ASD-sample were diagnosed by experienced clinicians and diagnoses were based on extensive multidisciplinary diagnostic procedures.

Additionally, another strength of our study is that parents completed the questionnaire prior to receiving a diagnostic evaluation. So parents were not biased by knowledge of an ASD diagnosis when answering the questions.

Future research

This study evaluated the screening accuracy of the BITSEA for ASD specifically. We recommend future studies to evaluate the screening accuracy of the BITSEA for a broader range of psychosocial problems.

Conclusions

Both the Problem and Competence scales and the Autism score have a good screening accuracy with regard to ASD for the total population and for boys and girls separately. The Autism score does not have added value to the already existing Competence score; for the screening of ASD, the Competence score is just as effective as the Autism score. Furthermore, the BITSEA is a short questionnaire and has in earlier research shown to have good reliability and validity. As mentioned before, in the introduction, early detection instruments that are used in preventive health care should cover a broad range of psychosocial problems. The BITSEA might therefore precede more extensive evaluations on ASD with other instruments, (e.g. the M-CHAT), by more specialized mental health care providers, when scores on the BITSEA indicate concern for ASD. The results of this study indicate that the BITSEA is suitable for use in the setting of (preventive) child health care for the early identification of ASD.

Author Contributions

Conceived and designed the experiments: HR WJ IK. Performed the experiments: IK. Analyzed the data: IK. Contributed reagents/materials/analysis tools: AC JV. Wrote the paper: IK. Provided expert input and advice: AC JV TB.

References

1. Laurent de Angulo MS, Brouwers-de Jong EA, Bulk A (2005) Ontwikkelingsonderzoek in de jeugdgezondheidszorg. Assen: Koninklijke Van Gorcum.
2. American Psychiatric Association (2013) Diagnostic and Statistical Manual of Mental Disorders (5th ed.). Arlington, VA: American Psychiatric Publishing.
3. Baron-Cohen S, Scott FJ, Allison C, Williams J, Bolton P, et al. (2009) Prevalence of autism-spectrum conditions: UK school-based population study. British Journal of Psychiatry 194: 500–509.
4. Kogan MD, Blumberg SJ, Schieve LA, Boyle CA, Perrin JM, et al. (2009) Prevalence of Parent-Reported Diagnosis of Autism Spectrum Disorder Among Children in the US, 2007. Pediatrics 124: 1395–1403.
5. Chakrabarti S, Fombonne E (2005) Pervasive developmental disorders in preschool children: Confirmation of high prevalence. American Journal of Psychiatry 162: 1133–1141.
6. Dawson G (2008) Early behavioral intervention, brain plasticity, and the prevention of autism spectrum disorder. Development and Psychopathology 20: 775–803.
7. Seida JK, Ospina MB, Karkhaneh M, Hartling L, Smith V, et al. (2009) Systematic reviews of psychosocial interventions for autism: an umbrella review. Developmental Medicine and Child Neurology 51: 95–104.
8. Dietz C, Swinkels S, van Daalen E, van Engeland H, Buitelaar JK (2006) Screening for autistic spectrum disorder in children aged 14–15 months. II: Population screening with the early screening of autistic traits questionnaire (ESAT). Design and general findings. Journal of Autism and Developmental Disorders 36: 713–722.
9. Filipek PA, Accardo PJ, Ashwal S, Baranek GT, Cook EH, et al. (2000) Practice parameter: Screening and diagnosis of autism - Report of the Quality Standards Subcommittee of the American Academy of Neurology and the Child Neurology Society. Neurology 55: 468–479.
10. Sandler AD, Brazdziunas D, Cooley WC, de Pijem LG, Hirsch D, et al. (2001) The pediatrician's role in the diagnosis and management of autistic spectrum disorder in children. Pediatrics 107: 1221–1226.
11. Baron-Cohen S, Allen J, Gillberg C (1992) Can autism be detected at 18 months - The needle, the haystack, and the CHAT. British Journal of Psychiatry 161: 839–843.
12. Robins DL, Fein D, Barton ML, Green JA (2001) The Modified Checklist for Autism in Toddlers: An initial study investigating the early detection of autism and pervasive developmental disorders. Journal of Autism and Developmental Disorders 31: 131–144.
13. Sunita, Bilszta JL (2012) Early identification of autism: A comparison of the Checklist for Autism in Toddlers and the Modified Checklist for Autism in Toddlers. Journal of Paediatrics and Child Health.
14. Briggs-Gowan MJ, Carter AS, Bosson-Heenan J, Guyer AE, Horwitz SM (2006) Are infant-toddler social-emotional and behavioral problems transient? Journal of the American Academy of Child and Adolescent Psychiatry 45: 849–858.
15. Egger HL, Angold A (2006) Common emotional and behavioral disorders in preschool children: presentation, nosology, and epidemiology. Journal of Child Psychology and Psychiatry 47: 313–337.
16. Scheeringa MS (2001) The differential diagnosis of impaired reciprocal social interaction in children: A review of disorders. Child Psychiatry and Human Development 32: 71–89.
17. Bornstein MH, Hahn CS, Haynes OM (2010) Social competence, externalizing, and internalizing behavioral adjustment from early childhood through early adolescence: Developmental cascades. Development and Psychopathology 22: 717–735.
18. Yirmiya N, Charman T (2010) The prodrome of autism: early behavioral and biological signs, regression, peri- and post-natal development and genetics. Journal of Child Psychology and Psychiatry 51: 432–458.
19. Briggs-Gowan MJ, Carter AS, Irwin JR, Wachtel K, Cicchetti DV (2004) The brief infant-toddler social and emotional assessment: Screening for social-emotional problems and delays in competence. Journal of Pediatric Psychology 29: 143–155.
20. Briggs-Gowan MJ, Carter AS (2002) Brief Infant-Toddler Social and Emotional Assessment (BITSEA) mannual, version 2.0. New Haven: CT: Yale University.

21. Haapsamo H, Ebeling H, Soini H, Joskitt L, Larinen K, et al. (2009) Screening infants with social and emotional problems: A pilot study of the Brief Infant Toddler Social and Emotional Assessment (BITSEA) in Northern Finland. International Journal of Circumpolar Health 68: 386–393.

22. Karabekiroglu K, Rodopman-Arman A, Ay P, Ozkesen M, Akbas S, et al. (2009) The reliability and validity of the Turkish version of the brief infant-toddler social emotional assessment (BITSEA). Infant Behavior & Development 32: 291–297.

23. Kruizinga I, Jansen W, de Haan CL, van der Ende J, Carter AS, et al. (2012) Reliability and validity of the dutch version of the brief infant-toddler social and emotional assessment (BITSEA). PLoS ONE 7.

24. Nunnally JC, Bernstein IH (1994) Psychometric theory. New York: McGraw-Hill.

25. Terwee CB, Bot SDM, de Boer MR, van der Windt D, Knol DL, et al. (2007) Quality criteria were proposed for measurement properties of health status questionnaires. Journal of Clinical Epidemiology 60: 34–42.

26. Karabekiroglu K, Briggs-Gowan MJ, Carter AS, Rodopman-Arman A, Akbas S (2010) The clinical validity and reliability of the Brief Infant-Toddler Social and Emotional Assessment (BITSEA). Infant Behavior & Development 33: 503–509.

27. Kruizinga I, Jansen W, Mieloo CL, Carter AS, Raat H (2013) Screening accuracy and clinical application of the Brief Infant-Toddler Social and Emotional Assessment (BITSEA). PLoS ONE 8(8): e72602. doi:10.1371/journal.pone.0072602.

28. Achenbach TM, Rescorla LA (2000) Manual for the ASEBA Preschool Forms & Profiles. Burlington: VT: University of Vermont, Research Center for Children, Youth, and Families.

29. Briggs-Gowan MJ, Carter AS (1998) Preliminary acceptability and psychometrics of the Infant-Toddler Social and Emotional Assessment (ITSEA): A new adult-report questionnaire. Infant Mental Health Journal 19: 422–445.

30. Carter AS, Briggs-Gowan MJ, Jones SM, Little TD (2003) The Infant-Toddler Social and Emotional Assessment (ITSEA): Factor structure, reliability, and validity. Journal of Abnormal Child Psychology 31: 495–514.

31. Briggs-Gowan MJ, Carter AS (2008) Social-emotional screening status in early childhood predicts elementary school outcomes. Pediatrics 121: 957–962.

32. Wet medisch-wetenschappelijk onderzoek met mensen [Dutch Act on research involving human subjects] (1998). Bwb-id:BWBR0009408. Available: http://wetten.overheid.nl/BWBR0009408/geldigheidsdatum_05-02-2010.

33. Oosterling IJ, Wensing M, Swinkels SH, van der Gaag RJ, Visser JC, et al. (2010) Advancing early detection of autism spectrum disorder by applying an integrated two-stage screening approach. Journal of Child Psychology and Psychiatry 51: 250–258.

34. Swinkels SHN, Dietz C, van Daalen E, Kerkhof I, van Engeland H, et al. (2006) Screening for autistic spectrum in children aged 14 to 15 months. I: The development of the early screening of autistic traits questionnaire (ESAT). Journal of Autism and Developmental Disorders 36: 723–732.

35. Oosterling IJ, Swinkels SH, van der Gaag RJ, Visser JC, Dietz C, et al. (2009) Comparative Analysis of Three Screening Instruments for Autism Spectrum Disorder in Toddlers at High Risk. Journal of Autism and Developmental Disorders 39: 897–909.

36. Swets JA (1988) Measuring the accuracy of diagnostic systems. Science 240: 1285–1293.

37. Akobeng AK (2007) Understanding diagnostic tests 3: receiver operating characteristic curves. Acta Paediatrica 96: 644–647.

38. Fischer JE, Bachmann LM, Jaeschke R (2003) A readers' guide to the interpretation of diagnostic test properties: clinical example of sepsis. Intensive Care Medicine 29: 1043–1051.

39. Cohen J (1988) Statistical power analysis for the behavioral sciences (2nd ed.). Hillsdale, NJ: Lawrence Erblaum Associates.

Effect of Familiarity on Reward Anticipation in Children with and without Autism Spectrum Disorders

Katherine K. M. Stavropoulos*, Leslie J. Carver

Psychology Department, University of California San Diego, La Jolla, California, United States of America

Abstract

Background: Previous research on the reward system in autism spectrum disorders (ASD) suggests that children with ASD anticipate and process social rewards differently than typically developing (TD) children—but has focused on the reward value of unfamiliar face stimuli. Children with ASD process faces differently than their TD peers. Previous research has focused on face processing of unfamiliar faces, but less is known about how children with ASD process familiar faces. The current study investigated how children with ASD anticipate rewards accompanied by familiar versus unfamiliar faces.

Methods: The stimulus preceding negativity (SPN) of the event-related potential (ERP) was utilized to measure reward anticipation. Participants were 6- to 10-year-olds with ($N = 14$) and without ($N = 14$) ASD. Children were presented with rewards accompanied by incidental face or non-face stimuli that were either familiar (caregivers) or unfamiliar. All non-face stimuli were composed of scrambled face elements in the shape of arrows, controlling for visual properties.

Results: No significant differences between familiar versus unfamiliar faces were found for either group. When collapsing across familiarity, TD children showed larger reward anticipation to face versus non-face stimuli, whereas children with ASD did not show differential responses to these stimulus types. Magnitude of reward anticipation to faces was significantly correlated with behavioral measures of social impairment in the ASD group.

Conclusions: The findings do not provide evidence for differential reward anticipation for familiar versus unfamiliar face stimuli in children with or without ASD. These findings replicate previous work suggesting that TD children anticipate rewards accompanied by social stimuli more than rewards accompanied by non-social stimuli. The results do not support the idea that familiarity normalizes reward anticipation in children with ASD. Our findings also suggest that magnitude of reward anticipation to faces is correlated with levels of social impairment for children with ASD.

Editor: Gabriel S. Dichter, UNC Chapel Hill, United States of America

Funding: This work was supported by an Autism Speaks Dennis Weatherstone Predoctoral Fellowship awarded to KKMS (grant 7844). The funders had no rule in study design, data collection and analysis, decision to publish, or preparation of the manuscript.

Competing Interests: The authors have declared that no competing interests exist.

* Email: kmeltzoff@gmail.com

Introduction

Autism spectrum disorder (ASD) is a disorder defined by social-communicative deficits and repetitive and restricted behaviors. ASD is estimated to effect up to 1 in 68 children in the US (Centers for Disease Control and Prevention [CDC], 2014). Children with ASD have well documented difficulties in multiple aspects of social communication, including eye contact [1,2], language [3], and joint attention [1], in addition to having repetitive behaviors and restricted interests.

Several theories have emerged concerning why individuals with ASD are impaired relative to their neurotypical peers in social abilities. One is the social motivation hypothesis [4–9]. According to this idea, children with ASD are less intrinsically motivated to attend to and engage with others, which leads to downstream social deficits. The social motivation hypothesis might predict, then, that children with ASD need to be more motivated than TD children in order to find faces rewarding. In the current study, we

tested the hypothesis that, although unfamiliar faces may not be rewarding for children with ASD, a socially important familiar face, such a caregiver's face, may have greater reward value than an unfamiliar face.

There is reason to believe that children with autism might respond differently to a caregiver's face than to other, unfamiliar faces. Previous literature has investigated how children with and without ASD react to their caregivers, and whether attachment relationships differ between the two groups. The attachment literature suggests that children with ASD show somewhat typical and secure attachment relationships to their caregivers [10,11], although a recent meta-analysis suggested that children with ASD are less likely to be securely attached compared to TD children and those with other developmental disorders [12]. Given the suggestion that children with ASD may react to their parents similarly to TD children despite their social impairments, it is possible that familiar faces may be particularly salient to children with ASD, and may "normalize" the neural responses of people with ASD [13]. While this is an intriguing possibility, no prior study has directly investigated the effect of face familiarity on the brain's reward system in ASD. The current study was designed to investigate whether familiar faces would increase reward anticipation in children with ASD compared to their TD peers.

Previous literature has documented different neural responses in individuals with ASD compared to their TD peers when viewing unfamiliar faces [14–16]. The relatively small literature on the effect of familiarity in ASD has been limited to the effect of familiarity on face processing [13,17–25]. The studies on familiarity have varied results, likely due to inter-study differences in participants' age, methodologies, and stimuli. Previous literature on the reward system in ASD has also had mixed results, with some studies finding reward deficits in social rewards only, and others finding global reward deficits. One recent study has integrated these two lines of research and investigated familiar versus unfamiliar faces, as well as monetary rewards in a behavioral paradigm and found that both face and monetary rewards improved behavioral performance for individuals with and without ASD in a go/no-go task [26]. In order to setup and motivate the current study, we next briefly review the research on the reward system in ASD individuals using electrophysiology, functional neuroimaging, and combined methodologies, and then review previous research on the effect of familiar faces in ASD.

Reward System in ASD

Electrophysiological studies. Event-related potentials (ERP) are brain potentials recorded at the surface of the scalp. These recordings reflect synchronous firing of groups of synapses, and have been used to measure the time course of brain activity related to the anticipation or processing of specific discrete events.

ERPs have been used to study the reward system in ASD. Three studies have compared reward anticipation between TD individuals and those with ASD [27–29]. One study used a probabilistic learning task with monetary rewards and found that children with ASD and ADHD demonstrated larger neural responses than TD children when anticipating positive outcomes, but equivalent responses when anticipating negative outcomes [27]. A second study measured attentional ERP components in response to cues triggering trials with social vs. nonsocial rewards and found that TD children exhibited larger attentional components during reward versus non-reward conditions, but children with autism did not. In addition, children with autism exhibited smaller attentional components after cues initiating social reward anticipation trials [28]. A third study measured neural correlates of reward anticipation in a guessing game task with social and nonsocial rewards and found group differences such that children with ASD showed reduced brain activity when anticipating rewards accompanied by intact versus scrambled faces [29]. Taken together, ERP studies of social reward anticipation provide evidence that individuals with ASD elicit less brain activity when anticipating social rewards compared to their TD peers.

Previous ERP studies have also investigated electrophysiological correlates of reward processing in ASD. In studies examining reward processing in ASD, two studies have utilized a guessing game with monetary rewards. Both studies found similar activation patterns in children with ASD and TD [30,31], suggesting that children with ASD do not demonstrate deficits in reward feedback processing when the rewards are monetary. Our previous investigation of social versus non-social rewards revealed group differences in reward processing between TD children and those with ASD—especially for social stimuli [29].

Functional neuroimaging studies. Previous research on social versus nonsocial rewards in ASD has also utilized functional

magnetic resonance imaging (fMRI). The fMRI literature on social versus nonsocial rewards in ASD vs. TD is mixed. Some studies have suggested that individuals with ASD may elicit reduced neural activation for monetary rewards compared to TD children, but have similar neural activation for social rewards [32]; others have found reduced brain activity in response to social rewards in ASD [33].

Behavioral studies. One recent study has investigated reward responsiveness to both familiar versus unfamiliar faces, as well as nonsocial rewards, in both TD children and those with ASD using a modified go/no-go task [26]. Children either received auditory or visual indicators of reward after successful response inhibition. The authors found that both monetary and social (both familiar and unfamiliar faces) rewards increased performance versus a control (no-reward) condition. The authors did not find evidence of decreased responsiveness to social rewards in children with ASD, but found that parents' practices with rewards and contingencies at home strongly predicted performance in the ASD group [26].

Effects of Familiarity in ASD

Electrophysiological studies. We now turn to previous research investigating the effects of familiarity on face processing in ASD. Several ERP studies have measured responses to familiar and unfamiliar faces. Some investigations have found that individuals with ASD are less responsive to familiar faces compared to their typically developing peers [18,25], yet others have found that responsiveness to familiarity may be typical, but delayed, in ASD [24], or may increase after exposure to social skills groups [17]. Conversely, other investigations found no differences between adults with and without ASD in responsiveness to familiar faces [23], or in children at high versus low risk for ASD [20,34]. The ERP literature on the effects of familiarity on face processing in ASD is widely varied, and likely depends on a variety of factors, including cognitive functioning, age of participants, and the tasks utilized.

Functional Neuroimaging Studies. Two studies have investigated recognition of face familiarity using functional neuroimaging with individuals with and without ASD [13,22]. In a study of adults, both typical and ASD groups showed increased neural activation in response to familiar versus unfamiliar faces. [22]. In a study of school-aged children with and without ASD, children with ASD demonstrated similar brain activity to their TD peers when viewing pictures of children or familiar adults, but reduced activation when viewing pictures of unfamiliar adults [13]. In contrast to these findings, many studies in which brain responses are elicited to novel faces suggest that people with ASD do not activate face-processing brain areas to the same degree that TD controls do [16,35]. Thus, the results of recent face processing studies that have manipulated familiarity using fMRI measures suggest that brain responses might be normalized when familiar faces are used as stimuli.

Summary

Previous research on the *reward* system in ASD has been mixed, likely due to the wide variety of methodologies and procedures utilized. However, several studies have found that individuals with ASD have differences in the neural correlates of the reward system compared to TD individuals. Similarly, previous investigations of *familiar faces* on face processing have met with mixed findings. While previous literature has investigated the effects of familiar faces on face processing, as well as the effects of social versus nonsocial stimuli on the reward system in ASD, only one study has directly investigated the effect of familiar faces on reward responsiveness in ASD [26]. No previous studies have investigated the effects of familiarity on *neural correlates* of reward in TD versus ASD.

Current Study

The aim of the current study was to utilize electrophysiology to investigate the effect of familiarity on reward anticipation in response to faces versus non-faces in children with and without ASD. While previous studies have investigated the effects of familiarity on face processing, none have directly explored how the neural reward system is affected by familiarity in ASD. Specifically, we wanted to investigate reward anticipation for familiar versus unfamiliar faces, and scrambled versions of those images.

Previous investigations using electrophysiology to measure reward anticipation focused on the stimulus preceding negativity (SPN) component [29,36,37] The SPN is a component of the ERP that reflects brain activity occurring before expected feedback about one's performance [38]. SPN reflects the *expectation* of reward, and related activity of the dopaminergic reward system [39]. Our previous study of the SPN in children with ASD versus their TD peers revealed differences in how children with ASD anticipate social stimuli (pictures of faces) [29]. However, this previous study utilized a variety of unfamiliar faces.

The current study utilized one familiar and one unfamiliar face in order to determine whether familiar faces accompanying reward stimuli normalized reward anticipation in children with ASD. This design allowed us to gain information about both the effect of familiar faces on reward anticipation, and also whether the use of only one face in each condition may lead to habituation effects over time. In the current study, we also investigated whether brain activity and behavioral measures of ASD (via the SRS-2) were correlated, and whether children with more severe social impairments had reduced reward anticipation for face stimuli. We hypothesized that TD children would have an increased SPN response to face versus arrow stimuli—and that this effect would be most pronounced for familiar versus unfamiliar faces. We hypothesized that children with ASD would not have increased SPN responses to face versus arrow stimuli overall, but would have larger SPN responses to a familiar versus unfamiliar face. Lastly, we hypothesized that we would find a specific brain-behavior correlation—children with more severe social impairments (as measured with the SRS-2) would have decreased SPN amplitude to faces.

Methods

Participants

To estimate the needed sample size for the current study, we ran a power analysis on data from our previous study which used the same paradigm [29]. The resulting power value of .86 yielded a sample size of 26. Therefore, we recruited 28 participants for the current study: TD children ($N = 14$) and children with ASD ($N = 14$). Each child that was tested provided an adequate number of ERP trials for analysis and was included in the final sample. Exclusionary criteria for participants with ASD included history of seizures, brain injury, neurological disorders, genetic causes of ASD (e.g. Fragile X), or any concurrent psychiatric condition (other than ASD), based on parent report. Exclusionary criteria for TD participants included all of the above criteria, plus an immediate family history of ASD. None of the children in the TD group were taking psychoactive medications. One child in the ASD group was taking medication to improve concentration, and one was taking medication to decrease aggression and stabilize mood. Participants were recruited from a UC San Diego subject pool and through postings on websites for parents of children on the autism spectrum. All participants had normal hearing and normal or corrected to normal vision. Procedures were approved by the University of California, San Diego institutional review board, and written consent was obtained from caregivers. All children over 7 years of age signed an assent form.

Table 1 provides detailed participant information. IQ scores [40] were available for all participants. TD children were matched with children with ASD on mental age (full scale IQ/100 * chronological age). No differences were found between groups on mental age, $F(1,26) = .01$. Children in the ASD group had been previously diagnosed with ASD through various sources (e.g. formal evaluations through an autism center, or school diagnosis). Diagnosis was confirmed for the current study with Module 3 of the ADOS-2 [41]. The ADOS-2 was administered by an individual trained to research reliability on administration, scoring, and interpretation of the measure.

Behavioral Measures

Participants' caregivers completed the Social Responsiveness Scales (SRS-2) [42], which measures social responsiveness and behavior. We also tested for overt motivation or affective differences between groups for each condition. To accomplish this, children ($N = 9$ TD, 13 ASD) completed a 1–7 Likert rating scale of how much they enjoyed the game (1 = "I do not like this game", and 7 = "I love this game") after each block. This was used in order to gather more information about whether one group felt more or less motivated to engage in the task. Previous research suggests that the presence of reward versus no reward affects SPN amplitude—with greater SPN amplitude in reward versus no-reward conditions [43]—and we wished to assess whether both groups felt equally invested in the game. Participants also completed a 1–7 Likert scale about their perception of answering correctly (1 = "I never got correct answers", and 7 = "I always got correct answers"). In reality, the correct versus incorrect answers was predetermined, equated for individuals, and controlled by experimental design; the rating was used to verify that the groups did not differ in their perception that they were obtaining correct answers.

Stimuli and Task

The task was identical to that described in previous studies [29,37], but the stimuli differed in order to include different blocks of trials with a familiar or an unfamiliar face. The task was a guessing game that presented blocks of trials that used left and right visual stimuli (question marks). Participants were asked to indicate their guess via button press whether the left or right stimulus was "correct." After this choice, the left and right question marks were replaced with an arrow in the middle pointing towards whichever question mark the participant chose. This was done to reinforce the idea that participants had control over the task and their responses were being recorded.

There were four blocked feedback conditions: *familiar social, familiar nonsocial, unfamiliar social, and unfamiliar nonsocial*. The incidental stimulus in the familiar social condition was a picture of the child's caregiver that was smiling for "correct" answers and frowning for "incorrect" answers (photographs obtained via digital camera in our lab, and modeled after the NimStim stimulus set) [44]. The incidental stimulus in the unfamiliar social condition was a picture of another child's caregiver that was smiling for "correct" answers and frowning for "incorrect" answers. Incidental stimuli in the nonsocial conditions were composed of scrambled face elements from the social conditions formed into an arrow that pointed upwards for

Table 1. Participant characteristics including: IQ (WASI), chronological age, mental age (WASI/100 * chronological age), gender, SRS-2 T-score, and ADOS-2 severity scores for the ASD group.

Group	Participants	WASI (full-scale)	Chron. Age	Mental Age	Gender	SRS-2 SCI T-Score	SRS-2 RBB T-Score	ADOS-2 Severity Score
ASD	14	$M = 99.42_a$ $SE = 4.10$	$M = 8.85$ $SE = .39$	$M = 8.86$ $SE = .57$	11 M 3 F	$M = 77.50_b$ $SE = 1.94$	$M = 80.07_c$ $SE = 2.30$	$M = 7.14$ $SE = .46$
TD	14	$M = 112.64_a$ $SE = 4.10$	$M = 7.94$ $SE = .39$	$M = 8.96$ $SE = .57$	11 M 3 F	$M = 43.53_b$ $SE = 2.01$	$M = 46.38_c$ $SE = 2.39$	N/A

$_aP = .03$, 95% CI [−1.28 − 25.14].
$_bP < .0001$, 95% CI [39.72 28.20].
$_dP < .0001$, 95% CI [40.52 26.84].

WASI Wechsler Abbreviated Scale of Intelligence, SRS-2 Social Responsiveness Scale, second edition, SCI Social Communication and Interaction, RBB Restricted Interests and Repetitive Behavior, ADOS-2 Autism Diagnostic Observation Schedule Second Edition.

"correct" answers and downwards for "incorrect" answers (e.g. the stimulus in the familiar nonsocial condition was an arrow composed from the familiar social photograph, and stimulus in the unfamiliar nonsocial condition was an arrow composed from the unfamiliar social photograph). The face images and scrambled-face images were individually created from photographs taken in our lab with a digital camera. The face in the unfamiliar condition was chosen for each subject to match his or her caregiver's face on ethnicity, gender, and presence or absence of glasses. The use of scrambled faces to construct the arrow controlled for low-level visual features of the stimuli. Presented stimuli subtended a horizontal visual angle of 14.5 degrees, and a vertical visual angle of 10.67 degrees. The order in which children saw the four blocks of trials was counterbalanced between participants.

Participants were told that the reward for each correct answer was a goldfish cracker, or if they preferred, fruit snacks. They were told that if they guessed correctly, they would see a ring of intact goldfish crackers, and the goldfish would be crossed out for incorrect answers. Participants were told that the computer would sum their total of correct responses, and they would receive a goldfish cracker for each correct answer they gave, but would not lose any goldfish crackers for incorrect answers. Importantly, in both the familiar and unfamiliar social and nonsocial feedback trials, the face/arrow information was incidental. A computer program predetermined correct versus incorrect answers in pseudorandom order such that children got 50% "correct" and 50% "incorrect," with no more than three of the same answer in a row.

The four feedback conditions were tested in separate blocks, each composed of 60 trials. There were four conditions that composed the trials (familiar face/"familiar social"; unfamiliar face/"unfamiliar social"; familiar arrow/"familiar nonsocial"; and unfamiliar arrow/ "unfamiliar nonsocial" trials). Within each block of 60 trials, there were 10-s breaks every 15 trials. During breaks, participants were asked to relax, or move if they felt restless. Between blocks, a longer break (2–5 min.) was taken. To control for attentional effects, children were observed via webcam, and trials in which they were not attending to the stimulus were marked and discarded during analysis. Of the final sample, none of the children had any trials discarded for this reason.

EEG Recording

Participants wore a standard, fitted cap (Electrocap International) with 33 silver/silver-chloride (Ag/AgCl) electrodes placed according to the extended international 10–20 system. Continuous EEG was recorded with a NeuroScan 4.5 System with a reference electrode at Cz and re-referenced offline to the average activity at left and right mastoids. Electrode resistance was kept under 10 kOhms. Continuous EEG was amplified with a low pass filter (70 Hz), a directly coupled high pass filter (DC), and a notch filter (60 Hz). The signal was digitized at a rate of 250 samples per second via an Analog-to-Digital converter. Eye movement artifacts and blinks were monitored via horizontal electrooculogram (EOG) placed at the outer canthi of each eye and vertical EOG placed above and below the left eye. ERP trials were time locked to the onset of the feedback stimulus. The baseline period was −2200 to −2000 ms, and the data were epoched from −2200 to 100 ms. The interval between trials was varied between 1,800–2,000 ms. Trials with no behavioral response, or containing electrophysiological artifacts, were excluded from the averages.

Artifacts were removed via a four-step process. Data were visually inspected for drift exceeding +/−200 mV in all electrodes, high frequency noise visible in all electrodes larger than 100 mV, and flatlined data. Following inspection, data were epoched and

Effect of Familiarity on Reward Anticipation in Children with and without Autism Spectrum Disorders
139

eyeblink artifacts were identified using independent component analysis (ICA). Individual components were inspected alongside epoched data, and blink components were removed. To remove additional artifacts, we utilized a moving window peak-to-peak procedure in ERPlab [45], with a 200 ms moving window, a 100 ms window step, and a 150 mV voltage threshold. Participants with less than 10 artifact-free trials in any block of testing were excluded ($N = 0$). Thus, our final analysis includes 14 children with ASD and 14 TD children.

Results

Data were analyzed using JMP (version 10.0). For our initial analysis, we separated familiarity (familiar, unfamiliar) from condition (face, arrow). We used mixed model (between and within subjects) analysis of variance (ANOVA) to test for differences between group, condition, familiarity, and caudality (anterior-posterior scalp locations).

Behavioral Measures

As expected, SRS-2 T-scores (which reflect more severe social impairments) were significantly higher for the ASD group than the TD group for the social communication subscale $F(1, 32) = 215$, $p < .0001$, and the repetitive and restricted behavior subscale $F(1,32) = 158.55$, $p < .0001$. Means and standard deviations between groups on the SRS-2 are shown in *Table 1*. No significant differences were found between groups on children's Likert ratings of liking the game for any of the four conditions, (all $ps > .2$), or perception of generating correct answers, (all $ps > .1$)

ERP

SPN. The mean amplitude of the SPN was measured between -210 and -10 ms, prior to feedback onset, as defined in previous research [29,37,46]. Electrode sites F3/F4, C3/C4, P3/P4, and T5/T6, which are typically maximum amplitude sites for SPN [43], were analyzed. Artifact-free trials were analyzed for each of the four conditions between groups. No significant differences were found between groups for any of the four conditions (all $ps > .15$). Mean amplitude and trial numbers for each group in all 4 conditions are shown in *Table 2*.

A 2 (Group) ×2 (Condition) ×2 (Familiarity) ×4 (Electrode location) ANOVA did not reveal a significant effect of familiarity, $F(1, 32.06) = .23$, *n.s*, or any interactions with familiarity and other variables of interest. It is possible that over the course of each block, children's response to the single repeated stimulus habituated. In order to explore this possibility, we analyzed the first and second half of each participant's accepted trials for all four blocks in a 2 (Time) ×2 (Group) 2 (Familiarity) ×2 (Condition) ×4 (Electrode location) ANOVA. There was a marginal main effect of time such that the first half of trials elicited a larger SPN than the second half, regardless of group or condition $F(25.9) = 3.72$, $p = .064$, 95% CI $[-2.31$ to $4.99]$. No other interactions with time were significant.

Given previous reports of differences in brain responses to familiar versus unfamiliar faces in TD children, but not those with ASD we conducted a planned 4 (Condition) ×2 (Group) ×4 (Electrode location) ANOVA for faces. We found a significant effect of group × electrode. Subsequent pairwise comparisons were non-significant. In order to better understand the effects of the different conditions on each group, a 4 (Condition) ×4 (Electrode location) ANOVA was conducted for the TD group and ASD groups separately. For TD children there was a main effect of condition, $F(3, 37.55) = 2.76$, $p = .055$, such that the familiar and unfamiliar face conditions elicited larger responses

Table 2. Descriptive statistics of trial numbers and amplitude of the SPN for typically developing (TD) individuals and those with autism spectrum disorder (ASD).

Group	Familiar Faces		Unfamiliar Faces		Familiar Arrows		Unfamiliar Arrows	
	Trials	Amplitude	Trials	Amplitude	Trials	Amplitude	Trials	Amplitude
TD	30.15 (2.67)	−6.58 (2.97)	30.21 (2.72)	−3.91 (2.89)	29.92 (3.01)	−.28 (2.97)	30.14 (2.31)	−.12 (2.89)
ASD	25.07 (2.57)	−3.65 (2.89)	30.28 (2.72)	−3.74 (2.89)	28.14 (2.90)	−2.21 (2.89)	25.21 (2.31)	−5.73(2.89)

Means are displayed, followed by standard error in parentheses (SE). Amplitude is the average magnitude of the SPN over the last 200 ms before reward stimulus onset (measured in microvolts).

than the familiar and unfamiliar arrow conditions. Follow-up contrasts between the familiar face condition and the other three conditions (alpha corrected = .016) revealed marginally significant differences between the familiar face condition and the unfamiliar arrow condition ($p = .018$, 95% CI [1.15 to 11.82]) as well as a marginally significant difference between the familiar face and unfamiliar arrow conditions ($p = .02$, 95% CI [.90 to 11.82]). No other pairwise comparisons were significant. For the ASD group, there was no effect of condition $F(3, 36.24) = .53$, n.s. Figure 1 shows grand averages of all four conditions for each group.

Because there was no main effect of familiarity within or between groups, nor interactions involving familiarity, we collapsed across familiarity for each condition (face, arrow) separately and conducted a 2 (Group) ×2 (Condition) ×4 (Electrode location) ANOVA. This analysis resulted in a significant group × condition interaction, $F(1, 26.03) = 5.97$, $p = .021$. Pairwise comparisons (alpha corrected = .012) revealed a significant effect of condition for the TD group, such that faces elicited a larger SPN than arrows for TD children, $F(1, 25.75) = 8.36$, $p > .01$, 95% CI [1.70 to 8.75], but not for children with ASD. Figure 2 shows grand averages of the face and arrow conditions for each group.

There was a significant effect of electrode position, $F(3, 77.28) = 2.72$, $p = .05$, such the SPN was larger over central and parietal electrodes than frontal or temporal electrode sites. Follow-up Tukey's HSD showed that central electrode sites showed a significantly larger SPN than frontal electrode sites ($p = .04$, 95% CI [.1 to 7.67]). No other pairs of electrode sites were significantly different. There was a Condition × Electrode interaction, $F(3, 75.59) = 2.72$, $p = .05$. Pairwise comparisons (alpha corrected = .008) revealed that the significant effect of electrode was largely driven by the face condition, $F(3, 140.7) = 4.31$, $p = .006$, such that faces elicited a larger SPN than arrows differentially over various electrode sites. Pairwise comparisons also revealed a significant effect of the parietal electrode position, $F(1, 76.74) = 8.53$, $p = .004$ 95% CI [1.29 9.20], such that the face condition elicited a larger SPN than the arrow conditions at this electrode site regardless of group. There was a Group × Condition × Electrode interaction, $F(3, 75.59) = 3.40$, $p = .02$. In order to investigate the Group × Condition interaction at each electrode site, we performed contrasts at all four electrode sites. These contrasts showed a significant Group × Condition interaction (alpha corrected = .012) at both the central, $F(1, 78.57) = 6.51$, $p = .012$, 95% CI [1.07 to 8.20], and frontal electrodes, $F(1, 78.57) = 11.24$, $p = .001$, 95% CI [2.53 to 9.66], such that for the TD group, faces elicited a larger SPN than arrows, whereas for the ASD group arrows elicited a larger SPN than faces.

Nc. Visual inspection of our waveforms in Figure 1 suggested a potential difference between groups in anticipation of face stimuli in a middle latency negative component (similar to an Nc) that occurred about 400 ms after the stimulus that signaled the choice of the participant in the guessing game. The Nc is traditionally thought to reflect attention and salience in frontal and central midline electrodes, and has previously been described as a response to a presented stimulus [47,48]. Our waveforms suggest an *anticipatory* Nc that occurred prior to the onset of face stimuli, but after children made their response. To investigate this possibility, we conducted a 2 (Group) ×2 (Familiarity) ×3 (Electrode) ANOVA for face stimuli between −1700 and −1550 ms (before the reward stimulus onset) in electrodes Fz, FCz, and Cz. Children's responses via button pad occur at −2000 ms— suggesting that this component occurred around 300 to 450 ms after the response. This time-frame (300 to 450 ms after response) is consistent with the time course of the Nc in previous

investigations [47]. The ANOVA revealed a marginally significant effect of electrode, $F(2, 52.47) = 3.10$, $p = .053$. However, Tukey HSD follow-up tests did not reveal any significant differences between electrode pairs. We found a significant main effect of group, $F(1, 26.06) = 4.91$, $p = .035$, 95% CI [2.50 to 10.81], such that the face stimulus elicited a larger Nc component for TD children compared to children with ASD. No significant effects of familiarity were found, $F(1, 25.66) = 1.8$, n.s. We re-ran the ANOVA collapsed across familiarity and our significant effects remained. Grand averages for both groups for the face condition are seen in Figure 3.

Brain-Behavior Correlations

We also investigated the relationship between brain activity and behavioral measures of ASD. Specifically, we asked whether magnitude of autism symptoms in the ASD group, as measured by the SRS-2, could predict the magnitude of SPN ERP response in the face condition (collapsed across familiarity). We found a significant correlation between T-scores on the SRS-2 and magnitude of SPN in response to faces, such that children with lower T-scores (and thus less severe social impairments as reported by caregivers), showed larger SPNs in response to faces, $F(1, 12) = 6.95$, $p = .021$, Cohen's $f^2 = .577$. Figure 4 shows a scatter-plot of SRS-2 scores and amplitude in the face condition. However, it is can be noted that one subject elicited a particularly large SPN response, and thus may be considered an outlier, and when this subject was removed, the correlation no longer reached statistical significance, $F(1,11) = 1.5$, n.s.

Discussion

ERP

SPN. The current study suggests that there is not a significant difference in anticipation of a familiar versus an unfamiliar face for either children with ASD or their TD peers. However, TD children showed differences between conditions such that familiar faces elicited larger SPN compared to either of the arrow conditions, whereas unfamiliar faces were numerically larger (but not significantly different from) either arrow condition. This suggests that for TD children between the ages of 6–11 years old, familiar faces elicit a larger reward anticipation response compared to non-face stimuli. For children with ASD, we did not find any significant differences between conditions. Because we did not find the expected familiarity differences, we also explored whether the use of one repeated stimulus in each block would lead to habituation effects in either or both groups. We found a marginal effect of time, such that the first half of trials in each block elicited larger SPN responses than the second half, regardless of stimulus type or group. This suggests that although there is likely some habituation in the SPN response to a large number of repetitions of a single stimulus, it does not differ between groups or social versus nonsocial stimuli. Thus, it is unlikely that differences in the SPN response observed between groups are due to differences in how children with and without ASD habituate to stimuli, although habituation effects may explain the lack of familiarity effects in the present study.

Our results differ from several previous investigations [13,17,18,22,24,25]. Key differences in our task compared to previous studies may explain this. Whereas previous studies have utilized passive viewing tasks, or tasks in which participants attend directly to images and respond to a target stimulus, the current study was designed such that pictures of faces (and scrambled versions of those images) were incidental to the task. In other words, participants did not need to attend to the face or arrow

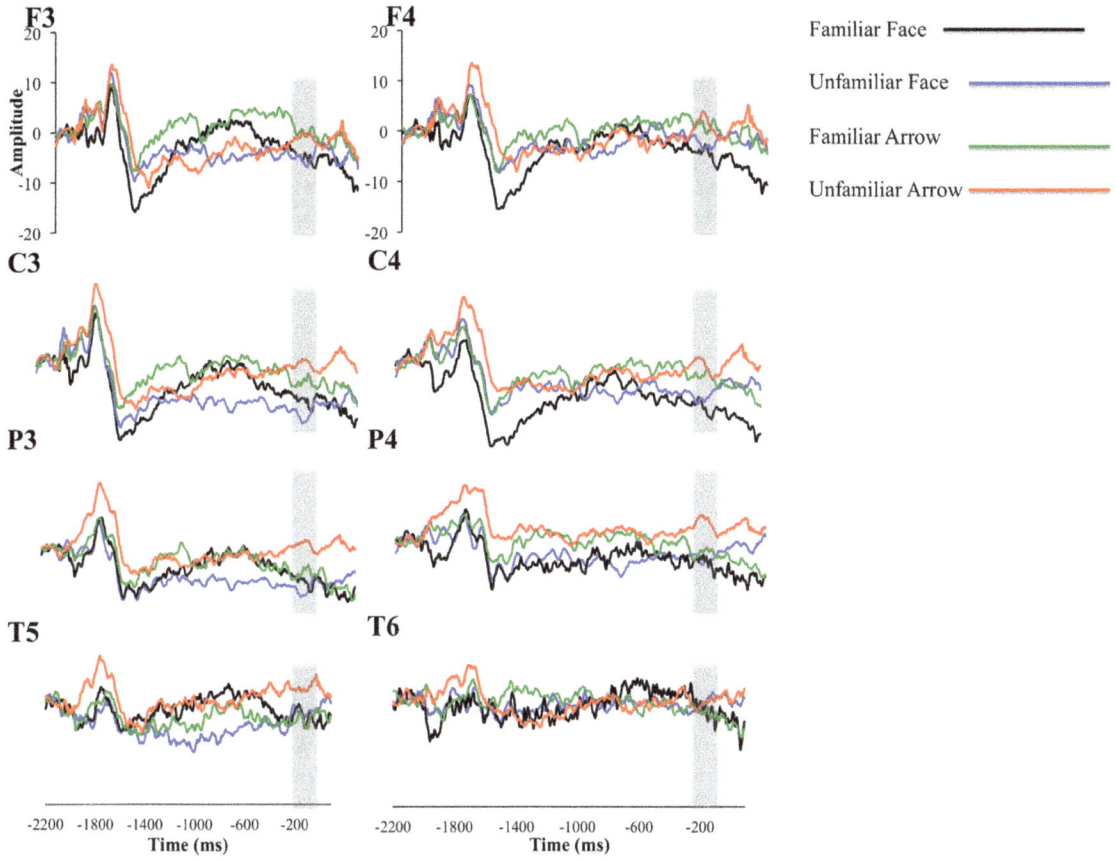

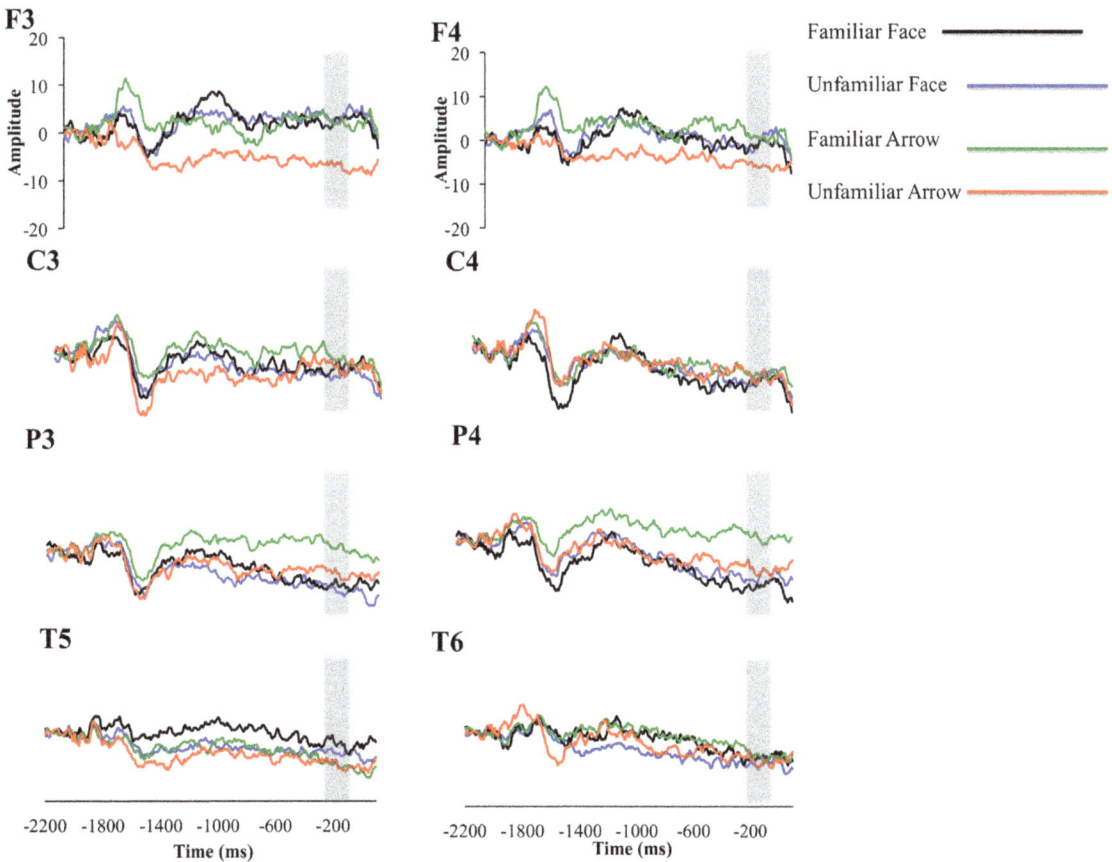

Figure 1. Grand averaged waveforms for the Stimulus Preceding Negativity (SPN). (A) Grand averaged waveforms for TD children from the Stimulus Preceding Negativity (SPN) prior to familiar faces, unfamiliar faces, familiar arrows, and unfamiliar arrows. (B) Grand averaged waveforms for children with ASD from the Stimulus Preceding Negativity (SPN) in ancitipation of familiar faces, unfamiliar faces, familiar arrows, and unfamiliar arrows. The area between -210 and -10 ms, used for statistical analysis, is highlighted with a grey box.

stimulus in order to gain information about whether their responses were "correct" or "incorrect." Although this paradigm allowed us to directly control for physical stimulus properties and tangibility between conditions, it is difficult to directly compare our results with those found in previous studies.

In previous research, one group of authors found that children with ASD showed differential neural activity in response to familiar versus unfamiliar faces [13], and another group of authors found that a small subset of children with ASD began to show differential neural activity in response to familiar face after social skills training [17]. One potential reason for this discrepancy in previous literature may be due to stimulus differences between studies. Previous studies used multiple familiar and unfamiliar faces (rather than just one familiar and one unfamiliar face) [13]. With the exception of [17], which investigated neural activation after social skills training, Pierce and Redcay [13] was the only study to find differences between familiar and unfamiliar faces in children with ASD. One possibility is that children with ASD are more likely to differentiate between familiar versus unfamiliar faces when viewing multiple exemplars from each category. The finding in the current study that there was a marginal tendency for children across groups to habituate to the repeated presentation of a single stimulus supports this idea. Previous research suggests the fusiform face area (FFA) may be involved in determining the identity of individual faces [49]—thus, presenting multiple different faces may activate the FFA to a greater degree than presentations of single faces. It is possible that in previous research, presentation of multiple different familiar faces was adequate to normalize brain responses to faces in ASD. This is an interesting direction for future research, and future studies may wish to compare within subjects whether children with ASD elicit differential neural activity when viewing multiple faces versus one face.

Importantly, although we did not find a main effect of familiarity or interactions between group and familiarity, when we collapsed across familiarity for both groups, we found a group by condition interaction such that TD children showed a larger SPN component in response to faces versus arrows, while children with ASD demonstrated the opposite pattern. This replicates our previous work [29] with a novel group of participants and novel stimuli. These results are in line with the social motivation hypothesis—that TD children are more rewarded by social versus nonsocial stimuli, while children with ASD do not demonstrate this pattern.

Our results are consistent with previous studies that examined reward anticipation in these populations [27,28], in that we found TD children and those with ASD elicited a statistically equivalent SPN response to *non*social feedback. Similarly, while the current study investigated reward anticipation of social versus nonsocial stimuli, and other ERP studies of the reward system in ASD have focused on reward processing of monetary stimuli only [30,31], our results are consistent with these investigations insofar as we found that children with ASD elicit similar reward anticipation to their TD peers for nonsocial stimuli. Our results differ with regards to TD children, however, because we found that TD children elicited a larger SPN response to social versus nonsocial stimuli, whereas [28] found the opposite pattern. Our results also differ from behavioral measures of response inhibition for social versus

monetary rewards [26], as those authors found that both TD children and those with ASD have increased performance for all reward types. However, the authors also found no difference in performance for familiar versus unfamiliar social stimuli in either group, which is consistent with the current findings [26].

One important difference between our current and previous findings is that current pairwise comparisons did not reveal a significant difference between the ASD and TD [29] groups for face stimuli. That is, while TD children had a significantly larger SPN to faces versus non-faces, there was not a significant difference between TD children and those with ASD for the face stimuli. This differs from our previous findings, where in addition to differences between face and non-face stimuli, TD children also had larger SPN responses to faces than children with ASD. One potential reason for this is stimulus variation. In our previous study, children saw a variety of unfamiliar faces, whereas in the current study they saw just one unfamiliar and one familiar face. When comparing our current results to our previous findings, TD children have a smaller SPN response in the face condition, while children with ASD have a larger SPN response in the face condition. In contrast, for the arrow condition, both groups are largely unchanged between studies. This raises the possibility that while TD children show larger SPN responses when viewing multiple faces, children with ASD demonstrate the opposite pattern. The current study was not designed to investigate this, and thus these possibilities remain conjecture, but future studies could manipulate the number of faces in the stimulus set, and measure resulting effects on the SPN.

Nc. We found an Nc-like component after participant's response, but before feedback. This component differentiated TD children from those with ASD. The component occurred at about the time ($\sim$400 msec after the participant's button press) and had a similar scalp distribution (prominent at frontal electrode sites) as the Nc component that has typically been investigated in response to visual stimuli [50]. These findings provide novel information about the Nc component—in effect that the Nc can act as an anticipatory waveform. Previous findings have examined the Nc as a component related to salience and attention in response to a stimulus in infants and young children (e.g. [25]). Our findings, however, suggest that the Nc is also sensitive to anticipation of upcoming stimuli and/or the testing context (i.e., blocks of familiar and unfamiliar faces vs. arrows), and differentiates between diagnostic groups. It is important to note, however, that the current study was not designed to investigate anticipatory effects of the Nc component, as most studies on the Nc do not involve overt responses by the participant. Thus, while our results have interesting implications for the Nc, it is necessary for future studies to look directly at the effect of anticipation on the Nc between children with and without ASD.

Brain and Behavior Correlations

The present results provide evidence that magnitude of reward anticipation response to faces in children with ASD can be predicted by reported levels of social impairments (as measured by the social responsiveness scales). This provides evidence that is in line with the social motivation hypothesis, insofar as children with lower levels of reported social impairments showed larger reward anticipation responses to faces compared to children with higher

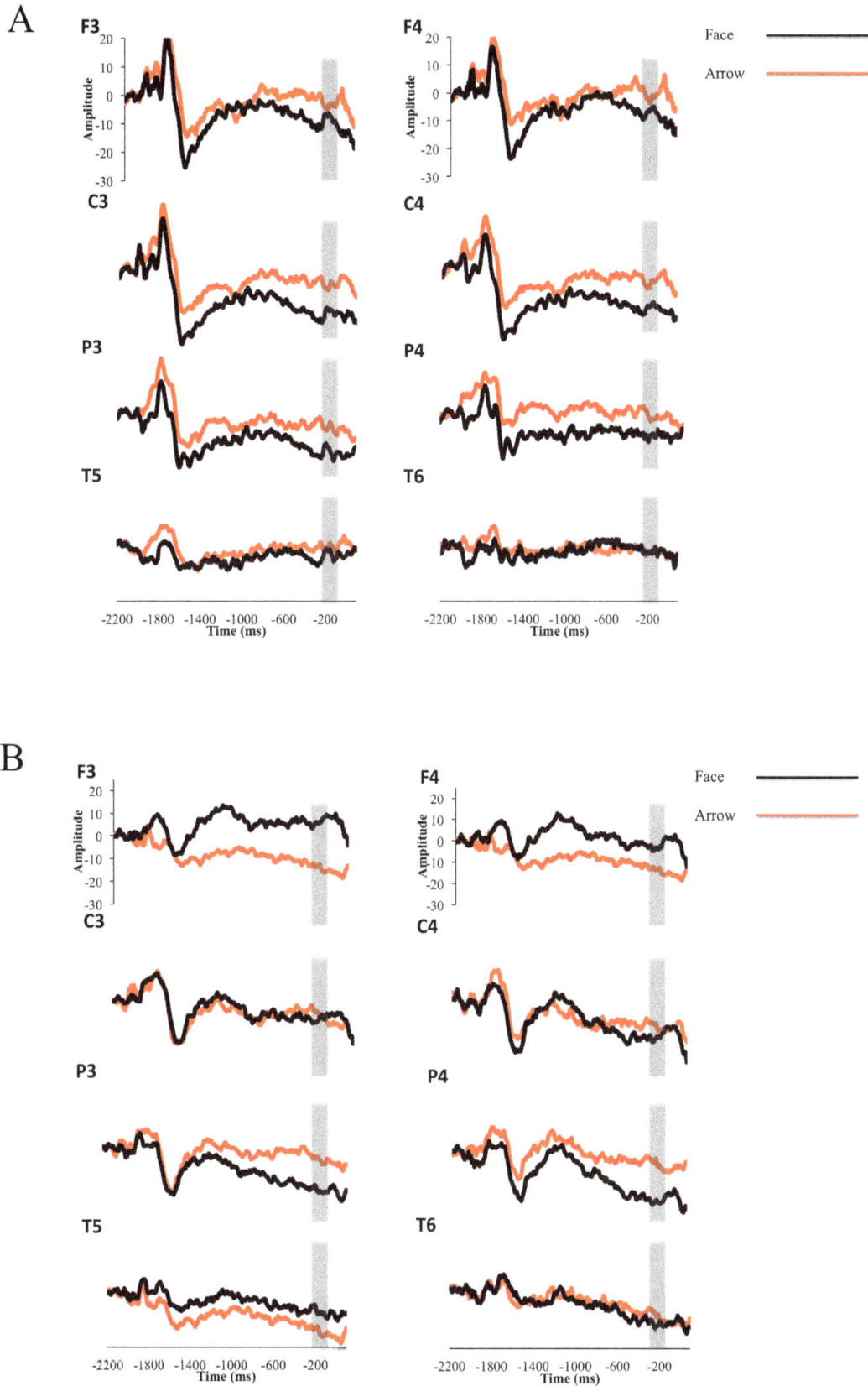

Figure 2. Grand averaged waveforms collapsed across familiarity. (A) Grand averaged waveforms for TD children from the Stimulus Preceding Negativity (SPN) prior to faces and arrows (collapsed across familiarity). The area between −210 and −10 ms, used for statistical analysis, is highlighted with a grey box. (B) Grand averaged waveforms for children with ASD from the Stimulus Preceding Negativity (SPN) prior to faces and arrows (collapsed across familiarity). The area between −210 and −10 ms, used for statistical analysis, is highlighted with a grey box.

Familiar Faces

Fz

FCz

Cz

Unfamiliar Faces

Fz

FCz

Cz

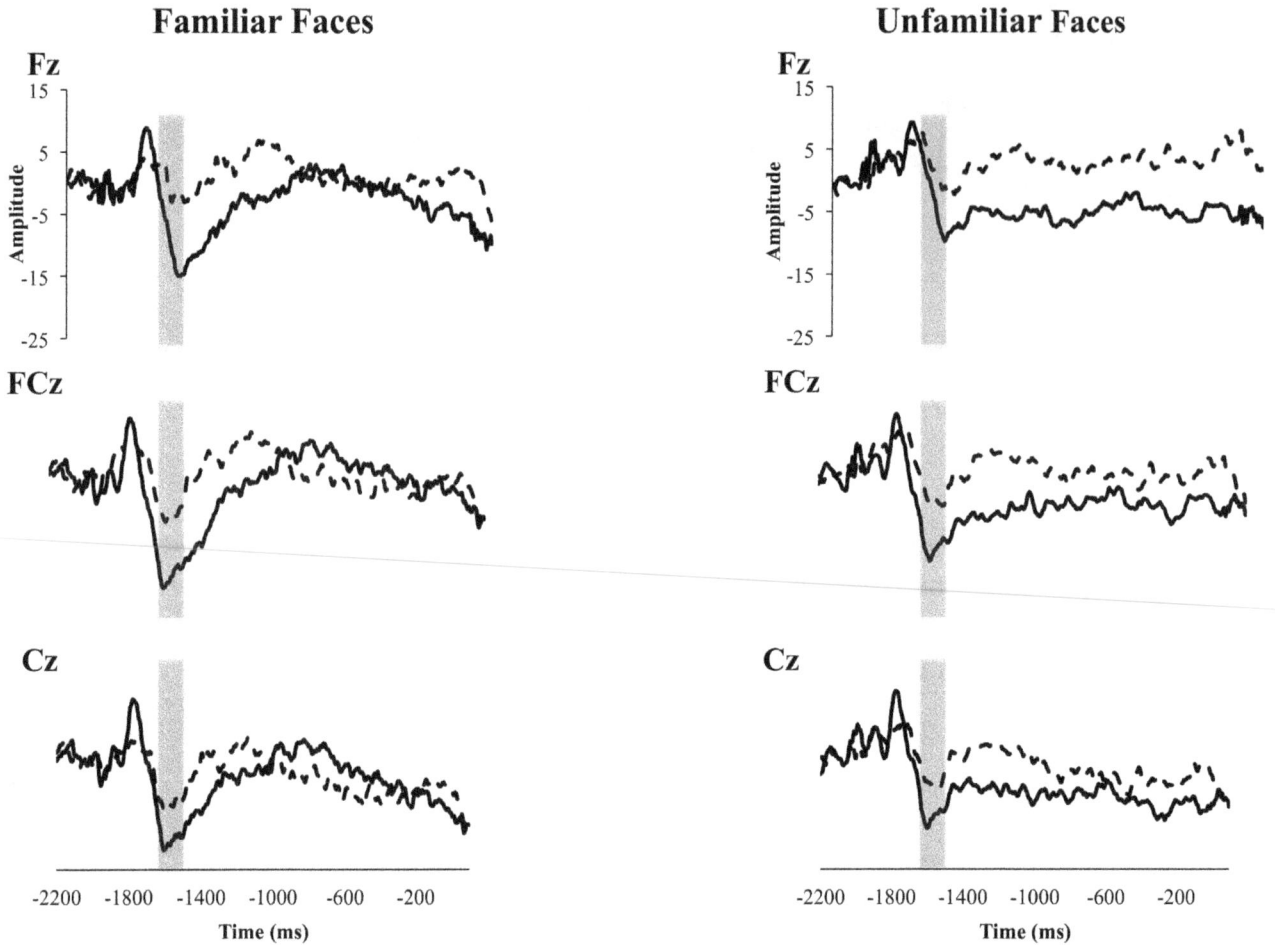

Figure 3. Grand averaged waveforms for both groups from the Nc component prior to familiar and unfamiliar faces. TD children are represented with a solid line, and children with ASD with a dashed line. The area between −1700 and −1550 ms, used for statistical analyses, is highlighted with a grey box.

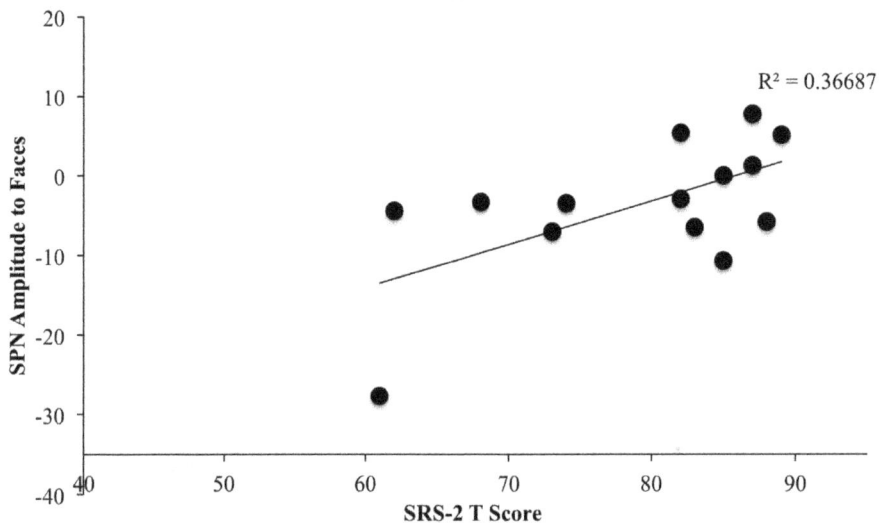

Figure 4. Scatter plot of SPN amplitude to faces (collapsed across familiarity) by SRS-2 T-score for children with ASD. Higher SRS-2 T-scores indicate more severe social impairments. As the SPN is a negative ERP component, more negative values indicate a larger response. Note that one participant had a particularly large SPN response and thus may be considered an outlier; and when this subject was removed, the correlation no longer reached statistical significance, $F(1,11) = 1.5$, ns.

levels of reported impairments. We note, however, that this effect may have been driven by a single participant in the current study, so it is not advisable to draw large-scale conclusions from this analysis. Future studies should look into these types of correlations with a larger sample of children with ASD.

The current study has some limitations that should be noted. First, our sample size ($N = 14$ in each of the TD and ASD groups) is relatively small (although within the estimates provided by our power analysis). This makes it difficult to draw broad and generalized inferences. Further, we did not obtain information about treatment history from participants. Given previous findings about the effect of social skills training on face processing [17], as well as parent attitudes towards reward contingencies on behavioral sensitivity to rewards [26], this limitation should be taken into consideration when interpreting the current findings.

Conclusions and Broader Implications

We examined reward anticipation of incidental familiar versus unfamiliar faces and scrambled versions of those images in children with and without ASD. Although we did not find evidence for an effect of familiar versus unfamiliar faces in either group, the current study adds to the body of literature supporting the social motivation hypothesis, and replicates previous findings using different stimuli and participants. The current study also provides evidence that magnitude of reward anticipation to faces is significantly correlated with levels of parent-reported social impairments. This suggests that our paradigm is sensitive to social impairments as measured by questionnaires, which provides evidence that we are accurately capturing social motivation in children with ASD.

Our findings provide interesting implications for future work on the Nc-like component, which we observed as a measure of anticipation in children, and suggest that for TD children, anticipation of face stimuli elicits a larger Nc-like component than for children with ASD. While our study was not designed to directly address this question, we feel it is an important future direction. The current study also suggests intriguing areas for

future research in regards to whether children with and without ASD are differentially affected by viewing one versus multiple unfamiliar faces. The current study and previous work suggest that perhaps TD children show larger reward anticipation for multiple unfamiliar faces, while children with ASD show the opposite pattern. However, because the current and previous studies utilized different participants and stimuli, we suggest this as an important future direction.

The current study suggests that social motivation deficits in ASD are not ameliorated by viewing familiar faces when face stimuli are incidental to the task. Future research is necessary to determine whether task specifications or number of faces within a stimulus set affects these findings. The current study provides further evidence for the social motivation hypothesis, and suggests that levels of social impairment in ASD are correlated with magnitude of reward anticipation to faces. This paradigm could be utilized as a biomarker of social motivation, and could be used before and after behavioral or pharmacological interventions designed to improve social motivation. In this way, individual children's levels of reward anticipation to faces could be tracked over time along with behavioral levels of social impairment, in order to see changes throughout the course of intervention.

Acknowledgments

We thank the children and their parents for their participation, and the members of the Developmental Neuroscience lab for their assistance. We thank Dr. Sara Webb for her recommendations about analysis strategies, and Kevin Smith, Dr. Julian Parris, and Dr. Mark Appelbaum, for assistance with statistics. We thank Dr. Eric Courchesne for assistance with study conceptualization, and Dr. Steven Hillyard for sharing his expertise concerning anticipatory ERP components.

Author Contributions

Conceived and designed the experiments: KKMS LJC. Performed the experiments: KKMS. Analyzed the data: KKMS. Contributed reagents/materials/analysis tools: KKMS LJC. Contributed to the writing of the manuscript: KKMS LJC.

References

1. Mundy P, Sigman M, Ungerer J, Sherman T (1986) Defining the social deficits of autism: the contribution of non-verbal communication measures. J Child Psychol Psychiatry 27: 657–669. doi: 10.1111/j.1469-7610.1986.tb00190.x.

2. Walters AS, Barrett RP, Feinstein C (1990) Social relatedness and autism: current research, issues, directions. Res Dev Disabil 11: 303–326. doi: 10.1016/0891-4222(90)90015-Z.

3. Charman T, Swettenham J, Baron-Cohen S, Cox A, Baird G, et al. (1998) An experimental investigation of social-cognitive abilities in infants with autism: Clinical implications. Infant Ment Health J 19: 260–275. doi: 10.1002/(SICI)1097-0355(199822)19:2<260::AID-IMHJ12>3.0.CO;2-W.

4. Chevallier C, Kohls G, Troiani V, Brodkin ES, Schultz RT (2012) The social motivation theory of autism. Trends Cogn Sci 16: 231–239. doi:10.1016/j.tics.2012.02.007.

5. Dawson G (2008) Early behavioral intervention, brain plasticity, and the prevention of autism spectrum disorder. Dev Psychopathol 20: 775–803. doi:10.1017/S0954579408000370.

6. Dawson G, Carver L, Meltzoff AN, Panagiotides H, McPartland J, et al. (2002) Neural correlates of face and object recognition in young children with autism spectrum disorder, developmental delay, and typical development. Child Dev 73: 700–717. doi: 10.1111/1467-8624.00433.

7. Dawson G, Webb SJ, Wijsman E, Schellenberg G, Estes A, et al. (2005) Neurocognitive and electrophysiological evidence of altered face processing in parents of children with autism: implications for a model of abnormal development of social brain circuitry in autism. Dev Psychopathol 17: 679–697. doi:10.1017/S0954579405050327.

8. Grelotti D, Gauthier I, Schultz RT (2002) Social Interest and the Development of Cortical Face Specialization: What Autism Teaches Us About Face Processing. Dev Psychobiol 40: 213–225. doi:10.1002/dev.10028.

9. Schultz RT (2005) Developmental deficits in social perception in autism: the role of the amygdala and fusiform face area. Int J Dev Neurosci 23: 125–141. doi:10.1016/j.ijdevneu.2004.12.012.

10. Sigman M, Mundy P (1989) Social attachments in autistic children. J Am Acad Child Adolesc Psychiatry 28: 74–81. doi: 10.1097/00004583-198901000-00014.

11. Sigman M, Ungerer JA (1984) Attachment behaviors in autistic children. J Autism Dev Disord 14: 231–244.

12. Rutgers AH, van Ijzendoorn MH, Bakermans-Kranenburg MJ, Swinkels SHN, van Daalen E, et al. (2007) Autism, attachment and parenting: a comparison of children with autism spectrum disorder, mental retardation, language disorder, and non-clinical children. J Abnorm Child Psychol 35: 859–870. doi:10.1007/s10802-007-9139-y.

13. Pierce K, Redcay E (2008) Fusiform function in children with an autism spectrum disorder is a matter of "who". Biol Psychiatry 64: 552–560. doi:10.1016/j.biopsych.2008.05.013.

14. McPartland J, Dawson G, Webb SJ, Panagiotides H, Carver LJ (2004) Event-related brain potentials reveal anomalies in temporal processing of faces in autism spectrum disorder. J Child Psychol Psychiatry 45: 1235–1245. doi:10.1111/j.1469-7610.2004.00318.x.

15. Dawson G, Webb SJ, Carver L, Panagiotides H, McPartland J (2004) Young children with autism show atypical brain responses to fearful versus neutral facial expressions of emotion. Dev Sci 7: 340–359. doi: 10.1111/j.1467-7687.2004.00352.x.

16. Schultz RT, Gauthier I, Klin A, Fulbright RK, Anderson AW, et al. (2000) Abnormal ventral temporal cortical activity during face discrimination among individuals with autism and Asperger syndrome. Arch Gen Psychiatry 57: 331–340. doi: 10.1001/archpsyc.57.4.331.

17. Gunji A, Goto T, Kita Y, Sakuma R, Kokubo N, et al. (2013) Facial identity recognition in children with autism spectrum disorders revealed by P300 analysis: a preliminary study. Brain Dev 35: 293–298. doi:10.1016/j.braindev.2012.12.008.

18. Gunji A, Inagaki M, Inoue Y, Takeshima Y, Kaga M (2009) Event-related potentials of self-face recognition in children with pervasive developmental disorders. Brain Dev 31: 139–147. doi:10.1016/j.braindev.2008.04.011.

19. Key APF, Stone WL (2012) Processing of novel and familiar faces in infants at average and high risk for autism. Dev Cogn Neurosci 2: 244–255. doi:10.1016/j.dcn.2011.12.003.

20. Kylliäinen A, Wallace S, Coutanche MN, Leppänen JM, Cusack J, et al. (2012) Affective-motivational brain responses to direct gaze in children with autism spectrum disorder. J Child Psychol Psychiatry 53: 790–797. doi:10.1111/j.1469-7610.2011.02522.x.

21. Luyster RJ, Wagner JB, Vogel-Farley V, Tager-Flusberg H, Nelson CA (2011) Neural correlates of familiar and unfamiliar face processing in infants at risk for autism spectrum disorders. Brain Topogr 24: 220–228. doi:10.1007/s10548-011-0176-z.

22. Pierce K, Haist F, Sedaghat F, Courchesne E (2004) The brain response to personally familiar faces in autism: findings of fusiform activity and beyond. Brain 127: 2703–2716. doi:10.1093/brain/awh289.

23. Webb SJ, Jones EJH, Merkle K, Murias M, Greenson J, et al. (2010) Response to familiar faces, newly familiar faces, and novel faces as assessed by ERPs is intact in adults with autism spectrum disorders. Int J Psychophysiol 77: 106–117. doi:10.1016/j.ijpsycho.2010.04.011.

24. Webb SJ, Jones EJH, Merkle K, Venema K, Greenson J, et al. (2011) Developmental change in the ERP responses to familiar faces in toddlers with autism spectrum disorders versus typical development. Child Dev 82: 1868–1886. doi:10.1111/j.1467-8624.2011.01656.x.

25. Dawson G, Carver L, Meltzoff AN, Panagiotides H, McPartland J, et al. (2002) Neural correlates of face and object recognition in young children with autism spectrum disorder, developmental delay, and typical development. Child Dev 73: 700–717. doi: 10.1111/1467-8624.00433

26. Pankert A, Pankert K, Herpertz-Dahlmann B, Konrad K, Kohls G (2014) Responsivity to familiar versus unfamiliar social reward in children with autism. J Neural Transm. doi:10.1007/s00702-014-1210-6.

27. Groen Y, Wijers AA, Mulder LJM, Waggeveld B, Minderaa RB, et al. (2008) Error and feedback processing in children with ADHD and children with Autistic Spectrum Disorder: an EEG event-related potential study. Clin Neurophysiol 119: 2476–2493. doi:10.1016/j.clinph.2008.08.004.

28. Kohls G, Peltzer J, Schulte-Rüther M, Kamp-Becker I, Remschmidt H, et al. (2011) Atypical brain responses to reward cues in autism as revealed by event-related potentials. J Autism Dev Disord 41: 1523–1533. doi:10.1007/s10803-011-1177-1.

29. Stavropoulos KKM, Carver LJ (2014) Reward anticipation and processing of social versus nonsocial stimuli in children with and without autism spectrum disorders. J Child Psychol Psychiatry. doi:10.1111/jcpp.12270.

30. McPartland JC, Crowley MJ, Perszyk DR, Mukerji CE, Naples AJ, et al. (2012) Preserved reward outcome processing in ASD as revealed by event-related potentials. J Neurodev Disord 4: 16. doi:10.1186/1866-1955-4-16.

31. Larson MJ, South M, Krauskopf E, Clawson A, Crowley MJ (2011) Feedback and reward processing in high-functioning autism. Psychiatry Res 187: 198–203. doi:10.1016/j.psychres.2010.11.006.

32. Dichter GS, Richey JA, Rittenberg AM, Sabatino A, Bodfish JW (2012) Reward circuitry function in autism during face anticipation and outcomes. J Autism Dev Disord 42: 147–160. doi:10.1007/s10803-011-1221-1.

33. Scott-Van Zeeland AA, Dapretto M, Ghahremani DG, Poldrack RA, Bookheimer SY (2010) Reward processing in autism. Autism Res 3: 53–67. doi:10.1002/aur.122.

34. Luyster RJ, Wagner JB, Vogel-Farley V, Tager-Flusberg H, Nelson CA (2011) Neural correlates of familiar and unfamiliar face processing in infants at risk for autism spectrum disorders. Brain Topogr 24: 220–228. doi:10.1007/s10548-011-0176-z.

35. Pierce K, Müller RA, Ambrose J, Allen G, Courchesne E (2001) Face processing occurs outside the fusiform "face area" in autism: evidence from functional MRI. Brain 124: 2059–2073. doi: 10.1093/brain/124.10.2059.

36. Ohgami Y, Kotani Y, Tsukamoto T, Omura K, Inoue Y, et al. (2006) Effects of monetary reward and punishment on stimulus-preceding negativity. Psychophysiology 43: 227–236. doi:10.1111/j.1469-8986.2006.00396.x.

37. Stavropoulos KKM, Carver LJ (2013) Reward sensitivity to faces versus objects in children: an ERP study. Soc Cogn Affect Neurosci. doi:10.1093/scan/nst149.

38. Brunia CHM, Hackley SA, van Boxtel GJM, Kotani Y, Ohgami Y (2011) Waiting to perceive: reward or punishment? Clin Neurophysiol 122: 858–868. doi:10.1016/j.clinph.2010.12.039.

39. Boxtel GJM Van, Böcker KBE (2004) Cortical Measures of Anticipation. J Psychophysiol 18: 61–76. doi:10.1027/0269-8803.18.2.

40. Wechsler D (1999) Wechsler Abbreviated Scale of Intelligence. San Antonio. TX: Pearson.

41. Lord C, Rutter M, DiLavore PC, Risi S, Gotham K (2012) ADOS-2: autism diagnostic observation schedule. Los Angeles: Western Psychological Services.

42. Constantino JN, Gruber CP (2012) Social Responsiveness Scale, Second Edition. Los Angeles: Western Psychological Services.

43. Kotani Y, Kishida S, Hiraku S, Suda K, Ishii M, et al. (2003) Effects of information and reward on stimulus-preceding negativity prior to feedback stimuli. Psychophysiology 40: 818–826. doi: 10.1111/1469-8986.00082.

44. Tottenham N, Tanaka JW, Leon AC, McCarry T, Nurse M, et al. (2009) The NimStim set of facial expressions: judgments from untrained research participants. Psychiatry Res 168: 242–249. doi:10.1016/j.psychres.2008.05.006.

45. Lopez-Calderon J, Luck SJ (2014) ERPLAB: an open-source toolbox for the analysis of event-related potentials. Front Hum Neurosci 8: 1–14. doi:10.3389/fnhum.2014.00213.

46. Kotani Y, Hiraku S, Suda K, Aihara Y (2001) Effect of positive and negative emotion on 10.1111/j.1467-7687.2005.00452.x.

47. Courchesne E (1978) Neurophysiological correlates of cognitive development: Changes in long-latency event-related potentials from childhood to adulthood. Electroencephalogr Clin Neurophysiol 45: 468–482. doi: 10.1016/0013-4694(78)90291-2.

48. Webb SJ, Long JD, Nelson CA (2005) A longitudinal investigation of visual event-related potentials in the first year of life. Dev Sci 8: 605–616. doi: 10.1111/j.1467-7687.2005.00452.x.

49. Haxby JV, Hoffman EA, Gobbini MI (2000) The distributed human neural system for face perception. Trends Cogn Sci 4: 223–233. doi:10.1111/j.1467-7687.2005.00452.x.

50. De Haan M, Johnson MH, Halit H (2003) Development of face-sensitive event-related potentials during infancy: a review. Int J Psychophysiol 51: 45–58. doi:10.1016/S0167-8760(03)00152-1.

Assessing the Impact of Copy Number Variants on miRNA Genes in Autism by Monte Carlo Simulation

Maurizio Marrale[1], Nadia Ninfa Albanese[1], Francesco Calì[2], Valentino Romano[1,2]*

1 Dipartimento di Fisica e Chimica, Università di Palermo, Palermo, Italy, **2** U.O.C. di Genetica Medica Laboratorio di Genetica Molecolare, Associazione Oasi Maria SS. (I.R.C.C.S.), Troina, Italy

Abstract

Autism Spectrum Disorders (ASDs) are childhood neurodevelopmental disorders with complex genetic origins. Previous studies have investigated the role of *de novo* Copy Number Variants (CNVs) and microRNAs as important but distinct etiological factors in ASD. We developed a novel computational procedure to assess the potential pathogenic role of microRNA genes overlapping *de novo* CNVs in ASD patients. Here we show that for chromosomes # 1, 2 and 22 the actual number of miRNA loci affected by *de novo* CNVs in patients was found significantly higher than that estimated by Monte Carlo simulation of random CNV events. Out of 24 miRNA genes over-represented in CNVs from these three chromosomes only hsa-mir-4436b-1 and hsa-mir-4436b-2 have not been detected in CNVs from non-autistic subjects as reported in the Database of Genomic Variants. Altogether the results reported in this study represent a first step towards a full understanding of how a dysregulated expression of the 24 miRNAs genes affect neurodevelopment in autism. We also propose that the procedure used in this study can be effectively applied to CNVs/miRNA genes association data in other genomic disorders beyond autism.

Editor: Jeong-Sun Seo, Seoul National University College of Medicine, Korea, Republic of

Funding: The authors acknowledge funding from University of Palermo and from the Italian Ministry of Health: "Ricerca corrente 2013" entitled: "Ritardo mentale, epilessia e autismo: studio genetico, clinico e neurofisiologico". The funders had no role in study design, data collection and analysis, decision to publish, or preparation of the manuscript.

Competing Interests: The authors have declared that no competing interests exist.

* E-mail: valentino.romano@unipa.it

Introduction

The Autism Spectrum Disorders (ASDs, MIM: 209850) are a heterogeneous group of childhood diseases characterized by abnormalities in social behaviour and communication, as well as patterns of restricted and repetitive behaviors [1]. The spectrum of autism reflects dimensional variability of each core symptom as well as the occurrence of co-morbid conditions (intellectual disability, epilepsy, dysmorphisms etc.). Like an epidemic, in part due to improved diagnostic tools, the global prevalence of autism and other pervasive developmental disorders has increased over the years reaching the current, impressive, figure of 1/160 children [2]. Twin studies have demonstrated a much higher concordance rates for the disease in monozygotic twins (92%) than in dizygotic twins (10%) [3,4], indicating a strong genetic basis for autism susceptibility, also supported by the presence of autistic features in several monogenic disorders (e.g., Fragile X syndrome, Tuberous sclerosis). However, despite these progresses the identity of genetic factors still remains unknown in the majority of patients and it is likely, that overall, the causes of autism are more complex than previously thought involving an interaction of genetic, epigenetic and environmental factors all interfering with the normal course of neurodevelopment [5–7].

In 2007 Copy Number Variants (CNVs) were for the first time recognized as important genetic factors in ASD [8]. CNVs are a class of inherited or *de novo* genomic mutations duplicating ("Gains") or deleting ("Losses") DNA segments >1 Kb, thus altering the normal dosage of the overlapping genes. According to

their frequency they can be divided into unique, rare (<1%) or recurrent. Since 2007, many studies have investigated CNVs in autism, to assess their functional impact, the biological networks where the genes in these CNVs are involved and the general burden of CNVs in these individuals (*e.g.* see references [9–11]). Extended, multiplex families are more likely to carry heritable risk factors while, in contrast, sporadic ASD families have demonstrated a higher rate of *de novo* CNVs [8,12]. A striking observation was the high prevalence of *de novo* CNVs in both sporadic and familial cases of ASD compared with controls. Rare, *de novo* or inherited CNVs were observed in 5–10% of idiopathic ASD cases.

Studies performed so far have highlighted the pathogenic role of CNVs in terms of dosage change for protein-coding genes [10,13–15], without taking into account the potential involvement of non-coding RNA, particularly microRNAs genes (see reference [16] for a recent exception).

miRNAs are an important class of post-trascriptional regulators each governing the expression of tens or even hundreds of proteins in both differentiated cells and during development. miRNA transcripts undergo several processing steps occurring first in the nucleus, then in the cytoplasm where the mature 22–25 nucleotide-long miRNA [17,18] enacts mRNA translational repression or cleavage by binding to the 3′-untranslated region of their respective target mRNAs [19]. Only a few studies have investigated the ASD transcriptome in *post-mortem* brain samples, so far [20–22]. Other studies have used mRNA from lymphoblastoid cell lines or peripheral blood cells isolated from patients [23–26]. Disruption of miRNA expression has been repeatedly reported in several microarray studies and believed to be linked to pathogenesis in autism [27–31]. However, lymphoblastoid cell lines are not the best proxy for neural tissue and only very few miRNAs displayed consistent dysregulation among different studies and patients.

In this paper, we aim to expand our knowledge on the pathogenic role of miRNA in autism by investigating the associations between *de novo* CNVs and miRNA genes. For this reason we developed a novel and powerful computational procedure based on Monte Carlo randomization [32] and applied it to several published *de novo* CNV datasets from patients. Our positive findings consist in the identification of 24 miRNA genes over-represented in *de novo* CNV from chromosomes nos. 1, 2 and 22 and therefore likely to play a pathogenic role in autism.

Results

Study design and preliminary analyses

The general strategy and steps of our study are outlined in the flow chart of Figure 1. We developed the MAPCNVMIR programme to map all human miRNA genes from miRBase to 178 *de novo* CNVs from 192 autistic patients ("APL datasets", see Table S1). Only 64 out of 178 CNVs were found to overlap at least one miRNA gene. In addition, 145 miRNA genes were identified within distinct or partly overlapping *de novo* CNVs (Table S1) spread over 20 chromosomes. No miRNA genes included in *de novo* CNVs were detected in chromosomes # 11, 13, 14, Y.

For each chromosome we compared the number and the length of all human microRNA genes reported so far in miRBase with the length of the chromosome. The fractional length of miRNA genes over the size of the chromosome (R_1 ratios) are of the order of 10^{-5} for all chromosomes except for chromosome 19 ($> 10^{-4}$) (see Table 1). This result shows that the fraction of the length of the chromosome covered by microRNA genes is very similar for all chromosomes (except chr. 19). On the other hand, the

fractional length of CNVs over the size of the chromosome (R_2 ratios),computed separately for CNV_Gains and CNV_Losses (Table 1) using the MAPCNVMIR software developed by us (see below), largely differ among the various chromosomes, from a value of 0.0006 up to value of 0.2618. This highlights that the fractional length of chromosomes covered by CNVs can be very dissimilar among chromosomes. Indeed, there are several instances (e.g., chr. # 10, 12, 15 and 22 for CNV_Gains and chr. # 7, 12, 16, 18, 21 and 22 for CNV_Losses) of CNVs affecting large regions of a particular chromosome. Therefore, an analysis was performed between the number of miRNA genes overlapping *de novo* CNVs and the R2 ratios in order to find possible correlations. Furthermore, the number of miRNA genes is also variable. Figures 2a and 2b show that, for many chromosomes, the number of miRNA genes included in CNVs follow a linear trend as function of the total length of both CNV_Gains and CNV_Losses. In order to quantify this kind of correlation, values of correlation coefficients were calculated and were found to be larger for CNV_Gains ($r = 0.75765$) than CNV_Losses ($r = 0.32732$). This finding is consistent with the larger spread of CNV_Losses compared to CNV_Gains. On the other hand, some chromosomes do not follow the linear trend and are characterized by a large number of miRNA genes associated to CNVs (see Figure 2 and Table 1). For example,chromosome 22 for CNV_Gains and chromosome 2 for CNV_Losses appear as "outliers" since they include a much higher number of miRNA genes in *de novo* CNVs than expected. However, the latter analysis does not allow us to classify the observed dissimilarities according to a statistically significant criterion.

Monte Carlo randomization

In order to assess which "outliers" with a high number of overlaps are actually significantly different from the other chromosomes, we developed the SIMCNVMIR programme which implements a numerical analysis procedure for the identification of all instances (*i.e.*, chromosomes) where the number of miRNA genes overlapping *de novo* CNVs is significantly higher than expected in case of random distribution of (simulated) CNVs. The steps of our computational analysis are reported in Figure 3. The results of this analysis are reported in Figure 4 and Table 2 and show that for chromosomes # 1, 2, and 22 the actual number of miRNA loci affected by *de novo* CNVs in patients is significantly higher (FDR-adjusted p-values < 0.05) than that estimated by the simulated random CNV events. Specifically, CNV_Gains in chromosome # 22 and CNV_Losses in chromosomes 1 and 2 display an over-representation of microRNA genes (see Table 2 and Figures 4). In Table 2, note that for CNV_Loss in chromosome # 2 the number. of "hits" is higher than the number of distinct miRNA genes ("Unique"), implying that the same miRNA gene is involved. Overall, there are 24 miRNA genes overlapping *de novo* CNVs in the three positive chromosomes (see Table 3). Only two, hsa-mir-4436b-1 and hsa-mir-4436b-2, have not yet been detected in CNVs from the general population (*i.e.*, the DGV database).

Code scripts of the MAPCNVMIR and SIMCNVMIR programmes are available to readers from the following URL: http://fisicaechimica.unipa.it/cnvmirna/

Pathway analysis

The two autism-specific miRNA genes (hsa-mir-4436 b-1 and has-mir-4436b-2), are deleted in a patient who bears one CNV of 332,304 bp. Interestingly, they encode the same 3p and 5p mature microRNAs. According to Mirwalk [33], no validated targets are yet known for these two miRNAs. We therefore performed a

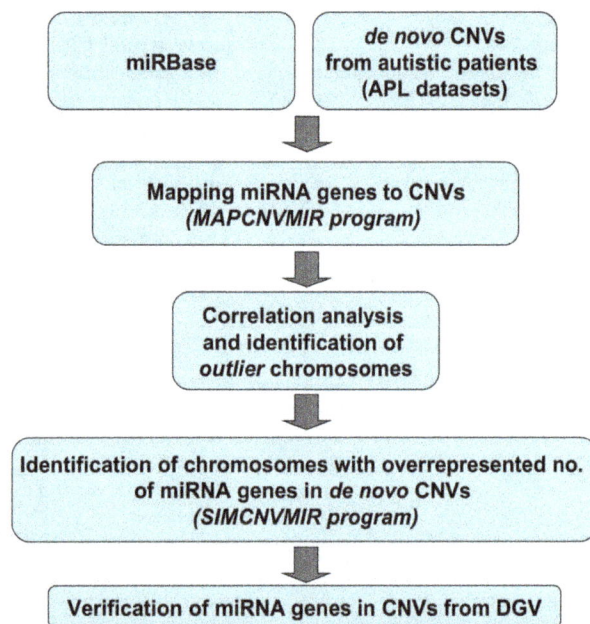

Figure 1. Overview of this study and source data. In this study we have used previously published data from 192 autistic patients (the "APL datasets" of Table S1) bearing overall 178 *de novo* CNVs (118 CNV_Losses and 60 CNV_Gains) with unique start and end positions.

Table 1. Fractional lengths of miRNA genes and CNVs in relation to chromosome's size.

Chromosome		# of miRNA genes	Ratio #1	Gain		Loss	
#	Length (bp)			Ratio #2	#hits	Ratio #2	#hits
1	249250621	127	4.05×10^{-5}	0.0241	5	0.0050	5
2	243199373	98	3.10×10^{-5}	0.0009	0	0.0314	17
3	198022430	76	3.21×10^{-5}	0.0041	1	0.0923	12
4	191154276	56	2.31×10^{-5}	N/A	N/A	0.0886	4
5	180915260	67	3.03×10^{-5}	N/A	N/A	0.0763	7
6	171115067	54	2.56×10^{-5}	0.0019	0	0.0187	2
7	159138663	67	3.41×10^{-5}	0.0103	4	0.1425	7
8	146364022	70	3.54×10^{-5}	0.0068	0	0.0088	1
9	141213431	71	3.95×10^{-5}	0.0371	9	0.0297	1
10	135534747	61	3.66×10^{-5}	0.0822	4	0.0005	0
11	135006516	69	4.03×10^{-5}	0.0002	0	0.0410	0
12	133851895	57	3.48×10^{-5}	0.1691	13	0.1013	3
13	115169878	37	2.62×10^{-5}	0.0009	0	0.0169	0
14	107349540	88	6.58×10^{-5}	0.0006	0	N/A	N/A
15	102531392	57	4.68×10^{-5}	0.1254	39	0.0742	7
16	90354753	48	4.40×10^{-5}	0.0320	2	0.1032	9
17	81195210	83	7.89×10^{-5}	0.0317	8	0.0256	1
18	78077248	30	2.74×10^{-5}	0.0006	0	0.2618	2
19	59128983	108	1.47×10^{-4}	N/A	N/A	0.0145	2
20	63025520	40	5.16×10^{-5}	N/A	N/A	0.0301	2
21	48129895	15	2.65×10^{-5}	0.0074	1	0.1183	3
22	51304566	36	5.59×10^{-5}	0.0893	18	0.1473	24
X	155270560	108	5.77×10^{-5}	0.0304	8	0.0406	1

Ratio #1: The ratio between the sum of lengths of all miRNA genes in a chromosome and the total length of the chromosome; Ratio #2: The ratio between the sum of lengths of all *de novo* CNVs in a chromosome and the total length of the chromosome; # hits: For each chromosome, the total no. of identical and/or different miRNA genes included in all *de novo* CNVs detected in patients.

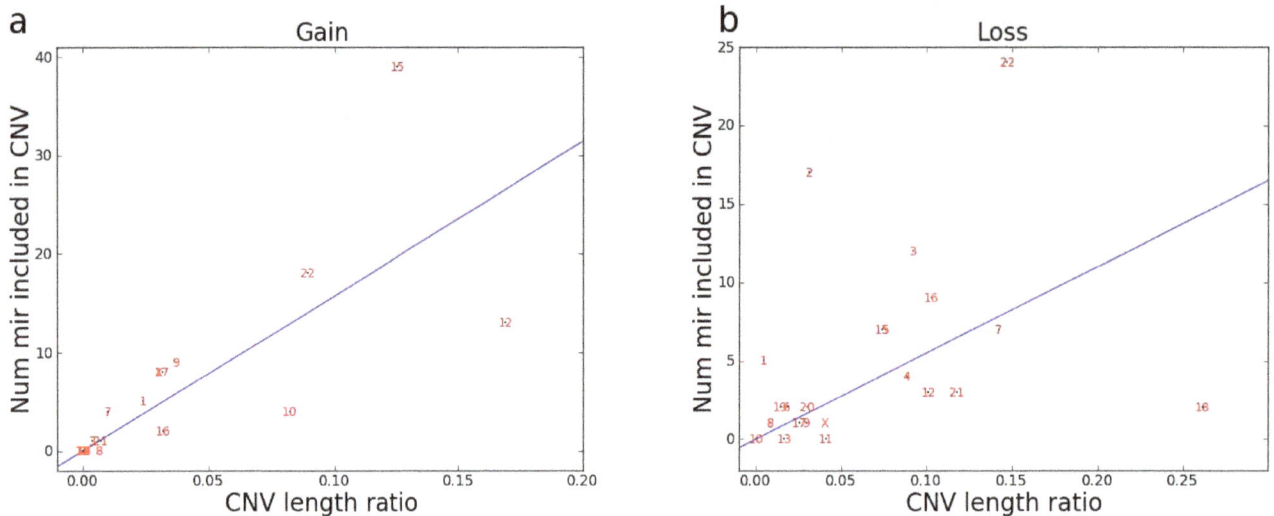

Figure 2. Correlation graph between the no. of miRNA genes in *de novo* CNVs and the CNV/Chr. lengths ratio (Ratio #2) For each chromosome, the number of miRNA genes associated to CNVs is plotted as a function of the fractional length of CNV over the chromosome's size for Gains (a) and Losses (b), respectively. The graphs show that whereas the majority of data points lay very close to the best-fit line, indicating that the two variables are positively correlated, few chromosomes instead behave as outliers in which certain CNVs appear to affect a no. of miRNA genes higher than expected (data used for the graphs were taken from Table 1).

functional enrichment analysis on the predicted target mRNAs to highlight the significance of these two microRNAs in ASD pathogenesis. The results of this latter analysis, reported in Table 4, show that several pathways identified by miRPath have been already implicated in autism by previous studies, (in bold in Table 4): Lysine degradation [34], Drug metabolism - cytochrome P450 [35], Notch signaling pathway [31,36], HIF-1 signaling pathway [37], Vasopressin-regulated water reabsorption [38], Natural killer cell mediated cytotoxicity [39]. 2NSD1 [40] and AMT [41] have been previously identified as autism candidate genes.

Discussion

In recent years, Copy Number Variants and microRNAs have emerged as potentially important etiological factors in ASD. However, until recently, in nearly all the studies, these two topics have been investigated separately in the context of the research of autism. The pathogenic role of CNVs has been interpreted in terms of their effect on the function of the overlapping protein-coding genes. On the other hand, miRNAs have been studied with the aim of uncovering changes in their level of expression in cells isolated from patients (see the Introduction for references) vs. control cells. In our study the focus is on the potential pathogenic role played by miRNA genes/de novo CNVs, instead. For this reason, we developed a new computational procedure implemented in a Fortran-written programme which allows to detect over-representation of miRNA genes in *de novo* CNVs in each chromosome. By this computational analysis based on Monte Carlo simulations we found that in positive chromosomes (FDR-adjusted p values <0.05, see Table 2 for details) there is a probability of less than 5% to find, by chance, a number of miRNA genes included in CNVs (gain and/or loss) higher than that actually detected in patients. Overall, twenty-four candidate susceptible miRNA genes of autism were identified in our study.

Hereafter, we discuss several potentially critical aspects of this new procedure that may have biased our results and interpretation. Firstly, the results do not appear to be biased by the different distribution of miRNA genes in chromosomes as all chromosomes display very similar miRNA genes length/chromosomes€length ratios. The only exception was chr. 19 which has the highest ratio (1.47×10^{-4}), but was not scored positive in a simulation analysis. Secondly, we considered if different ratios between the length of *de novo* CNVs and the length of the chromosome may have accounted for the detection of positive chromosomes. In general, we would expect the number of miRNA genes duplicated or deleted by a CNV to increase linearly with CNV size. However, such a linearity is not always followed, even for chromosomes displaying very similar ratios. Typical examples of this latter situation include CNV_Gains in chromosome 10 (ratio = 0.0822) vs. CNV_Gains in chromosome 22 (ratio = 0.0893) pair consisting of one negative (chr. 10) and one positive (chr. 22) chromosome. Thirdly, we could not perform a simulation analysis, to be used as a negative control, for CNVs detected in individuals from the general population, since the data stored in the Database of Genomic Variants generally refer to blood donors only and not to their parents, thus preventing ascertainment of *de novo* CNVs. However, it is worth mentioning here the results of a recent study by Marcinkowska et al [42], which are consistent with our findings. Indeed, these Authors found that miRNA loci are under-represented in highly polymorphic and well-validated CNVs from the general population (*i.e.*, the Database of Genomic Variants). Fourthly, in Table 1 the absence of "hits" for both CNV_Gain and CNV_Loss for chromosomes # 11, 13, 14, Y is simply due to the lack of autistic patients bearing *de novo* CNVs (Loss or Gain) overlapping miRNA genes (see Table S1). In turn, it can be speculated that, the lack of this type of patient may be ascribed to various factors such as the sample size, the use of low-resolution aCGH platforms, the occurrence of "protective" miRNA loci for autism in these chromosomes. Finally, a more suitable analysis could have involved more homogeneous CNV data from subjects (patients AND unaffected individuals) of the same ethnicity analyzed with aCGH platforms with similar resolution. This was indeed the case for the autistic sample (APL) we have used which was homogenous in relation to ethnicity in that all patients from the APL dataset were "Caucasians" (white north Americans and Europeans). In

a)   b)   c)

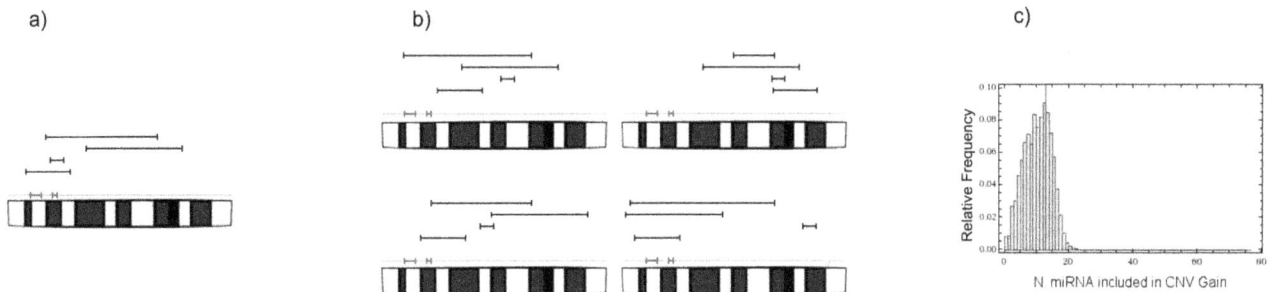

Figure 3. Schematic representation of the counting process of miRNA genes included in *de novo* CNVs of autistic patients. The small black rectangles close to chromosome are the miRNA genes, whereas the various segments above represent the various CNVs within the chromosome. An "hit" is an overlap between a CNV and a miRNA gene. In a) four "hits" are shown. b) Four examples of random distributions of simulated CNVs within the chromosome, keeping fixed the lenght of each CNV and changing its start/end positions. Clockwise from top left, the numbers of "hits" are 2, 0, 6 and 1, respectively. For each chromosome we carried out 10^6 simulations. c) Finally, the histograms displaying the relative frequency of miRNA genes included in randomly located CNVs ("hits") are obtained and the comparison between experimental data and computed Monte Carlo distribution is performed. Red lines correspond to the no. of miRNA genes detected in *de novo* CNVs from patients. p-values reported in Table 2 are the areas of the histogram to the right side of the red line. (See also Figure 4).

our study, the use of heterogeneous data concerns instead the different aCGH platforms used (APL and DGV datasets) and the mixed ethnicity of individuals reported in the Database of Genomic Variants. We decided to use such heterogeneous data to increase the chance of collecting a higher number of patients with *de novo* CNVs. This decision had its strengths and drawbacks. For instance, the use of different aCGH platforms may have caused an under-estimation of the number of CNV/miRNA genes associations in positive chromosomes from the APL dataset. In contrast, the use of samples with mixed ethnicity from the DGV database does not seem to have limited the identification of miRNA genes/CNV association in common between DGV and APL datasets. In conclusion, though the use of heterogeneous CNV data may have limited the identification of additional

miRNA/CNV associations, it did not prevent the identification of chromosomes with an enrichment of CNVs overlapping miRNA genes.

In our study, the occurrence of the same 22 deleted or duplicated miRNA genes detected in both patients and unaffected individuals (*i.e.*, DGV) strongly suggest that they are low-penetrant risk factors for autism. Difference in penetrance for such duplicated/deleted miRNA genes would be explained by a variety of factors including: (i) prenatal exposure to enviromental risk factors [43], (ii) presence/absence of functional SNPs in susceptibility protein-coding genes of autism [44], (iii) epistasis [45], (iv) epigenetic factors [6], (v) number and type of protein-coding genes co-existing in different CNVs overlapping the same miRNA. It is reassuring that other CNV studies have linked several miRNA

a)   b)

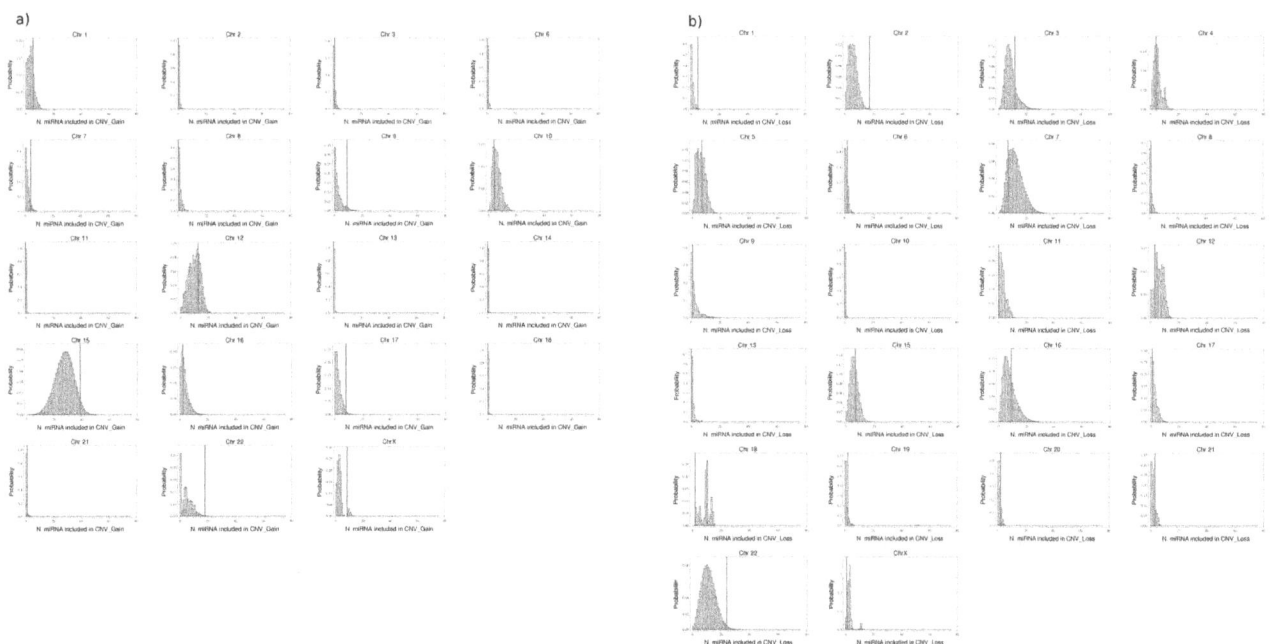

Figure 4. Histograms displaying the relative frequency of miRNA genes included in randomly located CNVs. For each chromosome, the SIMCNVMIR program computes the no. of miRNA genes affected by each randomly distributed CNV realizations and plots the frequency distribution corresponding to 10^6 realizations. The analyses were performed separately for CNV_Gains (a) and CNV_Losses (b).

Table 2. *de novo* CNVs from autistic patients with an overrepresented no. of miRNA genes.

chr	GAIN			LOSS		
	Unique	Hits	FDR-adjusted p-value	Unique	Hits	FDR-adjusted p-value
1	5	5	0.45204	5	5	**0.02309**
2	0	0	0.84211	10	17	**0.00449**
3	1	1	0.45642	10	12	0.64896
4	N/A	N/A	N/A	4	4	0.98516
5	N/A	N/A	N/A	7	7	0.73942
6	0	0	0.84211	2	2	0.70911
7	2	4	0.17818	6	7	1
8	0	0	0.84211	1	1	0.70911
9	9	9	0.17818	1	1	0.98516
10	3	4	0.84211	0	0	1
11	0	0	0.84211	0	0	1
12	13	13	0.46568	3	3	1
13	0	0	0.84211	0	0	1
14	0	0	0.84211	N/A	N/A	N/A
15	11	39	0.17818	6	7	0.70911
16	2	2	0.84211	8	9	0.70911
17	8	8	0.13920	1	1	1
18	0	0	0.84211	2	2	1
19	N/A	N/A	N/A	2	2	0.64896
20	N/A	N/A	N/A	2	2	0.64896
21	1	1	0.17818	3	3	0.64896
22	9	18	**0.04349**	9	24	0.07785
X	8	8	0.19599	1	1	1

Unique: the no. of distinct miRNA genes overlapping *de novo* CNVs in patients. Hits: the no. of identical or distinct miRNA genes overlapping *de novo* CNVs in patients. FDR-adjusted p-value: probability of obtaining a number of miRNA genes overlapping randomly-distributed CNVs larger than hits after correction for multiple testing. In bold, chromosomes displaying significant FDR-adjusted p-values (<0.05). N/A: no *de novo* CNVs are present in the APL dataset. For several chromosomes, the no. of unique is smaller than the no. of hits indicating that the same microRNA genes are affected by different *de novo* CNVs.

genes from this group to autism, and include: hsa-mir-1306, hsa-mir-185, hsa-mir-1286 and hsa-mir-649 genes [16,46], hsa-mir-200a and hsa-mir-429 [16,47], hsa-mir-200b and hsa-mir-149 [16]. Furthermore, hsa-miR-185 displays an 1.44-fold upregulation in lymphoblastoid cell lines from autistic patients [48]. Interestingly, this latter finding is consistent with the presence of 3 copies of the hsa-mir-185 gene in the 2 patients from our APL dataset.

To avoid an over-interpretation of our results we have adopted a stringent, conservative criterion according to which we propose that the 22 miRNA genes shared by unaffected individuals and patients should be considered as provisional candidates miRNA genes in ASD. On the other hand, hsa-mir-4436b-1 and hsa-mir-4436b-2, appear at the present time as strong pathogenic candidates in ASD. Unforunately, no validated targets have yet been identified for these two miRNAs. However, functional annotation analysis carried out on predicted mRNA targets for these two miRNAs revealed, that 43% (6/14) of the statistically significant KEGG pathways obtained with hsa-miR-4436b-3p have been already implicated in autism in previous studies (referenced in Table 4), a finding which supports a pathogenic role for this miRNA.

During the preparation of our manuscript, Vaishnavi et al published an article also addressing the impact of microRNAs present in autism-associated Copy Number Variants [16]. Despite, several differences (methodological, type of CNV data used) distinguishing our study from that of Vaishnavi et al., it is worth noting that 8 miRNA genes have been found in common between the two studies (chr. 1: hsa-mir-429, hsa-mir-200a, hsa-mir-200b; chr. 2: hsa-mir-149; chr. 22: hsa-mir-185, hsa-mir-1306, hsa-mir-1286, hsa-mir-649).

Conclusions

Summing up, positive findings of our study include the identification of 24 miRNA genes over-represented in *de novo* CNVs from 3 chromosomes. Two miRNA genes from this group, hsa-mir-4436b-1 and hsa-mir-4436b-2, are likely to play a significant pathogenic role in autism since they have not been found in CNVs from unaffected individuals. We hope these results will lead experimental research towards a better understanding on the role played by miRNAs in autism. Finally, we propose that the novel procedure used in this study can be effectively applied to CNV/miRNA genes association data from other genomic disorders beyond autism.

Table 3. List of 24 microRNA genes overrepresented in *de novo* CNVs.

miRNA gene name	Chr	Cytoband	Coordinates (GRCh37) start	Coordinates (GRCh37) end	strand +/-	Size (bp)	Clustered miRNA genes	DGV	no. of Patients	Gain/Loss in Patients	Gain/Loss in positive chr.	Intra/Intergenic miRNA loci
hsa-mir-2682	1	1p21.3	98510798	98510907	−	110	hsa-mir-137; hsa-mir-2682.	+	1	Loss	L	none (miRNA gene) / none
hsa-mir-137	1	1p21.3	98511626	98511727	−	102	hsa-mir-137; hsa-mir-2682.	+	1	Loss	L	(miRNA gene)
hsa-mir-200b	1	1p36.33	1102484	1102578	+	95	hsa-mir-200b; hsa-mir-200a; hsa-mir-429.	+	1	Loss	L	Intergenic
hsa-mir-200a	1	1p36.33	1103243	1103332	+	90	hsa-mir-200b; hsa-mir-200a; hsa-mir-429.	+	1	Loss	L	Intergenic
hsa-mir-429	1	1p36.33	1104385	1104467	+	83	hsa-mir-200b; hsa-mir-200a; hsa-mir-429.	+	1	Loss	L	Intergenic
hsa-mir-2467	2	2q37.3	240273419	240273499	−	81	-	+	2	Loss	L	HDAC4 intron 2
hsa-mir-3133	2	2q37.3	242417320	242417397	+	78	-	+	2	Loss	L	FARP2 intron 2 - 19
hsa-mir-4436b-2	2	2q13	111042430	111042520	+	91	-	−	1	Loss	L	Intergenic
hsa-mir-4440	2	2q37.3	239990513	239990610	−	98	-	+	2	Loss	L	HDAC4 intron 1 - 16 - 22
hsa-mir-4441	2	2q37.3	240007523	240007622	−	100	-	+	2	Loss	L	HDAC4 intron 5 - 13 - 19
hsa-mir-4786	2	2q37.3	240882432	240882511	−	80	-	+	2	Loss	L	NDUFA10 intron 4
hsa-mir-4267	2	2q13	110827538	110827619	−	82	-	+	1	Loss	L	Intergenic
hsa-mir-4436b-1	2	2q13	110844010	110844100	−	91	-	−	1	Loss	L	MALL intron 1 - 3-4 (antisense)
hsa-mir-4269	2	2q37.3	240227157	240227240	+	84	-	+	2	Loss	L	HDAC4 intron 1 - 2
hsa-mir-149	2	2q37.3	241395418	241395506	+	89	-	+	2	Loss	L	GPC1 intron 1
hsa-mir-3618	22	22q11.21	20073269	20073356	+	88	hsa-mir-3618; hsa-mir-1306.	+	2/3	Gain/Loss	L, G	DGCR8 3'UTR exon 1 - 2
hsa-mir-1306	22	22q11.21	20073581	20073665	+	85	hsa-mir-3618; hsa-mir-1306.	+	2/3	Gain/Loss	L, G	DGCR8 3'UTR exon 1 - 2
hsa-mir-301b	22	22q11.21	22007270	22007347	+	78	hsa-mir-301b; hsa-mir-130b	+	2	Gain	L, G	PPIL2 intron 1
hsa-mir-130b	22	22q11.21	22007593	22007674	+	82	hsa-mir-301b; hsa-mir-130b	+	2	Gain	L, G	PPIL2 exon 2
hsa-mir-4761	22	22q11.21	19951276	19951357	+	82	-	+	2/3	Gain/Loss	L, G	COMT 3'UTR exon 1 - 2 - 4 - 5
hsa-mir-185	22	22q11.21	20020662	20020743	+	82	-	+	2/3	Gain/Loss	L, G	C22orf25 intron 1 - 2
hsa-mir-1286	22	22q11.21	20236657	20236734	−	78	-	+	2/3	Gain/Loss	L, G	RTN4R intron 1 - 2
hsa-mir-649	22	22q11.21	21388465	21388561	−	97	-	+	2/3	Gain/Loss	L, G	Intergenic
hsa-mir-650	22	22q11.22	23165270	23165365	+	96	-	+	2	Gain	L, G	IGLV2-8 3'UTR exon 1

Information on miRNA gene coordinates, size, gene clustering, intergenic/intragenic loci are as reported in miRBase; no. of patients: number of patients bearing a CNV (including a given miRNA gene), CNVs among patients may have identical or different start/end; Gain/Loss in patients: CNV type overlapping miRNA genes detected in patients (from Table S1); Gain/Loss in positive chr.: CNV type overlapping miRNA genes detected in simulation.

Table 4. KEGG pathways enriched for targets of miRNAs hsa-mir-4436b-3p and -5p identified by mirPath[1].

	KEGG PATHWAY	p-value	# genes	Target Genes
hsa-mir-4436b-3p	**Lysine degradation**	3.30×10^{-8}	5	NSD1, KMT2D, PIPOX, KMT2A, KMT2E.
	Drug metabolism - cytochrome P450	6.73×10^{-6}	1	CYP3A43.
	Other glycan degradation	0.000197	1	NEU1.
	Glycerophospholipid metabolism	0.00029	4	PNPLA7, PGS1, LPCAT3, MBOAT2.
	Notch signaling pathway	0.000942	4	CTBP1, APH1A, NOTCH2, MAML1.
	HIF-1 signaling pathway	0.006618	5	PGF, EGLN3, PLCG1, ENO3, SLC2A1.
	Vasopressin-regulated water reabsorption	0.00847	1	AQP2.
	Glycine, serine and threonine metabolism	0.01361	3	SHMT2, **AMT**, PIPOX.
	Renal cell carcinoma	0.016804	3	PGF, EGLN3, SLC2A1.
	One carbon pool by folate	0.01935	2	SHMT2, **AMT**.
	Pathogenic Escherichia coli infection	0.04271	3	TUBA1A, TUBA8, TUBA1C.
	Graft-versus-host disease	0.04271	3	KIR3DL2, KIR2DL3, KIR3DL1.
	Antigen processing and presentation	0.044381	5	NFYA, NFYB, KIR3DL2, KIR2DL3, KIR3DL1.
	Natural killer cell mediated cytotoxicity	0.048633	5	KIR3DL2, KIR2DL3, TNFRSF10B, PLCG1, KIR3DL1.
hsa-mir-4436b-5p	Prion diseases	2.16×10^{-73}	1	PRNP.
	Sulfur relay system	2.63×10^{-9}	1	NFS1.
	Thiamine metabolism	0.002145	1	NFS1.
	Lysine degradation	0.008932	1	WHSC1.
	Transcriptional misregulation in cancer	0.023567	2	NCOR1, WHSC1.

[1]In bold pathways or genes previouly implicated in autism, see main text.

Methods

Data and databases used

Data on *de novo* CNVs detected in autistic patients were downloaded from three different sources: (i) 71 CNVs from the Autism Chromosome Rearrangements Database [49,50], (ii) 51 CNVs from Suppl. Table 8 of [10] and (iii) 75 CNVs from Table S1 (document S2) of [13]. Throughout our paper the combined three above sets of data will be named "APL datasets". CNV ("APL datasets") data used in this study are reported in the Table S1. CNVs and indels detected in individuals of the general population were downloaded from the Database of Genomic Variants (DGV vers. July 2013) [51]. In our paper this latter dataset is named by the acronym "DGV". Names, genomic coordinates and chromosomal position for 1,523 human microRNA genes, were obtained from miRBase (vers. 2012). Readers are referred to the article of Griffiths-Jones et al. [52] for an explanation of symbols and nomenclature used for miRNAs and their genes. Genomic coordinates for start and end of CNVs, indels and miRNAs genes were all from Build 37. When necessary, conversion of genomic coordinates between different genome versions was done using the Liftover tool of the UCSC Genome browser [53,54]. Finally, the list of potentially pathogenic miRNAs was obtained by excluding miRNA genes over-represented in *de novo* CNVs from patients, but not overlapping CNVs from the Database of Genomic Variants (DGV). miRWalk software was used to look for experimentally validated mRNA targets for miRNAs [33]. miRPath [55,56] was used to identify statistically significant KEGG pathways enriched in the list of predicted miRNA targets (p<0.05; p-values were corrected to account for the False Discovery Rate).

MAPCNVMIR program (Python)

Data pre-processing included: (i) computation of the total DNA length accounted for by all miRNA genes (L_1) and CNVs (L_2) in each chromosome; (ii) computation of R_1 ($R_1 = L_1$/chromosome length) and R_2 ($R_2 = L_2$/chromosome length); (iii) counts of the number of miRNA loci overall included in distinct or overlapping CNVs ("hits"). This analysis is performed separately for CNV_Gains and CNV_Losses. Thus, for a given chromosome, "hits" may consist of distinct and/or identical miRNA genes associated to CNVs; on the other hand, we indicate as "unique" the distinct miRNA genes overlapping de novo CNVs in patients.

We developed the MAPCNVMIR programme in Python language to achieve a two-fold task: (i) to calculate for each chromosome the total length of DNA corresponding to the *de novo* CNV regions and (ii) to map the microRNA genes within the *de novo* CNVs detected in patients using their genomic coordinates (Build 37). In order to achieve the first task this programme considers the overlapping DNA regions of different CNVs once only. The programme first initializes for each chromosome an empty array and put the numeric values corresponding to the first (C_{s1}) and last (C_{e1}) nucleotide positions ("start" and "end") of the first CNV (of the total list of CNVs reported in Table S1) into a sub-array. Afterwards, the code considers another CNV and compares its initial (C_{s2}) and final (C_{e2}) nucleotide positions with those of the first CNV. Three different cases can occur:

1. the first CNV is totally included in the second one (i.e. $C_{s2} < C_{1s}$ and $C_{e2} > C_{e1}$) and the values inside the sub-array are replaced by these new ones;

2. the second CNV is partially or totally included in the first one [i.e. $(C_{s2} < C_{s1}$ and $C_{e2} < C_{e1})$ or $(C_{s1} < C_{s2}$ and $C_{e1} < C_{e2})$ or $(C_{s1} < C_{s2}$ and $C_{e2} > C_{e1})]$ and the sub-array is composed of the minimum between C_{s2} and C_{s1} and the maximum between C_{e1} and C_{e2};

3. the second CNV does not overlap the first one and in this case a new sub-array with the C_{s2} and C_{e2} is added to the initial array.

Then another CNV is analyzed and its C_{s3} and C_{e3} values are compared with the values of the first and second CNVs and the values of the array are modified according the above-described procedure. This procedure is carried out for all CNVs and finally an array with the "start" and "end" values of non-overlapping DNA regions covered by different CNVs is achieved. The total length of CNVs in each chromosome is the sum of the lengths of the corresponding DNA regions. Regarding the mapping of the microRNA genes within the *de novo* CNVs detected in patients, for each chromosome, the programme first initializes a variable to zero and then compares the initial and final nucleotide positions of each CNV with the corresponding nucleotide positions of each miRNA gene. Let us name C_s, C_e, M_s, M_e the numeric values corresponding to the first and last nucleotide positions of each CNV and microRNA gene (M), respectively, in a particular chromosome. If the condition $C_s < M_s$ and $C_e > M_e$ is verified then the count of the number of miRNA genes is increased by one, otherwise the variable remains unchanged. By repeating this procedure for each CNV and each miRNA gene, the total number of microRNA genes overlapping a CNV is obtained for each chromosome.

Correlation analysis

On the data obtained by the MAPCNVMIR programme (see above) we performed an analysis to evaluate possible correlation between the number of miRNA genes overlapping *de novo* CNVs ("hits") and the fractional length of CNVs in relation to the size of the chromosome (R_2 ratios). Briefly, for each chromosome the number of "hits" was plotted against the R_2 ratios, thus obtaining the linear best fit functions and correlation coefficients were calculated. These analyses were performed separately for CNV_Gains and CNV_Losses.

SIMCNVMIR program (FORTRAN)

The SIMCNVMIR programme was developed to perform Monte Carlo randomization analyses, separately for CNV_Gains and CNV_Losses in each chromosome. These analyses included: (i) simulation of random CNV events, (ii) generation of a frequency distribution of "hits" in simulated CNVs, (iii) computation of p-values and FDR-adjusted p-values and (iv) selection of chromosomes displaying over-representation of miRNA genes in *de novo* CNVs from patients.

The analysis aimed at evaluating an over-representation of miRNA genes in CNVs was carried out by means of a computational simulation procedure implemented by a home-made written FORTRAN code. The null hypothesis underlying our investigation is that the distribution of CNVs within the chromosome is absolutely random, that is, they can occur anywhere throughout the whole length of a chromosome. Therefore, for each chromosome, the sizes (number of nucleotides) of all CNVs reported in the APL datasets (Table S1) are computed and various realizations of random distributions of these CNV regions within each chromosome are simulated. Once a new distribution of CNVs is obtained, the programme then computes the number of miRNA genes overlapping the simulated CNVs. This procedure was repeated 10^6 times for each chromosome. Data are then plotted as histograms displaying the occurrence frequency of miRNA genes associated to each CNV. These histograms provide information on the number of times a certain number of miRNAs genes are found to overlap CNVs randomly-distributed in each chromosome. These distributions take into account many factors such as the size of the chromosome, the number and positions of miRNA genes inside the chromosomes, and the size of CNVs. For each chromosome, the number of miRNA genes overall associated to the experimentally observed CNVs (*i.e.*, the CNVs reported in the APL datasets) was compared to the corresponding histogram obtained by the simulation. In order to evaluate whether the number of miRNA genes included in *de novo* CNV in patients is significantly larger than expected with a random distribution of CNVs in each chromosome, we estimated the probability (p-value) of obtaining a number of miRNA genes associated to the simulated CNVs larger than that seen with experimental CNVs. This probability is calculated by summing the area under the histogram for a number of miRNA genes included in CNVs larger than or equal to the experimental value. The p-value is very small if the number of miRNA genes included in experimental CNVs is much larger than the mean value. This means that if the distribution of the CNVs on a given chromosome was random (see the above-mentioned null hypothesis) we would have a low probability of finding a greater number of miRNA genes associated to CNVs. In other words, in autistic patients, CNVs tend to be more frequent in chromosomal regions where the miRNA genes are present than in other regions of the chromosome. The analyses described above have been performed twice: (i) for CNV_Gains and (ii) for CNV_Losses respectively. In our analysis we used a false discovery rate procedure (as multiple hypothesis testing) developed by Benjamini and Hochberg to control the expected proportion of incorrectly rejected null hypotheses [57]. In particular, we exploited a spreadsheet available on-line [58] which calculates FDR-adjusted pvalues from the knowledge of the p-values for the various chromosomes. We set acceptable FDR 0.05 as a maximum (which is the default value of the spreadsheet).

Author Contributions

Conceived and designed the experiments: MM VR. Performed the experiments: MM NNA FC. Analyzed the data: MM VR. Contributed reagents/materials/analysis tools: MM. Wrote the paper: VR.

References

1. Abrahams B, Geschwind D (2008) Advances in autism genetics: On the threshold of a new neurobiology. Nature Reviews Genetics 9: 341–355.

2. Elsabbagh M, Divan G, Koh YJ, Kim Y, Kauchali S, et al. (2012) Global Prevalence of Autism and Other Pervasive Developmental Disorders. Autism Research 5: 160–179.

3. Bailey A, Le Couteur A, Gottesman I, Bolton P, Simonoff E, et al. (1995) Autism as a strongly genetic disorder: Evidence from a British twin study. Psychological Medicine 25: 63–77.

4. Steffenburg S, Gillberg C, Hellgren L, Andersson L, Gillberg I, et al. (1989) A twin study of autism in Denmark, Finland, Iceland, Norway and Sweden. Journal of Child Psychology and Psychiatry and Allied Disciplines 30: 405–416.

5. Schaaf C, Zoghbi H (2011) Solving the Autism Puzzle a Few Pieces at a Time. Neuron 70: 806–808.

6. Miyake K, Hirasawa T, Koide T, Kubota T (2012) Epigenetics in autism and other neurodevelopmental diseases. Advances in Experimental Medicine and Biology 724: 91–98.

7. LaSalle J (2011) A genomic point-of-view on environmental factors influencing the human brain methylome. Epigenetics 6: 862–869.

8. Sebat J, Lakshmi B, Malhotra D, Troge J, Lese-Martin C, et al. (2007) Strong association of de novo copy number mutations with autism. Science 316: 445–449.

9. Glessner J, Wang K, Cai G, Korvatska O, Kim C, et al. (2009) Autism genome-wide copy number variation reveals ubiquitin and neuronal genes. Nature 459: 569–572.

10. Pinto D, Pagnamenta A, Klei L, Anney R, Merico D, et al. (2010) Functional impact of global rare copy number variation in autism spectrum disorders. Nature 466: 368–372.

11. Sanders S, Ercan-Sencicek A, Hus V, Luo R, Murtha M, et al. (2011) Multiple Recurrent De Novo CNVs, Including Duplications of the 7q11.23 Williams Syndrome Region, Are Strongly Associated with Autism. Neuron 70: 863–885.

12. Morrow E, Yoo SY, Flavell S, Kim TK, Lin Y, et al. (2008) Identifying autism loci and genes by tracing recent shared ancestry. Science 321: 218–223.

13. Levy D, Ronemus M, Yamrom B, Lee YH, Leotta A, et al. (2011) Rare De Novo and Transmitted Copy-Number Variation in Autistic Spectrum Disorders. Neuron 70: 886–897.

14. Cuscó I, Medrano A, Gener B, Vilardell M, Gallastegui F, et al. (2009) Autism-specific copy4 number variants further implicate the phosphatidylinositol signaling pathway and the glutamatergic synapse in the etiology of the disorder. Human Molecular Genetics 18: 1795–1804.

15. Ronemus M, Iossifov I, Levy D, Wigler M (2014) The role of de novo mutations in the genetics of autism spectrum disorders. Nature Reviews Genetics 15: 133–141.

16. Vaishnavi V, Manikandan M, Tiwary BK, Munirajan AK (2013) Insights on the Functional Impact of MicroRNAs Present in Autism-Associated Copy Number Variants. PLoS one 8: e56781:1–13.

17. Bartel D (2004) MicroRNAs: Genomics, Biogenesis, Mechanism, and Function. Cell 116: 281–297.

18. Lee Y, Ahn C, Han J, Choi H, Kim J, et al. (2003) The nuclear RNase III Drosha initiates microRNA processing. Nature 425: 415–419.

19. van den Berg A, Mols J, Han J (2008) RISC-target interaction: Cleavage and translational suppression. Biochimica et Biophysica Acta - Gene Regulatory Mechanisms 1779: 668–677.

20. Abu-Elneel K, Liu T, Gazzaniga F, Nishimura Y, Wall D, et al. (2008) Heterogeneous dysregulation of microRNAs across the autism spectrum. Neurogenetics 9: 153–161.

21. Garbett K, Ebert P, Mitchell A, Lintas C, Manzi B, et al. (2008) Immune transcriptome alterations in the temporal cortex of subjects with autism. Neurobiology of Disease 30: 303–311.

22. Purcell A, Jeon OH, Pevsner J (2001) The Abnormal Regulation of Gene Expression in Autistic Brain Tissue. Journal of Autism and Developmental Disorders 31: 545–549.

23. Baron C, Liu S, Hicks C, Gregg J (2006) Utilization of lymphoblastoid cell lines as a system for the molecular modeling of autism. Journal of Autism and Developmental Disorders 36: 973–982.

24. Gregg J, Lit L, Baron C, Hertz-Picciotto I, Walker W, et al. (2008) Gene expression changes in children with autism. Genomics 91: 22–29.

25. Hu V, Nguyen A, Kim K, Steinberg M, Sarachana T, et al. (2009) Gene expression profiling of lymphoblasts from autistic and nonaffected sib pairs: Altered pathways in neuronal development and steroid biosynthesis. PLoS ONE 4.

26. Nishimura Y, Martin C, Vazquez-Lopez A, Spence S, Alvarez-Retuerto A, et al. (2007) Genome-wide expression profiling of lymphoblastoid cell lines distinguishes different forms of autism and reveals shared pathways. Human Molecular Genetics 16: 1682–1698.

27. Chan AW, Kocerha J (2012) The path to microRNA therapeutics in psychiatric and neurodegenerative disorders. Frontiers in Genetics 3.

28. Sarachana T, Zhou R, Chen G, Manji H, Hu V (2010) Investigation of post-transcriptional gene regulatory networks associated with autism spectrum disorders by microRNA expression profiling of lymphoblastoid cell lines. Genome Medicine 2.

29. Talebizadeh Z, Butler M, Theodoro M (2008) Feasibility and relevance of examining lymphoblastoid cell lines to study role of microRNAs in autism. Autism research : official journal of the International Society for Autism Research 1: 240–250.

30. Abu-Elneel K, Liu T, Gazzaniga FS, Nishimura Y, Wall DP, et al. (2008) Heterogeneous dysregulation of micrornas across the autism spectrum. Neurogenetics 9: 153–161.

31. Ghahramani Seno MM, Hu P, Gwadry FG, Pinto D, Marshall CR, et al. (2011) Gene and mirna expression profiles in autism spectrum disorders. Brain research 1380: 85–97.

32. Kalos M, Whitlock P (2008) Monte Carlo Methods. Wiley.

33. Dweep H, Sticht C, Pandey P, Gretz N (2011) MiRWalk - Database: Prediction of possible miRNA binding sites by "walking" the genes of three genomes. Journal of Biomedical Informatics 44: 839–847.

34. James S, Shpyleva S, Melnyk S, Pavliv O, Pogribny I (2013) Complex epigenetic regulation of engrailed-2 (en-2) homeobox gene in the autism cerebellum. Translational psychiatry 3: e232.

35. Correia C, Almeida J, Santos P, Sequeira A, Marques C, et al. (2009) Pharmacogenetics of risperidone therapy in autism: association analysis of eight candidate genes with drug efficacy and adverse drug reactions. The pharmacogenomics journal 10: 418–430.

36. Griswold AJ, Ma D, Cukier HN, Nations LD, Schmidt MA, et al. (2012) Evaluation of copy number variations reveals novel candidate genes in autism spectrum disorder-associated pathways. Human molecular genetics 21: 3513–3523.

37. Burstyn I, Wang X, Yasui Y, Sithole F, Zwaigenbaum L (2011) Autism spectrum disorders and fetal hypoxia in a population-based cohort: Accounting for missing exposures via estimation-maximization algorithm. BMC medical research methodology 11: 2.

38. Miller M, Bales KL, Taylor SL, Yoon J, Hostetler CM, et al. (2013) Oxytocin and vasopressin in6 children and adolescents with autism spectrum disorders: Sex differences and associations with symptoms. Autism Research.

39. Bressler JP, Gillin PK, O'Driscoll C, Kiihl S, Solomon M, et al. (2012) Maternal antibody reactivity to lymphocytes of offspring with autism. Pediatric neurology 47: 337–340.

40. Buxbaum JD, Cai G, Nygren G, Chaste P, Delorme R, et al. (2007) Mutation analysis of the nsd1 gene in patients with autism spectrum disorders and macrocephaly. BMC medical genetics 8: 68.

41. Yu TW, Chahrour MH, Coulter ME, Jiralerspong S, Okamura-Ikeda K, et al. (2013) Using whole-exome sequencing to identify inherited causes of autism. Neuron 77: 259–273.

42. Marcinkowska M, Szymanski M, Krzyzosiak W, Kozlowski P (2011) Copy number variation of microRNA genes in the human genome. BMC Genomics 12.

43. Gardener H, Spiegelman D, Buka S (2009) Prenatal risk factors for autism: Comprehensive meta-analysis. British Journal of Psychiatry 195: 7–14.

44. Sanders S, Murtha M, Gupta A, Murdoch J, Raubeson M, et al. (2012) De novo mutations revealed by whole-exome sequencing are strongly associated with autism. Nature 484: 237–241.

45. Coutinho A, Sousa I, Martins M, Correia C, Morgadinho T, et al. (2007) Evidence for epistasis between SLC6A4 and ITGB3 in autism etiology and in the determination of platelet serotonin levels. Human Genetics 121: 243–256.

46. Xu B, Karayiorgou M, Gogos JA (2010) Micrornas in psychiatric and neurodevelopmental disorders. Brain research 1338: 78–88.

47. Qiao Y, Badduke C, Mercier E, Lewis SM, Pavlidis P, et al. (2013) mirna and mirna target genes in copy number variations occurring in individuals with intellectual disability. BMC genomics 14: 544.

48. Sarachana T, Zhou R, Chen G, Manji HK, Hu VW (2010) Investigation of post-transcriptional gene regulatory networks associated with autism spectrum disorders by microrna expression profiling of lymphoblastoid cell lines. Genome Med 2: 23.

49. Marshall C, Noor A, Vincent J, Lionel A, Feuk L, et al. (2008) Structural Variation of Chromosomes in Autism Spectrum Disorder. American Journal of Human Genetics 82: 477–488.

50. Autism Chromosome Rearrangements Database (version 2012). Available: http://projects.tcag.ca/autism/1.7

51. Zhang J, Feuk L, Duggan G, Khaja R, Scherer S (2006) Development of bioinformatics resources for display and analysis of copy number and other structural variants in the human genome. Cytogenetic and Genome Research 115: 205–214.

52. Griffiths-Jones S, Grocock R, van Dongen S, Bateman A, Enright A (2006) miRBase: microRNA sequences, targets and gene nomenclature. Nucleic acids research 34: D140–144.

53. James Kent W, Sugnet C, Furey T, Roskin K, Pringle T, et al. (2002) The human genome browser at UCSC. Genome Research 12: 996–1006.

54. Liftover Accessed June 2012 (2002). Tool of the UCSC Genome browser. Available: http://genome.ucsc.edu/cgi-bin/hgLiftOver.

55. Vlachos IS, Kostoulas N, Vergoulis T, Georgakilas G, Reczko M, et al. (2012) Diana mirpath v. 2.0: investigating the combinatorial effect of micrornas in pathways. Nucleic acids research 40: W498–W504.

56. miRPath version 20 (2012) Available: http://diana.imis.athena-innovation.gr/DianaTools/index.php?r=mirpath/index. Accessed 2013 Dec.

57. Benjamini Y, Hochberg Y (2000) On the adaptive control of the false discovery rate in multiple testing with independent statistics. Journal of Educational and Behavioral Statistics 25: 60–83.

58. Pike N. Spreadsheet for calculating the FDR-adjusted p-values starting from p-values. Available: http://users.ox.ac.uk/~npike/#programs. Accessed 2013 Oct 26.

Are Maternal Social Networks and Perceptions of Trust Associated with Suspected Autism Spectrum Disorder in Offspring? A Population-Based Study in Japan

Takeo Fujiwara[1]*, Ichiro Kawachi[2]

1 Department of Social Medicine, National Research Institute for Child Health and Development, Setagaya-ku, Tokyo, Japan, **2** Department of Society and Behavioral Sciences, Harvard School of Public Health, Boston, Massachusetts, United States of America

Abstract

Objective: To investigate the associations of maternal social networks and perceptions of trust with the prevalence of suspected autism spectrum disorders in 18-month-old offspring in Japan.

Methods: Questionnaires included measurements of maternal social networks (number of relatives or friends they could call upon for assistance), maternal perceptions of trust, mutual assistance (i.e. individual measures of "cognitive social capital"), and social participation (i.e. individual measures of "structural social capital") as well as the Modified Checklist for Autism in Toddlers to detect suspected autism spectrum disorder (ASD). These tools were mailed to all families with 18-month-old toddlers in Chiba, a city near Tokyo (N = 6061; response rate: 64%). The association between social capital or social network indicators and suspected ASD were analyzed, adjusted for covariates by logistic regression analysis.

Results: Low maternal social trust was found to be significantly positively associated with suspected ASD in toddlers compared with high maternal social trust (adjusted odds ratio [OR]: 1.82, 95% confidence interval [CI]: 1.38 to 2.40); mutual aid was also significantly positively related (low vs. high: OR, 1.82, 95% CI: 1.38 to 2.40). However, maternal community participation showed U-shape association with suspected ASD of offspring. Maternal social network showed consistent inverse associations with suspected ASD of offspring, regardless of the type of social connection (e.g., relatives, neighbors, or friends living outside of their neighborhood).

Conclusions: Mothers' cognitive social capital and social networks, but not structural social capital, might be associated with suspected ASD in offspring.

Editor: Kenji J. Tsuchiya, Hamamatsu University School of Medicine, Japan

Funding: This study was supported by grants from a Grant-in-aid for Scientific Research on Innovative Areas, Ministry of Education, Culture, Sports, Science and Technology KAKENHI (21119003). The funders had no role in study design, data collection and analysis, decision to publish, or preparation of the manuscript.

Competing Interests: The authors have declared that no competing interests exist.

* Email: fujiwara-tk@ncchd.go.jp

Introduction

Autism, or autism spectrum disorder (ASD), is a developmental disorder typified by impaired communication and social skills [1]. Genetic factors may play a significant role in causing ASD [2], however, they do not entirely explain all cases [1]. For example, the California Autism Twins Study showed that the rates of ASD among identical twins were 77% for male and 50% for female, and for fraternal twins, 31% for male and 36% for female [3], suggesting that environmental factors may contribute to the development of ASD. Several studies investigated the association between environmental factors and ASD, including toxin exposure [4–8], zinc deficiency [9–12], or infection during pregnancy [13,14]. However, few studies have investigated the association between social environment and ASD, or even autistic traits such as suspected ASD. Impairment of social behavior is one of the characteristics of ASD, therefore it seems plausible that characteristics of the social environment – such as the social networks surrounding the parent or the quality of social connections in the broader environment, referred to as "social capital" – might contribute to the development of ASD in the offspring. Few studies have investigated the association between social networks/social capital and autistic traits.

The term 'social capital' describes the resources accessed by individuals through their social networks in settings such as the community, school, or work [15]. Three key types of resources include: (a) levels of trust between individuals, (b) mutual aid, and (c) the ability to undertake coordinated, collective action. For example, a community with high social capital is one in which members frequently help each other and exchange favors. Mutual aid relies on high levels of interpersonal trust in the social network (i.e., trust that a recipient of a good deed will return the favor in the future). Therefore, social capital might have an effect on the social behaviors of children, directly or indirectly through guardians. Social capital can be assessed at both the community and individual levels: community-level social capital refers to aggregated social resources of individuals in the community, while individual-level social capital refers to each individual's perception of the quality of social interactions in the surrounding community. Recent studies have demonstrated links between oxytocin secretion and individual perceptions of social capital (i.e. individual assessments of the trustworthiness of their social connections) [15]. Moreover, oxytocin has been proposed as a treatment for autism [16]. In this context, we hypothesized that individual-level social capital as perceived by mothers and maternal social networks can be related to autistic traits in their children, even in a cross-sectional study.

Thus, the purpose of this study was to investigate the association of maternal social networks and individual perceptions of social capital with the prevalence of suspected ASD in their children in Japan.

Methods

Participants

The study was approved by the Ethics Committee of the National Institute for Child Health and Development. A questionnaire was mailed to all families with 18-month-old toddlers in Chiba (N = 95 000). Chiba is the capital city of Chiba Prefecture, located east of Tokyo. It is composed of six wards and has a population of around 963 000. It covers an area of 272 km^2, making the population density around 3540 person/km^2. Under the Japanese health care system, all mothers of newborn babies are followed up with "well baby" checkups through the local health centers. The mothers of the toddlers were requested to fill out the questionnaire and bring it to their 18-month health checkup at one of six health centers, from January to December 2011. In total, 8350 toddlers participated in the health checkup (participation rate: 87.9%), and 6106 mothers returned the questionnaires to their local health center, of which 6061 were valid for inclusion in the study (valid response rate: 63.8%).

Measures

Maternal perceptions of social capital were assessed in both cognitive and structural domains [17–20]. Indicators of cognitive social capital included items inquiring about social trust and availability of mutual aid among neighbors. Social trust was assessed through a single item: "Do you think that people in your neighborhood trust each other?" Mutual aid was also assessed with a single item: "Do you think that people in your neighborhood help each other?" Response choices for both items followed a 4-point Likert-scale ("yes," "somewhat yes," "somewhat no," and "no"), with each response labeled as "high," "high-middle," "low-middle," and "low" trust and mutual aid, respectively [17,18,20].

We assessed structural social capital by asking participants about their participation in the community, which was determined by the total number of organizations in which the respondent participated. Previous studies have used this measure to demonstrate associations with health status [20,21]. The types of organizations with which participants reported being affiliated included parenting groups, parent-teacher associations, civic organizations, consumers' cooperative societies, unions/religious groups, or other community groups [15]. Based on the distribution of responses, we classified community participation into three categories: no organizations, one organization, and more than one organizations. In addition, frequency of community participation was explored and categorized into four groups: no participation, not regularly, 1–3 times per month, and 4 or more times per month.

Social networks were assessed with the following question: "How many relatives or friends are you able to easily consult with to obtain support?" We then divided participants by the number

of relatives or friends the respondents consulted with, forming three categories: 0–3, 4 or 5, and 6 or more. Further, to identify the person consulted, the following questions were asked: "Among them, how many are relatives? How many are neighbors? How many are friends who are not living near you?" Participants were again divided into three categories according to their answers.

Suspected ASD was evaluated using the Japanese version of the Modified Checklist for Autism in Toddlers (M-CHAT), which is validated [22], rated by mothers. Following the cutoff of the original M-CHAT [23], children who failed two or more of the six critical items or three or more of any of the items were considered to have suspected ASD.

The association between social capital or social network and suspected ASD was of primary interest; therefore, possible confounders identified from previous studies [24–27] were also evaluated through the questionnaire. These included maternal characteristics, (age, self-rated health, employment status, and marital status), family characteristics (parental education, annual household income, living with grandparents or other relatives, and number of children) and child characteristics (low birth weight, preterm, and day care attendance). Self-rated health was assessed using the following question: "How would you rate your health in general?" Response choices followed a 5-point Likert scale (excellent, very good, good, fair, or poor), but were dichotomized for analysis as: poor/fair vs. all other. Maternal and paternal educational level was categorized as junior high school graduate, high school graduate, some college/vocational school, college, or graduate school. Annual household income was assessed in increments of 2 million yen up to 10 million yen, (i.e., less than 2, 2.1–4, 4.1–6, 6.1–8, 8.1–10, 10.1–15, and 15.1 or more million yen). At current exchange rates, 1 million yen is equivalent to 10,000 USD. The median annual household income in Japan was 4.5 million yen in 2008 [28].

Analysis

Logistic regression was used to calculate the odds ratios (OR) of suspected ASD for each social capital or social network indicator. The models adjusted for each socioeconomic status (SES) measure (i.e. parental education and income) and other potential confounders. Missing cases were treated as dummy variables to maximize statistical power. All statistical analyses were performed using the Stata MP 12, and the level of statistical significance was set at 0.05 (two-tailed).

Results

Table 1 shows the demographic characteristics of the participants. Regarding maternal characteristics, the mean age of mothers was 32.8 years (SD = 4.8); 97.5% were married, 25.9% had graduated high school or less, 95.3% rated their health as "good", and 68.9% were not working. As for household characteristics, 8.9% were living with grandparents or relatives, 53.9% had only one child, and annual income was distributed as follows: ≤4 million yen, 23.4%; 4.1–6 million yen, 32.8%; 6.1–8 million yen, 18.4%; ≥8.1 million yen, 14.0%; and missing, 11.4%. Regarding child characteristics, 7.9% had low birth weight and 26.1% attended nursery school. Suspected ASD was found in 13.5% of the sample.

The distribution of social capital and social network indicators are shown in Table 2. Social trust was found to be high for 17.9% of participants, and low for 11.5%. Similarly, high and low mutual aid was found in 18.2% and 11.5% of participants, respectively. In addition, 71.3% of participants did not participate in any community organization, while 10.4% participated in two or

Table 1. Characteristics of sample (N = 6061).

			N	%
Maternal characteristics	Age	<25 y	276	4.6
		25–29 y	1,220	20.1
		30–34 y	2,236	36.9
		35–39 y	1,756	29.0
		40+y	493	8.1
		Missing	80	1.3
	Marital status	Married	5,903	97.4
		Not married	151	2.5
		Missing	7	0.1
	Maternal education	HS or less	1,572	25.9
		Some college	2,670	44.1
		College+	1,658	27.4
		Missing	161	2.7
	Self-rated health	Good/very good/excellent	5,774	95.3
		Fair/poor	238	3.9
		Missing	49	0.8
	Employment status	Full-time	1,068	17.6
		Part-time	749	12.4
		Not working	4,176	68.9
		Missing	68	1.1
Household characteristics	Paternal education	HS or less	1,582	26.1
		Some college	1,210	20.0
		College+	2,978	49.1
		Missing	291	4.8
	Living with grandparents or other relatives	Yes	542	8.9
		No	5,516	91.0
		Missing	3	0.1
	Number of children	1	3,269	53.9
		2	2,135	35.2
		3+	657	10.8
	Annual household income	<400 m	1,418	23.4
		400–600 m	1,987	32.8
		600–800 m	1,117	18.4
		800 m+	851	14.0
		Missing	688	11.4
Child characteristics	Low birth weight	Yes	476	7.9
		No	5,428	89.6
		Missing	157	2.6
	Preterm birth	Yes	316	5.2
		No	5,383	88.8
		Missing	362	6.0
	Nursery school attendance	Yes	1,583	26.1
		No	4,416	72.9
		Missing	62	1.0
	Autism spectrum disorder	Suspected positive	815	13.5
		Suspected negative	5,246	86.6

Table 2. Distribution of maternal perception of social capital and social network indicators (N = 6061).

			N	%
Cognitive social capital	Social trust	High	1,085	17.9
		High-middle	3,121	51.5
		Low-middle	957	15.8
		Low	697	11.5
		Missing	201	3.3
	Mutual aid	High	1,101	18.2
		High-middle	2,929	48.3
		Low-middle	1,149	19.0
		Low	694	11.5
		Missing	188	3.1
Structural social capital	Number of community organizations affiliated with	0	4,322	71.3
		1	1,050	17.3
		2+	608	10.4
		Missing	81	1.3
	Frequency of participation in community organization	No participation	4,320	71.3
		Not regularly	476	7.9
		1–3 times per month	900	14.9
		4+ times per month	266	4.4
		Missing	99	1.6
Social network	Number of relatives or friends who are easy to consult with	0 to 3	1,981	32.7
		4 to 5	1,864	30.8
		6+	1,959	32.3
		Missing	257	4.2
	Number of relatives who are easy to consult with	0 to 1	1,851	30.5
		2	2,197	36.3
		3+	1,763	29.1
		Missing	250	4.1
	Number of neighbors who are easy to consult with	0	1,166	19.2
		1 to 2	2,431	40.1
		3+	1,624	26.8
		Missing	840	13.9
	Number of friends outside of neighborhood who are easy to consult with	0	1,159	19.1
		1 to 2	2,494	41.2
		3+	1,318	21.8
		Missing	1,090	18.0

more community organizations. Regarding the frequency of participation, 7.9% were not regular, 14.9% participated 1–3 times per month, and 4.4% participated 4 or more times per month. The distribution of the number of relatives or friends with whom the respondents could consult easily was as follows: 0 to 3, 32.7%; 4 to 5, 30.8%; and 5 or more, 32.3%.

The ORs of suspected ASD for social capital and social network indicators are shown in Table 3. Low maternal social trust was found to be significantly positively associated with having a toddler with suspected ASD in comparison with high maternal social trust (crude model: odds ratio [OR]: 1.97, 95% confidence interval [CI]: 1.51 to 2,57). Results were similar even after adjustment of maternal, household, and infant characteristics (adjusted OR: 1.82, 95% CI: 1.38 to 2.40). The gradient effect of social trust on having a toddler with suspected ASD was also found to be significant (p for trend <0.001). Similarly, mutual aid was also significantly associated with having a toddler with suspected ASD (low vs. high: adjusted OR, 1.82, 95% CI: 1.38 to 2.40) with a significant gradient effect (p for trend <0.001). By contrast, community participation had a marginally significant association with having a toddler with suspected ASD in the crude model (p for trend = 0.049), which became non-significant in the adjusted model (p for trend = 0.094). Interestingly, frequency of community participation showed a U-shape association with having suspected ASD offspring. It was found that mothers who participated in community activities 1–3 times per month were 25% less likely to have a toddler with suspected ASD (adjusted OR: 0.75, 95% CI: 0.60 to 0.95) in comparison with the no-community-participation group. On the other hand, participating 4 or more times per month was not associated with having a

Table 3. Odds ratio of maternal perception of social capital and social network indicators for offspring's suspected ASD.

			Crude		Adjusted	
			OR	95% CI	OR	95% CI
Cognitive social capital	Social trust	High	Reference		Reference	
		High-middle	1.10	0.88 to 1.36	1.09	0.87 to 1.36
		Low-middle	**1.60**	**1.23 to 2.06**	**1.54**	**1.19 to 2.00**
		Low	**1.97**	**1.51 to 2,57**	**1.82**	**1.38 to 2.40**
		P for trend	**<0.001**		**<0.001**	
	Mutual aid	High	Reference		Reference	
		High-middle	1.12	0.90 to 1.40	1.11	0.89 to 1.39
		Low-middle	**1.40**	**1.09 to 1.80**	**1.35**	**1.05 to 1.74**
		Low	**2.24**	**1.72 to 2.91**	1.82	1.38 to 2.40
		P for trend	**<0.001**		**<0.001**	
Structural social capital	Number of community organizations affiliated with	0	Reference		Reference	
		1	0.89	0.73 to 1.09	0.91	0.74 to 1.11
		2+	0.79	0.60 to 1.03	0.81	0.62 to 1.07
		P for trend	**0.049**		0.094	
	Frequency of participation in community organization	No participation	Reference		Reference	
		Not regularly	1.05	0.80 to 1.37	1.12	0.85 to 1.47
		1–3 times per month	**0.75**	**0.60 to 0.94**	**0.75**	**0.60 to 0.95**
		4+ times per month	0.97	0.67 to 1.39	0.96	0.66 to 1.39
		P for trend	0.072		0.096	
Social network	Number of relatives or friends to consult with	0 to 3	Reference		Reference	
		4 to 5	**0.66**	**0.55 to 0.79**	**0.66**	**0.55 to 0.79**
		6+	**0.55**	**0.45 to 0.66**	**0.56**	**0.46 to 0.67**
		P for trend	**<0.001**		**<0.001**	
	Number of relatives to consult with	0 to 1	Reference		Reference	
		2	**0.65**	**0.55 to 0.78**	**0.65**	**0.55 to 0.78**
		3+	**0.58**	**0.48 to 0.71**	**0.58**	**0.48 to 0.71**
		P for trend	**<0.001**		**<0.001**	
	Number of neighbors to consult with	0	reference		reference	
		1 to 2	**0.68**	**0.56 to 0.82**	**0.71**	**0.58 to 0.86**
		3+	**0.57**	**0.46 to 0.71**	**0.61**	**0.49 to 0.77**
		P for trend	**<0.001**		**<0.001**	
	Number of friends outside of neighborhood to consult with	0	reference		reference	
		1 to 2	**0.75**	**0.62 to 0.92**	**0.74**	**0.60 to 0.90**
		3+	**0.74**	**0.59 to 0.93**	**0.71**	**0.57 to 0.90**
		P for trend	**0.009**		**0.007**	

toddler with suspected ASD (adjusted OR: 0.96, 95% CI: 0.66 to 1.39).

Maternal social network showed consistent inverse associations with having offspring with suspected ASD, regardless of relatives, neighbors, or friends living outside of their neighborhood. For example, participants who had 4 to 5 relatives or friends to consult with were 34% less likely to have a toddler with suspected ASD (adjusted OR: 0.66, 95% CI: 0.55 to 0.79). Similarly, participants who had 6 or more relatives or friends to consult with were 44%

less likely to have a toddler with suspected ASD (adjusted OR: 0.56, 95% CI: 0.46 to 0.67), and the gradient was statistically significant (p for trend <0.001).

Discussion

The current study showed that a mother with low social trust is more likely to have a toddler with suspected ASD in comparison with a mother with high social trust. The results were similar in the case of mutual aid. However, structural social capital (i.e., maternal membership of community organizations) showed no linear association with having a child with suspected ASD, although a U-shaped association was found for frequency of community participation. Maternal social network showed consistent inverse association with having a child with suspected ASD, regardless of types of consultants, relatives, neighbors, or friends living outside their neighborhood.

To the best of our knowledge, this is the first study to show an association between social capital and prevalence of suspected ASD. However, because this study was a cross-sectional study, the causality of social capital on having a toddler with suspected ASD could not be determined—in other words, we could not explore whether having offspring with autistic traits directly induces low social capital or low social networks of parents. Moreover, previous studies including a study from Japan reported that parents who had children with ASD were less likely to have poor social relationships [29,30]. Nonetheless, the possibility of social causation remains. Previous studies reported associations of toxin exposure [4–8], zinc deficiency [9–12], and infection during pregnancy [13,14] with ASD, suggesting that mothers living in disadvantaged communities might be more likely to be exposed to toxic pollutants, or zinc deficiency due to poor access to food. Because low social capital communities are more likely to be disadvantaged [31], exposure to these risk factors might contribute to the association between maternal social capital and ASD. Possibly, characteristics of social environment – viz., the strength of social networks or local social capital – could enhance the quality of interaction between infants and caregivers [32], which might have an effect on the development of autistic traits [33].

Alternatively, the association found in this study might be confounded by shared genetic predisposition between mothers and infants. Mothers with a predisposition for autistic traits may be more likely to end up in less socially interactive community settings, such as rented housing [34], in which social capital is low. Due to the heritable component of ASD [2], mothers with an autistic predisposition are more likely to have offspring with autistic traits. Further study is needed to confirm the association between social capital and toddlers with suspected ASD, with adjustment for maternal autistic traits. Nonetheless, the current finding is significant because low social capital can be a marker to identify communities with a higher proportion of toddlers with suspected ASD, which might be useful from a needs assessment standpoint.

We found a U-shape association between frequency of community participation and having suspected ASD offspring. This finding is important because mothers who are frequent participants in community organizations are less likely to have autistic traits. However, it is also important to consider that maternal autistic traits are not necessarily linearly associated with having offspring with autistic traits. In addition, this finding suggests that appropriate frequency of community participation (1–3 times per month) for mothers is important for the social development of children, in comparison with a lack of community participation or too much community participation. A previous study reported that participation in education or support groups is beneficial for self-esteem, parenting skills, and communication with children [35]. Thus, frequency of community participation

can be considered as a factor affecting the social development of offspring indirectly by affecting the parents' social and parenting skills. Alternatively, mothers who have a child with suspected ASD may be more likely to participate in several community programs or attend parenting support groups for children with developmental problems. Further research is needed to elucidate the causation of the association between maternal community participation and autistic traits of offspring.

We investigated different sources of maternal network support, including relatives, neighbors, and friends not living in the neighborhood, and found that all three types were consistently inversely associated with having a child with suspected ASD. This suggests that mothers who have a child with suspected ASD are less likely to have high social skills, probably due to maternal autistic traits. A previous study reported that the physical distance of a friend affects people's happiness [36]. By contrast, it was found that in Chiba city, physical distance did not matter in terms of the prevalence of suspected ASD. This might be due to technology such as mobile phones, cars, or the internet, which may help individuals to stay in touch with social contacts irrespective of distance.

In addition to the previously mentioned points, other limitations of this study need to be addressed. First, as the M-CHAT screening scale was used to detect suspected ASD, misclassification of suspected ASD (i.e., false positive) might have resulted in underestimation of the association of social capital or social network with having a child with suspected ASD. However, as the prevalence of suspected ASD in our study (13.5%) was equivalent to the prevalence of suspected ASD among 18-month-old toddlers who were identified for follow-up in a previous study (i.e. 14.3%) [37], the assessment of suspected ASD is considered acceptable. Second, information on paternal characteristics such as age or occupation was not assessed, although previous studies reported that they might be independently associated with ASD [38,39]. However, paternal age could be correlated with maternal age, and we found no association with maternal age and suspected ASD in offspring (data not shown). In addition, although occupation was not considered, paternal education was adjusted for in the analysis.

In conclusion, maternal cognitive social capital and social networks, but not structural social capital, was associated with having a child with suspected ASD. Maternal social network was also associated with having a child with suspected ASD, regardless of types of social contacts. Further research is needed to elucidate the association between maternal cognitive social capital and the development of autistic traits in offspring.

Acknowledgments

We thank Ms Akiko Okada at Chiba City Health Center for her arrangements of this study. We also thank Dr. Emma L. Barber of the Department of Education for Clinical Research, National Center for Child Health and Development, for editing this manuscript.

Author Contributions

Conceived and designed the experiments: TF. Performed the experiments: TF. Analyzed the data: TF. Contributed reagents/materials/analysis tools: TF. Wrote the paper: TF IK.

References

1. Grabrucker AM (2012) Environmental factors in autism. Front Psychiatry 3: 118.
2. Abrahams BS, Geschwind DH (2010) Connecting genes to brain in the autism spectrum disorders. Arch Neurol 67: 395–399.
3. Hallmayer J, Cleveland S, Torres A, Phillips J, Cohen B, et al. (2011) Genetic heritability and shared environmental factors among twin pairs with autism. Arch Gen Psychiatry 68: 1095–1102.

4. Moore SJ, Turnpenny P, Quinn A, Glover S, Lloyd DJ, et al. (2000) A clinical study of 57 children with fetal anticonvulsant syndromes. J Med Genet 37: 489–497.

5. Stromland K, Nordin V, Miller M, Akerstrom B, Gillberg C (1994) Autism in thalidomide embryopathy: a population study. Dev Med Child Neurol 36: 351–356.

6. Karr CJ, Solomon GM, Brock-Utne AC (2007) Health effects of common home, lawn, and garden pesticides. Pediatr Clin North Am 54: 63–80.

7. Roberts EM, English PB, Grether JK, Windham GC, Somberg L, et al. (2007) Maternal residence near agricultural pesticide applications and autism spectrum disorders among children in the California Central Valley. Environ Health Perspect 115: 1482–1489.

8. Gardener H, Spiegelman D, Buka SL (2009) Prenatal risk factors for autism: comprehensive meta-analysis. Br J Psychiatry 195: 7–14.

9. Lakshmi Priya MD, Geetha A (2011) Level of trace elements (copper, zinc, magnesium and selenium) and toxic elements (lead and mercury) in the hair and nail of children with autism. Biol Trace Elem Res 142: 148–158.

10. Faber S, Zinn GM, Kern JC 2nd, Kingston HM (2009) The plasma zinc/serum copper ratio as a biomarker in children with autism spectrum disorders. Biomarkers 14: 171–180.

11. Yasuda H, Yoshida K, Yasuda Y, Tsutsui T (2011) Infantile zinc deficiency: association with autism spectrum disorders. Sci Rep 1: 129.

12. Golub MS, Keen CL, Gershwin ME, Hendrickx AG (1995) Developmental zinc deficiency and behavior. J Nutr 125: 2263S–2271S.

13. Libbey JE, Sweeten TL, McMahon WM, Fujinami RS (2005) Autistic disorder and viral infections. J Neurovirol 11: 1–10.

14. Pardo CA, Vargas DL, Zimmerman AW (2005) Immunity, neuroglia and neuroinflammation in autism. Int Rev Psychiatry 17: 485–495.

15. Fujiwara T, Kubzansky LD, Matsumoto K, Kawachi I (2012) The association between oxytocin and social capital. PLoS One 7: e52018.

16. Modahl C, Green L, Fein D, Morris M, Waterhouse L, et al. (1998) Plasma oxytocin levels in autistic children. Biol Psychiatry 43: 270–277.

17. Fujiwara T, Kawachi I (2008) A prospective study of individual-level social capital and major depression in the United States. J Epidemiol Community Health 62: 627–633.

18. Fujiwara T, Kawachi I (2008) Social capital and health a study of adult twins in the U.S. Am J Prev Med 35: 139–144.

19. Ueshima K, Fujiwara T, Takao S, Suzuki E, Iwase T, et al. (2010) Does social capital promote physical activity? A population-based study in Japan. PLoS One 5: e12135.

20. Fujiwara T, Takao S, Iwase T, Hamada J, Kawachi I (2012) Does Caregiver's Social Bonding Enhance the Health of their Children?: The Association between Social Capital and Child Behaviors. Acta Med Okayama 66: 343–350.

21. Murayama H, Fujiwara Y, Kawachi I (2012) Social capital and health: a review of prospective multilevel studies. J Epidemiol 22: 179–187.

22. Inada N, Koyama T, Inokuchi E, Kuroda M, Kamio Y (2011) Reliability and validity of the Japanese version of the Modified Checklist for autism in toddlers (M-CHAT). Research in Autism Spectrum Disorders 5: 330–336.

23. Robins DL, Fein D, Barton ML, Green JA (2001) The Modified Checklist for Autism in Toddlers: an initial study investigating the early detection of autism and pervasive developmental disorders. J Autism Dev Disord 31: 131–144.

24. Sullivan A, Winograd G, Verkuilen J, Fish MC (2012) Children on the autism spectrum: grandmother involvement and family functioning. J Appl Res Intellect Disabil 25: 484–494.

25. Lampi KM, Hinkka-Yli-Salomaki S, Lehti V, Helenius H, Gissler M, et al. (2013) Parental Age and Risk of Autism Spectrum Disorders in a Finnish National Birth Cohort. J Autism Dev Disord 43: 2526–2535.

26. Krakowiak P, Walker CK, Bremer AA, Baker AS, Ozonoff S, et al. (2012) Maternal metabolic conditions and risk for autism and other neurodevelopmental disorders. Pediatrics 129: e1121–1128.

27. Rai D, Lewis G, Lundberg M, Araya R, Svensson A, et al. (2012) Parental socioeconomic status and risk of offspring autism spectrum disorders in a Swedish population-based study. J Am Acad Child Adolesc Psychiatry 51: 467–476.

28. Ministry of Health Labor and Welfare (2012) Income distribution. Tokyo: Ministry of Health Labor and Welfare.

29. Mugno D, Ruta L, D'Arrigo VG, Mazzone L (2007) Impairment of quality of life in parents of children and adolescents with pervasive developmental disorder. Health Qual Life Outcomes 5: 22.

30. Yamada A, Kato M, Suzuki M, Suzuki M, Watanabe N, et al. (2012) Quality of life of parents raising children with pervasive developmental disorders. BMC Psychiatry 12: 119.

31. Kawachi I, Kennedy BP, Lochner K, Prothrow-Stith D (1997) Social capital, income inequality, and mortality. Am J Public Health 87: 1491–1498.

32. Aoyama M, Wei CN, Harada K, Ueda K, Takano M, et al. (2013) Community factors to promote parents' quality of child-nurturing life. Environ Health Prev Med 18: 57–70.

33. Wan MW, Green J, Elsabbagh M, Johnson M, Charman T, et al. (2013) Quality of interaction between at-risk infants and caregiver at 12–15 months is associated with 3-year autism outcome. J Child Psychol Psychiatry 54: 763–771.

34. Brugha TS, McManus S, Bankart J, Scott F, Purdon S, et al. (2011) Epidemiology of autism spectrum disorders in adults in the community in England. Arch Gen Psychiatry 68: 459–465.

35. Lipman EL, Kenny M, Jack S, Cameron R, Secord M, et al. (2010) Understanding how education/support groups help lone mothers. BMC Public Health 10: 4.

36. Fowler JH, Christakis NA (2008) Dynamic spread of happiness in a large social network: longitudinal analysis over 20 years in the Framingham Heart Study. BMJ 337: a2338.

37. Honda H, Shimizu Y, Nitto Y, Imai M, Ozawa T, et al. (2009) Extraction and Refinement Strategy for detection of autism in 18-month-olds: a guarantee of higher sensitivity and specificity in the process of mass screening. J Child Psychol Psychiatry 50: 972–981.

38. Parner ET, Baron-Cohen S, Lauritsen MB, Jorgensen M, Schieve LA, et al. (2012) Parental age and autism spectrum disorders. Ann Epidemiol 22: 143–150.

39. Windham GC, Fessel K, Grether JK (2009) Autism spectrum disorders in relation to parental occupation in technical fields. Autism Res 2: 183–191.

## 15

Atypical Mismatch Negativity in Response to Emotional Voices in People with Autism Spectrum Conditions

Yang-Teng Fan[1], Yawei Cheng[1,2,3]*

1 Institute of Neuroscience and Brain Research Center, National Yang-Ming University, Taipei, Taiwan, **2** Department of Rehabilitation, National Yang-Ming University Hospital, Yilan, Taiwan, **3** Department of Research and Education, Taipei City Hospital, Taipei, Taiwan

Abstract

Autism Spectrum Conditions (ASC) are characterized by heterogeneous impairments of social reciprocity and sensory processing. Voices, similar to faces, convey socially relevant information. Whether voice processing is selectively impaired remains undetermined. This study involved recording mismatch negativity (MMN) while presenting emotionally spoken syllables *dada* and acoustically matched nonvocal sounds to 20 subjects with ASC and 20 healthy matched controls. The people with ASC exhibited no MMN response to emotional syllables and reduced MMN to nonvocal sounds, indicating general impairments of affective voice and acoustic discrimination. Weaker angry MMN amplitudes were associated with more autistic traits. Receiver operator characteristic analysis revealed that angry MMN amplitudes yielded a value of 0.88 ($p < .001$). The results suggest that people with ASC may process emotional voices in an atypical fashion already at the automatic stage. This processing abnormality can facilitate diagnosing ASC and enable social deficits in people with ASC to be predicted.

Editor: Piia Susanna Astikainen, University of Jyväskylä, Finland

Funding: The study was funded by the Ministry of Science and Technology (MOST 103-2401-H-010-003-MY3), National Yang-Ming University Hospital (RD2014-003), Health Department of Taipei City Government (10301-62-009), and Ministry of Education (Aim for the Top University Plan). The funders had no role in the study design, data collection and analyses, decision to publish, or preparation of the manuscript.

* Email: ywcheng2@ym.edu.tw

Introduction

In Autism Spectrum Conditions (ASC), abnormalities in social skills usually coexist with atypical sensory processing and aberrant attention. Social deficits are characterized by difficulty in understanding others' mental status, including the recognition of emotional expressions through voices [1,2]. Sensory dysfunction includes abnormalities in auditory processing, indicative of hyposensitivity or hypersensitivity to sounds [3,4]. Aberrant attention typically shifts orientation from social to nonsocial stimuli [5]. To comprehensively understand the pathophysiology of autism, determining whether voice processing is selectively impaired in people diagnosed with ASC and whether this impairment is associated with sensory dysfunction and attention abnormalities is necessary.

Previous studies have suggested that ASC causes difficulty in encoding and representing the sensory features of physically complex stimuli [6]. Such a deficit causes people with autism to have a disadvantage when processing social information, because affective facial and vocal expressions are multifaceted. However, ASC does not cause certain types of complex auditory inputs, such as music, loudness, and pitch discrimination, to be misperceived [7,8,9]. Furthermore, people with ASC are considered to exhibit a fragmented mental representation and lack causative association because of slow voluntary attention shifting [10,11]. A highly dynamic and interactive social realm should be highly susceptible to such impairments. However, studies on social-stimulus-specific deficits resulted from ASC have not distinguished sensory from attention processes nor have they evaluated the effects of physical stimulus complexity on their brain responses [5,12].

Voice communication, a part of social interaction, is critical for survival [13,14]. During the first few weeks following birth, infants can recognize the intonational characteristics of the languages spoken by their mothers [15,16]. Typically developing infants can discriminate affective prosodies at 5 months of age [17] and react to affective components in vocal tones by 6 months of age [18]. However, young children with ASC do not show a preference for their mother's voice to other auditory stimuli [12,19]. Adults with ASC exhibit difficulty in extracting mental state inferences from voices [1] and prosodies [20]. In a study of adults with ASC, the superior temporal sulcus, a voice-selective region, failed to activate in response to vocal sounds; however, the adults exhibited a normal activation pattern in response to nonvocal sounds [21]. Neurophysiological processing of emotional voices is atypical among people with ASC [22,23].

Regarding superior temporal resolution, electroencephalographic event-related brain potentials (ERPs) enable the distinct stages of sensory and attentional processing to be examined. Mismatch negativity (MMN), which is elicited by perceptibly distinct sounds (deviants) in a sequence of repetitive sounds (standards), can be used to investigate the neural representation underlying automatic central auditory perception [24,25]. Compared with standard stimuli, deviant stimuli evoke a more pronounced response at 100 to 250 ms and maximal amplitudes elicited over frontocentral regions [24]. The amplitude and latency of MMN indicate how effectively sound changes are discriminated from auditory background [26,27,28]. Recent studies have reported that MMN can be used as an index of the salience of emotional voice processing [29,30,31,32].

Previous MMN findings regarding ASC are mixed [33]. When children with ASC were exposed to pitch changes in previous studies, the MMN responses were early peak latencies, [34], strong amplitudes [35], weak amplitudes [36], and no abnormality [11,37,38]. MMN was preserved when children with ASC attended to stimuli, but decreased in unattending conditions [39]. When presented with frequency deviants in streams of synthesized vowels, children with high-functioning ASC yielded MMN amplitudes compatible with those of controls [10]. MMN was preserved in response to nonspeech sounds, but diminished in response to speech syllables [19]. When elicited by one-word utterances, MMN in response to the neutral syllable as the standard, compared with the commanding, sad, and scornful deviants, was diminished in adults with Asperger's syndrome [23], whereas MMN elicited by commanding relative to tender voices in boys with Asperger's syndrome yielded the opposite result [22]. These discrepant findings may be related to population characteristics, stimulus features, and task designs. In particular, the corresponding acoustic parameters have not been controlled to a degree.

P3a that follows MMN is an ERP index of attentional orienting [40]. If deviants are perceptually salient, then an involuntary attention switch is generated to elicit P3a responses [10]. In a previous study, people with ASC exhibited P3a amplitudes similar to those of people with mental retardation and controls when inattentively listening to pure tones [34,35]. Children with ASC exhibited P3a comparable to nonspeech sounds [41], but diminished responses to speech sounds [10,11,42]. Impaired attention orienting to speech-sound changes might affect social communication [10]. ASC cause speech-specific deficits in involuntary attention switching as well as normal orienting to nonspeech sounds.

To quantitatively control physical stimulus complexity, we presented meaningless emotionally spoken syllables, *dada*, and acoustically matched nonvocal sounds, representing the most and least complex stimuli, respectively, in a passive oddball paradigm, to people with ASC and matched controls. We hypothesized that people with ASC produce impaired MMN responses to emotional syllables and nonvocal sounds when general deficits in auditory processing are present. When the deficits are selective for voices, emotional syllables rather than nonvocal sounds diminish MMN responses among people with ASC. When involuntary attention orienting among people with ASC is speech-sound specific, P3a relevant to emotional syllables rather than nonvocal sounds would becomes atypical. In addition, to examine the relationship between electrophysiological responses and autistic traits, we conducted correlation analyses to determine the extent to which emotional MMN covaried with the Autism Spectrum Quotient (AQ) and receiver operating characteristic (ROC) analyses to evaluate the diagnostic utility of emotional MMN.

Materials and Methods

Participants

22 people with ASC and 21 matched controls participated in this study. Because of poor electroencephalogram (EEG) qualities, such as excessive eye movements and blink artifacts, 20 people

with ASC and 20 controls were included in the data analysis. The participants with ASC, aged between 18 and 29 years (21.5±3.8 y, one female participant), were recruited from a community autism program. We reconfirmed the diagnosis of Asperger's syndrome and high-functioning autism by using Diagnostic and Statistical Manual of Mental Disorders (DSM)-IV diagnostic criteria as well as the Autism Diagnostic Interview-Revised (ADI-R) [43]. The participants in the age-, gender-, intelligence quotient (IQ)-, and handedness-matched control group, aged between 18 and 29 years (22.0±3.7 y, one female participant), were recruited from the local community and screened for major psychiatric illness by conducting structured interviews. The participants did not participate in any intervention or drug programs during the experimental period. Participants with a comorbid psychiatric or medical condition, history of head injury, or genetic disorder associated with autism were excluded. All of the participants exhibited normal peripheral hearing bilaterally (pure tone average thresholds <15 dB HL) at the time of testing. All of the participants or parents of the participants provided written informed consent for this study, which was approved by the Ethics Committee of Yang-Ming University Hospital and conducted in accordance with the Declaration of Helsinki.

Auditory Stimuli

The stimulus materials were divided into two categories: emotional syllables and acoustically matched nonvocal sounds (Table S1 and Figure S1 in File S1). For emotional syllables, a female speaker from a performing arts school produced the meaningless syllables *dada* with three sets of emotional (neutral, angry, happy) prosodies. Within each set of emotional syllables, the speaker produced the syllables dada for more than ten times (see [29,30,31,32] for validation). Emotional syllables were edited to become equally long (550 ms) and loud (min: 57 dB; max: 62 dB; mean 59 dB) using Sound Forge 9.0 and Cool Edit Pro 2.0. Each set was rated for emotionality on a 5-point Likert-scale. Two emotional syllables that were consistently identified as 'extremely angry' ad 'extremely happy' and one neutral syllables rated as the most emotionless were selected as the stimuli. The Likert-scale (mean ± SD) of angry, happy, and neutral syllables were 4.26±0.85, 4.04±0.91, and 2.47±0.87, respectively.

To create a set of control stimuli that retained acoustic correspondence, we synthesized nonvocal sounds by using Praat [44] and MATLAB (The MathWorks, Inc., Natick, MA, USA). The fundamental frequencies (f0) of emotional (angry, happy, neutral) syllables were extracted to produce the nonvocal sounds using a sine waveform and then multiplied by the syllable envelope. In this way, nonvocal sounds retained the temporal and spectral features of emotional syllables. All of the stimuli were controlled with respect to their length (550 ms) and loudness (min: 57 dB; max: 62 dB; mean 59 dB).

Procedures

Before the EEG recordings were performed, each participant completed a self-administered questionnaire, the AQ, used for assessing autistic traits [45]. During the EEG recordings, participants were required to watch a silent movie with Chinese subtitles while task-irrelevant emotional syllables or nonvocal sounds in oddball sequences were presented. The passive oddball paradigm for emotional syllables involved employing happy and angry syllables as deviants and neutral syllables as standards. The corresponding nonvocal sounds were applied in the same paradigm but were presented as separate blocks. Each stimulus category comprised two blocks, the order of which was counterbalanced and randomized among the participants. Each block consisted of 600 trials, of which 80% were neutral syllables or tones, 10% were angry syllables or tones, and the remaining 10% were happy syllables or tones. The sequences of blocks and stimuli were quasirandomized such that the blocks of an identical stimulus category and the deviant stimuli were not presented successively. The stimulus-onset asynchrony was 1200 ms, including a stimulus length of 550 ms and an interstimulus interval of 650 ms.

Electroencephalography Apparatus and Recordings

The EEG was continually recorded at 32 scalp sites. Please refer to Supplementary Materials (File S1) for details. The number of accepted standard and deviant trials between groups did not differ significantly irrespective of emotional syllables (ASC – Neutral: 750±149, Happy: 81±15, Angry: 83±11; Controls – Neutral: 746±112, Happy: 85±11, Angry: 83±13) or nonvocal sounds (745±189, 78±15, 76±17; 781±170, 78±11, 80±10). The paradigm was edited using MATLAB. Each event in the paradigm was associated with a digital code that was transmitted to the continual EEG, enabling offline segmentation and averages of selected EEG periods to be obtained for analysis. The ERPs were processed and analyzed using Neuroscan 4.3 (Compumedics Ltd., Australia).

MMN source distributions were qualitatively explored using current source density (CSD) mapping (http://psychophysiology. cpmc.columbia.edu/software/CSDtoolbox/index.html). The CSD method, as a measure of the strength of extracellular current generators underlying the recorded EEG potentials [46], computes the surface Laplacian over the surface potentials implying the dipole sources oriented normal to local skull [31,47].

Statistical Analysis

The MMN and P3a amplitudes were analyzed as an average within a 100-ms time window surrounding the peak latency at the electrode sites, Fz, Cz, and Pz according to previous knowledge [31,32,48]. The MMN peak was defined as the highest negativity in the subtraction between the deviant and standard sound ERPs, during a period of 150 to 250 ms after sound onset. Only the standards before the deviants were included in the analysis. The P3a peak was defined as the highest positivity during a period of 300 to 450 ms.

Statistical analyses were conducted, separately for each category (emotional syllables or nonvocal sounds), using a mixed ANOVA with deviant type (angry, happy), and electrode (Fz, Cz, or Pz) as the within-subject factors, and the group (ASC vs. control) as the between-subject factor with additional *a priori* group by deviant type ANOVA contrasts calculated within each electrode site [49]. The dependent variables were the mean amplitudes and peak latencies of the MMN and P3a components. Cohen's d was calculated to estimate the effect size (i.e., the standardized difference between means). Degrees of freedom were corrected using the Greenhouse-Geisser method. Bonferroni testing was conducted when preceded only by significant main effects.

To determine whether electrophysiological responses were associated with the severity of autistic traits, we conducted Pearson correlation analyses between MMN amplitudes and AQ scores. To examine the degree to which the MMN and P3a amplitudes could be used to differentiate between the participants with ASC and the controls, we conducted ROC analyses, which can identify optimal thresholds in diagnostic decision making.

Results

Demographics and Dispositional Measures

Table 1 lists the demographics and clinical variables of the participants. The ASC group, compared with the control group, scored higher on the AQ [$t(34) = 5.08$, $p<.001$, Cohen's $d = 1.69$] as well as on the subscales of social skill, attention switch, communication and imagination.

Neurophysiological Measures

ERP amplitudes were subjected to an ANOVA in which the category (emotion syllables or nonvocal sounds), stimulus (happy, angry, or neutral), and electrode (Fz, Cz, or Pz) were repeated measure factors and the group (ASC vs. control) was the between-subject factor. The stimulus [$F(2, 76) = 69.31$, $p<.001$, $d = 2.71$] produced a main effect. The deviants elicited significantly stronger amplitudes than the standards did, regardless of whether they were emotional syllables or nonvocal sounds. In addition, significant interactions between the stimulus and group [$F(2, 76) = 8.08$, $p = .001$, $d = 0.92$], the category and stimulus [$F(2, 76) = 6.93$, $p = .002$, $d = 0.85$], the stimulus and electrode [$F(4, 152) = 21.49$, $p<.001$, $d = 1.50$], and the category, stimulus, and group [$F(2, 76) = 3.25$, $p = .044$, $d = 0.58$] were observed.

Emotional and Nonvocal Mismatch Negativity. Automatic discrimination of emotional voices was examined using MMN, which was determined by subtracting the neutral ERP from angry and happy ERPs (Table S2 in File S1). According to the ANOVA model of emotional MMN amplitudes, the group [$F(1, 38) = 6.69$, $p = .014$, $d = 0.84$], deviant type [$F(1, 38) = 21.03$, $p<.001$, $d = 1.49$], and electrode site [$F(2, 76) = 13.25$, $p<.001$, $d = 1.18$] produced main effects. Participants with ASC exhibited weaker emotional MMN than the controls did. MMN in response to angry syllables (angry MMN) yielded stronger amplitudes than did MMN in response to happy syllables (happy MMN). Fz and Cz exhibited more negative deflections than did Pz. In addition, an interaction between the deviant type and the group [$F(1, 38) = 15.13$, $p<.001$, $d = 1.26$] was observed (Figure 1A). A post hoc analysis revealed that angry MMN were stronger than did happy MMN among the controls ($p<.001$), whereas no such difference was observed among the participants with ASC ($p = .67$).

To determine whether the MMN amplitude effects elicited by angry versus happy deviants between subject groups stemmed from differences in acoustic features, an additional MMN analysis was conducted by subtracting the neutral-derived ERP from the angry- and happy-derived ERPs. The ANOVA model indicated that the group [$F(1, 38) = 4.38$, $p = .043$, $d = 0.68$], deviant type [$F(1, 38) = 52.22$, $p<.001$, $d = 2.35$], and electrode site [$F(2, 76) = 22.12$, $p<.001$, $d = 1.52$] produced main effects. The people with ASC exhibited weaker MMN responses to nonvocal sounds than did the controls. Regardless of the group, MMN induced by angry-derived sounds (angry-derived MMN) was stronger than that elicited by happy-derived sounds (happy-derived MMN). Fz and Cz exhibited more negative deflections than did Pz. In addition, an interaction was observed between the deviant type and the electrode site [$F(2, 76) = 11.08$, $p<.001$, $d = 1.08$] (Figure 1B). A post hoc analysis indicated that the topographical distribution of angry-derived MMN yielded the most negative deflections at Fz and the least negative deflections at Pz. The happy-derived MMN exhibited no differential topography. Unlike emotional syllables, no interaction between the deviant type and the group was observed among nonvocal sounds ($p = .65$).

The ANOVA on the peak latency of MMN revealed that, regardless of the group, MMN in response to angry deviants peaked significantly later than did MMN in response to happy

Table 1. Demographic and clinical variables of study participants.

	ASC (*N*=20)		Controls (*N*=20)		
	Mean	SD	Mean	SD	*p* value
Age (yrs)	21.5	3.8	22.0	3.7	.65
IQ (WAIS)	105	13.7	107	13.0	.61
AQ	29.4	5.6	21	4.8	<.001
Social skill	6.4	2.6	4.3	2.5	.013
Attention switch	6.9	1.6	5.7	1.5	.021
Attend to detail	5.8	1.9	5.1	2.0	.24
Communication	5.9	1.8	3.2	2.1	<.001
Imagination	4.4	1.5	2.5	1.8	.001

Abbreviations: IQ (WAIS), intelligence quotient assessed using the Wechsler Adult Intelligence Scale-Forth Edition (WAIS-IV) [68]; AQ, Autism Spectrum Quotient [45].

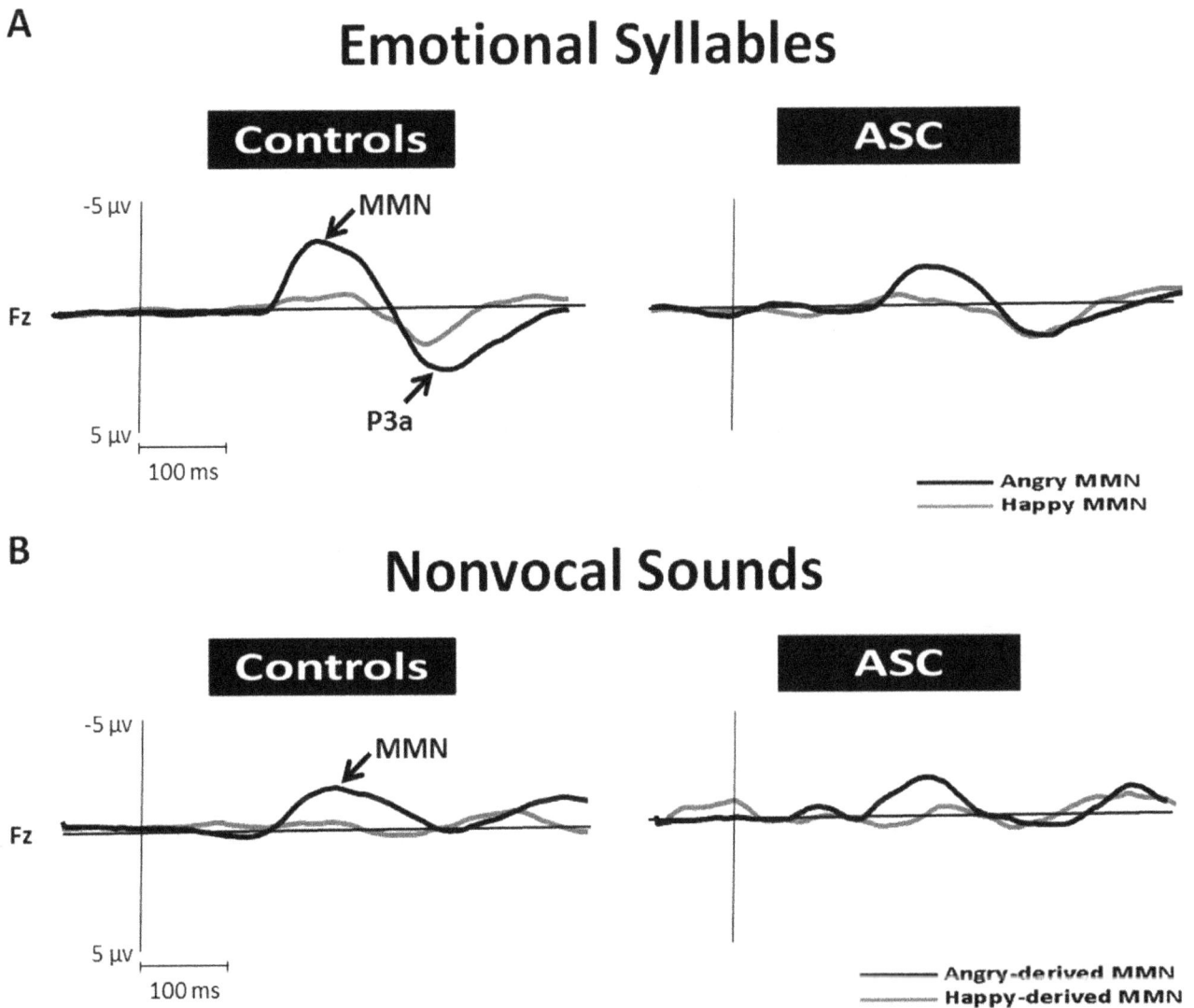

Figure 1. MMN amplitudes to emotional syllables and acoustically matched nonvocal sounds in people with ASC and controls at the electrode site Fz. MMN to angry deviants (black line) was significantly stronger in amplitude than MMN to happy deviants (gray line) in the controls (*p*<.001), whereas no differentiation was identified in people with ASC (*p* = .67). Nonvocal deviants that retained the acoustic features of emotional syllables were derived from angry (angry-derived) and happy (happy-derived) syllables. People with ASC exhibited weaker emotional-derived MMN than did the controls.

deviants [F (1, 38) = 13.38, p = .001, d = 1.19], but no such difference occurred in response to nonvocal deviants (p = .32). No significant MMN latency effect involving the group factor was observed in response to either emotional (p = .25) or nonvocal deviants (p = .55).

Emotional P3a. According to visual inspection, a P3a component was observed for only emotional syllables. The deviant type (angry or happy) and electrode site (Fz, Cz, or Pz) were the within-subject factors and the group (ASC vs. control) was the between-subject factor (Table S3 in File S1). The ANOVA revealed main effects in the deviant type [F (1, 38) = 13.49, p = .001, d = 1.19] and electrode site [F (2, 76) = 31.93, p<.001, d = 1.83]. P3a in response to angry syllables (angry P3a) yielded stronger amplitudes than did P3a in response to happy syllable (happy P3a). Fz exhibited the most positive deflections than did Cz and Pz. In addition, an interaction among the group, deviant type, and electrode site [F (2, 76) = 3.66, p = .029, d = 0.62]. A post hoc analysis revealed that angry P3a produced an interaction between the group and the electrode site [F (2, 76) = 3.89, p = .025, d = 0.64], but happy P3a did not (p = .96). People with ASC exhibited weaker angry P3a amplitudes than did the controls at Fz (p = .009). Figure 2 illustrates the ERP waveforms for standard and deviant responses.

Current Source Density Analyses. The scalp topographies for absolute voltages of MMN for emotional syllables and nonvocal sounds in both groups were consistent with the MMN amplitudes results (Figure 3A). The exploratory source distribution analyses based on CSDs indicated that MMN received a major contribution from the auditory cortex (Figure 3B). In the ASC group, there was a trend toward an additional posterior temporal source.

Correlation Among Mismatch Negativity and Autistic Traits. When the two groups were combined, lower amplitudes of angry MMN at Fz were coupled with higher total scores on the AQ [r (36) = 0.36, p = .03, d = 0.77] (Figure 4). However, such a correlation was not observed in either the ASC group or the control group. MMN induced by nonvocal sounds did not exhibit any correlation. Also, there was no age-related correlation.

Relationship Between Sensitivity and Specificity for Angry Mismatch Negativity. The area under the ROC curve (AUC) is indicative of the overall accuracy of the measurement, representing the probability that a randomly selected "true-positive" person scores higher according to the measure than a randomly selected "true-negative" person does. Separated ROC analyses for comparing the ASC participants with the controls were conducted for angry MMN, happy MMN, and angry-derived MMN, and happy-derived MMN. When determining optimal thresholds, we used Youden's index. This value corresponds with the point on the ROC curve farthest from the diagonal line. The diagonal line (sensitivity = 0.5 and specificity = 0.5) represents performance no better than chance. The ROC analysis of angry MMN yielded an AUC value of 0.88 (p<.001) (Figure 5). According to Youden's index, the most appropriate cutoff point for angry MMN amplitudes exhibiting a sensitivity of 95% and a specificity of 50% was −2.34 µV. By contrast, the AUC values of happy MMN, angry-derived MMN, and happy-derived MMN were not significant (p = .63; p = .14; p = .17).

Discussion

This study investigated whether people with ASC exhibit selective deficits during emotional voice processing. The results indicated that people with ASC failed to exhibit differentiation between angry MMN and happy MMN. By contrast, in response to acoustically matched nonvocal sounds, people with ASC differentiated angry-derived MMN from happy-derived MMN to a low degree. P3a specific to emotional voices was reduced in people with ASC, indicating atypically involuntary attention switching. The significant correlation between the MMN amplitudes elicited by angry syllables and the total scores on the AQ indicated that angry MMN amplitudes were associated with autistic traits. ROC analyses revealed that angry MMN amplitudes yielded an AUC value of 0.88 (p<.001) for diagnosing ASC.

People with ASC failed to exhibit negativity bias in responses to emotional voices. In a previous study involving the same paradigm, we determined that negativity bias to affective voice

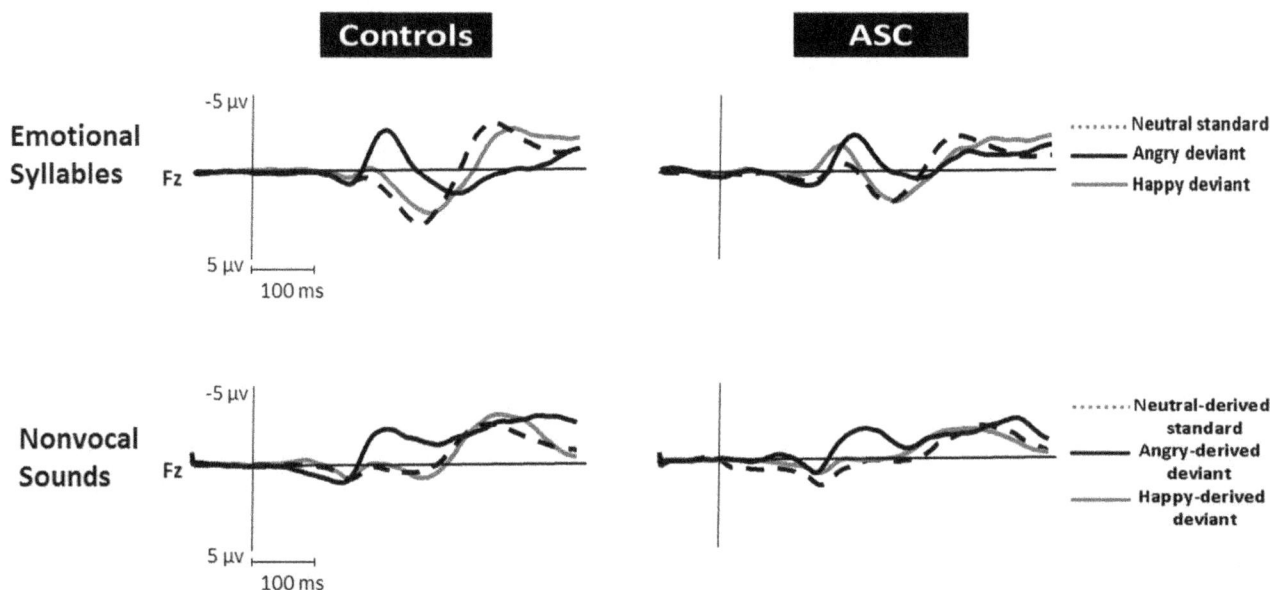

Figure 2. Grand average standard and deviant ERP waveforms for emotional syllables and acoustically matched nonvocal sounds in people with ASC and controls.

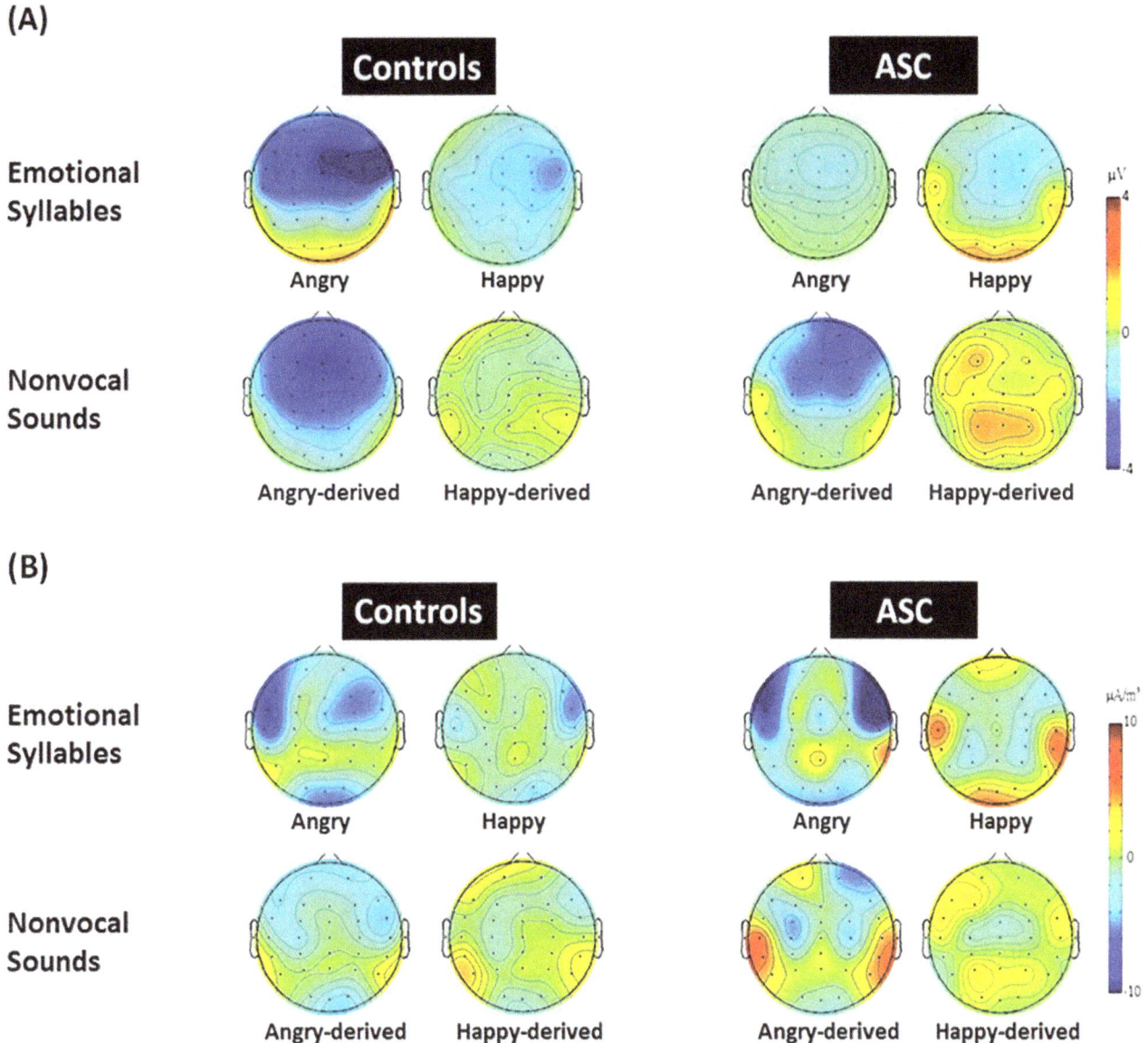

Figure 3. The MMN scalp potential distribution and the respective current source density (CSD) maps in people with ASC and controls. (A) A frontocentral minimum (or peak negativity) was similarly identified across the groups and categories. (B) The exploratory source distribution analyses on CSDs indicated that MMN received a major distribution from the bilateral auditory cortex. Additionally, for MMN to angry and angry-derived deviants, there was a trend toward a posterior temporal source in the ASC group.

emerges early in life [30]. Angry prosodies elicited a more negative-going ERP and stronger activation in the temporal voice area than did happy or neutral prosodies among infants [50]. Angry and fearful syllables evoked greater MMN than did happy or neutral syllables among adults and infants [30,51]. A recent visual MMN study determined that an early difference occurred during 70 ms to 120 ms after stimulus onset for only fearful deviants under unattended conditions [52]. From an evolutionary perspective, threat-related emotion processing (e.g., anger and fear) is particularly strong and indicates independence of attention [53]. Negativity bias in affective processing occurs as early as evaluative categorization into valence classes does [54]. In this study, the stronger amplitudes observed in angry MMN compared with happy MMN among the controls were obscured among the people with ASC.

The human voice not only contains speech information but can also carry a speaker's identity and emotional state [55]. One MMN study determined that the MMN amplitudes were higher in response to intensity change in vocal sounds than in response to intensity change in corresponding nonvocal sounds. Although vocal intensity deviants may call for sensory and attentional resources regardless of whether they are loud or soft, comparable resources are recruited for nonvocal intensity deviants only when they are loud [56]. Thus, emotional syllables are considered to be more complex than nonvocal sounds and beyond low-level acoustic features [29,30,31,32]. Because emotional MMN, instead of corresponding nonvocal sounds, exhibited a correlation with autistic traits and a positive predictive value for ASC, we speculated that low-level sensory deficits cannot be ascribed completely to social impairments in people with ASC.

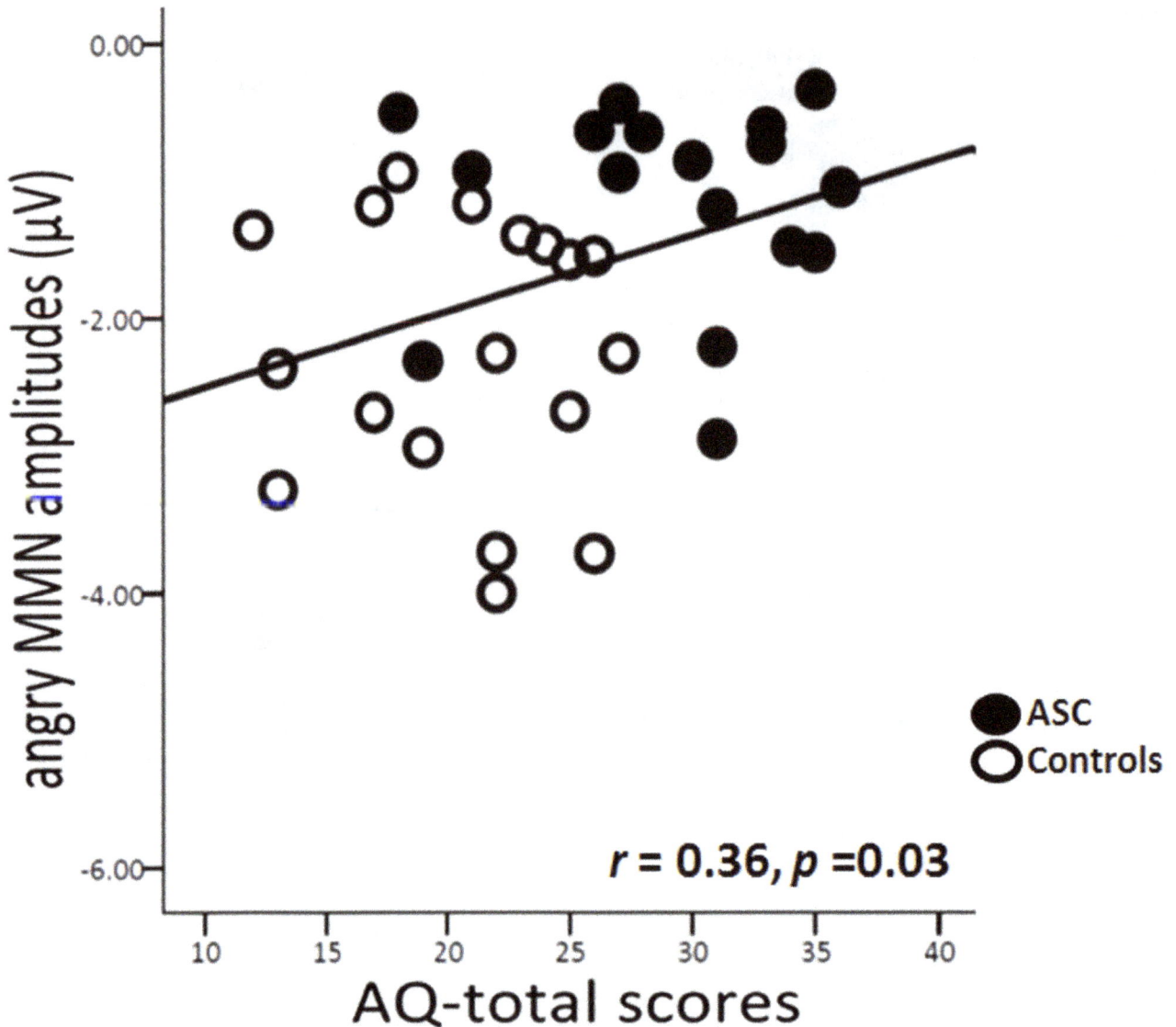

Figure 4. Correlation between angry MMN amplitudes and autistic traits.

In addition to lacking differentiation between angry and happy MMN, people with ASC exhibited reduced MMN in response to nonvocal sounds. The discrepancy between the results of this study and those of previous reports may be reflective of the heterogeneous characteristics of clinical participants, auditory stimuli, and task design [11,34,35]. For example, people with low-functioning autism might exhibit different MMN from those with high-functioning autism [35]. In one MMN study, basic acoustic features in the stimuli, specifically, emotional-neutral standards and emotional-laden deviants, were not controlled [23]. Furthermore, using one-word utterances or vowels as the auditory stimuli might cause variable familiarity or meaning, thus exerting potentially confounding effects on MMN responses [10,22].

Involuntary attention orienting to emotional voices was atypical in people with ASC, as indicated by diminished P3a amplitudes to angry syllables. P3a is reflective of the involuntary capture of attention to salient environmental events [57]. In a previous study, vowels compared with corresponding nonvocal sounds, produced stronger P3a [10]. The attention-eliciting effect may be particu-

larly pronounced when threat-related social information is involved [58]. We detected P3a for only emotional syllables, not for acoustically matched nonvocal sounds. Consistent with the results of previous studies [10,59,60,61], our results indicated weaker P3a to emotional syllables among people with ASC compared with controls, suggesting that attention orienting in people with ASC is more selectively impaired to social stimuli than to physical stimuli.

In consistent with previous MMN studies [31,62], our explorative CSD analyses suggested that the major contribution to deviance-standard difference responses comes from the bilateral auditory cortex. Furthermore, a slight trend toward to posterior enhancement observed in ASC for angry and angry-derived deviants could possibly reflect an additional posterior temporal source. The posterior lateral non-primary auditory cortex could be sensitive to emotion voices as indicated by functional neuroimaging [63]. However, given the known inaccuracies with EEG source localization, there CSD findings needs to be confirmed with more accurate source approaches.

Angry MMN Amplitudes

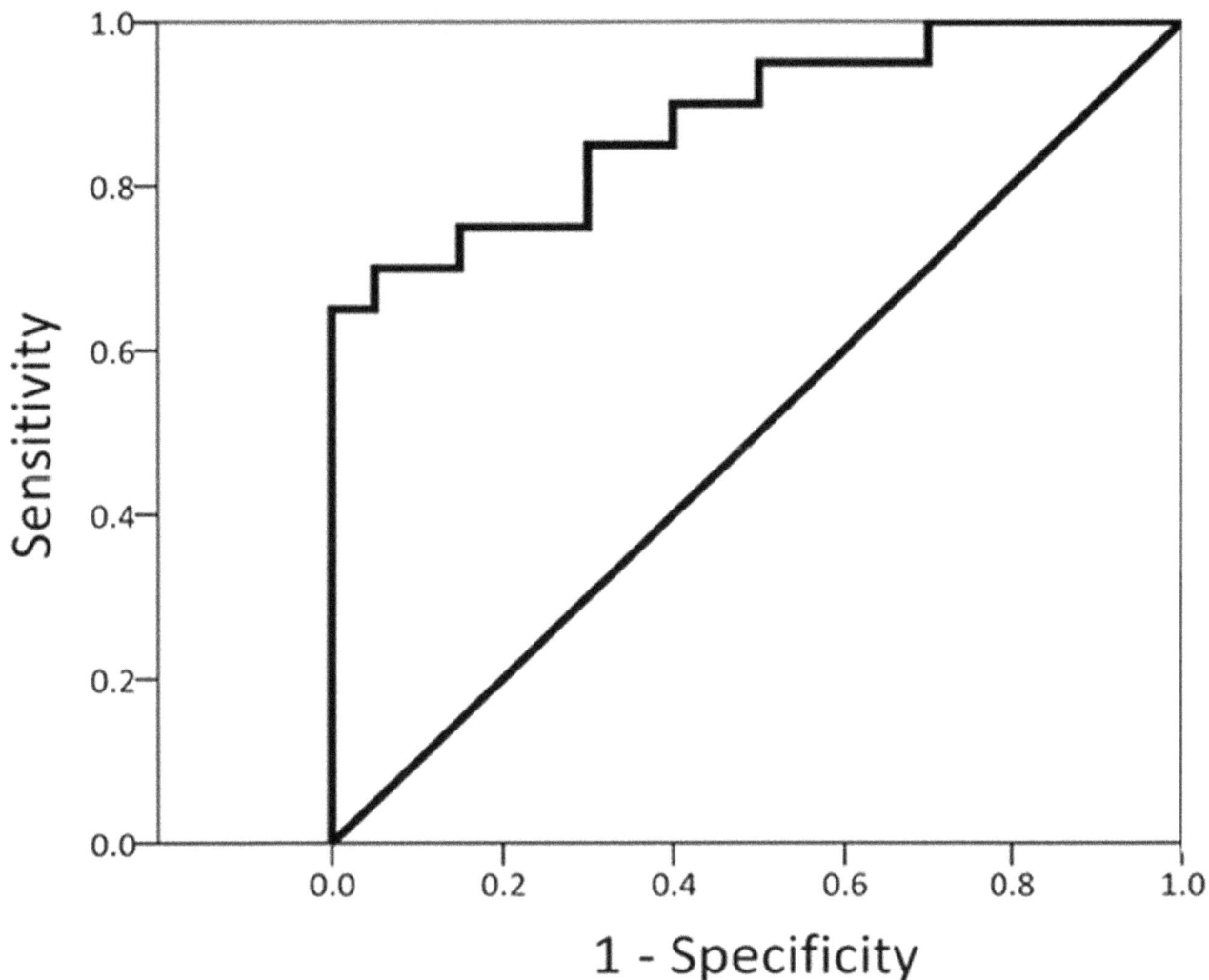

Figure 5. Receiver operator characteristic (ROC) analysis. The amplitude of angry MMN is suitable for predicting whether a person has a clinical diagnosis of ASC.

ROC analyses revealed that the amplitudes of angry MMN yielded a sensitivity of 95% and a specificity of 50% for diagnosing ASC. Strong amplitudes of angry MMN were coupled with low total scores on the AQ when the ASC and control groups were combined. MMN changes can be reliably observed in people with autism [34,64]. The AQ is a valuable instrument for rapidly determining where any given person is situated on the continuum from autism to normality [44]. AQ scores were determined to be associated with the ability to recognize mental state of others according to voices and eyes [65]. Thus, emotional MMM, particularly in response to angry syllables, is potentially useful as a neural marker for diagnosing autism.

Two limitations of this study must be acknowledged. First, regarding sample homogeneity, the generalizability of the results may be limited because people with low-functioning autism were not included. Second, stimuli that lack a quantitatively controlled function related to physical stimulus complexity, for instance, pure tones spectrally matching the fundamental frequency envelope of

emotional syllables [29,30,31,32], may limit the selectivity of emotional MMN. This may not be the optimal design, and future studies in which people with severe autism are recruited and a larger sample size and stimuli with greater acoustic correspondence are included are warranted.

Conclusions

This study revealed that ASC involves general impairments in affective voice discrimination as well as low-level acoustic distinction. In addition to reduced amplitudes of MMN in response to acoustically matched nonvocal sounds, people with ASC failed to differentiate between angry and happy syllables. Weak amplitudes of angry MMN were coupled with severe autistic traits. The ROC analysis revealed that the amplitude of angry MMN is suitable for predicting whether a person has a clinical diagnosis of ASC. The ability to determine the likelihood of an infant developing autism by using simple neurobiological measures would constitute a critical scientific breakthrough [66]. Considering the advantages of clinical population assessment [67] and the presence of emotional mismatch response in the human neonatal brain [30], future studies must examine the ability of emotional MMN to facilitate the early diagnosis of infants at risk for ASC.

Supporting Information

File S1 Electroencephalography apparatus and recordings, Figure S1, and Tables S1–S3. Figure S1. Acoustic properties of stimulus materials. **Table S1.** Physical and acoustic properties for the stimuli. **Table S2.** Mean amplitudes and peak latencies of MMN to emotional syllables and nonvocal sounds within a time window of 150 to 250 ms at predefined electrodes in each group (Mean ± SEM). **Table S3.** Mean amplitudes of P3a

to emotional syllables within a time window of 300 to 450 ms at predefined electrodes in each group (Mean ± SEM).

Acknowledgments

The authors deeply thank the participants and their parents who were included in the study.

Author Contributions

Conceived and designed the experiments: YC YTF. Performed the experiments: YTF. Analyzed the data: YTF YC. Contributed reagents/materials/analysis tools: YC. Contributed to the writing of the manuscript: YTF YC.

References

1. Rutherford MD, Baron-Cohen S, Wheelwright S (2002) Reading the mind in the voice: a study with normal adults and adults with Asperger syndrome and high functioning autism. J Autism Dev Disord 32: 189–194.

2. Hobson RP, Ouston J, Lee A (1989) Naming emotion in faces and voices: abilities and disabilities in autism and mental retardation. Brit J Dev Psychol 7: 237–250.

3. Mottron L (2011) Changing perceptions: The power of autism. Nature 479: 33–35.

4. Baron-Cohen S, Ashwin E, Ashwin C, Tavassoli T, Chakrabarti B (2009) Talent in autism: hyper-systemizing, hyper-attention to detail and sensory hypersensitivity. Philos Trans R Soc Lond B Biol Sci 364: 1377–1383.

5. Dawson G, Meltzoff AN, Osterling J, Rinaldi J, Brown E (1998) Children with autism fail to orient to naturally occurring social stimuli. J Autism Dev Disord 28: 479–485.

6. Dawson G, Lewy A (1989) Autism: Nature, Diagnosis, and Treatment; Dawson G, editor. New York: Guilford.

7. Mottron L, Peretz I, Menard E (2000) Local and global processing of music in high-functioning persons with autism: beyond central coherence? J Child Psychol Psychiatry 41: 1057–1065.

8. Jarvinen-Pasley A, Wallace GL, Ramus F, Happe F, Heaton P (2008) Enhanced perceptual processing of speech in autism. Dev Sci 11: 109–121.

9. Khalfa S, Bruneau N, Roge B, Georgieff N, Veuillet E, et al. (2004) Increased perception of loudness in autism. Hear Res 198: 87–92.

10. Čeponienė R, Lepistö T, Shestakova A, Vanhala R, Alku P, et al. (2003) Speech-sound-selective auditory impairment in children with autism: they can perceive but do not attend. Proc Natl Acad Sci USA 100: 5567–5572.

11. Lepistö T, Silokallio S, Nieminen-von Wendt T, Alku P, Naatanen R, et al. (2006) Auditory perception and attention as reflected by the brain event-related potentials in children with Asperger syndrome. Clin Neurophysiol 117: 2161–2171.

12. Klin A (1991) Young autistic children's listening preferences in regard to speech: a possible characterization of the symptom of social withdrawal. J Autism Dev Disord 21: 29–42.

13. Belin P, Grosbras MH (2010) Before speech: Cerebral voice processing in infants. Neuron 65: 733–735.

14. Grossmann T, Friederici AD (2012) When during development do our brains get tuned to the human voice? Soc Neurosci 7: 369–372.

15. Mehler J, Jusczyk P, Lambertz G, Halsted N, Bertoncini J, et al. (1988) A precursor of language acquisition in young infants. Cognition 29: 143–178.

16. Vouloumanos A, Werker JF (2007) Listening to language at birth: evidence for a bias for speech in neonates. Dev Sci 10: 159–164.

17. Flom R, Bahrick LE (2007) The development of infant discrimination of affect in multimodal and unimodal stimulation: The role of intersensory redundancy. Dev Psychol 43: 238–252.

18. Locke J (1993) The child's path to spoken language. Cambridge, MA: Harvard University Press.

19. Kuhl PK, Coffey-Corina S, Padden D, Dawson G (2005) Links between social and linguistic processing of speech in preschool children with autism: behavioral and electrophysiological measures. Dev Sci 8: F1–F12.

20. Paul R, Augustyn A, Klin A, Volkmar FR (2005) Perception and production of prosody by speakers with autism spectrum disorders. J Autism Dev Disord 35: 205–220.

21. Gervais H, Belin P, Boddaert N, Leboyer M, Coez A, et al. (2004) Abnormal cortical voice processing in autism. Nat Neurosci 7: 801–802.

22. Korpilahti P, Jansson-Verkasalo E, Mattila ML, Kuusikko S, Suominen K, et al. (2007) Processing of affective speech prosody is impaired in Asperger syndrome. J Autism Dev Disord 37: 1539–1549.

23. Kujala T, Lepistö T, Nieminen-von Wendt T, Näätänen P, Näätänen R (2005) Neurophysiological evidence for cortical discrimination impairment of prosody in Asperger syndrome. Neurosci Lett 383: 260–265.

24. Näätänen R, Paavilainen P, Rinne T, Alho K (2007) The mismatch negativity (MMN) in basic research of central auditory processing: a review. Clin Neurophysiol 118: 2544–2590.

25. Sussman ES, Chen S, Sussman-Fort J, Dinces E (2013) The Five Myths of MMN: Redefining How to Use MMN in Basic and Clinical Research. Brain Topogr.

26. Novitski N, Tervaniemi M, Huotilainen M, Näätänen R (2004) Frequency discrimination at different frequency levels as indexed by electrophysiological and behavioral measures. Brain Res Cogn Brain Res 20: 26–36.

27. Amenedo E, Escera C (2000) The accuracy of sound duration representation in the human brain determines the accuracy of behavioural perception. Eur J Neurosci 12: 2570–2574.

28. Kujala T, Kallio J, Tervaniemi M, Näätänen R (2001) The mismatch negativity as an index of temporal processing in audition. Clin Neurophysiol 112: 1712–1719.

29. Fan YT, Hsu YY, Cheng Y (2013) Sex matters: n-back modulates emotional mismatch negativity. Neuroreport 24: 457–463.

30. Cheng Y, Lee SY, Chen HY, Wang PY, Decety J (2012) Voice and emotion processing in the human neonatal brain. J Cogn Neurosci 24: 1411–1419.

31. Hung AY, Ahveninen J, Cheng Y (2013) Atypical mismatch negativity to distressful voices associated with conduct disorder symptoms. J Child Psychol Psychiatry 54: 1016–1027.

32. Hung AY, Cheng Y (2014) Sex differences in preattentive perception of emotional voices and acoustic attributes. Neuroreport 25: 464–469.

33. O'Connor K (2012) Auditory processing in autism spectrum disorder: a review. Neurosci Biobehav Rev 36: 836–854.

34. Gomot M, Giard MH, Adrien JL, Barthelemy C, Bruneau N (2002) Hypersensitivity to acoustic change in children with autism: electrophysiological evidence of left frontal cortex dysfunctioning. Psychophysiology 39: 577–584.

35. Ferri R, Elia M, Agarwal N, Lanuzza B, Musumeci SA, et al. (2003) The mismatch negativity and the P3a components of the auditory event-related potentials in autistic low-functioning subjects. Clin Neurophysiol 114: 1671–1680.

36. Seri S, Cerquiglini A, Pisani F, Curatolo P (1999) Autism in tuberous sclerosis: evoked potential evidence for a deficit in auditory sensory processing. Clin Neurophysiol 110: 1825–1830.

37. Kemner C, Verbaten MN, Cuperus JM, Camfferman G, van Engeland H (1995) Auditory event-related brain potentials in autistic children and three different control groups. Biol Psychiatry 38: 150–165.

38. Jansson-Verkasalo E, Čeponienė R, Kielinen M, Suominen K, Jäntti V, et al. (2003) Deficient auditory processing in children with Asperger Syndrome, as indexed by event-related potentials. Neurosci Lett 338: 197–200.

39. Dunn MA, Gomes H, Gravel J (2008) Mismatch negativity in children with autism and typical development. J Autism Dev Disord 38: 52–71.

40. Escera C, Alho K, Schröger E, Winkler I (2000) Involuntary attention and distractibility as evaluated with event-related brain potentials. Audiol Neurootol 5: 151–166.

41. Lincoln AJ, Courchesne E, Harms L, Allen M (1993) Contextual probability evaluation in autistic, receptive developmental language disorder, and control children: event-related brain potential evidence. J Autism Dev Disord 23: 37–58.

42. Lepistö T, Kajander M, Vanhala R, Alku P, Huotilainen M, et al. (2008) The perception of invariant speech features in children with autism. Biol Psychol 77: 25–31.

43. Lord C, Rutter M, Le Couteur A (1994) Autism Diagnostic Interview-Revised: a revised version of a diagnostic interview for caregivers of individuals with possible pervasive developmental disorders. J Autism Dev Disord 24: 659–685.

44. Boersma P (2001) Praat, a system for doing phonetics by computer. Glot International 5: 341–345.

45. Baron-Cohen S, Wheelwright S, Skinner R, Martin J, Clubley E (2001) The Autism-Spectrum Quotient (AQ): Evidence from Asperger Syndrome/High-Functioning Autism, Malesand Females, Scientists and Mathematicians. J Autism Dev Disord 31: 5–17.

46. Nicholson C (1973) Theoretical analysis of field potentials in anisotropic ensembles of neuronal elements. IEEE Trans Biomed Eng 20: 278–288.

47. Giard MH, Perrin F, Pernier J, Bouchet P (1990) Brain generators implicated in the processing of auditory stimulus deviance: a topographic event-related potential study. Psychophysiology 27: 627–640.

48. Duncan CC, Barry RJ, Connolly JF, Fischer C, Michie PT, et al. (2009) Event-related potentials in clinical research: guidelines for eliciting, recording, and quantifying mismatch negativity, P300, and N400. Clin Neurophysiol 120: 1883–1908.

49. Winer B, Brown D, Michels K (1991) Statistical Principles in Experimental Design.; McGrawhill, editor. New York.

50. Grossmann T, Oberecker R, Koch SP, Friederici AD (2010) The developmental origins of voice processing in the human brain. Neuron 65: 852–858.

51. Schirmer A, Escoffier N, Zysset S, Koester D, Striano T, et al. (2008) When vocal processing gets emotional: on the role of social orientation in relevance detection by the human amygdala. Neuroimage 40: 1402–1410.

52. Stefanics G, Csukly G, Komlosi S, Czobor P, Czigler I (2012) Processing of unattended facial emotions: A visual mismatch negativity study. Neuroimage 59: 3042–3049.

53. Vuilleumier P (2005) How brains beware: neural mechanisms of emotional attention. Trends Cogn Sci 9: 585–594.

54. Ito TA, Larsen JT, Smith NK, Cacioppo JT (1998) Negative information weighs more heavily on the brain: the negativity bias in evaluative categorizations. J Pers Soc Psychol 75: 887–900.

55. Belin P, Fecteau S, Bedard C (2004) Thinking the voice: neural correlates of voice perception. Trends Cogn Sci 8: 129–135.

56. Schirmer A, Simpson E, Escoffier N (2007) Listen up! Processing of intensity change differs for vocal and nonvocal sounds. Brain Res 1176: 103–112.

57. Escera C, Alho K, Schroger E, Winkler I (2000) Involuntary attention and distractibility as evaluated with event-related brain potentials. Audiol Neurootol 5: 151–166.

58. Pratto F, John OP (1991) Automatic vigilance: the attention-grabbing power of negative social information. J Pers Soc Psychol 61: 380–391.

59. Lepistö T, Kujala T, Vanhala R, Alku P, Huotilainen M, et al. (2005) The discrimination of and orienting to speech and non-speech sounds in children with autism. Brain Res 1066: 147–157.

60. Maestro S, Muratori F, Cavallaro MC, Pei F, Stern D, et al. (2002) Attentional skills during the first 6 months of age in autism spectrum disorder. J Am Acad Child Adolesc Psychiatry 41: 1239–1245.

61. Dawson G, Toth K, Abbott R, Osterling J, Munson J, et al. (2004) Early social attention impairments in autism: social orienting, joint attention, and attention to distress. Dev Psychol 40: 271–283.

62. Folstein JR, Van Petten C (2008) Influence of cognitive control and mismatch on the N2 component of the ERP: a review. Psychophysiology 45: 152–170.

63. Ethofer T, Bretscher J, Gschwind M, Kreifelts B, Wildgruber D, et al. (2012) Emotional voice areas: anatomic location, functional properties, and structural connections revealed by combined fMRI/DTI. Cereb Cortex 22: 191–200.

64. Roberts TP, Cannon KM, Tavabi K, Blaskey L, Khan SY, et al. (2011) Auditory magnetic mismatch field latency: a biomarker for language impairment in autism. Biol Psychiatry 70: 263–269.

65. Golan O, Baron-Cohen S, Hill JJ, Rutherford MD (2007) The 'Reading the Mind in the Voice' test-revised: a study of complex emotion recognition in adults with and without autism spectrum conditions. J Autism Dev Disord 37: 1096–1106.

66. Griffin R, Westbury C (2011) Infant EEG activity as a biomarker for autism: a promising approach or a false promise? BMC Med 9: 61.

67. Light GA, Braff DL (2005) Stability of mismatch negativity deficits and their relationship to functional impairments in chronic schizophrenia. Am J Psychiatry 162: 1741–1743.

68. Wechsler D (2008) Wechsler Adult Intelligence Scale-Fourth Edition. San Antonia, TX: Pearson.

## 16

Attenuation of Typical Sex Differences in 800 Adults with Autism vs. 3,900 Controls

Simon Baron-Cohen[1,2]*, Sarah Cassidy[1], Bonnie Auyeung[1,3], Carrie Allison[1], Maryam Achoukhi[1], Sarah Robertson[1], Alexa Pohl[1], Meng-Chuan Lai[1,2,4]*

1 Autism Research Centre, Department of Psychiatry, University of Cambridge, Cambridge, United Kingdom, 2 Cambridge Lifespan Asperger Syndrome Service (CLASS) Clinic, Cambridgeshire and Peterborough National Health Service Foundation Trust, Cambridge, United Kingdom, 3 Department of Psychology, University of Edinburgh, Edinburgh, United Kingdom, 4 Department of Psychiatry, National Taiwan University Hospital and College of Medicine, Taipei, Taiwan

Abstract

Sex differences have been reported in autistic traits and systemizing (male advantage), and empathizing (female advantage) among typically developing individuals. In individuals with autism, these cognitive-behavioural profiles correspond to predictions from the "extreme male brain" (EMB) theory of autism (extreme scores on autistic traits and systemizing, below average on empathizing). Sex differences within autism, however, have been under-investigated. Here we show in 811 adults (454 females) with autism and 3,906 age-matched typical control adults (2,562 females) who completed the Empathy Quotient (EQ), the Systemizing Quotient-Revised (SQ-R), and the Autism Spectrum Quotient (AQ), that typical females on average scored higher on the EQ, typical males scored higher on the SQ-R and AQ, and both males and females with autism showed a shift toward the extreme of the "male profile" on these measures and in the distribution of "brain types" (the discrepancy between standardized EQ and SQ-R scores). Further, normative sex differences are attenuated but not abolished in adults with autism. The findings provide strong support for the EMB theory of autism, and highlight differences between males and females with autism.

Editor: Valerie W. Hu, The George Washington University, United States of America

Funding: This study received funding from the UK Medical Research Council, the Wellcome Trust, and the Autism Research Trust. Meng-Chuan Lai was supported by the William Binks Autism Neuroscience Fellowship, the European Autism Interventions - A Multicentre Study for Developing New Medications (EU-AIMS), and Wolfson College, Cambridge. The funders had no role in study design, data collection and analysis, decision to publish, or preparation of the manuscript.

Competing Interests: The authors have declared that no competing interests exist.

* Email: sb205@cam.ac.uk (SBC); mcl45@cam.ac.uk (M-CL)

Introduction

Typical males on average score higher on measures of autistic traits (i.e., the individual features that comprise the quantitative variation in domains of cognition and behaviour associated with autism) [1] than do typical females [2–5]. In addition, the sex ratio of the prevalence for autism spectrum conditions (henceforth 'autism') is male-biased [6]. The *extreme male brain* (EMB) theory of autism explains these two findings by positing that there are typical male and female cognitive profiles ('brain types') in the general population, in two domains: empathizing (the drive and ability to identify a person's thoughts and feelings, and to respond to these with an appropriate emotion) [7] and systemizing (the drive and ability to analyse or build systems) [8]. Typical females, on average, exhibit more empathizing and less systemizing compared to typical males, and people with autism show an extreme of this 'male profile' [9,10].

One unresolved issue is whether normative sex differences in this cognitive profile in the general population are also observed in autism. This is important for identifying sex-specific autism phenotypes [11], understanding the biological basis of these phenotypes [12,13], and deepening our understanding of females with autism [9]. The few studies investigating cognitive and behavioural sex differences within autism show inconsistent results: some studies have found no significant sex differences in autism [14,15], whilst other studies have found some sex differences, on a

mixed set of measures [16–21]. For example, a meta-analysis (based on smaller-scale studies) [22] and large-scale studies [20,23] indicate that females show fewer repetitive, restricted behaviours and interests. Cognitively, most differences between males and females with autism (when compared respectively to neurotypical males and females) are observed in executive functions and visuospatial processing, whereas they tend to share similar levels of social-emotional cognitive difficulties [18,19,24]. It is unclear what the relevance of these is to the EMB theory as normative sex differences were not always tested, and these tasks may not load on to empathizing or systemizing. One study found females with autism had slightly but significantly higher scores on the Autism Spectrum Quotient (AQ) via self-report, even though they scored lower than males with autism on the Autism Diagnostic Observation Schedule (ADOS) [21]. This suggests they may have developed strategies to better 'camouflage' their social-communication difficulties. Overall, it remains unclear if autism abolishes or simply attenuates normative sex differences.

Most previous studies also suffer from relatively small sample sizes. An exception is the largest study to date using the Simons Simplex Collection, comparing autism symptoms in 304 female and 2,114 male children with 'simplex' autism, aged 4–18 years [25]. This study found that, compared to males, females have somewhat greater social communication impairments, fewer restricted interests (but not fewer repetitive behaviours and stereotypies), poorer adaptive skills, and higher level of externalizing problems. There is, however, no study with a comparative sample size in adults with autism. In many of the above studies there is a relative under-representation of females with autism, especially those with average or above-average intelligence [22]. Small and sex-unbalanced sample sizes may affect the statistical power to detect sex differences with small or medium effect sizes [26]. In addition, comparing studies testing very young children [17] with others including a broad age range [16] may obscure sex differences due to developmental changes. Furthermore, sex differences within autism may vary with IQ, and whilst some studies have matched for age and IQ, others have not. Previous studies have also varied in whether measures were retrospective parent-reports [16] or direct observation [17], and this could produce discrepant results [27,28].

To overcome these confounds, and to test the EMB theory directly, Lai et al. tested 33 male and 29 female adults with high-functioning autism or Asperger syndrome, matched for age and IQ, and found no sex differences on the EQ or SQ-R [21]. This suggests that normative sex differences on these measures are abolished in autism [7,8]. Wheelwright et al. investigated 69 males and 56 females with high functioning autism or Asperger syndrome, and also found typical sex differences on self-report scores of EQ or SQ-R were abolished in autism [29]. Auyeung et al. studied 46 girls and 219 boys with autism, and they too confirmed that typical sex differences in parent-reported empathizing and systemizing were abolished in autism [30]. These findings from studies of empathizing and systemizing are consistent with the EMB theory of autism [10].

In the present study, we attempt to overcome the issue of statistical power by investigating sex differences in the largest, and importantly, most sex-balanced sample in adults to date: over 800 individuals with autism. Again we focus on empathizing and systemizing because these have given the clearest results to date, both in terms of normative sex differences, and the predicted attenuation or absence of these sex differences in autism, based on the EMB theory. We selected individuals over 18 years of age since dispositional traits of empathy and systemizing, such as aspects of personality, are likely to be stabilized by adulthood. In addition, all individuals were high-functioning, so that sex differences could be investigated independent of learning disability. We used online self-report questionnaires to gather a very large sample, which increased statistical power in detecting sex differences, even if these were attenuated in autism.

Method

Participants

Participants were recruited online. After exclusions (see below), the autism group comprised 811 individuals (454 females, 357 males) who completed questionnaires at one of two websites (www.autismresearchcentre.com or www.cambridgepsychology.com) and reported having a formal clinical diagnosis of an autism spectrum condition. Diagnoses comprised Asperger Syndrome ($n = 506$), High Functioning Autism ($n = 41$), Autism ($n = 11$), Pervasive Developmental Disorder ($n = 15$), and Autism Spectrum Condition (participants who did not specify a subtype) ($n = 238$).

After exclusions (see below), the typical control group comprised 3,906 individuals (2,562 females, 1,344 males), who completed questionnaires and who reported they had no diagnosis of an autism spectrum condition, via www.cambridgepsychology.com. Anyone from this group who reported having a child or other family members with autism was excluded from the control group, to avoid inadvertently including those with the 'broader autism

phenotype' [31]. Individuals with a diagnosis of bipolar disorder, epilepsy, schizophrenia, attention-deficit/hyperactivity disorder (ADHD), obsessive-compulsive disorder (OCD), learning disability (LD), an intersex/transsexual condition, or psychosis were excluded from both groups. Outliers, defined as having a z-score of 3.29 or greater on each measure, were also excluded.

Participants were aged between 18 and 75 years old (see Table 1) and those in the autism group did not differ in age from the control group ($F(1, 4713) = .21$, $p = .63$). A majority of the individuals in the autism group provided information on type of education (mainstream, home, special) ($n = 769$), and of these individuals a majority reported having attended mainstream school ($n = 679$; 88.3%). A majority of the autism group also provided information on current occupation ($n = 676$), and of these a majority ($n = 471$; 69.7%) were currently employed, 115 (17%) individuals were in full time study, and 90 (13.3%) individuals were unemployed. In the control group, 1,709 individuals provided information on their education type, and of these 1,679 (98.2%) individuals reported having mainstream education. In total 2,648 control individuals provided information on their occupation, and of these 2,184 (82.5%) were currently employed, 424 (16%) were in full time study and 40 (1.5%) were unemployed.

Ethical Approval

Ethical approval was from the Psychology Research Ethics Committee (PREC), University of Cambridge, UK. There is no reason to question if adults with Asperger Syndrome (AS) or High-Functioning Autism (HFA) can give informed consent since by definition they have at least average, if not above-average IQ, and have normal intellectual competence. Consent was obtained online when participants registered to join the research database and where they had the opportunity to read the Terms and Conditions, which included how their data will be used for research and how their personal information is only seen by named database managers who take legal responsibility for data protection. This data covers both their questionnaire data but also performance data each participant provides, and their willingness to be re-contacted to hear about new studies. This consent procedure was approved by PREC as well.

Measures

We used the following four measures: (1) The Empathy Quotient (EQ) quantifies individual differences in empathizing [7]. (2) The Systemizing Quotient-Revised (SQ-R) [29] measures individual differences in systemizing [8]. (3) The Autism Spectrum Quotient (AQ) measures the degree to which an adult with an average or above-average IQ has autistic traits [2]. (4) D score/ 'Brain Type' is a measure of the standardized difference between an individual's empathizing and systemizing scores [30,32]. The raw SQ-R and EQ scores are standardized by subtracting the typical population mean (denoted by $<...>$) from the participant's score and then dividing this by the maximum possible score ($S = (SQ\text{-}R - <SQ\text{-}R>)/150$ and $E = (EQ - <EQ>)/80$). The control group means are used as estimations of the typical population means in this standardization procedure: EQ (*mean* $= 44.87$, *SD* $= 14.58$) and SQ-R (*mean* $= 59.66$, *SD* $= 22.15$). The difference (D) between the standardized EQ and SQ-R scores is then calculated by: $D = (S-E)/2$. Using the D score, individuals can be classed into one of five cognitive profiles, or 'brain types'. 'Brain types' based on D score are quantitatively defined in Table 2, based on a prior study [32] which classed the lowest and highest 2.5th percentiles of scores in a large population-based typically developing group as 'Extreme Type E' (E>>S) and 'Extreme Type S' (S>>E) respectively. Those scoring between the 2.5th and

Table 1. Mean scores for each measure (with standard deviations, SDs).

Group	Sex		Age	AQ	EQ	SQ-R	D
Autism	Female	Mean	34.5	32.9	26.4	71.7	0.15
		SD	13.1	11.5	17.2	25.7	0.17
		n	454	454	419	397	397
	Male	Mean	34.9	34.8	20.4	78.4	0.22
		SD	13.3	9.1	12.4	24.3	0.12
		n	357	357	307	295	295
Control	Female	Mean	34.4	17.1	48.5	55.1	−0.04
		SD	12.5	7.6	13.7	21.1	0.12
		n	2562	2562	2376	2261	2261
	Male	Mean	34.4	20.3	38	68.1	0.07
		SD	14.3	7.8	13.7	21.6	0.11
		n	1344	1344	1253	1197	1197

35th percentiles are classed as 'Type E' (E>S), those between the 35th and 65th percentile as 'Type B' (balanced, E≈S), and those between the 65th and 97.5^{th} percentile as 'Type S' (S>E).

Statistical Analysis

Large samples increase the robustness of ANOVA to violation of normality and homogeneity of variance. Separate two-way ANOVAs were conducted on AQ, EQ, SQ-R and D, with two between-subject factors of 'Diagnosis' (autism vs. control) and 'Sex' (female vs. male). Sex-by-diagnosis interaction effects indicate whether the effect of sex is dependent on the diagnostic status. Significant interaction effects are followed up by simple main effects analysis to establish whether significant sex differences exist in each diagnostic group and to reveal whether the interaction is ordinal or disordinal. Effect sizes were calculated using omega (ω) for main effects and interactions and Cohen's d for focused comparisons (simple main effects). For calculation of omega, the harmonic mean sample size (the average sample size) is used to correct for unequal sample size between groups. Omega has the same benchmarks for effect size as r: $0.1 =$ small effect, $0.3 =$ medium effect and $0.5 =$ large effect. As for Cohen's d: $0.2 =$ small effect, $0.5 =$ medium effect and $>0.8 =$ large effect.

Results

Table 1 shows the mean scores for AQ, EQ, SQ-R and D for males and females in the autism and control groups. Figures 1–3 show the distribution of scores for AQ, EQ and SQ-R in the control and autism male and female groups.

AQ

An ANOVA revealed significant main effects of Diagnosis ($F(1, 4713) = 2207$, $p<.001$, $\omega = .67$) and Sex ($F(1, 4713) = 63$, $p<.001$, $\omega = .11$). AQ scores were higher in the autism group than the control group, and higher in males than females. There was a significant ordinal interaction between Sex and Diagnosis ($F(1, 4713) = 3.94$, $p = .047$, $\omega = .02$), reflecting that sex differences were smaller in the autism than the control groups. Simple main effect analysis showed that typical males scored significantly higher than typical females ($F(1, 4713) = 133$, $p<.001$, $d = .41$), and males with autism scored significantly higher than females with autism, though with a small effect size ($F(1, 4713) = 10.87$, $p<.001$, $d = .18$). This indicates that normative sex differences were attenuated, but not absent in the autism group.

EQ

An ANOVA revealed significant main effects of Diagnosis ($F(1, 4351) = 1171.5$, $p<.001$, $\omega = .56$) and Sex ($F(1, 4351) = 202.6$, $p<.001$, $\omega = .23$). EQ scores were lower in the autism group than the control group, and higher in females than males. There was also a significant ordinal interaction between Sex and Diagnosis ($F(1, 4351) = 14$, $p<.001$, $\omega = .06$), again reflecting that sex differences were smaller in the autism than the control groups. Simple main effect analysis showed that typical females scored significantly higher than typical males ($F(1, 4351) = 455$, $p<.001$, $d = .76$), and females with autism scored significantly higher than males with autism, though with a relatively smaller effect size ($F(1, 4351) = 33.4$, $p<001$, $d = .40$). This also indicates that normative sex differences were attenuated, but not absent in the autism group.

SQ-R

An ANOVA revealed significant main effects of Diagnosis ($F(1, 4146) = 206.87$, $p<.001$, $\omega = .28$) and Sex ($F(1, 4146) = 11.97$, $p<$

Table 2. Brain type boundaries based on the D score, calculated from the current sample and a previous population-based adult sample.

Brain type	Brain type boundary	Brain type boundary[a]
Extreme E	D<−0.23	D<−0.21
Type E	−0.23≤D<−0.053	−0.21≤D<−0.041
Type B	−0.053≤D<0.048	−0.041≤D<0.040
Type S	0.048≤D<0.277	0.040≤D<0.21
Extreme S	D≥0.277	D≥0.21

[a]Data from [29].

.001, ω = .21). SQ-R scores were higher in the autism group than the control group, and higher in males than females. There was also a significant ordinal interaction between Sex and Diagnosis (F(1, 4146) = 11.6, p<.001, ω = .06), once again reflecting that sex differences were smaller in the autism than the control groups. Simple main effect analysis showed that males scored significantly higher than females in the control group (F(1, 4146) = 275.36, p< .001, d = .61), and in the autism group but to a lesser extent (F(1, 4146) = 15.6, p<.001, d = .27). This also indicates that the normative sex difference was attenuated, but not absent in the autism group.

D-score and Brain Types

Table 2 shows the brain type boundaries calculated from the current sample and a previous population-based adult sample [29]. Table 3 shows the percentage of participants with each brain type by group. In the control group more males than females were in Type S and Extreme Type S, and more females than males were in Type E and Extreme Type E. In the autism group, there was a shift towards Type S and Extreme Type S for both males and females, and there were more females than males with autism in Type B, Type E and Extreme Type E. This is shown in Figure 4, in which the D axis runs from the top left corner to the bottom right corner. It is clear that typical females cluster in the top left corner with the lowest D scores, followed by typical males,

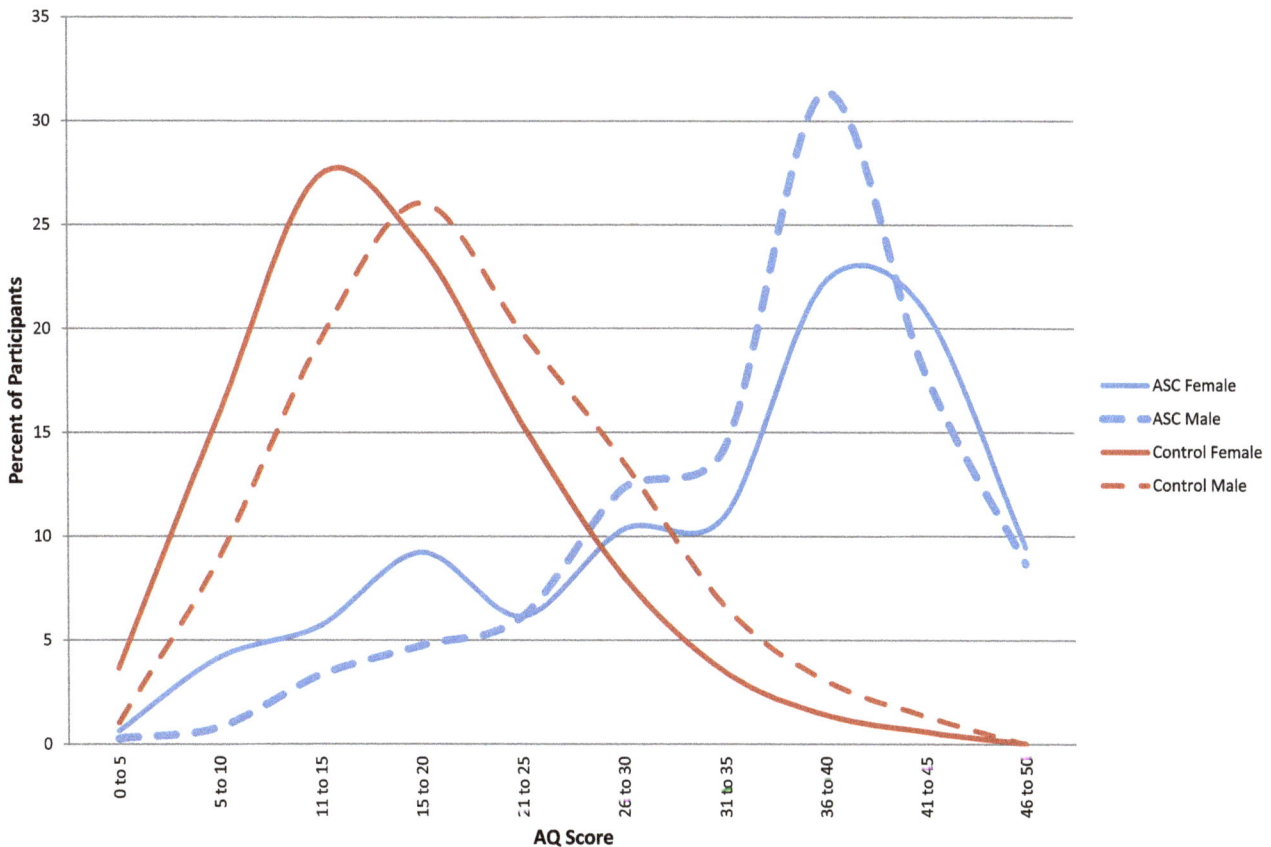

Figure 1. The distributions of Autism Spectrum Quotient (AQ) scores by the four groups: males and females with and without autism spectrum conditions.

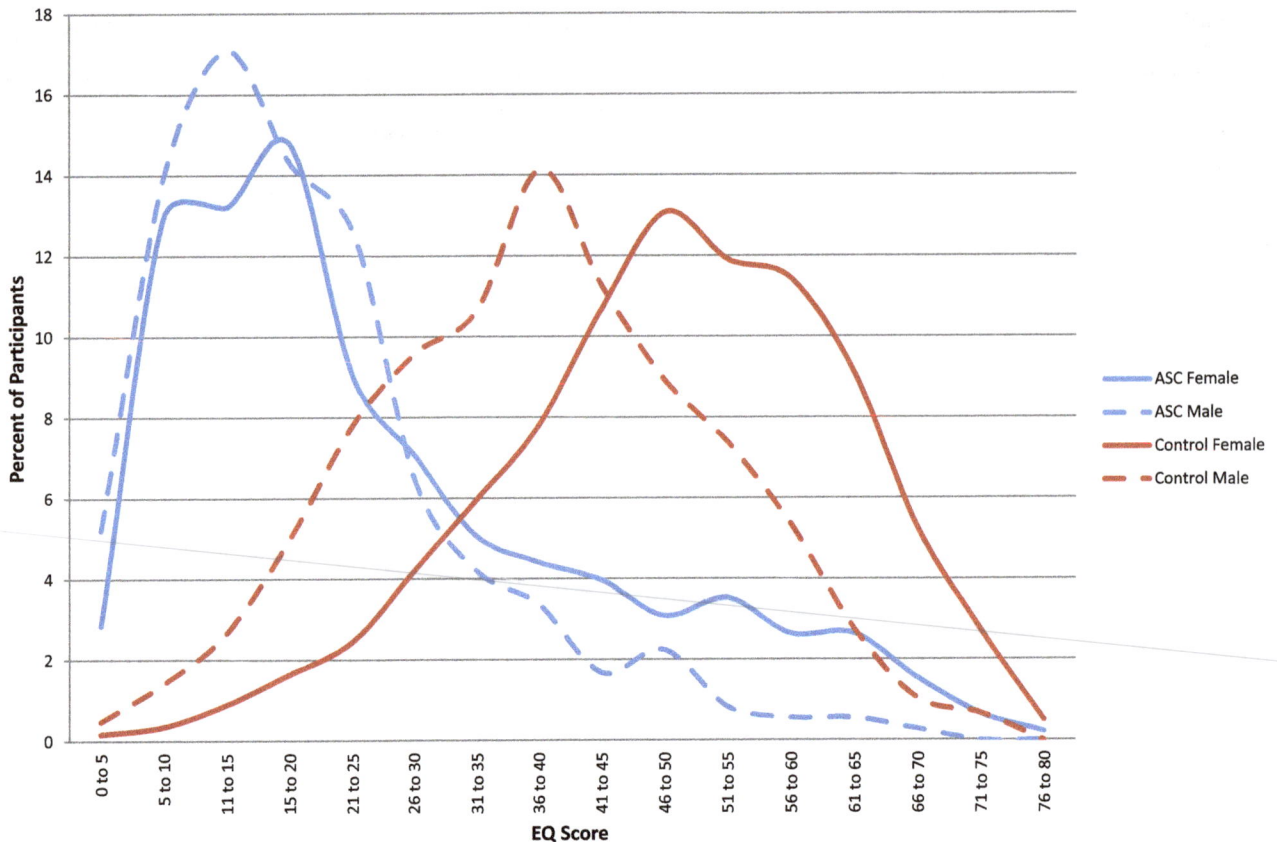

Figure 2. The distributions of Empathy Quotient (EQ) scores by the four groups: males and females with and without autism spectrum conditions.

followed by females with autism, and finally by males with autism in the bottom right corner, and with the highest D scores. Males and females with autism appear to have a greater scatter across the brain types than the typical control groups.

These findings were supported by an ANOVA on the D score, which revealed significant main effects of Diagnosis ($F_{(1, 4146)} = 1058.8$, $p<.001$, $\omega = .55$) and Sex ($F_{(1, 4146)} = 259.68$, $p<.001$, $\omega = .27$). D scores were higher in the autism group than the control group, and higher in males than females. There was a significant ordinal interaction between Sex and Diagnosis ($F_{(1, 4146)} = 21.59$, $p<.001$, $\omega = .07$), demonstrating that sex differences were smaller in the autism than the control group. Simple main effects analysis showed that males had significantly higher D scores than females in the control group ($F_{(1, 4146)} = 606$, $p<.001$, $d = .95$), and also in the autism group but to a lesser extent ($F_{(1, 4146)} = 39.99$, $p<.001$, $d = .41$). Again this indicates that normative sex differences were attenuated, but not absent, in the autism group.

Table 4 shows a comparison of demographic characteristics between individuals with two opposite sets of brain types ('Extreme Type S and Type S' vs. 'Extreme Type E, Type E and Type B') in the male and female autism groups. In the male autism group, individuals with 'Extreme Type E, Type E and Type B' brain types were significantly lower in mean age ($t(293) = 2.6$, $p = .01$), and were significantly more likely to be in full time education (odds ratio OR = 3.66, 95% confidence interval CI = [1.28, 10.42]; $\chi^2(1) = 6.6$, $p = .01$), than individuals with 'Extreme Type S and Type S' brain types. In the female autism group, individuals with

'Extreme Type E, Type E and Type B' brain types were significantly more likely to be employed (OR = 2.1, 95% CI = [1.1, 3.96]; $\chi^2(1) = 5.4$, $p = .02$), significantly less likely to be unemployed (OR = 0.25, 95% CI = [0.057, 1.08]; $\chi^2(1) = 3.97$, $p = .046$), and marginally significantly more likely to have had a mainstream education (OR = 2.45, 95% CI = [0.93, 6.48]; $\chi^2(1) = 3.49$, $p = .06$), than individuals with 'Extreme Type S and Type S' brain types.

Discussion

Consistent with previous smaller-scale studies [8,29,30] we confirmed that in a very large typical control group, females on average score higher on EQ, males on average scored higher on AQ and SQ-R, and that both males and females with autism show a shift to the extreme of the 'male profile'. Using EQ and SQ-R scores to calculate D score, which corresponds to specific cognitive 'brain types', Type E was the most frequent profile amongst typical females, Type S was the most frequent profile in typical males, and Type S and the Extreme Type S were the most common ones in the autism group for both males and females. A diagnosis of autism shifted the profiles of both males and females towards the 'extreme-male' end (indicated by the same direction of significant main effects of Diagnosis and Sex in the ANOVAs), and the patterns of normative sex differences were significantly attenuated in individuals with autism (indicated by the significant ordinal interaction between Sex and Diagnosis). These findings fit the predictions from the EMB theory of autism [10]. This likely reflects a more pronounced effect of 'masculinization' (i.e., shifting

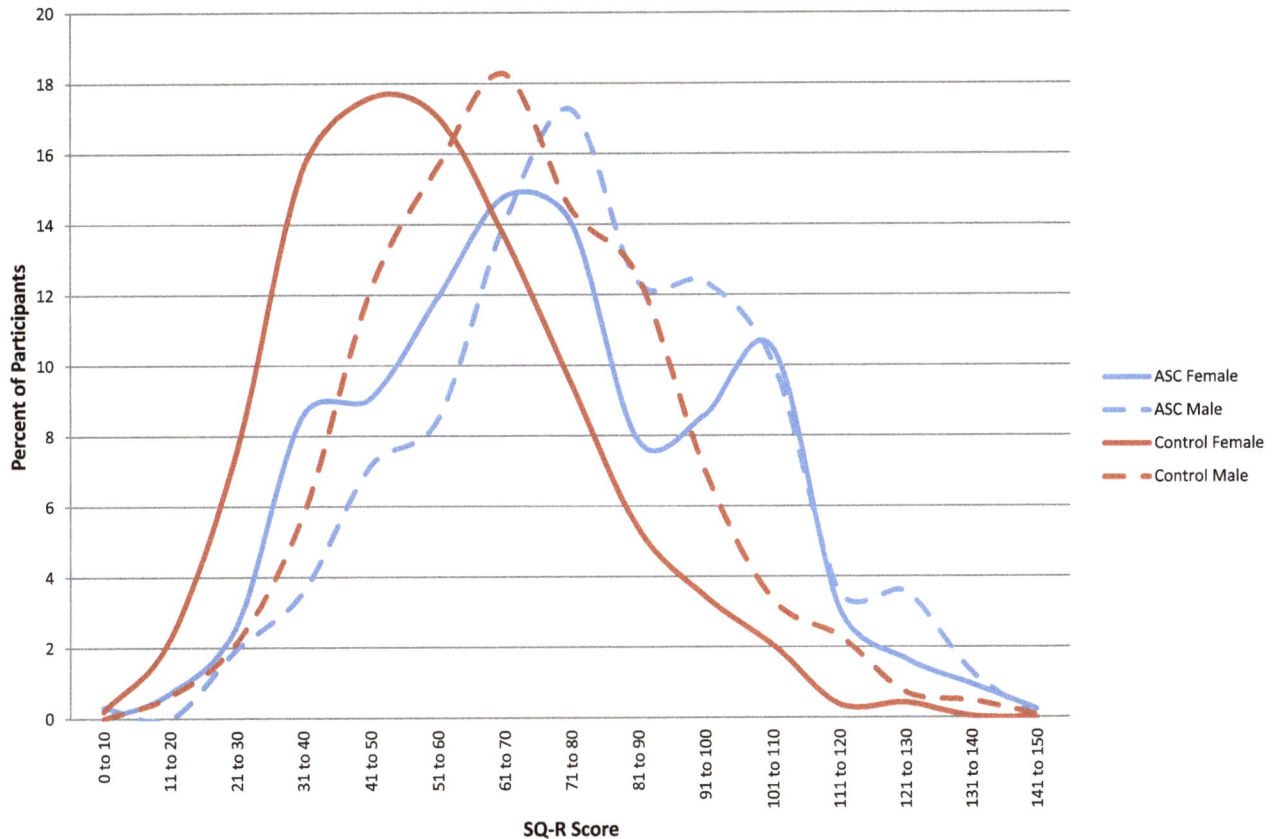

Figure 3. The distributions of Systemizing Quotient-Revised (SQ-R) scores by the four groups: males and females with and without autism spectrum conditions.

towards the typical male-end of the profile) in females with autism in these aspects. This is also in line with recent neuroimaging studies showing 'masculinization' of the brain in females with autism [12,33,34] and likely reflects sex-linked biological factors at work in autism, such as foetal testosterone [35,36].

Data from this large study also provide an adequately powered test of whether normative sex differences in autistic traits, empathizing, systemizing and cognitive 'brain type', previously documented in typical individuals, are also present in individuals with autism. Although the patterns of normative sex differences were attenuated in individuals with autism, significant sex differences were still evident, in the same direction as in the control group (indicated by the significant ordinal Sex-by-Diagnosis interaction and the significant differences shown by simple effect analyses). The fact that significant sex differences within autism were found in the present study is likely due to the substantially larger sample size (6.5 times larger than the largest of previous studies [29]), which provides greater power to detect small and medium effect size sex differences.

The persistence of normative sex differences in autism, found in this high-functioning adult cohort that is the largest to date, is notable and fits with recent reflections about what the field may have missed regarding females with autism. First, even though both sexes have been clinically diagnosed with autism, autism-related trait characteristics in males and females with autism distribute differently on average. These traits, continuously

distributed in the general population, have well-established sex-differential distributions [2,7,8]. Therefore, our finding here echoes the call to consider sex-differential thresholds for clinically diagnosing autism [1,37]. Second, the persistence of normative sex differences in autism corresponds with recent findings of less male-typical, possibly 'compensated', 'masked' or qualitatively different 'female phenotypes' of autism [18,20,21,25,38,39]. For example, in our sample there were a moderate proportion of females with autism having a Type B, Type E or even an Extreme Type E profile (25.7%, who were also more likely to be employed and had received mainstream education compared to those in Type S or Extreme Type S), in contrast to males with autism (8.4%), suggesting that there is substantial variability in 'brain type' profiles in this group. A less male-typical presentation of autism in females, especially in high-functioning individuals, may be related to the existing diagnostic bias towards males [39–41]. Further studies are needed to directly address the various presentations of autism in females and how they are similar to or different from those of males.

This study has several limitations. First, only individuals who were capable of self-reporting formal clinical diagnosis of an autism spectrum condition were investigated, so the observed sex differences may not generalize to subgroups with intellectual disability or with substantial communication difficulties. Generalizability could be tested via parent-report of children on the autistic spectrum, irrespective of the individual's age or IQ.

Table 3. Percentage of participants with each brain type in the present study, listed alongside a previous population-based study.

Brain Type	Autism Females (n = 397)	Autism Males (n = 295)	Control Females (n = 2,261)	Control Males (n = 1,197)	Autism Group[a] (n = 125)	Control Females[a] (n = 1,038)	Control Males[a] (n = 723)
Extreme E	1.5	0	3.7	0.3	0	4.3	0.1
Type E	11.6	1.0	43.1	12.9	0	44.8	15.1
Type B	12.6	7.4	30.6	28.4	6.4	29.3	30.3
Type S	46.8	60.3	21.2	53.7	32	20.7	49.5
Extreme S	27.4	31.3	1.4	4.7	61.6	0.9	5

[a]Data from [29].

Second, since the data were all collected online, it is unknown if the findings would generalize to individuals who cannot access the internet to volunteer for research. Third, individuals with certain co-occurring conditions or major psychiatric conditions were excluded, so it is unknown how these might modulate cognitive profiles. Fourth, there was no independent verification of diagnosis for the majority of the autism group since participants were recruited online. However, this approach did allow us to obtain a much larger sample than could otherwise have been investigated. Previous studies have shown high levels of agreement between self/parent-reported and clinician-reported diagnosis [42], and all individuals with autism in the present study provided the name of the clinician and the clinic where they were diagnosed, so there is no obvious reason to question their diagnoses. In addition, a subset (n = 64) attended the National Health Service Cambridge Lifespan Asperger Syndrome Service (CLASS) clinic in Cambridge, where diagnosis was independently confirmed in person.

Although there is a long-held view that the male-bias in prevalence is particularly extreme in the high-functioning end of the autism spectrum (e.g., up to 14:1 [43]), recent large-scale epidemiological data indicate that the sex ratio at the high-functioning end is not as extreme as previously believed, but rather falling between 2–5:1 [44–48]. This suggests that the earlier view may be due to under-recognition of high-functioning females in the past. With increased awareness and improved clinical recognition, increasing numbers of high-functioning females with autism volunteer for research to help our understanding of how autism manifests in females. This is probably one reason why, in the present study, we were able to recruit even more females than males with autism. Although this sex ratio may not be representative of the autism population at large, the comparable sample size of males and females with autism in the present study is desirable for a statistically robust investigation of sex differences within autism (which has not been attainable in earlier studies).

The growing evidence of 'masculinization' in females with autism now covers five different levels: behaviour, medical symptomatology, cognition, neural, and endocrine. At the behavioural level females with autism are shifted along the continuum from 'typical females' to 'typical males' with regard to gender-stereotyped behaviours [49–51]. At the medical symptomatology level, females with autism show higher rates of testosterone-driven conditions such as Polycystic Ovary Syndrome (PCOS) and severe acne [49,52]. At the cognitive level, females with autism are shifted beyond the 'male-end' along the 'typical females'—'typical males' continuum on the AQ, EQ, SQ-R (present data), and the Reading the Mind in the Eyes test (Baron-Cohen et al., in preparation). At the neural level, females with autism show a shift towards 'masculinization' in both grey and white matter brain morphology [12]. Finally, at the endocrine level, females with autism show elevated serum levels of androgens [53–55]. On the other hand, a recent large-scale population-based study shows that elevated levels *in utero* of all of the Δ4 sex steroid pathway (progesterone, 17α-hydroxy-progesterone, androstenedione, and testosterone), as well as cortisol, predict later diagnosis of autism in males [56]. It will be important to now test this in females who go on to develop autism, in order to understand early plausible developmental mechanisms associated with later 'masculinization' across multiple levels.

We conclude that when measuring empathizing, systemizing, and autistic traits in a large, adequately powered sample of high-functioning adults with autism via self-report, results provide

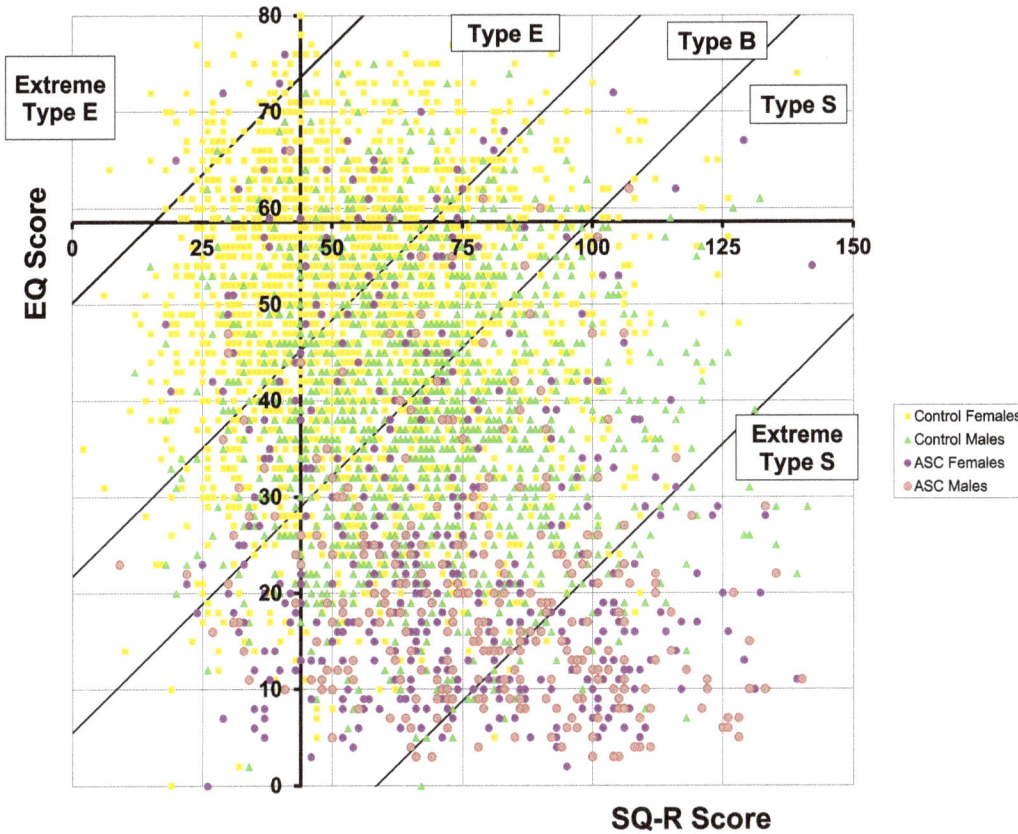

Figure 4. The distributions of males and females with and without autism spectrum conditions by 'brain type' (or cognitive style), in relation to their EQ and SQ-R scores.

strong support for predictions from the EMB theory [10] that the cognitive profiles of both males and females with autism are shifted towards and beyond the typical male-distribution, and normative sex differences in these profiles are attenuated in autism. However, significant sex differences within autism (with small to medium effect sizes) are evident, indicating a persistence of normative sex differences despite the clinical diagnoses of autism. Future research

needs to address what factors (e.g. prenatal hormonal effects, sex-linked genetic and epigenetic factors, and other mechanisms associated with the regulation of gene expression) [57,58] contribute to the emergence of the cognitive 'masculinization' in autism [9], and characterize the similarities and differences between males and females with autism [12,13,39] to help clarify the substantial heterogeneity of the spectrum [1].

Table 4. Comparison of demographic characteristics between the two opposite sets of brain types in the male and female autism groups.

Demographic Characteristics	Autism Females		Autism Males	
	Extreme Type E, Type E and Type B	Extreme Type S and Type S	Extreme Type E, Type E and Type B	Extreme Type S and Type S
Mean Age (n)	36.8 (102)	33.7 (295)	29.4** (25)	36** (270)
Employment Status	n = 84	n = 247	n = 20	n = 229
% Employed	83.33*	70.44*	60	67.69
% Unemployed	2.39*	8.91*	10	21.83
% In full time education	14.28	20.65	30**	10.48**
Education Type	n = 98	n = 283	n = 25	n = 220
% Mainstream education	94.8	88.34	80	88.6

*p<.05,
**p<.01.

Acknowledgments

This study was conducted in association with the National Institute for Health Research Collaborations for Leadership in Applied Health Research and Care (NIHR CLAHRC) East of England (EoE). This study was submitted in part fulfilment of the Degree of BSc by Maryam Achoukhi and Sarah Robertson to the Department of Psychology, University of Cambridge. We would like to thank Sally Wheelwright for assistance in the maintenance of the volunteer database, and Rebecca Kenny for assistance in the preparation of the manuscript.

Author Contributions

Conceived and designed the experiments: SBC SC BA CA MA SR AP M-CL. Performed the experiments: SBC SC BA CA MA SR AP M-CL. Analyzed the data: SC. Wrote the paper: SBC SC BA CA MA SR AP M-CL.

References

1. Lai MC, Lombardo MV, Chakrabarti B, Baron-Cohen S (2013) Subgrouping the Autism "Spectrum": Reflections on DSM-5. PLoS Biol 11: e1001544.
2. Baron-Cohen S, Wheelwright S, Skinner R, Martin J, Clubley E (2001) The autism-spectrum quotient (AQ): evidence from Asperger syndrome/high-functioning autism, males and females, scientists and mathematicians. J Autism Dev Disord 31: 5–17.
3. Allison C, Baron-Cohen S, Wheelwright S, Charman T, Richler J, et al. (2008) The Q-CHAT (Quantitative CHecklist for Autism in Toddlers): a normally distributed quantitative measure of autistic traits at 18–24 months of age: preliminary report. J Autism Dev Disord 38: 1414–1425.
4. Baron-Cohen S, Hoekstra RA, Knickmeyer R, Wheelwright S (2006) The Autism-Spectrum Quotient (AQ)–adolescent version. J Autism Dev Disord 36: 343–350.
5. Auyeung B, Baron-Cohen S, Wheelwright S, Allison C (2008) The Autism Spectrum Quotient: Children's Version (AQ-Child). J Autism Dev Disord 38: 1230–1240.
6. Lai MC, Lombardo MV, Baron-Cohen S (2014) Autism. Lancet 383: 896–910.
7. Baron-Cohen S, Wheelwright S (2004) The empathy quotient: an investigation of adults with Asperger syndrome or high functioning autism, and normal sex differences. J Autism Dev Disord 34: 163–175.
8. Baron-Cohen S, Richler J, Bisarya D, Gurunathan N, Wheelwright S (2003) The systemizing quotient: an investigation of adults with Asperger syndrome or high-functioning autism, and normal sex differences. Philos Trans R Soc Lond B Biol Sci 358: 361–374.
9. Baron-Cohen S, Lombardo MV, Auyeung B, Ashwin E, Chakrabarti B, et al. (2011) Why are autism spectrum conditions more prevalent in males? PLOS Biol 9: e1001081.
10. Baron-Cohen S (2002) The extreme male brain theory of autism. Trends Cogn Sci 6: 248–254.
11. Kirkovski M, Enticott PG, Fitzgerald PB (2013) A review of the role of female gender in autism spectrum disorders. J Autism Dev Disord 43: 2584–2603.
12. Lai MC, Lombardo MV, Suckling J, Ruigrok AN, Chakrabarti B, et al. (2013) Biological sex affects the neurobiology of autism. Brain 136: 2799–2815.
13. Werling DM, Geschwind DH (2013) Sex differences in autism spectrum disorders. Curr Opin Neurol 26: 146–153.
14. Holtmann M, Bolte S, Poustka F (2007) Autism spectrum disorders: sex differences in autistic behaviour domains and coexisting psychopathology. Dev Med Child Neurol 49: 361–366.
15. Pilowsky T, Yirmiya N, Shulman C, Dover R (1998) The Autism Diagnostic Interview-Revised and the Childhood Autism Rating Scale: differences between diagnostic systems and comparison between genders. J Autism Dev Disord 28: 143–151.
16. McLennan JD, Lord C, Schopler E (1993) Sex differences in higher functioning people with autism. J Autism Dev Disord 23: 217–227.
17. Carter AS, Black DO, Tewani S, Connolly CE, Kadlec MB, et al. (2007) Sex differences in toddlers with autism spectrum disorders. J Autism Dev Disord 37: 86–97.
18. Lai MC, Lombardo MV, Ruigrok AN, Chakrabarti B, Wheelwright SJ, et al. (2012) Cognition in males and females with autism: similarities and differences. PLOS One 7: e47198.
19. Bolte S, Duketis E, Poustka F, Holtmann M (2011) Sex differences in cognitive domains and their clinical correlates in higher-functioning autism spectrum disorders. Autism 15: 497–511.
20. Mandy W, Chilvers R, Chowdhury U, Salter G, Seigal A, et al. (2012) Sex differences in autism spectrum disorder: evidence from a large sample of children and adolescents. J Autism Dev Disord 42: 1304–1313.
21. Lai MC, Lombardo MV, Pasco G, Ruigrok AN, Wheelwright SJ, et al. (2011) A behavioral comparison of male and female adults with high functioning autism spectrum conditions. PLoS One 6: e20835.
22. Van Wijngaarden-Cremers PJ, van Eeten E, Groen WB, Van Deurzen PA, Oosterling IJ, et al. (2014) Gender and age differences in the core triad of impairments in autism spectrum disorders: a systematic review and meta-analysis. J Autism Dev Disord 44: 627–635.
23. Szatmari P, Liu XQ, Goldberg J, Zwaigenbaum L, Paterson AD, et al. (2012) Sex differences in repetitive stereotyped behaviors in autism: Implications for genetic liability. Am J Med Genet B Neuropsychiatr Genet 159B: 5–12.
24. Lemon JM, Gargaro B, Enticott PG, Rinehart NJ (2011) Executive functioning in autism spectrum disorders: a gender comparison of response inhibition. J Autism Dev Disord 41: 352–356.
25. Frazier TW, Georgiades S, Bishop SL, Hardan AY (2014) Behavioral and cognitive characteristics of females and males with autism in the Simons Simplex Collection. Journal of the American Academy of Child & Adolescent Psychiatry 53: 329–340.
26. Field A (2013) Discovering statistics using IBM SPSS statistics. London: SAGE Publications Ltd. 952 p.
27. Lemler M (2012) Discrepancy between parent report and clinician observation of symptoms in children with autism spectrum disorders. Discussions 8: 2 Available: http://wwwstudentpulsecom/a?id = 803. Accessed 2014 Jun 2.
28. Grantham CL, Gower MW, McCalla MK, Harris AN, O'Kelley SE, et al. (2011) Diagnosis of autism utilizing the ADOS and ADI-R: are there factors to account for discrepancies? International Meeting for Autism Research. San Diego, California Available: https://imfar.confex.com/imfar/2011/webprogram/Paper7956.html. Accessed 2014 Jun 2.
29. Wheelwright S, Baron-Cohen S, Goldenfeld N, Delaney J, Fine D, et al. (2006) Predicting Autism Spectrum Quotient (AQ) from the Systemizing Quotient-Revised (SQ-R) and Empathy Quotient (EQ). Brain Res 1079: 47–56.
30. Auyeung B, Wheelwright S, Allison C, Atkinson M, Samarawickrema N, et al. (2009) The children's Empathy Quotient and Systemizing Quotient: sex differences in typical development and in Autism Spectrum Conditions. J Autism Dev Disord 39: 1509–1521.
31. Wheelwright S, Auyeung B, Allison C, Baron-Cohen S (2010) Defining the broader, medium and narrow autism phenotype among parents using the Autism Spectrum Quotient (AQ). Mol Autism 1: 10.
32. Goldenfeld N, Baron-Cohen S, Wheelwright S (2005) Empathizing and systemizing in males, females and autism. Clinical Neuropsychiatry 2: 8.
33. Beacher FD, Minati L, Baron-Cohen S, Lombardo MV, Lai MC, et al. (2012) Autism attenuates sex differences in brain structure: a combined voxel-based morphometry and diffusion tensor imaging study. AJNR Am J Neuroradiol 33: 83–89.
34. Beacher FD, Radulescu E, Minati L, Baron-Cohen S, Lombardo MV, et al. (2012) Sex differences and autism: Brain function during verbal fluency and mental rotation. PLOS ONE 7: e38355.
35. Auyeung B, Baron-Cohen S, Ashwin E, Knickmeyer R, Taylor K, et al. (2009) Fetal testosterone and autistic traits. Br J Psychol 100: 1–22.
36. Baron-Cohen S, Knickmeyer RC, Belmonte MK (2005) Sex differences in the brain: implications for explaining autism. Science 310: 819–823.
37. Constantino JN, Charman T (2012) Gender bias, female resilience, and the sex ratio in autism. J Am Acad Child Adolesc Psychiatry 51: 756–758.
38. Gould J, Ashton-Smith J (2011) Missed diagnosis or misdiagnosis? Girls and women on the autism spectrum. Good Autism Practice 12: 34–41.
39. Kreiser N, White S (2014) ASD in females: are we overstating the gender difference in diagnosis? Clin Child Fam Psychol Rev 17: 67–84.
40. Dworzynski K, Ronald A, Bolton P, Happe F (2012) How different are girls and boys above and below the diagnostic threshold for autism spectrum disorders? J Am Acad Child Adolesc Psychiatry 51: 788–797.
41. Begeer S, Mandell D, Wijnker-Holmes B, Venderbosch S, Rem D, et al. (2013) Sex differences in the timing of identification among children and adults with autism spectrum disorders. J Autism Dev Disord 43: 1151–1156.
42. Daniels AM, Rosenberg RE, Law JK, Lord C, Kaufmann WE, et al. (2011) Stability of initial autism spectrum disorder diagnoses in community settings. J Autism Dev Disord: 110–121.
43. Wing L (1981) Sex ratios in early childhood autism and related conditions. Psychiatry Res 5: 129–137.
44. Idring S, Rai D, Dal H, Dalman C, Sturm H, et al. (2012) Autism spectrum disorders in the stockholm youth cohort: design, prevalence and validity. PLOS ONE 7: e41280.
45. Mattila ML, Kielinen M, Linna SL, Jussila K, Ebeling H, et al. (2011) Autism spectrum disorders according to DSM-IV-TR and comparison with DSM-5 draft criteria: An epidemiological study. J Am Acad Child Adolesc Psychiatry 50: 583–592 e511.
46. Hinkka-Yli-Salomaki S, Banerjee PN, Gissler M, Lampi KM, Vanhala R, et al. (2013) The incidence of diagnosed autism spectrum disorders in Finland. Nord J Psychiatry. doi: 10.3109/08039488.2013.861017.
47. Jensen CM, Steinhausen HC, Lauritsen MB (2014) Time trends over 16 years in incidence-rates of autism spectrum disorders across the lifespan based on nationwide Danish register data. J Autism Dev Disord. doi:10.1007/s10803-014-2053-6.

48. Saemundsen E, Magnusson P, Georgsdottir I, Egilsson E, Rafnsson V (2013) Prevalence of autism spectrum disorders in an Icelandic birth cohort. BMJ Open 3.

49. Ingudomnukul E, Baron-Cohen S, Wheelwright S, Knickmeyer R (2007) Elevated rates of testosterone-related disorders in women with autism spectrum conditions. Horm Behav 51: 597–604.

50. Knickmeyer RC, Wheelwright S, Baron-Cohen SB (2008) Sex-typical play: masculinization/defeminization in girls with an autism spectrum condition. J Autism Dev Disord 38: 1028–1035.

51. Bejerot S, Eriksson JM (2014) Sexuality and gender role in autism spectrum disorder: a case control study. PLoS One 9: e87961.

52. Pohl A, Cassidy S, Auyeung B, Baron-Cohen S (2014) Uncovering steroidopathy in women with autism: a latent class analysis. Mol Autism 5: 27.

53. Schwarz E, Guest PC, Rahmoune H, Wang L, Levin Y, et al. (2011) Sex-specific serum biomarker patterns in adults with Asperger's syndrome. Mol Psychiatry 16: 1213–1220.

54. Bejerot S, Eriksson JM, Bonde S, Carlstrom K, Humble MB, et al. (2012) The extreme male brain revisited: gender coherence in adults with autism spectrum disorder. Br J Psychiatry 201: 116–123.

55. Ruta L, Ingudomnukul E, Taylor K, Chakrabarti B, Baron-Cohen S (2011) Increased serum androstenedione in adults with autism spectrum conditions. Psychoneuroendocrino 36: 1154–1163.

56. Baron Cohen S, Auyeung B, Norgaard-Pedersen B, Hougaard DM, Abdallah MW, et al. (2014) Elevated fetal steroidogenic activity in autism. Mol Psychiatry. doi: 10.1038/mp.2014.48.

57. Sarachana T, Hu VW (2013) Genome-wide identification of transcriptional targets of RORA reveals direct regulation of multiple genes associated with autism spectrum disorder. Mol Autism 4: 14.

58. Schaafsma SM, Pfaff DW (2014) Etiologies underlying sex differences in Autism Spectrum Disorders. Front Neuroendocrinol. doi: 10.1016/j.yfrne.2014.03.006.

High Resolution Magnetic Resonance Imaging for Characterization of the Neuroligin-3 Knock-in Mouse Model Associated with Autism Spectrum Disorder

Manoj Kumar[1], Jeffery T. Duda[1], Wei-Ting Hwang[2], Charles Kenworthy[3], Ranjit Ittyerah[1], Stephen Pickup[1], Edward S. Brodkin[4], James C. Gee[1], Ted Abel[3], Harish Poptani[1]*

1 Department of Radiology, Perelman School of Medicine at the University of Pennsylvania, Philadelphia, Pennsylvania, United States of America, 2 Department of Biostatistics and Epidemiology, Center for Clinical Epidemiology and Biostatistics, Perelman School of Medicine at the University of Pennsylvania, Philadelphia, Pennsylvania, United States of America, 3 Department of Biology, University of Pennsylvania, Philadelphia, Pennsylvania, United States of America, 4 Center for Neurobiology and Behavior, Department of Psychiatry, Perelman School of Medicine at the University of Pennsylvania, Philadelphia, Pennsylvania, United States of America

Abstract

Autism spectrum disorders (ASD) comprise an etiologically heterogeneous set of neurodevelopmental disorders. Neuroligin-3 (NL-3) is a cell adhesion protein that mediates synapse development and has been implicated in ASD. We performed ex-vivo high resolution magnetic resonance imaging (MRI), including diffusion tensor imaging (DTI) and behavioral (social approach and zero maze) tests at 3 different time points (30, 50 and 70 days-of-age) on NL-3 and wild-type littermates to assess developmental brain abnormalities in NL-3 mice. MRI data were segmented in 39 different gray and white matter regions. Volumetric measurements, along with DTI indices from these segmented regions were also performed. After controlling for age and gender, the NL-3 knock-in animals demonstrated significantly reduced sociability and lower anxiety-related behavior in comparison to their wild type littermates. Significantly reduced volume of several white and gray matter regions in the NL-3 knock-in mice were also observed after considering age, gender and time point as covariates. These findings suggest that structural changes in the brain of NL-3 mice are induced by the mutation in the NL-3 gene. No significant differences in DTI indices were observed, which suggests that the NL-3 mutation may not have a profound effect on water diffusion as detected by DTI. The volumetric and DTI studies aid in understanding the biology of disrupting function on an ASD risk model and may assist in the development of imaging biomarkers for ASD.

Editor: Valerie W Hu, The George Washington University, United States of America

Funding: This study was supported by R01MH080718 (ESB), R21HD058237 (HP), 1P50MH096891 -subproject 6773 (ESB and TA), 5-T32-MH017168 (TA) and the Pennsylvania Department of Health (SAP # 4100042728, TA and ESB). The funders had no role in study design, data collection and analysis, decision to publish, or preparation of the manuscript.

Competing Interests: The authors have declared that no competing interests exist.

* Email: Harish.Poptani@uphs.upenn.edu

Introduction

Autism spectrum disorder (ASD) comprises a complex and etiologically heterogeneous group of neurodevelopmental disorders with an unknown unifying pathogenesis. While ASD is defined by the presence of deficits in social interaction as well as restricted and repetitive patterns of behavior, ASD is nevertheless highly heterogeneous in terms of behavior and genetic abnormalities [1–5]. The etiology of ASD is unknown in most cases, but monogenic heritable forms exist that have provided insights into ASD pathogenesis and have led to the notion of autism as a 'synapse disorder' [4]. Neuroligins are a family of postsynaptic cell-adhesion molecules that are ligands for neurexins, a class of synaptic cell-adhesion molecules [6], and Jamain et al. [7] reported an inherited mutation in the Neuroligin-3 (NL-3) gene in a family with two brothers having ASD. The point mutation at the amino acid position 451 (R451C) caused a decrease in the amount of NL-3 in patients with ASD. Later, the same point

mutation was introduced in a mouse to generate the NL-3 R451C knock-in mouse model of ASD [6]. The NL-3 knock-in mice have been reported to exhibit behavioral symptoms similar to those observed in human ASD [6]. However, a subsequent study did not observe behavioral phenotypes relevant to ASD in this model, and therefore raised concerns about the relevance of the model to ASD [8].

Magnetic Resonance Imaging (MRI) has been employed extensively to examine morphological changes in human ASD [9–11] as well as in mouse models relevant to ASD [2,3,12–14]. More recently, diffusion tensor imaging (DTI) has also been used to characterize ASD in humans [15–17] and animal models [2,3,12,14]. High resolution microscopic MRI studies have been used to characterize inbred (BALB/cJ, and BTBR) [12,14] as well as genetic models of ASD (NL-3 knock-in, 16p11.2) [3,13,14,18]. These studies have been primarily performed on isolated fixed brain specimens and have reported volumetric differences in several gray and white matter regions of the ASD brain relative to normal controls [3]. Recently a DTI study also reported a correlation between social abnormalities and fractional anisotropy (FA) in the pre-pubescent BALB/cJ mouse model [12].

High resolution MRI studies of the adult NL-3 knock-in mouse brain (108 day-old) indicated reduced volume in several regions of the brain, compared to wild-type (WT) littermates. Despite, volumetric differences, no differences were noted in any of the DTI parameters in this study [3]. Since reduced interest in social interaction (low sociability) is especially prominent in childhood ASD and the BALB/cJ mice exhibit low sociability and DTI abnormalities at a pre-pubescent age [2], we hypothesized that the lack of differences in DTI in the previous study of NL-3 mice may have been due to the adult age of the mice, as well as the smaller sample size used [3]. Thus in the current study behavioral assays (social approach and elevated zero maze tests) and high resolution MRI studies were performed on 28–30 (juvenile), 48–50 (peripubescent) and 68–70 (early adult) days old NL-3 knock-in mice in order to characterize the developmental brain changes in this model and to also look for correlations between behavior and MRI findings.

Methods

Animal housing and breeding

A breeding pair of NL-3 knock-in mice (JAX strain number 008475) was procured from The Jackson Laboratory (Bar Harbor, ME), bred in-house at the University of Pennsylvania, and offsprings were genotyped using protocols from Jackson Labs. All animal experiments were approved by the Institutional Animal Care and Use Committee (IACUC). At 2–4 days postnatally, litters were culled to two males and two females to ensure adequate nutrition for all pups and a more uniform social environment during development and to also ensure that litters were balanced in the numbers of males and females. Mice were group housed in a light and temperature controlled animal facility that is accredited by the Association for Assessment and Accreditation of Laboratory Animal Care. Males were removed from breeding cages prior to the birth of pups. All efforts were made to minimize animal pain and discomfort. Water and standard rodent chow were available *ad lib*. With the exception of a weekly cage change, mice were not handled until after the completion of all behavioral tests. To avoid any confounding effects, similar conditions for housing, feeding and handling were used throughout the study. This study was started during the spring of 2011 (4/2011) and completed by in the fall of 2011 (10/2011). A few animals were randomly selected after each time point (30, 50 and 70 day-of-age) for imaging. Details of the animal distributions including age, gender and strains for behavioral (social approach and elevated zero maze test) and imaging studies are summarized in Table S1. Due to the longitudinal nature of the study, some of the animals underwent behavioral study more than once but since the behavioral studies were separated by 3-weeks, any potential effects of repeated behavioral testing were minimized. Seasonal effects and cohort differences were further minimized by selecting the wild type and mutant animals from the same litter to randomize these effects between the groups. To reduce the effect of handling, only one person (R.I.) performed all behavioral assays throughout the study.

Social approach and anxiety tests

Social Approach Test (also known as the Social Choice Test) was performed on NL-3 knock-in mice and WT mice at 28 (juvenile), 48 (peri-pubescent) and 68 (early adult) days-of-age using a 3-chambered Plexiglas apparatus under dim lighting (<2 lux) during testing in order to minimize the general stress level of the mice, as described previously [2,12,19,20]. The social approach test was performed in the morning between 9:00 AM to 12:00 noon and all procedures were videotaped by using a Sony digital video camera with Night Shot (infrared) feature for recording in low light. The amount of time spent sniffing the stimulus mouse was used as the outcome variable for statistical analysis, with longer sniffing time indicating higher sociability.

Anxiety-related behavior was also assessed in these animals using the elevated zero maze test, which was performed a day after the social approach test (at 29, 49 and 69 days-of-age) at approximately the same time of the day. A circular variant of the elevated plus maze, the zero maze apparatus consists of a raised circular track divided into two open and two closed quadrants. The track had an internal diameter of 40.5 cm and a width of 5.1 cm and was elevated off the floor at a height of 40 cm. The closed quadrants had walls that were 11 cm high. The animal was placed into the center of a closed quadrant and observed for 5 min. Digitized video of each 5 min trial was scored manually to determine the total time spent in open and closed quadrants and the number of transitions between each open and closed quadrant [21,22]. Longer time spent in the open quadrants indicates lower anxiety-related behavior.

After completion of the zero maze tests, a subset of NL-3 knock-in mice [n = 25 (10 at 29 day-old, 10 at 49 day-old and 5 at 69 day-old)] and WT littermates [n = 24 (7 at 29 day-old, 9 at 49 day-old and 8 at 69 day-old)] were sacrificed at each time point to perform high resolution MRI on extracted brain samples. Because we randomly selected a subset of animals after the zero maze test for imaging, not all animals had behavioral data at all three time points. The distribution of age, gender and strain of all animals used in this study is summarized in Table S1. The animals were anesthetized with an intraperitoneal injection of ketamine. Following lack of deep tendon responses, the thoracic cavity was opened under aseptic conditions and the animals were perfused through the left ventricle with phosphate saline buffer (PBS), followed by 4% paraformaldehyde (PFA) solution. After perfusion, the brain was removed from the skull. The extracted perfused brains were stored at 4°C in 4% PFA solution for 2 weeks to fix the brain tissue prior to ex vivo high resolution DTI studies.

Sample preparation for *ex vivo* high resolution DTI

Prior to imaging, brain samples were removed from the fixative and switched back to PBS solution for 48 hours at 4°C to rehydrate the tissue. After 48 hours, the sample was removed and rinsed twice with fresh PBS solution and blotted using a soft tissue paper to remove any remaining PBS. The brain was then placed in a plastic tube filled with proton-free susceptibility-matching fluid (Fomblin, Ausimount, Thorofare; USA).

Ex vivo high resolution DTI

High resolution DTI was performed on a 9.4T, 8.9 cm vertical bore magnet equipped with a 55 mm inner-diameter 100 gauss/cm gradient tube and interfaced to a Direct Drive console (Agilent, Palo Alto, CA, USA) running the vnmrj 2.3.C software version. All MRI studies employed a horizontally mounted 2 turn, 11×20 mm (ID x length) solenoid RF coil for transmit and receive. The plastic tube containing the brain sample was placed inside the coil and the probe was mounted inside the magnet. Scout images were acquired in 3 orthogonal planes to localize the position and orientation of the brain sample. DTI data was then acquired using a 3D multi-echo pulsed-gradient spin echo sequence [23] with oval sampling in the two phase encoding directions. Acquisition parameters were: TR = 800 ms; TE = 29.50 ms; number of echoes $= 6$, number of averages $= 1$, b-value $= 902$ mm^2/s, FOV (field of view) $= 17$ mm$\times 8.5$ mm$\times 10$ mm; acquisition matrix size $= 136 \times 68 \times 80$, resulting in a 125 μm isotropic resolution. The diffusion-weighted images were acquired with diffusion weighting in 6 non-collinear directions with both positive and negative diffusion gradient amplitudes in addition to 2 reference scans with minimal diffusion weighting for a total of 14 data sets resulting in a total acquisition time of 13 hours and 19 minutes per sample.

DTI data processing and quantification

Image processing. Image reconstruction was performed offline using in-house custom software developed in the IDL programming environment (ITT Visual Information Solutions, Boulder, CO, USA). Following application of a Gaussian filter and 3D Fourier transformation, the magnitude images from each echo train were summed in order to improve SNR. Data sets acquired with opposite polarity diffusion weighting gradients were then combined in order to minimize contributions of background gradients to the diffusion data [24]. The resulting group of images was saved in DTI studio [25] format for further processing.

The b $= 0$ images for each mouse were registered to a general brain template in preparation for automated region based segmentation such that the same ROI was assessed from each specimen. The alignment and segmentation routines were performed using Advanced Normalization Tools (ANTs). The Camino Toolkit [26] was used to estimate the diffusion tensors via an unweighted linear least-squares to fit to the log measurements of the diffusion weighted data [27]. To obtain an anatomical labeling for each sample, a multi-atlas approach was used along with a publicly available data set consisting of five manually labeled mouse brains [27]. Diffeomorphic normalization was performed using the mutual information metric provided by ANTs [28] to map each sample's B0 image to each of the five manually labeled brains. The resulting transformations were used to warp the five anatomical label sets into each samples DTI space. Finally, STAPLE [29] was used to merge the multiple label sets to obtain a final set of probabilistic anatomical labels for each sample as shown in Figure 1. Using these methods, each mouse brain was segmented into 39 regions including the ventricles, gray and white matter regions (Figure 1). These probabilistic labels were then used to obtain regional volumes, as well as each region's averaged values for fractional anisotropy (FA), mean diffusivity (MD, $\times 10^{-3}$ mm^2/s), and radial diffusivity (RD). The regional brain volumes were computed and divided by the total brain volume from each individual sample to account for any differences in volumetric differences associated with extraction or fixation of the tissue.

Statistical analysis

Descriptive statistics were computed for all study variables. Because animals were subjected to social approach and elevated zero maze tests repeatedly over time, a linear mixed effect model was used to analyze the behavioral data which accounts for possible correlation in outcomes collected from the same animal over time. Three factors were considered in this model: group (WT vs NL-3), gender (male vs female) and age/time points (28–29, 48–49 and 68–69 day) as covariates. The three-way interaction effect was first tested using a Wald test followed by testing the two-way interaction effects using likelihood ratio tests. As there was no evidence for interaction in the social sniffing time, the results from the final model that included only the main effects terms are reported. For the anxiety data, the results from a model that contains the main effects terms and an interaction term between group and age are reported.

A linear regression model was used to analyze the cross-sectional volumetric and DTI data that included: group (NL-3 vs WT) as design factor and gender (male vs female), and the actual age (in days), as covariates. The interaction effect was first tested and each region was analyzed separately. Because multiple tests or regression analyses were done for each of the 39 regions for the outcomes of DTI indices and volumes, a false-discovery rate (FDR) was computed to control the type I error and a cut off value of 0.05 was used to determine statistical significance. None of the interaction terms reached statistical significance. Therefore, we reported the results from the model that only included main effects for the three factors. The adjusted mean volume in the significant region was computed from the final model using the predictive average volume of a 50-day male mouse for NL-3 and wild type animal respectively.

Using data from 28 animals that had both behavioral and imaging studies, the correlation between social, anxiety measures and segmented brain volumes were examined by calculating partial correlation coefficient through a linear regression model that have been adjusted for group, gender, and age. A p-value of <0.05 was considered significant. The correlation analysis was performed only on the selected brain regions which showed significant differences in volume between wild type and NL-3 mice. All statistical computations were performed using STATA 12 (StataCorp LP, College Station, Texas, USA) and statistical package for social sciences (SPSS, version 16.0 SPSS, Inc., Chicago, IL, USA).

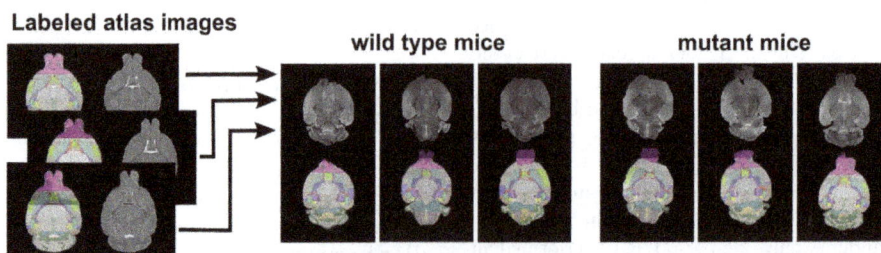

Figure 1. Demonstrating co-registration and segmentation approaches for the analysis of MRI images from the mouse brain. Each of the manually labeled brain was co-registered to each sample's B0 image. The corresponding labels (illustrated as a semi-transparent color overlay) were warped into the sample space and merged via STAPLE. Resulting anatomical labels are illustrated for single wild type and mutant type samples. The olfactory bulb was not included in this analysis due to the variability in extracting the brain tissue leading to incomplete extraction of the olfactory bulbs in some cases. While the resulting labels were probabilistic, the hard segmentations seen here were used for visualization and quality control, and were created by assigning the label of highest probability at each voxel. The color indicates the different regions of the brain.

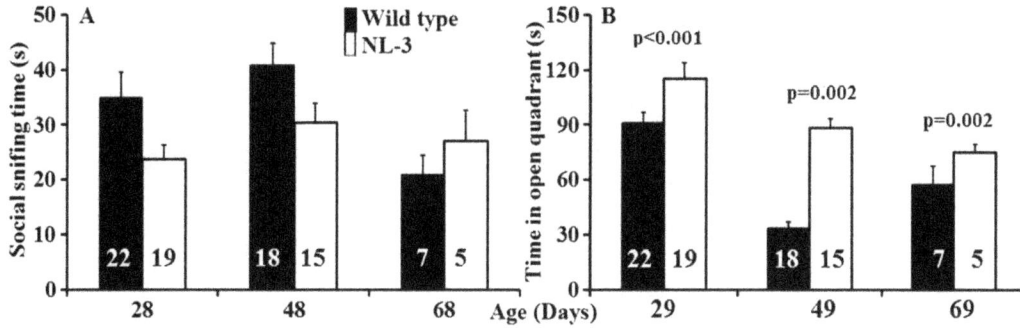

Figure 2. Bar graphs from the NL-3 knock-in and wild type littermates showing average social sniffing time (time spent by the test animal sniffing the stimulus mouse) at 3 different ages (A). Social sniffing test demonstrated significant differences at each time points between wild type and NL-3 mice (p = 0.019) based on a linear mixed effects model adjusting for gender and age and with no significant group interaction. Bar graph showing the average time spent by the animals in the open quadrant of the zero maze test in wild type littermates and NL-3 knock-in mice (B). Longer time spent in the open quadrants is thought to reflect lower anxiety-related behavior. Significant differences in anxiety scores were observed between wild type and NL-3 mice at each time point after adjusting for gender and age using a linear mixed effect model. A significant group interaction was also observed in anxiety score (p<0.05) based on a liner mixed effects model adjusting for gender and age. The numbers inside each bar show the number of animals while the error bars represent SEM.

Results

We found no evidence of 3-way and 2-way interaction effects in social approach behavior (all p-value>0.05). After controlling for gender and age, the NL-3 knock-in animals exhibited lower social preference than the WT animals. On an average, the NL-3 animals spent 8.7 seconds (95% CI: 1 to 15 seconds) less time

sniffing the stimulus mouse in comparison to their wild type littermates (p = 0.019) (Figure 2A). On the test of anxiety, the NL-3 mice spent significantly longer time in the open quadrant after controlling for gender and age, indicating lower anxiety (Figure 2B). There was a significant interaction effect between group and age (p = 0.006), with a larger difference in anxiety between NL-3 mice and wild type observed at 49-day time point

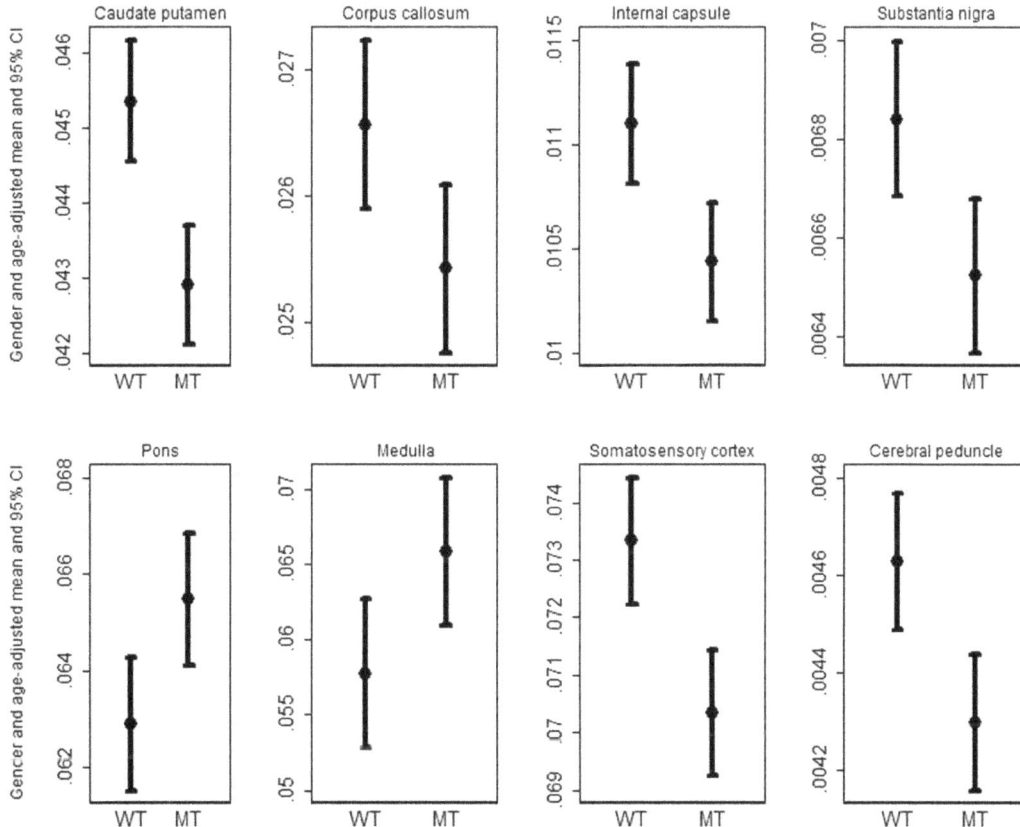

Figure 3. Average and 95% CI of the adjusted brain volume between NL-3 and wild type animals studied from eight out of the 39 regions that showed significant differences in volume.

Table 1. Average ±SD values from DTI indices (FA, MD, and RD) and normalized volume from gray and white matter regions of the brain between wild type (n = 7) and NL-3 (n = 10) mice at 30 days of age.

#	Regions	FA		MD×10^{-3}		RD		Normalize brain volume	
		WT	NL-3	WT	NL-3	WT	NL-3	WT	NL-3
1	Lat ventricle	0.36±0.03	0.32±0.03	0.25±0.02	0.26±0.03	0.21±0.02	0.23±0.03	0.20±0.02	0.19±0.02
2	Hippo CA3	0.26±0.01	0.26±0.01	0.25±0.02	0.25±0.02	0.23±0.02	0.23±0.02	0.20±0.02	0.20±0.01
3	Hippo CA1	0.29±0.02	0.29±0.02	0.26±0.01	0.26±0.01	0.23±0.01	0.23±0.01	0.17±0.01	0.19±0.09
4	Hippo dent gyr	0.26±0.02	0.25±0.01	0.26±0.02	0.27±0.01	0.24±0.02	0.25±0.01	0.18±0.02	0.19±0.01
5	Hippo gen	0.30±0.01	0.30±0.01	0.25±0.02	0.25±0.02	0.22±0.02	0.23±0.02	0.18±0.01	0.18±0.01
6	Olfact system	0.25±0.03	0.26±0.03	0.26±0.02	0.25±0.02	0.25±0.02	0.23±0.02	0.83±0.02	0.91±0.01
7	Frontal cortex	0.24±0.02	0.23±0.02	0.26±0.03	0.25±0.03	0.24±0.02	0.23±0.02	0.44±0.01	0.44±0.03
8	Perirh cortex	0.28±0.03	0.26±0.03	0.26±0.02	0.24±0.02	0.25±0.02	0.23±0.02	0.10±0.01	0.10±0.01
9	Entorhi cortex	0.22±0.02	0.20±0.02	0.27±0.01	0.26±0.01	0.25±0.01	0.24±0.01	0.27±0.01	0.27±0.02
10	Cortex general	0.26±0.03	0.25±0.03	0.26±0.02	0.25±0.02	0.24±0.02	0.23±0.01	0.81±0.02	0.78±0.04
11	Caud putamen	0.22±0.01	0.21±0.02	0.25±0.02	0.24±0.02	0.24±0.02	0.23±0.02	0.46±0.02	0.43±0.02
12	B gang general	0.26±0.02	0.25±0.02	0.23±0.02	0.23±0.02	0.21±0.02	0.22±0.02	0.26±0.01	0.25±0.01
13	Corpus callosum	0.51±0.03	0.50±0.03	0.20±0.03	0.19±0.03	0.16±0.02	0.15±0.02	0.27±0.01	0.25±0.02
14	Ant commissure	050±0.03	0.48±0.04	0.22±0.03	0.21±0.03	0.1 6±0.02	0.16±0.02	0.04±0.03	0.04±0.02
15	Lat olfact tract	0.29±0.04	0.31±0.03	0.26±0.03	0.25±0.02	0.24±0.02	0.22±0.02	0.05±0.06	0.05±0.03
16	Internal capsule	0.53±0.01	0.51±0.02	0.21±0.03	0.20±0.03	0.16±0.02	0.16±0.02	0.11±0.01	0.10±0.01
17	Amygdala	0.22±0.02	0.21±0.02	0.25±0.02	0.26±0.02	0.24±0.02	0.24±0.02	0.32±0.01	0.31±0.02
18	Third ventricle	0.25±0.03	0.24±0.03	0.26±0.02	0.27±0.03	0.24±0.01	0.25±0.03	0.09±0.01	0.09±0.01
19	Thalamus	0.33±0.02	0.32±0.02	0.23±0.03	0.22±0.03	0.21±0.03	0.21±0.03	0.44±0.02	0.44±0.02
20	Hypothalamus	0.26±0.02	0.25±0.04	0.23±0.03	0.21±0.02	0.21±0.03	0.20±0.02	0.20±0.01	0.20±0.01
21	Cereb aqueduct	0.24±0.05	0.25±0.04	0.33±0.10	0.26±0.05	0.31±0.10	0.26±0.05	0.29±0.02	0.31±0.01
22	Substantia nigra	0.38±0.03	0.36±0.02	0.22±0.03	0.22±0.02	0.19±0.02	0.19±0.02	0.07±0.01	0.07±0.01
23	Sup+Inf colli	0.25±0.02	0.25±0.01	0.24±0.02	0.23±0.02	0.23±0.02	0.22±0.02	0.36±0.01	0.36±0.02
24	Periaqued Gray	0.25±0.03	0.25±0.02	0.23±0.04	0.22±0.03	0.21±0.03	0.21±0.03	0.12±0.01	0.13±0.01
25	Midbrain general	0.32±0.02	0.31±0.02	0.23±0.03	0.22±0.02	0.21±0.02	0.20±0.02	0.38±0.01	0.38±0.01
26	Cereb general	0.32±0.03	0.31±0.02	0.22±0.02	0.21±0.02	0.20±0.03	0.19±0.02	0.57±0.02	0.58±0.03
27	Fourth ventricle	0.26±0.03	0.25±0.03	0.37±0.05	0.36±0.07	0.35±0.05	0.34±0.08	0.11±0.01	0.11±0.01
28	Pons	0.35±0.03	0.34±0.02	0.27±0.02	0.25±0.02	0.24±0.02	0.22±0.02	0.62±0.02	0.66±0.03
29	Medulla	0.30±0.02	0.30±0.02	0.26±0.03	0.25±0.02	0.24±0.02	0.23±0.02	0.60±0.09	0.65±0.09
30	Optic nerve	0.45±0.06	0.43±0.05	0.27±0.02	0.25±0.02	0.21±0.02	0.21±0.02	0.57±0.03	0.56±0.05
31	Fornix system	0.49±0.05	0.49±0.03	0.22±0.03	0.22±0.02	0.17±0.03	0.16±0.02	0.12±0.01	0.12±0.01
32	Pituitary	0.34±0.09	0.32±0.07	0.41±0.07	0.35±0.09	0.37±0.08	0.33±0.10	0.03±0.01	0.03±0.01
33	Septum	0.29±0.03	0.26±0.03	0.23±0.03	0.23±0.03	0.21±0.02	0.21±0.02	0.08±0.01	0.08±0.01

Table 1. Cont.

#	Regions	FA		MD×10^{-3}		RD		Normalize brain volume	
		WT	NL-3	WT	NL-3	WT	NL-3	WT	NL-3
34	Motor cortex	0.23±0.02	0.23±0.02	0.26±0.03	0.26±0.03	0.25±0.02	0.24±0.03	0.30±0.01	0.30±0.02
35	Somatosen cortex	0.23±0.02	0.22±0.02	0.26±0.02	0.25±0.02	0.25±0.02	0.24±0.02	0.75±0.02	0.71±0.02
36	Auditory cortex	0.25±0.02	0.24±0.02	0.26±0.02	0.25±0.02	0.24±0.02	0.23±0.02	0.13±0.01	0.13±0.01
37	Visual cortex	0.22±0.02	0.21±0.02	0.27±0.02	0.26±0.02	0.25±0.02	0.25±0.02	0.37±0.02	0.36±0.02
38	Cerebellar cortex	0.29±0.04	0.28±0.02	0.24±0.02	0.23±0.01	0.22±0.02	0.21±0.02	0.82±0.04	0.85±0.05
39	Cereb peduncle	0.52±0.03	0.51±0.04	0.27±0.02	0.26±0.02	0.21±0.02	0.21±0.02	0.45±0.01	0.41±0.02

FA = fractional anisotropy, MD = mean diffusivity, RD = radial diffusivity, WT = wild type. [Lat ventricle = lateral ventricle; Hippo CA3 = hippocampus CA3, Hippo CA1 = hippocampus CA1, Hippo dent gyr = hippocampus dentate gyrus, Hippo gen = hippocampus general, Olfact system = olfactory system, Perih cortex = perirhinal cortex, Entorhi cortex = entorhinal cortex, Caud putamen = caudate putamen, B gang general = basal ganglia general, Ant commissure = anterior commissure, Lat olfact tract = lateral olfactory tract, Cereb aqueduct = cerebral aqueduct, Sup+Inf colli = superior and inferior colliculus, Periaqued gray = periaqueductal gray matter, Cereb general = cerebellum general, Somatosen cortex = somatosensory cortex, Cereb peduncle = cerebral peduncle].

(83 seconds, 95% CI: 49 to 116 seconds, p = 0.002) and a smaller difference at day 28 (52 seconds, 95% CI: 34 to 70 seconds, p< 0.001) and day 69 (56 seconds, 95% CI: 21 to 90 seconds, p = 0.002).

Raw data on volume and DTI indices at each time points are summarized in Table 1, 2, 3. After FDR correction, no significant interaction was noted and some of the segmented brain regions demonstrated significantly reduced volume in NL-3 knock-in as compared to wild type mice in the adjusted analysis that included age and gender as covariate. However, the gender and age-adjusted volume of the pons and medulla were significantly larger in NL-3 knock-in mice than the wild type littermates (Figure 3). On the other hand, none of the DTI indices demonstrated any significant differences in NL-3 mice compared to wild type from any regions of the brain (Table 1, 2, 3).

Correlation between the brain regions which demonstrated significant differences in volume (8 regions) and behavioral data (social sniffing time and elevated zero maze tests) was also performed. No significant correlation between these brain regions and social sniffing time (partial correlations ranged from −0.014 to 0.313, all p>0.05) was observed. However, a significant correlation between the volume of internal capsule (partial correlation = −0.447, p = 0.025) and medulla (partial correlation = 0.407, p = 0.043) and elevated zero maze test score was observed after accounting for strain, gender and age as covariates.

Discussion

We observed significantly lower volume from 6 brain regions and higher volume from the pons and medulla in NL-3 knock-in mice compared to the wild type littermates after considering age and gender as covariates. These volumetric differences were found at all the three stages of development (juvenile, peri-pubescent and early adult) indicating that the NL-3 knock-in mutation causes alterations in these brain areas that are developmentally stable. While volumetric differences were observed, no significant differences in DTI parameters were observed between NL-3 knock-in and WT mice. These results are in agreement with a previously published MRI study on a smaller sample of 108-day-old male NL-3 knock-in mice [3]. Additionally, NL-3 knock-in mice demonstrated significantly reduced social approach and anxiety-related behavior compared to wild type litter-mates after considering age and gender as covariates.

The neuroligin and neurexin genes have been recognized in human autism association studies [7,30]. Jamain et al. [7], reported an inherited mutation in NL-3 gene within a highly conserved region of the gene in two male siblings, one with autism and severe intellectual disabilities and seizures and the other with Asperger syndrome. To gain insights into the possible mechanisms of ASDs, this genetic mutation was introduced in the R451C substitution mutation into a mouse to create the NL-3 R451C knock-in mouse model associated with autism [6]. However, conflicting results were reported from the behavioral studies on this model, with one group [6] reporting behavioral abnormalities and other group [8] not observing any autism relevant behavioral abnormalities in this model. We also observed significantly lower social approach behavior in NL-3 mice compared to wild type litter mates. While our findings may seem to be similar to the observations made by Tabuchi et al [6] and in contrast to the study by Chadman et al [8], it should be noted that our experiments and analysis were somewhat distinct from both studies in that we conducted Social Approach testing at multiple ages, and found the reduction in social approach behavior to be

Table 2. Average ± SD values from DTI indices (FA, MD, and RD) and normalized volume from gray and white matter regions of the brain between wild type (n = 9) and NL-3 (n = 10) mice at 50 days of age.

#	Regions	FA		MD×10^{-3}		RD		Normalize brain volume	
		WT	NL-3	WT	NL-3	WT	NL-3	WT	NL-3
1	Lat ventricle	0.34±0.04	0.32±0.04	0.24±0.03	0.26±0.03	0.21±0.02	0.24±0.03	0.20±0.01	0.20±0.02
2	Hippo CA3	0.27±0.02	0.28±0.02	0.24±0.02	0.25±0.02	0.22±0.02	0.23±0.02	0.21±0.02	0.21±0.01
3	Hippo CA1	0.30±0.02	0.30±0.02	0.25±0.01	0.27±0.03	0.23±0.01	0.24±0.02	0.18±0.01	0.17±0.01
4	Hippo dent gyr	0.27±0.03	0.27±0.03	0.26±0.02	0.28±0.02	0.24±0.02	0.26±0.02	0.19±0.02	0.19±0.01
5	Hippo gen	0.30±0.02	0.31±0.03	0.24±0.02	0.25±0.02	0.22±0.02	0.25±0.02	0.19±0.02	0.19±0.01
6	Olfact system	0.24±0.02	0.24±0.02	0.25±0.03	0.26±0.02	0.24±0.03	0.24±0.03	0.80±0.07	0.72±0.04
7	Frontal cortex	0.23±0.01	0.23±0.02	0.24±0.03	0.25±0.03	0.23±0.02	0.24±0.03	0.44±0.02	0.43±0.02
8	Perih cortex	0.26±0.02	0.26±0.03	0.24±0.03	0.26±0.03	0.22±0.02	0.24±0.02	0.10±0.01	0.10±0.01
9	Entorhi cortex	0.21±0.01	0.21±0.02	0.25±0.03	0.28±0.03	0.24±0.03	0.26±0.03	0.28±0.02	0.28±0.02
10	Cortex general	0.25±0.02	0.26±0.02	0.24±0.02	0.25±0.03	0.23±0.02	0.24±0.01	0.79±0.03	0.77±0.01
11	Caud putamen	0.22±0.02	0.22±0.01	0.24±0.02	0.24±0.02	0.23±0.02	0.23±0.02	0.47±0.02	0.44±0.01
12	B gang general	0.26±0.02	0.26±0.02	0.22±0.02	0.23±0.02	0.21±0.02	0.22±0.02	0.27±0.02	0.26±0.02
13	Corpus callosum	0.51±0.02	0.51±0.03	0.18±0.02	0.19±0.02	0.15±0.01	0.15±0.01	0.27±0.02	0.25±0.02
14	Ant commissure	0.48±0.03	0.46±0.02	0.20±0.02	0.20±0.02	0.1 5±0.01	0.16±0.02	0.036±0.01	0.035±0.01
15	Lat olfact tract	0.28±0.03	0.28±0.02	0.26±0.03	0.25±0.02	0.24±0.02	0.22±0.02	0.05±0.01	0.04±0.01
16	Internal capsule	0.53±0.04	0.52±0.02	0.20±0.02	0.20±0.02	0.15±0.02	0.15±0.02	0.12±0.01	0.11±0.01
17	Amygdala	0.21±0.01	0.22±0.02	0.24±0.04	0.26±0.03	0.23±0.03	0.24±0.02	0.34±0.02	0.32±0.02
18	Third ventricle	0.24±0.04	0.22±0.02	0.26±0.03	0.27±0.03	0.25±0.03	0.26±0.03	0.09±0.01	0.10±0.01
19	Thalamus	0.34±0.04	0.33±0.02	0.21±0.02	0.22±0.02	0.20±0.02	0.20±0.02	0.46±0.03	0.44±0.02
20	Hypothalamus	0.26±0.03	0.26±0.02	0.21±0.03	0.21±0.02	0.20±0.03	0.20±0.02	0.20±0.02	0.20±0.01
21	Cereb aqueduct	0.28±0.09	0.23±0.03	0.28±0.08	0.28±0.05	0.26±0.08	0.27±0.06	0.03±0.01	0.03±0.02
22	Substantia nigra	0.38±0.03	0.37±0.02	0.21±0.02	0.22±0.02	0.19±0.02	0.19±0.02	0.07±0.01	0.07±0.01
23	Sup+Inf colli	0.24±0.03	0.26±0.02	0.22±0.02	0.23±0.02	0.21±0.02	0.22±0.02	0.04±0.03	0.04±0.02
24	Periaqued Gray	0.27±0.06	0.26±0.03	0.20±0.03	0.22±0.02	0.19±0.03	0.21±0.02	0.03±0.01	0.03±0.01
25	Midbrain general	0.33±0.04	0.32±0.02	0.22±0.02	0.23±0.01	0.20±0.02	0.21±0.01	0.40±0.01	0.39±0.01
26	Cereb general	0.32±0.01	0.32±0.01	0.21±0.01	0.21±0.01	0.19±0.01	0.19±0.01	0.56±0.03	0.65±0.02
27	Fourth ventricle	0.25±0.03	0.23±0.03	0.36±0.01	0.39±0.01	0.34±0.01	0.38±0.01	0.10±0.02	0.11±0.01
28	Pons	0.35±0.02	0.34±0.02	0.24±0.02	0.25±0.02	0.21±0.02	0.23±0.02	0.64±0.04	0.66±0.02
29	Medulla	0.33±0.07	0.37±0.11	0.25±0.03	0.26±0.03	0.22±0.03	0.23±0.03	0.52±0.11	0.65±0.11
30	Optic nerve	0.44±0.03	0.43±0.05	0.26±0.02	0.25±0.02	0.21±0.02	0.21±0.02	0.06±0.01	0.06±0.01
31	Fornix system	0.50±0.03	0.49±0.02	0.20±0.02	0.20±0.02	0.15±0.02	0.15±0.01	0.13±0.02	0.13±0.04
32	Pituitary	0.29±0.04	0.28±0.05	0.38±0.01	0.42±0.01	0.36±0.01	0.40±0.01	0.03±0.01	0.03±0.01
33	Septum	0.29±0.03	0.27±0.04	0.22±0.02	0.24±0.02	0.20±0.02	0.22±0.02	0.08±0.01	0.08±0.01

Table 2. Cont.

#	Regions	FA		MD×10^{-3}		RD		Normalize brain volume	
		WT	NL-3	WT	NL-3	WT	NL-3	WT	NL-3
34	Motor cortex	0.21±0.01	0.22±0.02	0.25±0.03	0.25±0.03	0.24±0.03	0.24±0.03	0.32±0.02	0.30±0.02
35	Somatosen cortex	0.21±0.01	0.22±0.01	0.24±0.03	0.25±0.03	0.23±0.03	0.24±0.03	0.76±0.04	0.72±0.02
36	Auditory cortex	0.24±0.01	0.25±0.03	0.24±0.03	0.26±0.03	0.22±0.03	0.24±0.03	0.13±0.01	0.13±0.01
37	Visual cortex	0.20±0.02	0.22±0.02	0.25±0.03	0.25±0.03	0.24±0.03	0.24±0.03	0.36±0.03	0.35±0.03
38	Cerebellar cortex	0.29±0.01	0.27±0.02	0.23±0.01	0.24±0.02	0.21±0.01	0.23±0.02	0.81±0.04	0.84±0.03
39	Cereb peduncle	0.53±0.03	0.52±0.03	0.26±0.03	0.27±0.02	0.20±0.02	0.21±0.03	0.49±0.04	0.44±0.01

FA = fractional an sotropy, MD = mean diffusivity, RD = radial diffusivity, WT = wild type. [Lat ventricle = lateral ventricle; Hippo CA3 = hippocampus CA3, Hippo CA1 = hippocampus CA1, Hippo dent gyr = hippocampus dentate gyrus, Hippo gen = hippocampus general, Olfact system = olfactory system, Perirh cortex = perirhinal cortex, Entorhi cortex = entorhinal cortex, Caud putamen = caudate putamen, B gang general = basal ganglia general, Ant commissure = anterior commissure, Lat olfact tract = lateral olfactory tract, Cereb aqueduct = cerebral aqueduct, Sup+Inf colli = superior and inferior colliculus, Periaqued gray = periaqueductal gray matter, Cereb general = cerebellum general, Somatosen cortex = somatosensory cortex, Cereb peduncle = cerebral peduncle].

more striking at earlier ages whereas the other studies conducted Social Approach Testing only in adult mice.

MRI has been used for examining both volume changes and white matter structural integrity in patients with ASD [9,31] as well as in mouse models of ASD [2,3,12,14]. We observed significantly lower volume from the caudate putamen, substantia nigra, somatosensory cortex, corpus callosum, internal capsule and cerebral peduncles along with significantly higher volume from the pons and medulla in NL-3 knock-in mice compared to wild type litter mates. The volumetric differences observed in NL-3 mice in the current study suggest that the microstructural abnormality in this model is diffuse and affects several regions of the brain. A previous MRI study on NL-3 mice brains also reported lower volume in major white matter regions especially the corpus callosum, internal capsule and cerebral peduncles [3]. Specific structures, like the corpus callosum, have long been implicated in human autism and reduced corpus callosum volume has been reported in various mouse models of autism [3,12,20], suggesting decreased interhemispheric connectivity in these models. The corpus callosum enables communication between the two hemi-spheres and reduced corpus callosum size may indicate white matter deficits that result in impaired cortical connectivity [32]. The lower volume of the other white matter regions (internal capsule and cerebral peduncle) in NL-3 mice suggest a plausible neural basis for disrupted systems-level connectivity in this model [33]. These white matter regions have also been reported to be smaller in size in mouse models relevant to autism including NL-3 knock-in [3] and the integrin β3 [34] knockout models. Human autism MRI studies have also reported reduced internal capsule and cerebral peduncle volumes [35], however, many other studies indicate enlargement of brain and subcortical regions in ASD.

ASD comprises a set of neurodevelopmental disorders affecting socio-communicative behavior along with abnormalities in the sensorimotor skill learning, oculomotor control, and executive functioning. Some of these impairments may be related to abnormalities in the caudate nuclei, substantia nigra and somatosensory cortex as these regions have been reported to be abnormal in ASD. One of the core behavioral symptoms in autism is restricted and repetitive behaviors, and these behaviors have often been thought to be associated with the caudate putamen or striatum [36]. Structural imaging studies have also reported volumetric differences in the caudate putamen and cortex of humans with ASD [10,37]. Similar to a previous report, our results of reduced volume from these regions indicate that genetic differences due to the NL-3 knock-in mutation might be responsible for the volumetric changes in this model [3].

The link between neuroanatomical findings and behavioral symptoms is vital for understanding the role of structural changes in the etiology of ASD. Investigations of structural measures of the corpus callosum and other white matter regions have reported decreased size along with under connectivity associated with behavioral abnormalities in ASDs [12,20]. Overall reduction of whole brain volume in NL-3 mouse has also been reported previously using ex vivo MRI [18].

While our results of reduced volume in both gray and white matter of NL-3 knock-in agree with previous published reports in human ASD as well as in mouse models relevant to ASD, it is worth noting that there is significant heterogeneity in the literature with respect to volumetric differences in cortical thickness and morphology in ASD, with at times seemingly contradictory results, depending on the age, IQ, and clinical severity of the study population [38]. One potential reason for the variability in volumetric differences in human ASD studies could be due to its etiological and clinical heterogeneity. In the current study, we also

Table 3. Average ± SD values from DTI indices (FA, MD, and RD) and normalized volume from gray and white matter regions of the brain between wild type (n = 8) and NL-3 (n = 5) mice at 70 days of age.

#	Regions	FA		MD×10^{-3}		RD		Normalize brain volume	
		WT	NL-3	WT	NL-3	WT	NL-3	WT	NL-3
1	Lat ventricle	0.31±0.03	0.29±0.02	0.26±0.04	0.30±0.03	0.24±0.04	0.27±0.04	0.20±0.01	0.21±0.02
2	Hippo CA3	0.27±0.04	0.24±0.02	0.25±0.03	0.25±0.02	0.23±0.03	0.24±0.02	0.21±0.01	0.21±0.02
3	Hippo CA1	0.29±0.03	0.27±0.02	0.26±0.02	0.27±0.02	0.24±0.02	0.24±0.02	0.16±0.01	0.17±0.01
4	Hippo dent gyr	0.27±0.04	0.24±0.02	0.28±0.03	0.28±0.03	0.26±0.03	0.26±0.02	0.19±0.02	0.19±0.01
5	Hippo gen	0.30±0.03	0.28±0.02	0.25±0.02	0.25±0.02	0.22±0.02	0.23±0.02	0.18±0.01	0.19±0.01
6	Olfact system	0.23±0.02	0.25±0.02	0.25±0.02	0.25±0.02	0.23±0.02	0.23±0.02	0.81±0.17	0.89±0.15
7	Frontal cortex	0.22±0.02	0.23±0.02	0.25±0.02	0.24±0.02	0.23±0.02	0.23±0.02	0.42±0.02	0.43±0.01
8	Perirh cortex	0.26±0.03	0.26±0.03	0.25±0.02	0.24±0.02	0.24±0.02	0.23±0.02	0.09±0.01	0.10±0.01
9	Entorhi cortex	0.21±0.02	0.20±0.02	0.27±0.01	0.26±0.01	0.25±0.01	0.26±0.01	0.25±0.03	0.26±0.02
10	Cortex general	0.26±0.02	0.25±0.02	0.24±0.01	0.24±0.01	0.23±0.01	0.23±0.01	0.75±0.04	0.75±0.01
11	Caud putamen	0.21±0.02	0.21±0.02	0.24±0.02	0.23±0.02	0.23±0.02	0.22±0.02	0.44±0.02	0.44±0.01
12	B gang general	0.26±0.01	0.25±0.02	0.22±0.02	0.22±0.02	0.21±0.02	0.21±0.02	0.26±0.01	0.26±0.01
13	Corpus callosum	0.53±0.02	0.52±0.02	0.17±0.02	0.17±0.02	0.13±0.02	0.13±0.02	0.26±0.01	0.26±0.01
14	Ant commissure	0.48±0.02	0.48±0.03	0.19±0.02	0.20±0.03	0.1 5±0.01	0.15±0.02	0.04±0.03	0.04±0.03
15	Lat olfact tract	0.26±0.03	0.28±0.03	0.26±0.02	0.25±0.02	0.24±0.02	0.22±0.01	0.05±0.01	0.05±0.01
16	Internal capsule	0.53±0.03	0.51±0.03	0.19±0.03	0.18±0.03	0.14±0.02	0.14±0.02	0.11±0.01	0.10±0.02
17	Amygdala	0.21±0.02	0.21±0.02	0.25±0.01	0.25±0.02	0.24±0.01	0.24±0.02	0.32±0.02	0.32±0.02
18	Third ventricle	0.21±0.03	0.20±0.03	0.28±0.03	0.27±0.04	0.27±0.03	0.26±0.04	0.10±0.04	0.10±0.01
19	Thalamus	0.34±0.06	0.31±0.01	0.21±0.04	0.21±0.02	0.19±0.04	0.20±0.02	0.44±0.01	0.42±0.02
20	Hypothalamus	0.24±0.02	0.24±0.03	0.19±0.01	0.21±0.03	0.18±0.01	0.20±0.03	0.20±0.01	0.20±0.01
21	Cereb aqueduct	0.22±0.04	0.22±0.03	0.39±0.07	0.29±0.07	0.38±0.08	0.28±0.07	0.30±0.03	0.31±0.04
22	Substantia nigra	0.38±0.04	0.36±0.02	0.20±0.03	0.21±0.03	0.21±0.02	0.22±0.01	0.07±0.01	0.07±0.01
23	Sup-Inf colli	0.25±0.03	0.24±0.01	0.23±0.02	0.23±0.02	0.22±0.02	0.22±0.02	0.35±0.02	0.35±0.01
24	Periaqued Gray	0.25±0.05	0.23±0.01	0.20±0.03	0.22±0.03	0.19±0.03	0.21±0.03	0.13±0.01	0.13±0.01
25	Midbrain general	0.32±0.04	0.30±0.02	0.22±0.03	0.22±0.03	0.20±0.03	0.20±0.02	0.38±0.02	0.38±0.01
26	Cereb general	0.31±0.01	0.31±0.02	0.21±0.01	0.22±0.01	0.21±0.01	0.22±0.02	0.58±0.03	0.58±0.02
27	Fourth ventricle	0.22±0.02	0.23±0.02	0.44±0.06	0.38±0.05	0.43±0.06	0.38±0.05	0.11±0.01	0.12±0.02
28	Pons	0.33±0.02	0.33±0.03	0.25±0.02	0.24±0.03	0.22±0.02	0.22±0.02	0.64±0.02	0.66±0.03
29	Medulla	0.29±0.02	0.29±0.02	0.26±0.02	0.24±0.02	0.23±0.02	0.22±0.02	0.61±0.11	0.69±0.04
30	Optic nerve	0.41±0.02	0.41±0.04	0.27±0.02	0.24±0.03	0.23±0.02	0.20±0.02	0.06±0.01	0.06±0.01
31	Fornix system	0.51±0.03	0.49±0.03	0.19±0.03	0.19±0.03	0.14±0.02	0.15±0.02	0.13±0.01	0.13±0.01
32	Pituitary	0.28±0.05	0.27±0.06	0.19±0.03	0.19±0.03	0.14±0.02	0.15±0.02	0.03±0.01	0.03±0.01
33	Septum	0.26±0.03	0.24±0.03	0.22±0.03	0.22±0.02	0.20±0.03	0.21±0.02	0.08±0.01	0.08±0.01

Table 3. Cont.

#	Regions	FA		MD×10^{-3}		RD		Normalize brain volume	
		WT	NL-3	WT	NL-3	WT	NL-3	WT	NL-3
34	Motor cortex	0.22±0.01	0.21±0.02	0.24±0.02	0.25±0.01	0.28±0.02	0.23±0.01	0.29±0.02	0.29±0.01
35	Somatosen cortex	0.21±0.02	0.20±0.02	0.24±0.02	0.24±0.01	0.23±0.01	0.23±0.01	0.71±0.02	0.68±0.02
36	Auditory cortex	0.24±0.03	0.22±0.01	0.25±0.02	0.24±0.01	0.23±0.02	0.23±0.01	0.12±0.01	0.12±0.01
37	Visual cortex	0.20±0.02	0.19±0.01	0.25±0.01	0.24±0.01	0.24±0.01	0.23±0.01	0.34±0.01	0.32±0.01
38	Cerebelar cortex	0.27±0.01	0.27±0.02	0.25±0.02	0.24±0.01	0.24±0.02	0.23±0.01	0.84±0.04	0.83±0.04
39	Cereb peduncle	0.54±0.04	0.51±0.04	0.24±0.04	0.26±0.03	0.18±0.04	0.21±0.02	0.45±0.01	0.44±0.01

FA = fractional anisotropy, MD = mean diffusivity, RD = radial diffusivity, WT = wild type. [Lat ventricle = lateral ventricle; Hippo CA3 = hippocampus CA3, Hippo CA1 = hippocampus CA1, Hippo dent gyr = hippocampus dentate gyrus, Hippo gen = hippocampus general, Olfact system = olfactory system, Perirh cortex = perirhinal cortex, Entorhi cortex = entorhinal cortex, Caud putamen = caudate putamen, B gang general = basal ganglia general, Ant commissure = anterior commissure, Lat olfact tract = lateral olfactory tract, Cereb aqueduct = cerebral aqueduct, Sup+Inf colli = superior and inferior collicus, Periaqued gray = periaqueductal gray matter, Cereb general = cerebellum general, Somatosen cortex = somatosensory cortex, Cereb peduncle = cerebral peduncle].

observed these volumetric differences, which occurred at all three developmental stages of the animal, confirming that the differences were due to genetic mutation that stayed throughout the life span of the animal. Reduced brain volume from several gray and white matter regions of the brain in the NL-3 mice suggest that volumetric MRI can be used to better understand the biological basis of behavioral changes seen in this genetically defined model of ASD.

DTI is sensitive to the integrity of white matter and provides a better understanding of the neuroanatomical abnormalities in ASD. Several DTI studies have shed light on microstructural integrity of the white matter and developmental abnormalities in various brain regions in ASD in human [10,11,15–17,35,38] as well as mouse models relevant to ASD [2,12,14,34]. DTI has also been proposed as a surrogate imaging biomarker in the diagnosis of ASD in humans [35,39–41]. It has also been reported that DTI is not only sensitive for detection of microstructural abnormalities but also correlates with behavioral abnormalities in the BALB/cJ mouse model relevant for ASD [12]. However, recently Koldewyn et al. [42], reported no differences in major white matter structures between autistic children and healthy controls except in right inferior longitudinal fasciculus using DTI. The authors of this study suggested that the abnormalities in FA of ASD subjects reported in previously published studies may probably be due to an artifact from differential head motion during the scan of autistic children [42,43] raising concerns about the validity of DTI as an imaging biomarker for ASD. We also did not find any significant differences in DTI parameters between NL-3 knock-in and wild type animals in the current study, which may be due to the fact that the genotypic differences in NL-3 mutation may not have had a sufficient effect on water diffusion to affect DTI parameters in this model.

We did not observe any significant correlation between brain volumes and social behavior of the mice. However a significant correlation between volume from internal capsule and medulla with anxiety score was observed in these animals. These preliminary studies in a small set of behavior assays used for assessing rodent behaviors indicate that imaging and behavior tests may act as independent parameters for the diagnosis of ASD in mouse models. Although more studies are needed, we believe that developmental studies involving behavioral and imaging assays in a genetically defined model of ASD, as performed in the current study, will aid in further understanding the biology of ASD in relevant mouse models.

Our results should be interpreted with caution in light of limitations of the study, which include the following: 1) we have used only two behavioral assays - the social approach test and the elevated zero maze test, however other behavioral assays including studies of repetitive behaviors, ultrasonic vocalizations, social memory, open field locomotion, Morris water maze spatial learning and acquisition could provide a more detailed interpretation of behavioral phenotypes relevant to ASD as reported in previous studies [6,8,18]. 2) Another limitation is that we did not perform any histological studies on brain tissue to confirm the differences in volume of the various regions in the NL-3 mice. Histological measures of volume are time consuming and are confounded by the variabilities induced in tissue sectioning and fixation and thus image based segmentation, as reported here, is believed to provide more accurate volume estimates of brain anatomy. Nevertheless, future studies correlating histological assessments with MRI are warranted.

In summary, reduced volume of several white and gray matter areas in the brains of NL-3 knock-in mice suggests that these structural changes are induced by the mutation in the NL-3 gene.

Future imaging and behavior studies on NL-4 knock-in and knockout models, which have been suggested to be more relevant to ASD [44], may help in establishing the role of neuroligins in ASD.

References

1. Geschwind DH (2008) Autism: many genes, common pathways? Cell 135: 391–395.
2. Kumar M, Kim S, Pickup S, Chen R, Fairless AH, et al. (2012) Longitudinal in-vivo diffusion tensor imaging for assessing brain developmental changes in BALB/cJ mice, a model of reduced sociability relevant to autism. Brain Res 1455: 56–67.
3. Ellegood J, Lerch JP, Henkelman RM (2011) Brain abnormalities in a Neuroligin3 R451C knockin mouse model associated with autism. Autism Res 4: 368–376.
4. El-Kordi A, Winkler D, Hammerschmidt K, Kastner A, Krueger D, et al. (2013) Development of an autism severity score for mice using Nlgn4 null mutants as a construct-valid model of heritable monogenic autism. Behav Brain Res 251: 41–49.
5. Li X, Zou H, Brown WT (2012) Genes associated with autism spectrum disorder. Brain Res Bull 88: 543–552.
6. Tabuchi K, Blundell J, Etherton MR, Hammer RE, Liu X, et al. (2007) A neuroligin-3 mutation implicated in autism increases inhibitory synaptic transmission in mice. Science 318: 71–76.
7. Jamain S, Quach H, Betancur C, Rastam M, Colineaux C, et al. (2003) Mutations of the X-linked genes encoding neuroligins NLGN3 and NLGN4 are associated with autism. Nat Genet 34: 27–29.
8. Chadman KK, Gong S, Scattoni ML, Boltuck SE, Gandhy SU, et al. (2008) Minimal aberrant behavioral phenotypes of neuroligin-3 R451C knockin mice. Autism Res 1: 147–158.
9. Verhoeven JS, De Cock P, Lagae L, Sunaert S (2010) Neuroimaging of autism. Neuroradiology 52: 3–14.
10. Stigler KA, McDonald BC, Anand A, Saykin AJ, McDougle CJ (2011) Structural and functional magnetic resonance imaging of autism spectrum disorders. Brain Res 1380: 146–161.
11. Scheel C, Rotarska-Jagiela A, Schilbach L, Lehnhardt FG, Krug B, et al. (2011) Imaging derived cortical thickness reduction in high-functioning autism: key regions and temporal slope. Neuroimage 58: 391–400.
12. Kim S, Pickup S, Fairless AH, Ittyerah R, Dow HC, et al. (2012) Association between sociability and diffusion tensor imaging in BALB/cJ mice. NMR Biomed 25: 104–112.
13. Horev G, Ellegood J, Lerch JP, Son YE, Muthuswamy L, et al. (2011) Dosage-dependent phenotypes in models of 16p11.2 lesions found in autism. Proc Natl Acad Sci U S A 108: 17076–17081.
14. Ellegood J, Babineau BA, Henkelman RM, Lerch JP, Crawley JN (2013) Neuroanatomical analysis of the BTBR mouse model of autism using magnetic resonance imaging and diffusion tensor imaging. Neuroimage 70: 288–300.
15. Kleinhans NM, Pauley G, Richards T, Neuhaus E, Martin N, et al. (2012) Age-related abnormalities in white matter microstructure in autism spectrum disorders. Brain Res 1479: 1–16.
16. Walker L, Gozzi M, Lenroot R, Thurm A, Behseta B, et al. (2012) Diffusion tensor imaging in young children with autism: biological effects and potential confounds. Biol Psychiatry 72: 1043–1051.
17. Billeci L, Calderoni S, Tosetti M, Catani M, Muratori F (2012) White matter connectivity in children with autism spectrum disorders: a tract-based spatial statistics study. BMC Neurol 12: 148.
18. Radyushkin K, Hammerschmidt K, Boretius S, Varoqueaux F, El-Kordi A, et al. (2009) Neuroligin-3-deficient mice: model of a monogenic heritable form of autism with an olfactory deficit. Genes Brain Behav 8: 416–425.
19. Sankoorikal GM, Kaercher KA, Boon CJ, Lee JK, Brodkin ES (2006) A mouse model system for genetic analysis of sociability: C57BL/6J versus BALB/cJ inbred mouse strains. Biol Psychiatry 59: 415–423.
20. Fairless AH, Dow HC, Kreibich AS, Torre M, Kuruvilla M, et al. (2012) Sociability and brain development in BALB/cJ and C57BL/6J mice. Behav Brain Res 228: 299–310.
21. Ecker DJ, Stein P, Xu Z, Williams CJ, Kopf GS, et al. (2004) Long-term effects of culture of preimplantation mouse embryos on behavior. Proc Natl Acad Sci U S A 101: 1595–1600.
22. Stein JM, Bergman W, Fang Y, Davison L, Brensinger C, et al. (2006) Behavioral and neurochemical alterations in mice lacking the RNA-binding protein translin. J Neurosci 26: 2184–2196.
23. Mori S, van Zijl PC (1998) A motion correction scheme by twin-echo navigation for diffusion-weighted magnetic resonance imaging with multiple RF echo acquisition. Magn Reson Med 40: 511–516.
24. Neeman M, Freyer JP, Sillerud LO (1991) A simple method for obtaining cross-term-free images for diffusion anisotropy studies in NMR microimaging. Magn Reson Med 21: 138–143.
25. Jiang H, van Zijl PC, Kim J, Pearlson GD, Mori S (2006) DtiStudio: resource program for diffusion tensor computation and fiber bundle tracking. Comput Methods Programs Biomed 81: 106–116.
26. Cook PA, Bai Y, Nedjati-Gilani S, Seunarine KK, Hall MG, et al. (2006) Camino: Open-Source Diffusion-MRI Reconstruction and Processing. International Society for Magentic Resonance in Medicine. Seattle, WA, USA: International Society for Magentic Resonance in Medicine. pp. P2759.
27. Bai J, Trinh TL, Chuang KH, Qiu A (2012) Atlas-based automatic mouse brain image segmentation revisited: model complexity vs. image registration. Magn Reson Imaging 30: 789–798.
28. Avants BB, Yushkevich P, Pluta J, Minkoff D, Korczykowski M, et al. (2010) The optimal template effect in hippocampus studies of diseased populations. Neuroimage 49: 2457–2466.
29. Warfield SK, Zou KH, Wells WM (2004) Simultaneous truth and performance level estimation (STAPLE): an algorithm for the validation of image segmentation. IEEE Trans Med Imaging 23: 903–921.
30. Laumonnier F, Bonnet-Brilhault F, Gomot M, Blanc R, David A, et al. (2004) X-linked mental retardation and autism are associated with a mutation in the NLGN4 gene, a member of the neuroligin family. Am J Hum Genet 74: 552–557.
31. Beacher FD, Minati L, Baron-Cohen S, Lombardo MV, Lai MC, et al. (2012) Autism attenuates sex differences in brain structure: a combined voxel-based morphometry and diffusion tensor imaging study. AJNR Am J Neuroradiol 33: 83–89.
32. Just MA, Keller TA, Malave VL, Kana RK, Varma S (2012) Autism as a neural systems disorder: a theory of frontal-posterior underconnectivity. Neurosci Biobehav Rev 36: 1292–1313.
33. Ringo JL (1991) Neuronal interconnection as a function of brain size. Brain Behav Evol 38: 1–6.
34. Ellegood J, Henkelman RM, Lerch JP (2012) Neuroanatomical Assessment of the Integrin beta3 Mouse Model Related to Autism and the Serotonin System Using High Resolution MRI. Front Psychiatry 3: 37.
35. Travers BG, Adluru N, Ennis C, Tromp do PM, Destiche D, et al. (2012) Diffusion tensor imaging in autism spectrum disorder: a review. Autism Res 5: 289–313.
36. Sears LL, Vest C, Mohamed S, Bailey J, Ranson BJ, et al. (1999) An MRI study of the basal ganglia in autism. Prog Neuropsychopharmacol Biol Psychiatry 23: 613–624.
37. Amaral DG, Schumann CM, Nordahl CW (2008) Neuroanatomy of autism. Trends Neurosci 31: 137–145.
38. Baribeau DA, Anagnostou E (2013) A Comparison of Neuroimaging Findings in Childhood Onset Schizophrenia and Autism Spectrum Disorder: A Review of the Literature. Front Psychiatry 4: 175.
39. Alexander AL, Lee JE, Lazar M, Boudos R, DuBray MB, et al. (2007) Diffusion tensor imaging of the corpus callosum in Autism. Neuroimage 34: 61–73.
40. Barnea-Goraly N, Kwon H, Menon V, Eliez S, Lotspeich L, et al. (2004) White matter structure in autism: preliminary evidence from diffusion tensor imaging. Biol Psychiatry 55: 323–326.
41. Travers BG, Bigler ED, Tromp do PM, Adluru N, Froehlich AL, et al. (2014) Longitudinal processing speed impairments in males with autism and the effects of white matter microstructure. Neuropsychologia 53: 137–145.
42. Koldewyn K, Yendiki A, Weigelt S, Gweon H, Julian J, et al. (2014) Differences in the right inferior longitudinal fasciculus but no general disruption of white matter tracts in children with autism spectrum disorder. Proc Natl Acad Sci U S A 111: 1981–1986.
43. Yendiki A, Koldewyn K, Kakunoori S, Kanwisher N, Fischl B (2013) Spurious group differences due to head motion in a diffusion MRI study. Neuroimage 88C: 79–90.
44. Jamain S, Radyushkin K, Hammerschmidt K, Granon S, Boretius S, et al. (2008) Reduced social interaction and ultrasonic communication in a mouse model of monogenic heritable autism. Proc Natl Acad Sci U S A 105: 1710–1715.

Author Contributions

Conceived and designed the experiments: MK HP TA ESB. Performed the experiments: MK RI SP. Analyzed the data: MK WH JTD. Contributed reagents/materials/analysis tools: JCG CK JTD. Wrote the paper: MK HP.

Metabolomics as a Tool for Discovery of Biomarkers of Autism Spectrum Disorder in the Blood Plasma of Children

Paul R. West[1]*, David G. Amaral[2], Preeti Bais[3], Alan M. Smith[1], Laura A. Egnash[1], Mark E. Ross[1], Jessica A. Palmer[1], Burr R. Fontaine[1], Kevin R. Conard[1], Blythe A. Corbett[4], Gabriela G. Cezar[1¤], Elizabeth L. R. Donley[1], Robert E. Burrier[1]

1 Stemina Biomarker Discovery, Madison, Wisconsin, United States of America, 2 The M.I.N.D. Institute and Department of Psychiatry and Behavioral Sciences, University of California Davis, Davis, California, United States of America, 3 The Jackson Laboratory for Genomic medicine, University of Connecticut Health Center, Farmington, Connecticut, United States of America, 4 Department of Psychiatry, Psychology and Kennedy Center, Vanderbilt University, Nashville, Tennessee, United States of America

Abstract

Background: The diagnosis of autism spectrum disorder (ASD) at the earliest age possible is important for initiating optimally effective intervention. In the United States the average age of diagnosis is 4 years. Identifying metabolic biomarker signatures of ASD from blood samples offers an opportunity for development of diagnostic tests for detection of ASD at an early age.

Objectives: To discover metabolic features present in plasma samples that can discriminate children with ASD from typically developing (TD) children. The ultimate goal is to identify and develop blood-based ASD biomarkers that can be validated in larger clinical trials and deployed to guide individualized therapy and treatment.

Methods: Blood plasma was obtained from children aged 4 to 6, 52 with ASD and 30 age-matched TD children. Samples were analyzed using 5 mass spectrometry-based methods designed to orthogonally measure a broad range of metabolites. Univariate, multivariate and machine learning methods were used to develop models to rank the importance of features that could distinguish ASD from TD.

Results: A set of 179 statistically significant features resulting from univariate analysis were used for multivariate modeling. Subsets of these features properly classified the ASD and TD samples in the 61-sample training set with average accuracies of 84% and 86%, and with a maximum accuracy of 81% in an independent 21-sample validation set.

Conclusions: This analysis of blood plasma metabolites resulted in the discovery of biomarkers that may be valuable in the diagnosis of young children with ASD. The results will form the basis for additional discovery and validation research for 1) determining biomarkers to develop diagnostic tests to detect ASD earlier and improve patient outcomes, 2) gaining new insight into the biochemical mechanisms of various subtypes of ASD 3) identifying biomolecular targets for new modes of therapy, and 4) providing the basis for individualized treatment recommendations.

Editor: Subhabrata Sanyal, Biogen Idec, United States of America

Funding: Stemina funded this study. The funder provided support in the form of salaries for authors (PRW, LAE, AMS, MER, JAP, BRF, KRC, GGC, ELRD, and REB), but did not have any additional role in the study design, data collection and analysis, decision to publish, or preparation of the manuscript.

Competing Interests: All authors except Blythe Corbett have, within the past five years, received salary from, and/or hold stocks or stock options in, Stemina Biomarker Discovery, which as a company may gain or lose financially from the publication of this manuscript. PRW, LAE, AMS, MER, JAP, BRF, KRC, GGC, ELRD and REB are employees of Stemina, whose company funded this study and holds, or is currently, applying for patents relating to the content of the manuscript as follows: BIOMARKERS OF AUTISM SPECTRUM DISORDER; PCT App No. PCT/US2014/045397 and METABOLIC BIOMARKERS OF AUTISM; PCT Application No. PCT/US2011/034654. There are no further patents, products in development, or marketed products to declare.

* Email: pwest@stemina.com

¤ Current address: Pfizer Inc., São Paulo, Brazil

Introduction

Autism spectrum disorder (ASD) is a lifelong neurodevelopmental disorder characterized by social deficits, impaired verbal and nonverbal communication and repetitive movements or circumscribed interests [1]. About 1 in 68 children has been identified with autism spectrum disorder (ASD) according to estimates from CDC's Autism and Developmental Disabilities Monitoring (ADDM) Network. The current process for a clinical diagnosis includes establishing a developmental history and assessments of speech, language, intellectual abilities, and educational or vocational attainment. In practice, these methods lead to a diagnosis at an average age of 4 years [2] in the United States. It is recognized that establishing personalized therapy for children with ASD at the earliest age possible improves outcomes including a higher level of cognitive and social function and improved communication as well as decreased financial and emotional burden on families [3,4]. Development of blood-based diagnostic tests to aid in the assessment of risk for a diagnosis of ASD at an early age would facilitate implementing intensive behavioral therapy at the earliest age possible.

The etiology of the vast majority of cases of ASD are unknown and their genetics have proven to be incredibly complex [5,6]. There is now widespread appreciation that there will be many causes of ASD with varying combinations of genetic and environmental risk factors at play. Numerous studies have attempted to identify the causes of the disorder by studying transcriptomics and genomics, leading to the identification of multiple genes associated with ASD [6,7]. There are currently hundreds of observable genetic variants that account for about 20% of the cases of autism. These data are currently most useful in understanding the intra-familial genetics of autism. For this reason, clinical tests based on genomic measures often include genetic counseling to assess the chance of disease occurrence or recurrence within a family [8,9]. Prediction accuracies of ASD risk based on genomic approaches range from 56% to 70% depending largely on the population of patients assessed. Separate analyses of at least one of the genomic studies by Skafidas et al. has questioned whether the results have been confounded by biases due to ancestral origins [10,11]. An additional limitation of genomic studies is that the results of environmental influences on the child and/or mother are not discernible. Metabolomics is sensitive to biochemical changes caused by even subtle environmental influences and therefore can complement genomic approaches by addressing some of these factors that may be closer to phenotype.

Given the complexities of the genetic environment of ASD, metabolomic profiling may provide an alternative path to developing early diagnostic tests. Previous metabolic studies of ASD have used biological matrices such as cells, organelles, urine and blood, and have implicated a wide range of metabolites including fatty acids, sterols, intermediary metabolites, phospholipids, and molecules associated with oxidative stress [12–16]. Two recent reports highlight the potential use of metabolomic analysis of urine to identify signatures of ASD. One study used 1H-NMR methods and showed changes in metabolites associated with the tryptophan/nicotinic acid metabolic pathway, sulphur and amino acid pathways, as well as microbial metabolites implicating the involvement of microbial metabolism in the etiology of ASD [16]. Ming et al. used a combination of liquid- and gas-chromatography based mass spectrometry methods to identify changes in a number of amino acids and antioxidants such as carnosine, as well as confirming the changes associated with altered gut microbiomes [17].

Measurement of metabolites offers an excellent opportunity to identify differences in small molecule abundance that may have the ability to characterize some forms of ASD. High resolution mass spectrometry (HRMS) is not only a very sensitive detection method for small molecule metabolites, it also provides accurate mass data that aids in metabolite identification through molecular formulae determination [18]. HRMS offers an additional distinct advantage in the ability to distinguish between compounds with the same nominal mass (isobaric compounds), providing enhanced chemical formula and structure information [19]. Unfortunately there is not one universal chromatographic mass spectrometric technique capable of detecting all of the metabolites in blood. To identify novel potential biomarkers associated with ASD, it is necessary to facilitate broad metabolite detection coverage. Toward this goal, we applied an orthogonal approach to chromatographic separation, mass spectral ionization and detection [20]. The current study employed multiple chromatographic mass spectrometric metabolomic methods including gas chromatography-mass spectrometry (GC-MS) and liquid chromatography-high resolution mass spectrometry (LC-HRMS) to discover a wide range of metabolites in blood plasma samples that were able to differentiate TD individuals from those with ASD. Subsequently, tandem mass spectrometry (MS-MS) experiments were employed to aid in structural confirmation of the metabolites discovered by LC-HRMS.

The aim of the study was to perform a broad evaluation of small molecules in blood plasma to discover metabolites that may lead to biomarkers associated with ASD. Univariate, multivariate and machine learning methods were employed to discover metabolites or groups of metabolites exhibiting statistically significant abundance differences that can be used as biomarkers to distinguish children with ASD from TD individuals.

Materials and Methods

Subject Samples

The experimental subjects were initially recruited through the UC Davis M.I.N.D. Institute Clinic, Regional Centers, referrals from clinicians, area school districts and community support groups such as Families for Early Autism Treatment (FEAT). Subjects were limited to an age range of 4–6 years. Typically developing participants were recruited from area school districts and community centers. All facets of this study were approved by the University of California at Davis Institutional Review Board (IRB). Written informed consent was obtained from the parent or guardian of each participant and data were analyzed without personal information identifiers then subjects completed diagnostic and psychological measures. Study participants with ASD were enrolled under inclusion criteria consisting of a diagnosis of autism spectrum disorder based on the DSM-IV criteria determined by an experienced neuropsychologist (BAC), which was further corroborated by the following measures using research reliable clinicians: the Autism Diagnostic Observation Schedule-Generic (ADOS-G) provides observation of a child's communication, reciprocal social interaction, and stereotyped behavior including an algorithm with cutoffs for autism and autism spectrum disorder; the Autism Diagnostic Interview-Revised (ADI-R) is a comprehensive, semi-structured parent interview that assesses a child's developmental history and relevant ASD characteristic behaviors and generates a diagnostic algorithm for children with ASD. Based on the DSM-IV criteria [21], only children with strictly defined autistic disorder were enrolled whereas children with pervasive developmental disorder-not otherwise specified (PDD-NOS) or Asperger Syndrome were excluded from the study. The Social Communication Questionnaire (SCQ) was used as a screening tool to ensure the absence of symptoms of ASD in the TD children. The patients recruited for this study were primarily Caucasian and the ages were similar between groups. However, the participants with autism had lower IQ scores than the TD subjects [22,23].

The exclusion criteria for all subjects included the presence of Fragile X or other serious neurological (e.g., seizures), psychiatric (e.g., bipolar disorder) or known medical conditions such as autoimmune disease and inflammatory bowel diseases/celiac disease. All subjects were screened via parental interview for current and past physical illness. Children with known endocrine, cardiovascular, pulmonary, and liver or kidney disease were excluded from enrollment in the study. Dietary restriction for participation in the study was not required with the exception of an overnight fast. Participation in the study required two clinical visits for behavioral assessment and blood draws. After application of exclusion criteria, the final study group consisted of 104 children, 69 with ASD and 35 in the TD group.

Samples were collected on Thursday morning visits to the M.I.N.D. Institute over a period of 13 months. Blood was drawn into a 9.6 mL EDTA Vaccutainer tube by an experienced pediatric phlebotomist between the hours of 8 and 10 AM following an overnight fast. Tubes were immediately inverted 6–8 times to assure mixing with the anticoagulant and placed on ice. Immediately after plasma separation and aliquoting, samples were sent on the morning of the draw via courier with a barcode label, wrapped tube cap with a strip of parafilm; bubble wrapped then set in a biohazard bag which was placed inside a carrier between coolant packs. Samples were stored at −80°C.

Samples from 103 of the 104 children were sent to Stemina for metabolomic analyses on dry ice… Upon receipt, 5 samples were removed after visual inspection and observation of overt hemolysis and the remaining 98 samples were analyzed by mass spectrometry. Quality checks of the raw mass spectrometric data from the 98 samples were performed, resulting in removing data from 16 patient samples that did not contain MS data from all 5 methods from further analysis. The final 82 samples used in these studies originated from 52 children with ASD and 30 children in the TD group. The children were chosen so that the age and gender distributions were similar across the groups. There was no statistical difference in age between ASD cases and the TD children for the current study (Welch's t-test $p = 0.25$) (see Table 1).

Regarding patient medication, 18 out of 52 of the subjects with ASD in this study were taking medications which included Risperidone (5), Sertraline (3), Aripiprazole (2), antihistamines (2), antivirals (2), antifungals (2), and various other less frequent drugs. Three of the 30 typical subjects were taking medications, which included methylphenidate (1), albuterol (1) and loratadine (1). Ten of the 52 ASD subjects were on a gluten and/or casein-free (GFCF) diet. Importantly, blood draws were administered prior to eating and any morning administration of any medication.

Sample Preparation for LC-MS

Plasma samples were split into 50 μl aliquots and stored at −80°C prior to metabolite extraction. Samples were kept on ice

during these procedures. Samples were randomized into three batches for the LC-HRMS analysis such that diagnosis, IQ, age and ethnicity were equally distributed in each batch. Small molecules were extracted from 50 μL plasma aliquots using 450 μL of 8:1 methanol: water solution at −20°C [24]. The extraction solution also contained internal standards. The samples were agitated for 10 minutes at 2–8°C then centrifuged at 18,400×G for 20 minutes at 4°C to remove the precipitate. The supernatant was transferred to a fresh tube and the centrifugation step was repeated to remove any residual precipitate. After the final centrifugation, 450 μL of supernatant was transferred to a fresh tube then evaporated to dryness in a SpeedVac, then resolublized in 45 μL of a 50:50 mixture of 0.1% formic acid in acetonitrile: 0.1% formic acid, also containing internal standards. This solution was then transferred to a high performance liquid chromatograph (HPLC) autosampler injection vial for LC-HRMS analysis.

Mass Spectrometry

Both targeted GC-MS as well as untargeted LC-HRMS were employed for better metabolome coverage. Four untargeted LC-HRMS methods were used including C8 or HILIC chromatography coupled to electrospray ionization in both positive and negative ion polarities, resulting in 4 separate data acquisitions per sample. For each methodology and condition, only a single sample aliquot was assessed, due to limited material availability.. LC-HRMS methods were developed and tested prior to the evaluation of the clinical patient samples to optimize the breadth of coverage of small molecule metabolites.

Liquid Chromatography High Resolution Mass Spectrometry

LC-HRMS was performed using an Agilent G6540 Quadrupole Time of Flight (QTOF) system consisting of an Agilent 1290 HPLC coupled to a high resolution (QTOF) mass spectrometer. Electrospray ionization (ESI) in both positive and negative ion modes was employed using a dual ESI source under high-resolution exact mass conditions. 2 μL of sample was injected. A Waters Acquity ultra high performance liquid chromatography (UPLC) BEH Amide column with dimensions 2.1×150 mm, 1.7 μM particle size was used for Hydrophilic Interaction Liquid Chromatography (HILIC), and maintained at 40°C. Data was acquired for each sample for 29 minutes at a flow rate of 0.5 mL/minute using a solvent gradient with 0.1% formic acid in water and 0.1% formic acid in acetonitrile. An Agilent Zorbax Eclipse Plus C8 2.1×100 mm, 1.8 μM particle size column was used for C8 chromatography and data was acquired for each sample for

Table 1. Patient demographic information.

Demographic		TD	ASD	Overall
Group Size		30	52	82
Sex (male %)		86.67	78.85	81.7
Age (Years)	Range	4.17–6.92	4–6.92	4–6.92
	Average	5.6	5.37	5.46
	Std. Dev.	0.95	0.81	0.87
IQ	Range	88–137	40–110	40–137
	Average	114.3	67.48	80
	Std. Dev.	10.78	17.69	27.47

50 minutes at a flow rate of 0.5 mL/minute using a gradient with 0.1% formic acid in water and 0.1% formic acid in acetonitrile and maintained at 40°C.

Gas Chromatography - Mass Spectrometry

GC-MS analyses were performed at the West Coast Metabolomics Center at UC Davis as described in [25]. GC-MS data was acquired using an Agilent 6890 gas chromatograph coupled to a LECO Pegasus IV TOF mass spectrometer. Metabolite identification was done by comparing sample data to a database of over 1,000 compounds identified by GC-MS that includes mass spectra, retention indices, structures and links to external metabolic databases.

Metabolite chemical structure confirmation by LC-HRMS-MS

The chemical structures of key metabolites were further confirmed using tandem mass spectrometry (LC-HRMS-MS) methods with chromatographic conditions identical to those used for their discovery. LC-HRMS-MS analyses were performed on an Agilent QTOF mass spectrometer for patient samples and/or reference blood samples with collision energy conditions optimized to obtain the highest quality product ion spectra. The resulting product ion spectra were then compared to MS-MS spectra available in public spectral databases such as METLIN [26], MassBank [27] and Stemina's own SteminaMetDB database.

Data Analysis

LC-HRMS Data preprocessing. Raw mass spectral data and were initially examined for quality criteria established during method development such as abundance thresholds, retention time and peak shape consistency for total ion chromatograms, and extracted ion chromatograms for internal standards and markers. Data files exhibiting chromatograms that failed these quality criteria were removed from further analysis. A portion of these were retested, depending on the nature of the QC failure. Raw data were converted to open source mzData files [28]. Peak picking and feature creation were performed using XCMS [29] and then deviations in retention times were corrected using the obiwarp algorithm [30] based on a non-linear clustering approach to align the LC-HRMS data. Mass features were generated using the XCMS density based grouping algorithm. Missing features were integrated based on retention time and mass range of a feature bin using iterative peak filling. A "mass feature" (also abbreviated here as "feature") is a moiety detected by the mass spectrometer that is defined by 2 properties 1) the detected mass-to-charge ratio (*m/z*) and 2) the chromatographic retention time.

A series of data filters were then employed to remove features exhibiting low abundance levels, those resulting from background noise, ions with non-biological mass defects, and known contaminants from subsequent data analyses. To reduce LC-HRMS batch variations in feature detection, the abundance values were then normalized by sample to the experiment-wide median area of spiked-in internal reference standards. The integrated areas of the normalized mass features from the GC-MS and LC-HRMS platforms were combined into a single dataset. There were 4572 features for the training set of samples that passed preprocessing filters.

Training and Independent Validation Sets. The 82 patient samples (52 ASD and 30 TD samples) were split into two sets, (1) a training set of 61 samples (39 ASD and 22 TD) for identification of statistically significant features and classification modeling and (2) a 21-sample independent validation set (13 ASD and 8 TD) used to evaluate performance of the classification models. This was accomplished by randomizing the samples using the diagnosis, patient IQ, and gender in these training and validations sets so that each set contained a similar proportion of factors used in randomization. The validation sample set was withheld from the univariate filtering and model development process to act as an independent external sample set to evaluate model performance. Detailed patient demographics for the samples in the training and validation sets are provided in Table S4.

Univariate Filtering of Mass Features. T-tests were used to reduce the overall feature set, the potential for over-fitting, and increase the biological interpretability of the predictive signature [31]. The integrated areas of mass features normalized to internal standards (IS) from the GC-MS and LC-HRMS platforms were combined into a single dataset. The 4572 features passing the preprocessing filters for the training set of samples were further filtered using Welch T-tests under the null hypothesis that no difference in mean integrated areas of a mass feature is present between the experimental classes, and the alternative hypothesis that there is a difference in mean integrated areas between ASD and TD training set samples to identify differential features. For each feature that exhibited a statistically significant change with an uncorrected p-value <0.05, its extracted ion chromatogram (EIC) was reviewed for consistency of integration across samples, peak shape, and a minimum peak height requirement of >3000. Features passing this EIC quality review process were then utilized in the classification modeling. False discovery rates (FDRs) were calculated using the Benjamini Hochberg method of p-value correction [32].

Classification Modeling. Model development was performed with two primary goals: 1) to robustly rank the importance of metabolites in discriminating ASD using a VIP (Variable Importance in the Projection) score index and 2) to identify the minimum set of predictive metabolites needed to reach the highest levels of differentiation of the ASD and TD experimental classes. The final models were created by training a Partial Least Squares Discriminant Analysis (PLS-DA) or Support Vector Machine (SVM) classifier using the entire 61-sample training set. The modeling techniques PLS-DA as well as SVM with a linear kernel [33,34] were both utilized to demonstrate that the molecular signature can be predictive using multiple approaches. PLS and SVM classification models were created using the R package Classification and Regression Training "caret" version 5.17–7 [35]. Receiver operator Curve (ROC) analysis was performed using the R package ROCR version 1.0–5 [36].

A nested cross validation (CV) approach (Figure 1) was used to meet the first objective of model development - a robust measure of feature VIP scores. The 179 features from the 61 sample training set were analyzed using 100 resamples with an 80:20 split to weight the importance of each of the 179 statistically significant features. The tuning loop utilized 10-fold cross validation to tune model parameters (cost parameter C for SVM and the number of components for PLS-DA). The recursive feature elimination loop was used to identify the best performing feature subset from each iteration using steps of 20 features. The results from the 100 resamples were used to estimate model performance and create a robust biomarker VIP score index to rank the importance of each of the 179 features in classification of ASD from TD individuals.

Feature VIP robustness was measured by resampling the training set 100 times using an 80:20 split into 49-sample CV training and 12-sample CV test sets. VIP scores were calculated for each of the 100 resamples and the most informative features at each resample were identified by backwards recursive feature

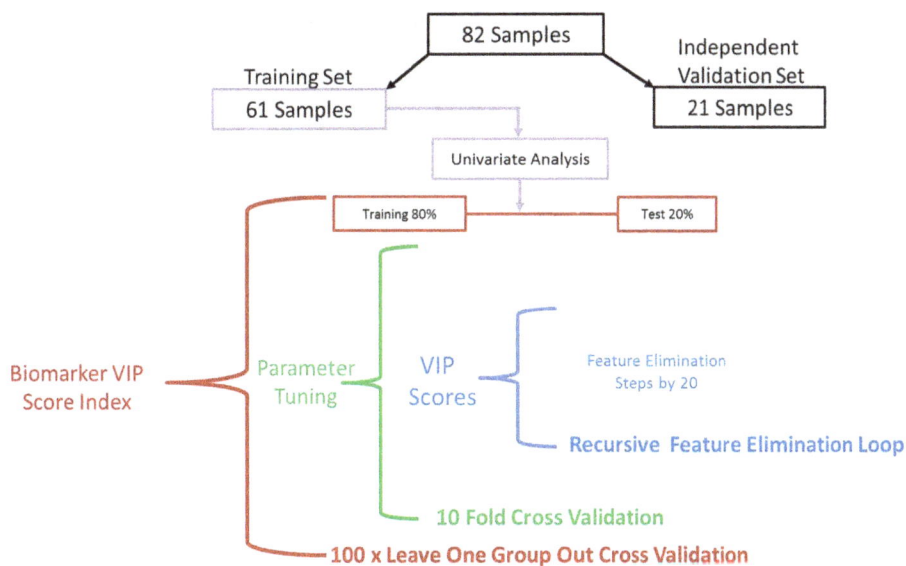

Figure 1. Classification modeling process. A three-layer nested cross-validation approach was applied using both PLS-DA and SVM modeling methods to determine significant features capable of classifying children with ASD from TD children. The 179 features of the training set were analyzed using a leave-one-group-out cross-validation loop as described. The results from this cross-validation process were used to estimate model performance and create a robust feature VIP score index to rank the ASD vs TD classification importance of each of the 179 features. These feature ranks were used to evaluate the performance of the molecular signature using an independent validation set.

elimination (in 20-feature steps) using the Area Under the ROC Curve (AUC). The most informative set of features was then used to predict each CV test set. The VIP scores were averaged across the 100 resamples to create the VIP index for each feature. The classification performance metrics of the CV test sets were averaged across resamples to understand potential future performance.

The second objective of the classification modeling approach was to identify the minimum number of features with the highest level of classification accuracy. This objective was met using feature subsets based on the ordered VIP score index and evaluating the subset performance in the validation set of samples. The classification models were created using the entire 61 sample training set and by stepping through features. The feature stepping process utilized the 20 top VIP features then added the next 20 highest weighted features until all 179 features were evaluated.

Performance metrics (Accuracy, Sensitivity, Specificity, and ROC analysis) were determined based on the prediction of the 21 sample independent validation set for assessment of the molecular signature at each feature subset bin size (Table S3). Accuracy is defined as the proportion of correctly classified participants and is calculated by dividing the number of correctly classified participants by the total number of participants in a sample set. Specificity is the proportion of correctly classified TD individuals out of all TD participants in a sample set. Sensitivity is the proportion of correctly classified ASD individuals out of all participants with ASD in a sample set. The top 179 features were also compared for rank between SVM and PLS modeling methods (Figure 2).

Feature Metabolite Annotations. Metabolite annotation (assignment of putative chemical structures) was carried out for each feature. Annotation was accomplished by comparing m/z value of each mass feature to the m/z value of common ESI adducts contained in public chemical databases and/or Stemina's internal metabolite database. All mass features that were annotated with chemical identities in that the measured exact

mass was consistent (within 20 ppm relative mass error) with one or more chemical structures. These annotations were considered to be putative until the chemical structure of the feature was further confirmed by LC-HRMS-MS.

The molecular formulae of the mass features with putative annotations were then input into the "Find by Formula" (FBF) algorithm in the Agilent Technologies MassHunter Qualitative Analysis software which tests whether the mass spectra for a given feature is a reasonable match with the proposed formula. In most cases, the annotations for any feature with a median FBF score of less than 70, a retention time difference greater than 35 seconds or which was present in less than 50% of the data files was not included for further analysis due to lack of confidence in the formula assignment of the annotation.

Features from the GC-MS analysis were identified as described by [25]. This procedure used comparison of the sample data to spectra of metabolite reference standards that had been previously acquired by the same identical GC-MS method. Therefore, the data analysis and confirmation of the metabolite chemical structures was performed by a simple comparison of the acquired patient sample data to the database. GC-MS data also contained peaks that remained unidentified and showed statistically significant changes depending on sample class.

Results

The use of multiple orthogonal analytical methods provided a broad coverage of the metabolome and each method contributed mass features to the model for classification of the children with ASD from the TD controls. Each analytical method was assessed for the unique features it provided. The HILIC LC-HRMS method resulted in the highest number of distinctive mass features in the models, followed by C8 LC-HRMS then GC-MS. Univariate analysis filtering was performed on the 4572 features that passed the preprocessing filters. About 60% of the LC-HRMS features were putatively annotated with a chemical structure and

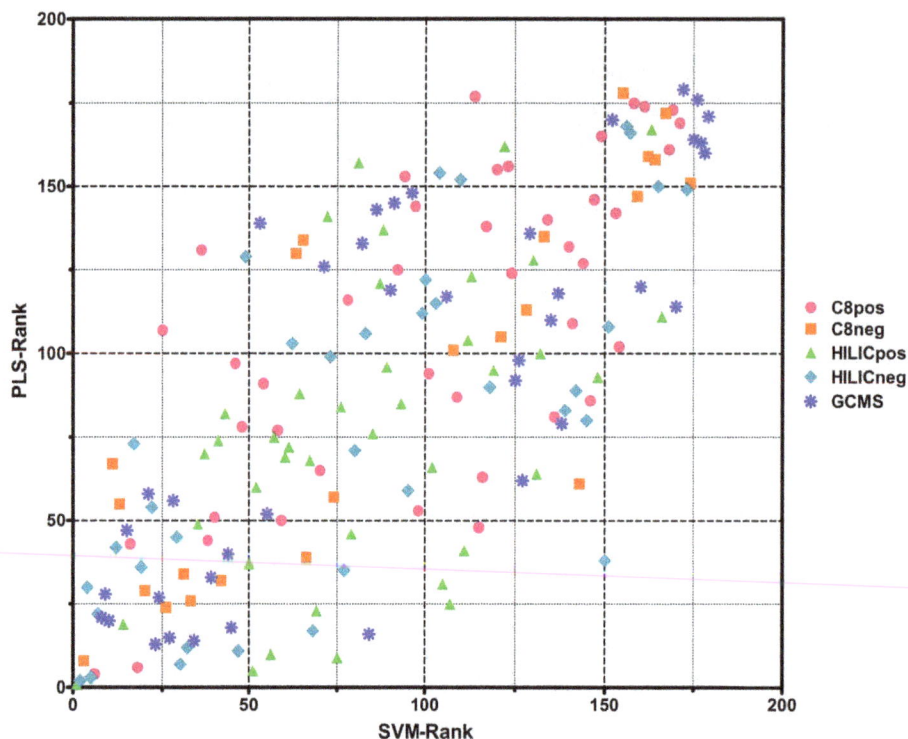

Figure 2. Feature Importance Rankings. The top 179 features were compared for rank between SVM and PLS modeling methods. The lowest rank scores represent the most important features.

8% (503) of the annotated features passed the FBF procedural criteria. Approximately 36% (142) of the targeted GC-MS features were confirmed metabolites. A breakdown of these results is contained in Table 2.

Data across the 61-sample training set from all analytical platforms were used to identify and robustly rank the features that could be utilized to discriminate plasma samples from children with ASD from samples from TD children. The univariate analysis filtering, as described in the methods, resulted in 389 statistically significant features. Following feature QC, 210 features were removed from the analysis due to poor quality EICs, leaving 179 features that were included in classification modeling. The 179 features comprised 3% of the LC-HRMS and 8% of the GC-MS preprocessed set of features and are shown in Table S1.

Training Set Model Performance

SVM and PLS classification methods were used to discriminate between samples from children with ASD and TD children using the 179 selected features as variables and each feature's contribution toward classification was evaluated for future biomarker development efforts. Based on the best performing model from each of the 100 nested CV resampling iterations, ROC plots were generated for the average of the 100 resamples to understand performance of each modeling method (SVM and PLS-DA). Both SVM and PLS modeling methods indicated that a metabolic signature could be detected that could classify children with ASD from TD individuals (Table S2). For the 61-sample training set, the average ASD prediction accuracy of the SVM model was 0.86, with AUC values of 0.95 (95% CI 0.94–0.96). The PLS model gave an average prediction accuracy of 0.84 with AUC values of 0.92 (95% CI 0.91–0.94). To confirm that the model classification accuracies were not random results, the

modeling process was repeated with random permutations of the diagnosis class labels. These results showed near random classification, with AUC values of 0.52 (95% CI 0.48–0.57) and 0.52 (95% CI 0.49–0.56) for SVM and PLS, respectively, indicating that the 179 features did not discriminate the classes by chance (Figure 3).

Anticipating that blood tests for ASD may be more efficient and less expensive if they measure an optimally lower number of metabolites, the classification modeling paradigm also included a feature number optimization in each model, based on the highest resulting AUC. The feature sets were evaluated using feature subsets based on the ordered VIP scores of individual features to identify the minimum number of features that maximized performance for each modeling method (Table S2). These data together indicate that not all of the features contributed equally to the models and that the number of features could be reduced by removing those that contributed less while still retaining model accuracy and robustness. As a result, the entire set of 179 features was not required for optimal model performance for either of the modeling methods (Figure 3). The results from the model training process indicated that SVM models that were trained using an 80 feature set exhibited the best combined classification performance metrics (when compared to PLS and other SVM results) with an average accuracy of 90%, an average sensitivity of 92%, an average specificity of 87%, and an average AUC of 0.95 (Table S2).

Validation Set Model Performance

Different subsets of features, created based on the weighted VIP scores, were evaluated independently of the outer cross-validation loop using the 21-sample independent validation set. The 80-feature SVM model described above had a classification predic-

Table 2. A breakdown of the numbers of features resulting from filtering and annotation processes, based on molecular formula.

Platform	Raw Features	Annotated Features	Unique Formula within a Platform	Features Passing Preprocessing Filters	Features Passing Univariate Filter
HILIC +	3207	1985	146	1527	40
HILIC−	1865	1061	140	950	35
C8+	3062	1902	140	1096	42
C8−	1568	847	77	514	23
GC-MS	485	178*	142*	485	39
Total	10187	5795	645	4572	179

This table also helps to illustrate the orthogonality and contribution of each of the 5 analytical platforms. Molecular formulae are being used here only to approximate the method orthogonality, since any given molecular formula may be associated with multiple chemical structures. *These annotations were confirmed in the GCMS platform and the formula were confirmed by using the KEGG database instead of the FBF procedure used in the 4 LCMS platforms.

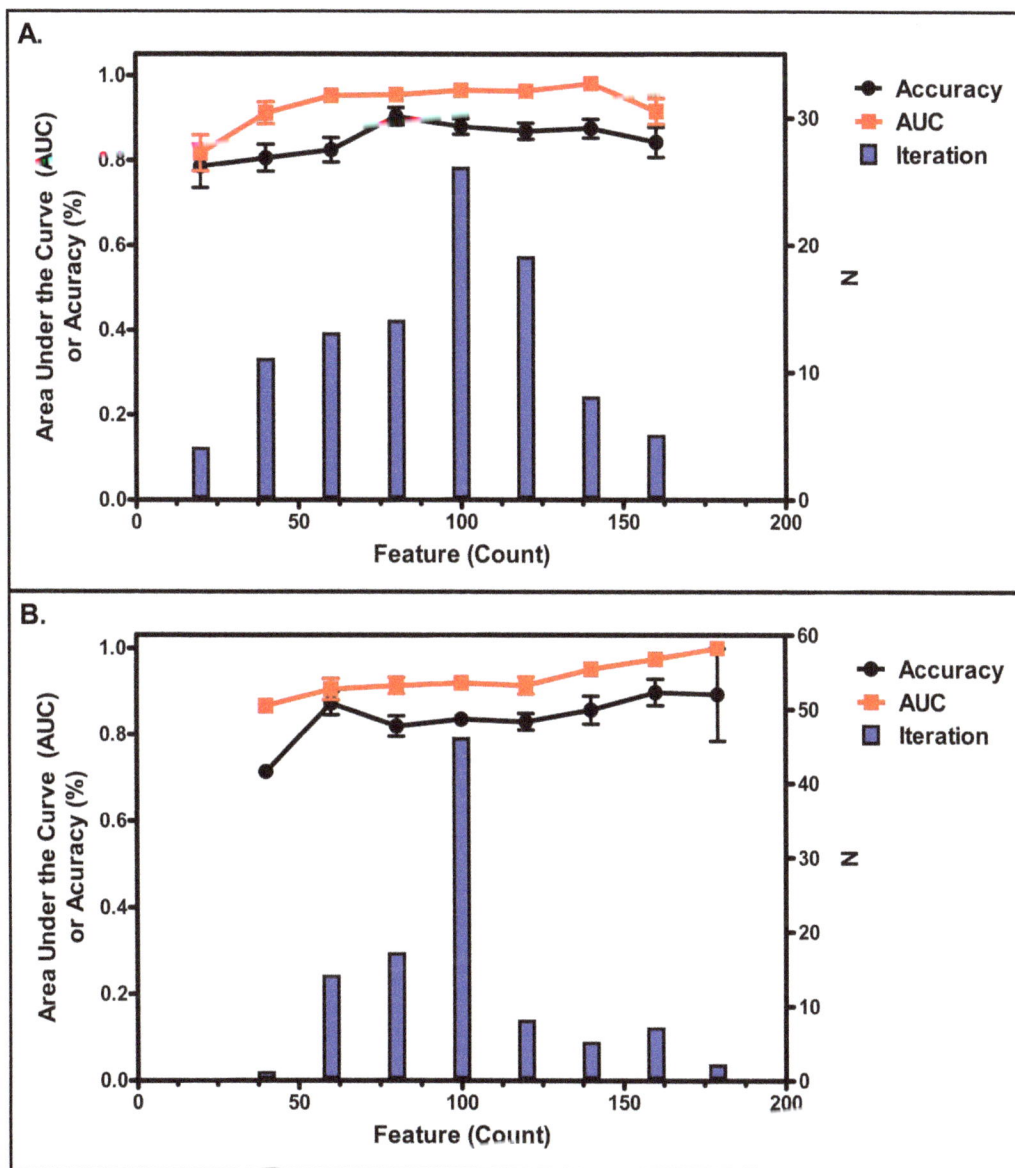

Figure 3. Performance of the SVM and PLS models. Average AUC and accuracy of the (a) SVM and (b) PLS models containing different numbers of features. The bar graphs show the number of optimal models which were derived from recursive feature elimination process that was included in the resampling process for the indicated number of features.

tion accuracy of 81%, a sensitivity of 85%, a specificity of 75% and an AUC of 84% (Figure 4, red line; Table 3). The best performing PLS model, comprised of 160 variables, had an accuracy of 81%, a sensitivity of 92%, a specificity of 63% and an AUC of 0.81% (Figure 4, blue line; Table 3). Detailed results are shown in Table S3. The results suggest that at least 40 features are needed to reach an accuracy of 70% and that a range of 80 to 160 features had the best performance with this independent validation sample set as well as the training set of samples.

Confirmation of Metabolite Chemical Structures

The chemical identities of the 7 LC-MS mass features that were confirmed by LC-HRMS-MS are shown in Table 4. Included in the metabolites confirmed by LC-HRMS-MS or targeted GC-MS was homocitrulline, which was decreased in ASD patients. Other metabolites showing significant up or down regulation in our study include: aspartate, glutamate, DHEAS, citric acid, succinic acid, methylhexa-, tetra- and hepta-decanoic acids, isoleucine, glutaric acid, 3-aminoisobutyric acid and creatinine. These are listed in Table 4 and represent a variety of molecular classes including amino acids, organic acids, sterols, and fatty acids.

Discussion

Our metabolomic approach was not biased toward possible biochemical pathways other than by the separation and detection limits of the analytical methods used. We used robust VIP scores and recursive feature elimination to estimate that between 80 and 160 mass features are required to produce an optimal predictive signature in this set of patients. The predictive signatures in this study are the result of modeling a 62-patient training set, then applying those models to predict a 21-patient validation set. This

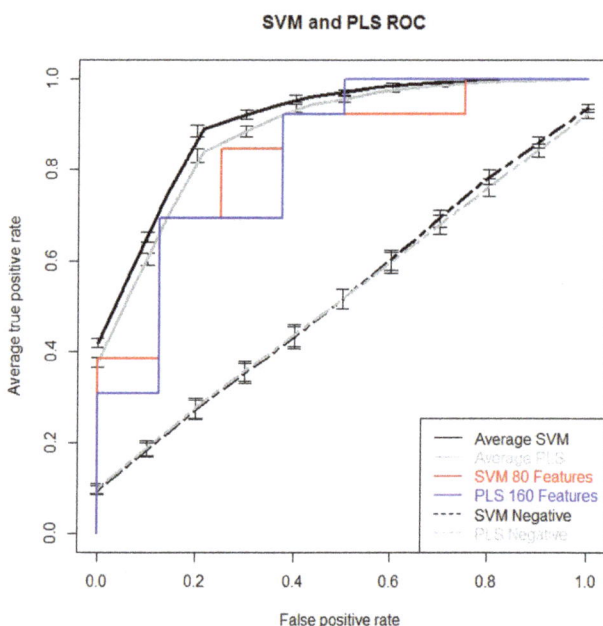

Figure 4. ROC curve performance of the classification models from the training and validation sets. The average of 100 iterations of the classifier for the best performing feature sets following recursive feature elimination comparing ASD vs. TD samples (Black and Grey Lines). The blue (PLS) and red (SVM) lines are ROC curves of the best performing validation feature subsets. Vertical bars represent the standard error of the mean.

approach has resulted in the discovery of a biochemically diverse set of metabolites that might be useful in distinguishing individuals at risk for ASD. It is difficult to determine how generalizable these predictive signatures will be in the broader population, given the small sample size. Larger studies need to be performed in order to assess and refine a signature into a clinical diagnostic. Several of the metabolites identified so far in these signatures point to biological mechanisms that have been previously identified as having a role in the etiology of ASD. Our signatures will most likely represent a portion of the metabolic changes that will be critical in the diagnosis of ASD through metabolic end points.

Identification of metabolites previously associated with ASD

Examples of metabolites showing significant up or down regulation in the current study that have been previously associated with autism include:

- Tricarboxylic acid cycle associated molecules including citric acid (decreased) and succinic acid (increased) were found to be significantly altered in the ASD participants. Elevations in urinary succinate [16,17] and decreased urinary citrate [37] in children with autism have been previously reported.
- Fatty acids have previously been observed to be decreased in the plasma of children with ASD, similar to our observations for methylhexa-, tetra- and hepta-decanoic acids [12]. Links between saturated fatty acid metabolism and oxidative stress have been reported in erythrocytes in children with ASD [38].
- 3-aminoisobutyric acid was increased in samples from participants with ASD. This is also consistent with previous findings [39].
- Creatinine was decreased in children with ASD and is consistent with the findings of Whitely et al, who observed similar changes in urinary creatinine in children diagnosed with PDD [40].

Evidence for a role in mitochondrial dysfunction in ASD

The goal of this study was to evaluate biomarkers in blood. When metabolism is disrupted, active transporters and tissue specific differences in metabolism can cause different levels of the same metabolites in different biological compartments (plasma, urine, CSF, etc.). When discussing individual metabolites in the context of autism, it is important to recognize that autism is a systemic disease that affects other organ systems besides the brain. For example, serotonin levels have been reported to be elevated in blood in some patients with autism, and other evidence suggests that intracerebral serotonergic activity is decreased in ASD. Serotonin does not cross the blood brain barrier, and the brain has different enzymes for serotonin synthesis than peripheral tissues [41].

Many of the confirmed metabolites that are associated with ASD are relevant to aspects of mitochondrial biology. Mitochondrial disease or dysfunction may be a risk factor for autism [42]. In addition, several other observed metabolites are associated with other processes already proposed to be involved in ASD including oxidative stress [43] and energy production [44].

- Aspartate and glutamate levels in blood were significantly elevated in ASD, as has been observed in previous studies [45,46]. Mutations in the aspartate/glutamate mitochondrial transporter, SLC25A12, have been previously associated with ASD [47]. This transporter is an important component of the malate/aspartate shuttle, a crucial system supporting oxidative

Table 3. Classifier performance metrics based on predictions on the independent 21-sample validation set, showing the feature sets with the highest accuracy.

Model	Feature No.	Accuracy	Sensitivity	Specificity	AUC
SVM	80	0.81	0.85	0.75	0.84
PLS	160	0.81	0.92	0.63	0.81

Feature No. corresponds to the number of the ordered, ranked VIP features that were evaluated. Table S3 shows the results for all feature sets.

phosphorylation, adenosine triphosphate production, and key metabolites for the urea cycle [47].

- DHEAS, the predominant plasma sterol, was increased in children with ASD. DHEA is known to affect mitochondrial energy production through inhibition of enzymes associated with the respiratory chain [48] with variable findings in children with ASD [49,50].
- The branched chain amino acid isoleucine was reduced in samples from children with ASD versus TD children as observed by others [51]. Possible molecular mechanisms would include mutation in the branched chain amino acid kinase dehydrogenase (BCKD-kinase), a mitochondrial enzyme [52] as well as amino acids in energy metabolism [53].
- Glutaric acid levels were elevated in children with ASD. Increased urinary glutaric acid occurs in a variety of neuronal deficiencies such as glutaryl-CoA dehydrogenase (GCDH) deficiency. A significant portion of the glutaric acid metabolism takes place in the mitochondria [54].

The potential relationship of the gut microbiome with ASD

This potential connection between the gut microbiome and ASD is also receiving considerable attention [55]. Metabolomic studies of urine from individuals with ASD have identified molecules associated with the microbiome such as dimethylamine, hippuric acid and phenylacetylglutamine [16,17]. We observed decreased plasma levels of p-hydroxyphenyllactate, a metabolite associated with bifidobacteria and lactobacilli that is known to serve as an antioxidant both in the circulation and tissues [56]. We have yet to identify other microbiome related metabolites.

Novel metabolic alterations in ASD

We identified novel statistically significant changes in some metabolites that had not been previously reported in other metabolomics profiling as well as identifying novel changes in metabolites that had never before been associated with ASD. Significant changes in the levels of aspartate, citrate, creatinine, DHEA-S, hydroxyphenyllactate, indoleacetate, isoleucine, glutamate and glutarate between ASD and TD individuals were identified in this study compared to previous metabolomics studies of urine metabolites where changes in these metabolites were not significant [17]. These differences could be related to transport and accumulation of metabolites in the urine compared to the blood, differences in the study populations, or application different LC-MS and GC-MS methodology allowing better detection of these metabolites in this study.

We also identified a new, previously undescribed potential ASD biomarker, homocitrulline. This metabolite was decreased in ASD patients and had the highest rank of all features in both SVM and PLS classification models. Homocitrulline is a poorly understood molecule which is known to be formed inside the mitochondria

from lysine and carbamoyl phosphate. The decreased homocitrulline levels in the blood suggests that homocitrulline metabolism in the brain may also be disrupted, Homocitrulline levels are increased in urine and blood in patients with ornithine translocase (SLC25A15) deficiency which diverts carbamyl phosphate to react with lysine. These patients can exhibit behavioral abnormalities similar to ASD such as developmental delay, ataxia, spasticity, learning disabilities, cognitive deficits and/or unexplained seizures [57]. Rats treated with intracerebroventricular administration of homocitrulline are also observed to have disrupted brain redox status and energy metabolism [58,59]. These observations suggest that elevated brain levels of homocitrulline are deleterious; however additional studies are needed to define the brain levels of homocitrulline and the potential role in the development of ASD.

Summary

The current study profiled metabolites in blood plasma using metabolomics methods to evaluate the possibility that differences in the metabolite abundances might provide a metabolic signature that could prove useful in distinguishing individuals at high risk for developing ASD. The cohort of subjects enrolled in this study was carefully assembled to reflect a diagnosis of ASD by strict research criteria. Beyond careful clinical diagnosis, great pains were taken to ensure that fasting blood collection was obtained at the same time for all study participants and that complicating factors such as illness were minimized. We consider the current work as a proof of concept that there are predictive metabolic signatures which can be used to distinguish ASD and TD individuals.

Two independent statistical classification methods (PLS and SVM) were employed to determine the most influential metabolites and mass features that could be used to discriminate between ASD and TD individuals. Both classification modeling methods yielded relatively similar results with respect to maximum prediction accuracy of about 81% as evaluated by an independent 21-sample validation sample set. This was followed by recursive feature elimination to establish the minimal numbers of features needed for a predictive model. Interestingly, several of the key features for classification, such as homocitrulline, were common between the two methods indicating their importance in the development of future blood based diagnostics. It is clear that access to a larger sample set will be required to further validate and confirm the annotations of the key features. Metabolomics determines changes in small molecule metabolites that are reactants and products of endogenous biochemical processes as well as small molecules derived from diet, the gut microbiome and contact with the environment. Perturbations in their abundance can result not only from genomic and proteomic influences, but from environmental and epigenetic influences as well. A metabolomic approach may therefore provide enhanced predictive results by keying in on common, end stage metabolites rather than on specific genomic or proteomic determinants.

Table 4. Confirmed metabolites.

Analytical Platform	Metabolite	Feature ID	HMDB ID [61]	Fold Change (ASD/TD)	p-value (ASD vs. TD)	FDR	SVM Rank	PLS Rank
HILICpos	homocitrulline	M190T512	HMDB00679	0.67	<0.001	0.059	1	1
C8neg	2-hydroxyvaleric acid	M117T127	HMDB01863	0.80	0.0289	0.53	33	26
HILICpos	cystine	M241T774	HMDB00192	0.91	0.0277	0.532	87	121
GCMS	aspartic acid	GCMS_aspartic.acid	HMDB00191	1.33	<0.001	0.086	34	14
HILICpos	isoleucine	M132T248	HMDB00172	0.76	0.0351	0.541	60	69
HILICpos	creatinine	M114T262	HMDB00562	0.88	0.0471	0.576	57	75
GCMS	serine	GCMS_serine	HMDB00187	1.16	0.00275	0.267	137	118
HILICneg	4-hydroxyphenyllactic acid	M181T66	HMDB00755	0.84	0.0344	0.541	47	11
GC-MS	citric acid	GCMS_citric.acid	HMDB00094	0.91	0.0492	0.580	84	16
GC-MS	glutamic acid	GCMS_glutamic.acid	HMDB00148	1.28	0.00144	0.188	15	47
GC-MS	lactic acid	GCMS_indol.3.lactate	HMDB00671	0.87	0.0181	0.457	55	52
C8neg	DHEA sulfate	M367T736	HMDB01032	2.55	0.00152	0.188	11	67
GC-MS	glutaric acid	GCMS_glutaric.acid	HMDB00661	1.36	0.00492	0.322	27	15
GC-MS	5-hydroxynorvaline	GCMS_X5. Hydroxy norvaline.NIST	HMDB31658	1.27	0.0457	0.576	177	163
GC-MS	heptadecanoic acid	GCMS_heptadecanoic.acid.NIST	HMDB02259	0.81	0.0270	0.527	135	110
GC-MS	5-aminovaleric acid lactam	GCMS_X5.aminovaleric.acid.lactame	HMDB11749	2.43	0.00211	0.22	127	62
GC-MS	succinic acid	GCMS_succinic.acid	HMDB00254	1.11	0.0457	0.576	175	164
GC-MS	myristic acid	GCMS_myristic.acid	HMDB00806	0.76	0.00892	0.371	24	27
GC-MS	2-hydroxyvaleric acid	GCMS_X2.hydroxyvaleric.acid	HMDB01863	1.41	0.0406	0.564	179	171
GC-MS	methylhexadecanoic acid	GCMS_methylhexadecanoic.acid	NA	0.82	0.0399	0.564	160	120
GC-MS	3-aminoisobutyric acid	GCMS_X3.aminoisobutyric.acid	HMDB02166	1.19	0.0473	0.576	176	176

Statistically significant metabolites from the 61-sample training set with chemical structures confirmed by LC-HRMS-MS or GC-MS.

Limitations

While the patient population was very well characterized, represented all severity levels of ASD and the blood samples were taken in a very systematic fashion, the total number of subjects (ASD = 52; TD = 30) was not large enough to definitively create a model for prediction of ASD or characterize metabolic differences that may be more highly associated with ASD subtypes.

Due to the small sample size, analysis of the data with respect to medication, sex, special diet, race, ethnicity or other potential confounding covariates was not conclusive. These are important considerations which require a larger sample size to address properly. A much larger study is currently in progress. Randomization methods were implemented to help prevent biasing the results based on any single covariate. The 4 misclassified patients in the 80 feature SVM model in the validation test set were Caucasian male and females whereas the Hispanic, Asian, and other ethnicity were predicted correctly.

Strong evidence of hemolysis, based on visual observation, was observed in 5 samples from ASD children. These samples were excluded from analysis Hemolysis can be a result of poor medical condition, but can also result from suboptimal blood collection and handling. However, Yin et. al found that if EDTA tubes were placed on ice immediately, as was done in this protocol, the metabolome was very stable. Therefore, it remains possible, but unlikely, that minor hemolysis may confound the data by effecting some of the metabolite fold changes that were observed [60].

Conclusions

This initial study provides proof of concept to further pursue development of metabolic biomarkers of ASD. We have demonstrated that a profile of altered metabolites in the blood plasma from a well-curated sample set from clinically diagnosed children with ASD and TD individuals between 4 and 6 years of age, can be detected by a combination of several MS-based metabolomic analyses. Statistical models developed from the derived metabolic data distinguished children with ASD from TD individuals with better than 80% accuracy in both the 61-sample training set and the 21 sample validation set.

The broad metabolite profiling methods developed here can also be employed to discover a wide variety of additional metabolites, leading to the determination of biochemical pathways and mechanisms that are involved in the etiologies of ASD, and advancing the understanding of autism in broader patient populations, eventually leading to new modes of therapy. Given the pronounced clinical and co-morbid features of ASD, it is possible that metabolic profiling of individual patients may enable individualized therapeutic approaches for improved outcomes.

Future Endeavors

Further research is currently being carried out in much larger and younger patient populations to confirm these results, discover and confirm additional diagnostic metabolites and determine which are the most robust for evaluating ASD risk. We are also comparing metabolite profiles in clinically defined subtypes of ASD to determine whether predictive accuracy can be increased through better phenotyping of the ASD population. Analysis and consequential stratification will be performed based on covariables such as medication, sex, special diet, race, ethnicity, onset and co-morbid features such as gastrointestinal distress or seizure disorders may lead to a more accurate set of diagnostic metabolic profiles.

Acknowledgments

The authors thank Agilent Technologies for providing instrumentation, software and assistance.

Author Contributions

Conceived and designed the experiments: PRW DGA PB AS JAP GC ELRD REB. Performed the experiments: PRW LE MR KC. Analyzed the data: PRW LE AS KC BF PB. Wrote the paper: PRW DGA PB LE AS BF BAC JAP ELRD REB.

References

1. American Psychiatric Association (2013) Desk Reference to the Diagnostic Criteria from DSM-5. 5th ed. Washington, D.C.: American Psychiatric Association.
2. Centers for Disease Control and Prevention (2014) Prevalence of autism spectrum disorder among children aged 8 years - autism and developmental disabilities monitoring network, 11 sites, United States, 2010. MMWR Surveill Summ 63: 1–21. Available: http://www.ncbi.nlm.nih.gov/pubmed/24670961.
3. Dawson G, Rogers S, Munson J, Smith M, Winter J, et al. (2010) Randomized, controlled trial of an intervention for toddlers with autism: the Early Start Denver Model. Pediatrics 125: e17–23. Available: http://www.ncbi.nlm.nih.gov/pubmed/19948568. Accessed 12 August 2013.
4. Ganz ML (2007) The lifetime distribution of the incremental societal costs of autism. Arch Pediatr Adolesc Med 161: 343–349. Available: http://www.ncbi.nlm.nih.gov/pubmed/17404130.
5. State MW, Šestan N (2012) Neuroscience. The emerging biology of autism spectrum disorders. Science 337: 1301–1303. Available: http://www.ncbi.nlm.nih.gov/pubmed/22984058. Accessed 27 February 2013.
6. Berg JM, Geschwind DH (2012) Autism genetics: searching for specificity and convergence. Genome Biol 13: 247. Available: http://www.pubmedcentral.nih.gov/articlerender.fcgi?artid=3491377&tool=pmcentrez&rendertype=abstract.
7. Huguet G, Ey E, Bourgeron T (2013) The genetic landscapes of autism spectrum disorders. Annu Rev Genomics Hum Genet 14: 191–213. Available: http://www.ncbi.nlm.nih.gov/pubmed/23875794. Accessed 11 December 2013.
8. Bucan M, Abrahams BS, Wang K, Glessner JT, Herman EI, et al. (2009) Genome-wide analyses of exonic copy number variants in a family-based study point to novel autism susceptibility genes. PLoS Genet 5: e1000536. Available: http://www.pubmedcentral.nih.gov/articlerender.fcgi?artid=2695001&tool=pmcentrez&rendertype=abstract. Accessed 7 August 2013.
9. Wang K, Zhang H, Ma D, Bucan M, Glessner JT, et al. (2009) Common genetic variants on 5p14.1 associate with autism spectrum disorders. Nature 459: 528–533. Available: http://www.pubmedcentral.nih.gov/articlerender.fcgi?artid=2943511&tool=pmcentrez&rendertype=abstract. Accessed 9 August 2013.
10. Belgard TG, Jankovic I, Lowe JK, Geschwind DH (2014) Population structure confounds autism genetic classifier. Mol Psychiatry 19: 405–407. doi: 10.1038/mp.2013.34.
11. Skafidas E, Testa R, Zantomio D, Chana G, Everall IP, et al. (2012) Predicting the diagnosis of autism spectrum disorder using gene pathway analysis. Mol Psychiatry in press. Available: http://www.ncbi.nlm.nih.gov/pubmed/22965006. Accessed 24 October 2012.

12. El-Ansary AK, Bacha AG Ben, Al-Ayahdi LY (2011) Plasma fatty acids as diagnostic markers in autistic patients from Saudi Arabia. Lipids Health Dis 10: 62. Available: http://www.pubmedcentral.nih.gov/articlerender.fcgi?artid=3107800&tool=pmcentrez&rendertype=abstract. Accessed 6 August 2013.

13. James SJ, Melnyk S, Fuchs G, Reid T, Jernigan S, et al. (2009) Efficacy of methylcobalamin and folinic acid treatment on glutathione redox status in children with autism 1–3. Am J Clin Nutr 89: 425–430.

14. Lee RWY, Tierney E (2011) Hypothesis: the role of sterols in autism spectrum disorder. Autism Res Treat 2011: 653570. Available: http://www.pubmedcentral.nih.gov/articlerender.fcgi?artid=3420784&tool=pmcentrez&rendertype=abstract. Accessed 23 August 2013.

15. Damodaran LPM, Arumugam G (2011) Urinary oxidative stress markers in children with autism. Redox Rep 16: 216–222. Available: http://www.ncbi.nlm.nih.gov/pubmed/22005342. Accessed 23 August 2013.

16. Yap IKS, Angley M, Veselkov K a, Holmes E, Lindon JC, et al. (2010) Urinary metabolic phenotyping differentiates children with autism from their unaffected siblings and age-matched controls. J Proteome Res 9: 2996–3004. Available: http://www.ncbi.nlm.nih.gov/pubmed/20337404.

17. Ming X, Stein TP, Barnes V, Rhodes N, Guo L (2012) Metabolic perturbance in autism spectrum disorders: a metabolomics study. J Proteome Res 11: 5856–5862. Available: http://www.ncbi.nlm.nih.gov/pubmed/23106572.

18. Dunn WB, Bailey NJC, Johnson HE (2005) Measuring the metabolome: current analytical technologies. Analyst 130: 606–625. Available: http://www.ncbi.nlm.nih.gov/pubmed/15852128. Accessed 19 August 2013.

19. Gross ML (1994) Accurate masses for structure confirmation. J Am Soc Mass Spectrom 5: 57. Available: http://link.springer.com/10.1016/1044-0305(94)85036-4.

20. Bruce SJ, Jonsson P, Antti H, Cloarec O, Trygg J, et al. (2008) Evaluation of a protocol for metabolic profiling studies on human blood plasma by combined ultra-performance liquid chromatography/mass spectrometry: From extraction to data analysis. Anal Biochem 372: 237–249. Available: http://www.ncbi.nlm.nih.gov/pubmed/17964273. Accessed 12 August 2013.

21. American Psychiatric Association (2000) Desk Reference to the Diagnostic Criteria from DSM IV. 4th ed. Washington, D.C.: American Psychiatric Association.

22. Corbett BA, Kantor AB, Schulman H, Walker WL, Lit L, et al. (2007) A proteomic study of serum from children with autism showing differential expression of apolipoproteins and complement proteins. Mol Psychiatry 12: 292–306. Available: http://www.ncbi.nlm.nih.gov/pubmed/17189958. Accessed 14 January 2013.

23. Ashwood P, Corbett BA, Kantor A, Schulman H, Van de Water J, et al. (2011) In search of cellular immunophenotypes in the blood of children with autism. PLoS One 6: e19299. Available: http://www.pubmedcentral.nih.gov/articlerender.fcgi?artid=3087757&tool=pmcentrez&rendertype=abstract. Accessed 21 January 2013.

24. Jiye A, Trygg J, Gullberg J, Johansson AI, Jonsson P, et al. (2005) Extraction and GC/MS analysis of the human blood plasma metabolome. Anal Chem 77: 8086–8094. Available: http://www.ncbi.nlm.nih.gov/pubmed/16351159.

25. Fiehn O, Wohlgemuth G, Scholz M, Kind T, Lee DY, et al. (2008) Quality control for plant metabolomics: reporting MSI-compliant studies. Plant J 53: 691–704. doi: 10.1111/j.1365-313X.2007.03387.x.

26. Smith CA, O'Maille G, Want EJ, Qin C, Trauger S a, et al. (2005) METLIN: a metabolite mass spectral database. Ther Drug Monit 27: 747–751. Available: http://www.ncbi.nlm.nih.gov/pubmed/16404815.

27. Horai H, Arita M, Kanaya S, Nihei Y, Ikeda T, et al. (2010) MassBank: a public repository for sharing mass spectral data for life sciences. J Mass Spectrom 45: 703–714. Available: http://www.ncbi.nlm.nih.gov/pubmed/20623627. Accessed 23 August 2013.

28. Orchard S, Montechi-Palazzi L, Deutsch EW, Binz P-A, Jones AR, et al. (2007) Five years of progress in the Standardization of Proteomics Data 4th Annual Spring Workshop of the HUPO-Proteomics Standards Initiative April 23-25, 2007 Ecole Nationale Supérieure (ENS), Lyon, France. Proteomics 7: 3436–3440. Available: http://www.ncbi.nlm.nih.gov/pubmed/17907277. Accessed 1 May 2014.

29. Smith CA, Want EJ, O'Maille G, Abagyan R, Siuzdak G (2006) XCMS: processing mass spectrometry data for metabolite profiling using nonlinear peak alignment, matching, and identification. Anal Chem 78: 779–787. Available: http://www.ncbi.nlm.nih.gov/pubmed/16448051.

30. Prince JT, Marcotte EM (2006) Chromatographic alignment of ESI-LC-MS proteomics data sets by ordered bijective interpolated warping. Anal Chem 78: 6140–6152. Available: http://www.ncbi.nlm.nih.gov/pubmed/16944896.

31. Haury A-C, Gestraud P, Vert J-P (2011) The influence of feature selection methods on accuracy, stability and interpretability of molecular signatures. PLoS One 6: e28210. Available: http://www.ncbi.nlm.nih.gov/pubmed/22205940. Accessed 1 May 2014.

32. Benjamini Y, Hochberg Y (1995) Controlling the false discovery rate: a practical and powerful approach to multiple testing. J R Stat Soc Ser B 57: 289–300.

33. Wold H (1985) Partial least squares. In: Kotz S, Johnson NL, editors. Encyclopedia of statistical sciences. New York: Wiley, Vol. 6. pp. 581–591.

34. Cortes C, Vapnik V (1995) Support-vector networks. Mach Learn 20: 273–297. Available: http://link.springer.com/article/10.1007/BF00994018. Accessed 1 May 2014.

35. Kuhn M (2008) Building predictive models in R using the caret package. J Stat Softw 28: 1–26.

36. Sing T, Sander O, Beerenwinkel N, Lengauer T (2005) ROCR: visualizing classifier performance in R. Bioinformatics 21: 3940–3941. Available: http://www.ncbi.nlm.nih.gov/pubmed/16096348. Accessed 29 April 2014.

37. Frye RE, Melnyk S, Macfabe DF (2013) Unique acyl-carnitine profiles are potential biomarkers for acquired mitochondrial disease in autism spectrum disorder. Transl Psychiatry 3: e220. Available: http://www.pubmedcentral.nih.gov/articlerender.fcgi?artid=3566723&tool=pmcentrez&rendertype=abstract. Accessed 9 January 2014.

38. Ghezzo A, Visconti P, Abruzzo PM, Bolotta A, Ferreri C, et al. (2013) Oxidative Stress and Erythrocyte Membrane Alterations in Children with Autism: Correlation with Clinical Features. PLoS One 8: e66418. Available: http://www.pubmedcentral.nih.gov/articlerender.fcgi?artid=3686873&tool=pmcentrez&rendertype=abstract. Accessed 7 August 2013.

39. Adams JB, Audhya T, McDonough-Means S, Rubin RA, Quig D, et al. (2011) Nutritional and metabolic status of children with autism vs. neurotypical children, and the association with autism severity. Nutr Metab (Lond) 8: 34. Available: http://www.pubmedcentral.nih.gov/articlerender.fcgi?artid=3135510&tool=pmcentrez&rendertype=abstract.

40. Whiteley P, Waring R, Williams L, Klovrza L, Nolan F, et al. (2006) Spot urinary creatinine excretion in pervasive developmental disorders. Pediatr Int 48: 292–297. Available: http://www.ncbi.nlm.nih.gov/pubmed/16732798. Accessed 22 July 2013.

41. Whitaker-Azmitia PM (2005) Behavioral and cellular consequences of increasing serotonergic activity during brain development: a role in autism? Int J Dev Neurosci 23: 75–83. Available: http://www.ncbi.nlm.nih.gov/pubmed/15730889. Accessed 12 November 2013.

42. Marazziti D, Baroni S, Picchetti M, Landi P, Silvestri S, et al. (2012) Psychiatric disorders and mitochondrial dysfunctions. Eur Rev Med Pharmacol Sci 16: 270–275. Available: http://www.ncbi.nlm.nih.gov/pubmed/22428481.

43. Rossignol DA, Frye RE (2012) A review of research trends in physiological abnormalities in autism spectrum disorders: immune dysregulation, inflammation, oxidative stress, mitochondrial dysfunction and environmental toxicant exposures. Mol Psychiatry 17: 389–401. Available: http://www.pubmedcentral.nih.gov/articlerender.fcgi?artid=3317062&tool=pmcentrez&rendertype=abstract. Accessed 5 February 2013.

44. Blaylock RL (2009) A possible central mechanism in autism spectrum disorders, part 2: immunoexcitotoxicity. Altern Ther Health Med 15: 60–67. Available: http://www.ncbi.nlm.nih.gov/pubmed/19161050.

45. Shinohe A, Hashimoto K, Nakamura K, Tsujii M, Iwata Y, et al. (2006) Increased serum levels of glutamate in adult patients with autism. Prog Neuropsychopharmacol Biol Psychiatry 30: 1472–1477. Available: http://www.ncbi.nlm.nih.gov/pubmed/16863675. Accessed 15 July 2013.

46. Moreno-Fuenmayor H, Borjas L, Arrieta A, Valera V, Socorro-Candanoza L (1996) Plasma excitatory amino acids in autism. Invest Clin 37: 113–128.

47. Napolioni V, Persico AM, Porcelli V, Palmieri L (2011) The mitochondrial aspartate/glutamate carrier AGC1 and calcium homeostasis: physiological links and abnormalities in autism. Mol Neurobiol 44: 83–92.

48. Safiulina D, Peet N, Seppet E, Zharkovsky A, Kaasik A (2006) Dehydroepiandrosterone inhibits complex I of the mitochondrial respiratory chain and is neurotoxic in vitro and in vivo at high concentrations. Toxicol Sci 93: 348–356. Available: http://www.ncbi.nlm.nih.gov/pubmed/16849397. Accessed 9 January 2014.

49. Strous RD, Golubchik P, Maayan R, Mozes T, Tuati-Werner D, et al. (2005) Lowered DHEA-S plasma levels in adult individuals with autistic disorder. Eur Neuropsychopharmacol 15: 305–309. Available: http://www.ncbi.nlm.nih.gov/pubmed/15820420. Accessed 23 August 2013.

50. Tordjman S, Anderson GM, McBride PA, Hertzig ME, Snow ME, et al. (1995) Plasma androgens in autism. J Autism Dev Disord 25: 295–304. Available: http://www.ncbi.nlm.nih.gov/pubmed/7559294.

51. Arnold GL, Hyman SL, Mooney RA, Kirby RS (2003) Plasma amino acids profiles in children with autism: potential risk of nutritional deficiencies. J Autism Dev Disord 33: 449–454. Available: http://www.ncbi.nlm.nih.gov/pubmed/12959424.

52. Novarino G, El-Fishawy P, Kayserili H, Meguid N a, Scott EM, et al. (2012) Mutations in BCKD-kinase lead to a potentially treatable form of autism with epilepsy. Science 338: 394–397. Available: http://www.ncbi.nlm.nih.gov/pubmed/22956686. Accessed 24 October 2012.

53. Valerio A, D'Antona G, Nisoli E (2011) Branched-chain amino acids, mitochondrial biogenesis, and healthspan: an evolutionary perspective. Aging (Albany NY) 3: 464–478. Available: http://www.pubmedcentral.nih.gov/articlerender.fcgi?artid=3156598&tool=pmcentrez&rendertype=abstract.

54. Müller E, Kölker S (2004) Reduction of lysine intake while avoiding malnutrition–major goals and major problems in dietary treatment of glutaryl-CoA dehydrogenase deficiency. J Inherit Metab Dis 27: 903–910. Available: http://www.ncbi.nlm.nih.gov/pubmed/15505398.

55. Mulle JG, Sharp WG, Cubells JF (2013) The gut microbiome: a new frontier in autism research. Curr Psychiatry Rep 15: 337. Available: http://www.ncbi.nlm.nih.gov/pubmed/23307560. Accessed 7 August 2013.

56. Beloborodova N, Bairamov I, Olenin A, Shubina V, Teplova V, et al. (2012) Effect of phenolic acids of microbial origin on production of reactive oxygen species in mitochondria and neutrophils. J Biomed Sci 19: 89. Available: http://www.pubmedcentral.nih.gov/articlerender.fcgi?artid=3503878&tool=pmcentrez&rendertype=abstract. Accessed 6 August 2013.

57. Palmieri F (2004) The mitochondrial transporter family (SLC25): physiological and pathological implications. Pflugers Arch 447: 689–709.

58. Viegas CM, Busanello ENB, Tonin AM, de Moura AP, Grings M, et al. (2011) Dual mechanism of brain damage induced in vivo by the major metabolites accumulating in hyperornithinemia-hyperammonemia-homocitrullinuria syndrome. Brain Res 1369: 235–244. Available: http://www.ncbi.nlm.nih.gov/pubmed/21059345. Accessed 26 August 2014.

59. Sokoro A a H, Lepage J, Antonishyn N, McDonald R, Rockman-Greenberg C, et al. (2010) Diagnosis and high incidence of hyperornithinemia-hyperammo-nemia-homocitrullinemia (HHH) syndrome in northern Saskatchewan. J Inherit Metab Dis 33 Suppl 3: S275–81. Available: http://www.ncbi.nlm.nih.gov/pubmed/20574716. Accessed 26 August 2014.

60. Yin P, Peter A, Franken H, Zhao X, Neukamm SS, et al. (2013) Preanalytical aspects and sample quality assessment in metabolomics studies of human blood. Clin Chem 59: 833–845. Available: http://www.ncbi.nlm.nih.gov/pubmed/23386698. Accessed 18 August 2014.

61. Kanehisa M (1997) A database for post-genome analysis. Trends Genet 13: 375–376.

## 19

Views on Researcher-Community Engagement in Autism Research in the United Kingdom: A Mixed-Methods Study

Elizabeth Pellicano[1]*, Adam Dinsmore[1,2], Tony Charman[3]

1 Centre for Research in Autism and Education (CRAE), Department of Psychology and Human Development, Institute of Education, University of London, London, United Kingdom, **2** Wellcome Trust, Strategic Planning & Policy Unit, London, United Kingdom, **3** Department of Psychology, King's College London, Institute of Psychiatry, London, United Kingdom

Abstract

There has been a substantial increase in research activity on autism during the past decade. Research into effective ways of responding to the immediate needs of autistic people is, however, less advanced, as are efforts at translating basic science research into service provision. Involving community members in research is one potential way of reducing this gap. This study therefore investigated the views of community involvement in autism research both from the perspectives of autism researchers and of community members, including autistic adults, family members and practitioners. Results from a large-scale questionnaire study (n = 1,516) showed that researchers perceive themselves to be engaged with the autism community but that community members, most notably autistic people and their families, did not share this view. Focus groups/interviews with 72 participants further identified the potential benefits and remaining challenges to involvement in research, especially regarding the distinct perspectives of different stakeholders. Researchers were skeptical about the possibilities of dramatically increasing community engagement, while community members themselves spoke about the challenges to fully understanding and influencing the research process. We suggest that the lack of a shared approach to community engagement in UK autism research represents a key roadblock to translational endeavors.

Editor: Sassy Molyneux, University of Oxford, Kenya

Funding: This work was funded by the Inge Wakehurst Foundation, the Charles Wolfson Foundation, and The Waterloo Foundation. The funders had no role in the design of the study, collection and analysis of the data, or preparation and review of the manuscript.

Competing Interests: Dr. Charman has received grant or research support from the UK Medical Research Council, European Commission FP7, European Science Foundation, Autism Speaks, the Simons Foundation, Autistica, Research Autism, and the Waterloo Foundation. He has received royalties from Guilford Press and Sage. Dr Pellicano has received grant or research support from the Medical Research Council, the Australian Research Council, the Nuffield Foundation, Research Autism, and the Waterloo Foundation.

* Email: l.pellicano@ioe.ac.uk

Introduction

Basic scientific research is fundamental to improving human health. Yet the application of major scientific breakthroughs to where they are most needed, in clinics and communities, is often not swiftly forthcoming [1]. Translational research has therefore become a high priority for biomedical research policy around the world. Research centres have been established, grant programmes launched and scientists have been urged to think anew about the potential impact of their research. These initiatives have been motivated to accelerate "the translation of discoveries from basic laboratory and clinical science into benefits for human health [2] and to ensure public accountability for the investment in basic science. But whatever the precise driver, the core intention of translational research is clear: to close the gap between fundamental biomedical research and clinical, educational and related practice [3–5].

The potential benefits of translational research are nowhere greater than in the field of autism. There has been a dramatic increase in the recorded prevalence of autism in the past few decades [6–7]. Recent figures estimate that approximately 1% of the population in the United Kingdom has an autism spectrum condition [8–9], with similar estimates recorded in other parts of the world [10]. There has also been a dramatic expansion of research, particularly on neural and cognitive systems, genetics and other causal pathways both in the UK and abroad [11–12]. This surge in basic autism science promises to enhance the life chances of autistic people and their families. Yet the translational potential of this work remains unfulfilled, partly because only a minority of UK research funding is directed towards identifying effective treatments, interventions and services for individuals with autism [13]. As a result, the opportunities and life-chances for autistic people remain often severely limited in comparison with the non-autistic population. It has thus become imperative for autism researchers to reduce the translational gap.

In biomedical research more broadly, models of translational research have moved beyond a unidirectional bench-to-bedside approach to ones that also encourage *backwards translation*, with knowledge "from the bedside" informing research in the laboratory [5]. There is growing recognition, however, that even these bi-directional approaches can be overly simplistic; that the translational process is instead multidirectional and dynamic, including multiple points of knowledge exchange not only between researcher and practitioner communities but also, critically, between researcher and "patient" communities. That appears to be rarely the case in practice, however. Despite good intentions, in many current models [14] engagement of stakeholders is usually restricted to the dissemination and implementation phases – the very ends of the "translational pipeline". Yet it is plausibly argued that translation will only be successful when scientific discoveries are more thoroughly *relevant* to "patients" and communities, are sufficiently *tailored* to the realities of their everyday lives and are consistent with their values [15–18].

In response, there has been a deliberate expansion of public participation across the UK's National Health Service (www.invo.org.uk), where health and social care researchers are encouraged to involve "patients" and members of the public as partners in the research process – working actively *with* community members rather than on or for them [19]. Such community engagement might be thought to be particularly important with regard to autism, given the long history of controversial claims by autism scientists – from "refrigerator mothers" [20] to the vaccine furore [21] – and the growing distrust of mainstream autism science by autistic self-advocates [22–24]. This entails that efforts to engage the broader autism community have advantages beyond any practical use they may or may not have in directly translating research findings into concrete changes in clinical and other practice. Engagement can potentially help overcome distrust between professionals and others, can strengthen the self-esteem and self-respect of researched communities and can help ensure that the research process properly responds to the interests and entitlements of autistic people [25–26].

Despite the potential importance of such efforts, almost nothing is formally known about the extent to which the autism community is engaged in research, beyond being involved as 'subjects'. We simply do not know how commonplace formal or informal engagement practices are in autism research and whether a lack of community engagement represents a barrier to the translational endeavour. This study aimed to address these issues by asking both researchers and members of the autism community about their experiences of engagement in research. The autism community, however, is not homogenous and seldom speaks with a singular voice [25]. We therefore also examined potential differences in the degree and nature of the engagement experiences of distinct groups within the autism community. Rather than the more commonly used terms such as "patients", "service user" or "stakeholder", we use the term "autism community" to reflect the varied nature of this group, which includes those who are autistic themselves and those who care for, or who work with, children, young people and adults on the autism spectrum.

Method

Focus groups and interviews

Seventy-two participants took part in 11 focus groups and 10 individual interviews, including 14 autistic adults (2 female), 27 parents of autistic children (all mothers), 20 practitioners (18 female; 2 speech and language therapists; 16 teachers, 2 educational psychologists), 11 autism researchers (5 female; 6 early career researchers). Of the mothers, their children ranged in age from 5 to 19 years and also ranged in ability from those who had limited spoken language (n = 10) to those who they considered to be cognitively able or "high functioning" (n = 27). These groups were selected because they each held a "stake" in autism research. Autistic adults, parents and practitioners were recruited through community contacts across the UK. Researchers were recruited through personal contacts.

The focus groups and semi-structured interviews followed the same format. Discussion focused on participants' perceptions of current UK autism research and their priorities for future research (analysis of these data are presented in [13]). Towards the end of these discussions, we elicited participants' views and perspectives about the degree and nature of the autism community's engagement in research. Specifically, we asked about their experiences of being involved in research (or, in the case of researchers, involving the autism community in their research) and how they would like to be involved in the future.

Each focus group was kept exclusive (e.g., autistic adults only) and was conducted face-to-face in a location convenient for participants. Groups were led by a facilitator, who from time-to-time summarised the key points to the group and confirmed the interpretation of comments. Focus groups ranged from 44 to 124 mins (M = 93 mins). Interviews were conducted either face-to-face (n = 4), over Skype (n = 2) or on the telephone (n = 4), and lasted between 32 and 104 mins (M = 51 mins).

Where possible, focus groups/interviews were audiotaped and subsequently transcribed and analysed using the NVivo software package (Version 9). The resulting data were analysed using thematic analysis [27]. We adopted an inductive approach, providing descriptive overviews of the key features of the semantic content of data within an essentialist framework. Two of the authors (LP and AD) independently familiarised themselves with the data, meeting regularly to discuss preliminary themes and make a list of provisional codes. Each author then independently applied an exhaustive list of codes to the transcript of each interview/focus group. The authors met several times to review the results, resolve discrepancies and decide how the codes could be collapsed into themes and subthemes. All authors approached the coding and discussions from the perspective of autism scientists with an interest in public and community engagement in research.

Online questionnaire

To reach a larger sample of the UK's autism community, we then developed an online questionnaire to gauge people's experiences of autism research in the UK. To encourage participation, this questionnaire was brief (11 questions), following a very similar structure to the focus groups/interviews. The design of the questionnaire was informed by the results of the focus groups/interviews, yielding changes to specific wording of items and the inclusion of the category 'dissemination' in our levels of engagement question (see below). This latter modification was in response to parents' wide-ranging experiences of hearing about autism research being conducted in the UK.

The questionnaire began with a series of background items (UK resident, primary interest in autism research, age, gender) followed by questions relating to participants' research priorities and their perspectives on the pattern of UK funding for autism research [13]. The final three questions related to the degree of engagement in research between the autism/research communities. Specifically, we asked participants (1) to indicate how often they had experienced three levels of 'engagement' (public dissemination, dialogue and partnership) between autism researchers and the broader autism community (on a 5-point scale from 'very rarely' (score of 1) to 'very frequently' (score of 5)), (2) to rate how satisfied they were with the level of engagement they had experienced (on a 5-point scale from 'very dissatisfied' (score of 1) to 'very satisfied' (score of 5)), and (3) to provide a reason for their stated level of satisfaction (open comment).

Respondents were told that engagement between researchers and the broader autism community could occur in a variety of ways including through:

1. *Dissemination*, where researchers provide information about the results of completed research through newsletters, online blogs, public events, etc.

2. *Dialogue*, where researchers communicate directly or consult with members of the autism community for their views about the research being conducted.

3. *Partnership*, where researchers and members of the autism community collaborate, as partners, in the research process, working together to set research goals and coming up with ways of realising them.

Our three levels of engagement differed somewhat from those advocated by INVOLVE (which include (1) consultation, (2) collaboration, and (3) lay control; see www.invo.org.uk and [28]) because (a) our initial results from the focus groups suggested that several community members had no previous experience of engaging in autism research (see below) and (b) instances of user-controlled autism research are extremely rare. Our levels of engagement therefore might be conceived of as lower down the rungs of a 'ladder of participation' [29] than those of INVOLVE but nevertheless reflected the current range of engagement activities in this particular field of research.

Participants were recruited through extensive community canvassing, including through autistic organisations, parent advocacy groups, practitioner and researcher networks, and via social media (Twitter, Facebook) and online fora. 1,632 people completed the engagement items of the questionnaire. To facilitate comparisons with the focus groups/interviews, analysis focused upon the 1,516 respondents aged 18 and over who could be divided into four key stakeholder groups: autistic adults, immediate family members, practitioners and researchers (see Table 1). The remaining 107 participants, who had labeled themselves as 'other' (e.g., student, "interested in autism"), were not considered further. For parents and carers (n = 825), the mean age of their child with autism was 13.4 years (SD = 9.0; range = 2–57; 142 females) and, for sons, daughters or siblings (n = 24), the mean age of their autistic family member was 27.1 years (SD = 16.3; range = 4–65; 6 females).

To ensure that our study was accessible as possible, autistic adults were invited to take part in the study using a range of formats (focus group, individual face-to-face interview, telephone/ Skype interview and email); both the questions for discussion and the survey questions were offered to autistic participants so that they could review them in advance, if required; and two autistic adults acted as pilot participants and worked with the research team to make sure that discussion and survey items were comprehensible and easy to respond to.

Ethics Statement

Ethical approval for this study was granted by the Faculty of Policy and Society's Research Ethics Committee at the Institute of Education, University of London. All participants gave written informed consent prior to participation and all data were collected anonymously.

Results

Focus groups/interviews: Researcher views

Uncertainty towards community involvement. The first subtheme related to the *limits of involvement* (see Figure 1A). For some researchers there was a strong sense of the need for real participation in research: "we have to involve them from the very start, in helping to define and shape the research". Others felt that people making judgments about research and research funding "have to be other scientists" but that the viewpoints of different stakeholders should nevertheless be consulted: "I don't think that we want it to, the decision making, to move away from the scientists but I think they should at least get input from relevant stakeholders". Others still were wary about involving autistic people and their families in decisions about research because (a) they might not be the appropriate people to decide what and how issues should be researched and (b) it risks "politicizing" scientific issues.

The second subtheme was *contesting partnership*. While there was consensus that involving members of the autism community as partners in research was not commonplace in autism research, researchers nevertheless differed in what they meant by "partnership". Some researchers understood it as members of the autism community being involved in priority-setting exercises, while others talked of such members "contributing feedback" and "being on steering groups". There were also suggestions that the nature and degree of involvement depended on the type of research being conducted: "People are much more likely to be better at involvement or engagement with people when there's a very direct patient interaction … whereas if you're dealing with anonymized urine samples or DNA samples then you're less likely to directly try and engage with stakeholders."

The final subtheme related to the *obstacles to, but potential rewards of, community engagement*. Some researchers acknowledged the potential costs of community involvement, including the considerable time, money and effort spent in building and

Table 1. Descriptives for respondents to the online survey for each of the four key stakeholder groups (total n = 1516).

	Autistic[a] person (n = 122)	Immediate family member (n = 849)	Professional (n = 426)	Researcher (n = 119)
Chronological age				
M (SD)	39.4 (12.9)	45.1 (9.8)	42.2 (11.8)	40.6 (13.8)
Range	18–72	18–83	21–70	22–87
Gender				
Female	56	765	350	81
Male	60	83	74	38
Other/would rather not say	6	1	2	1

Note: [a] The term "autistic person" is the preferred language of many people on the spectrum [50]. In this paper, we use this term as well as person-first language to respect the wishes of all individuals on the spectrum.

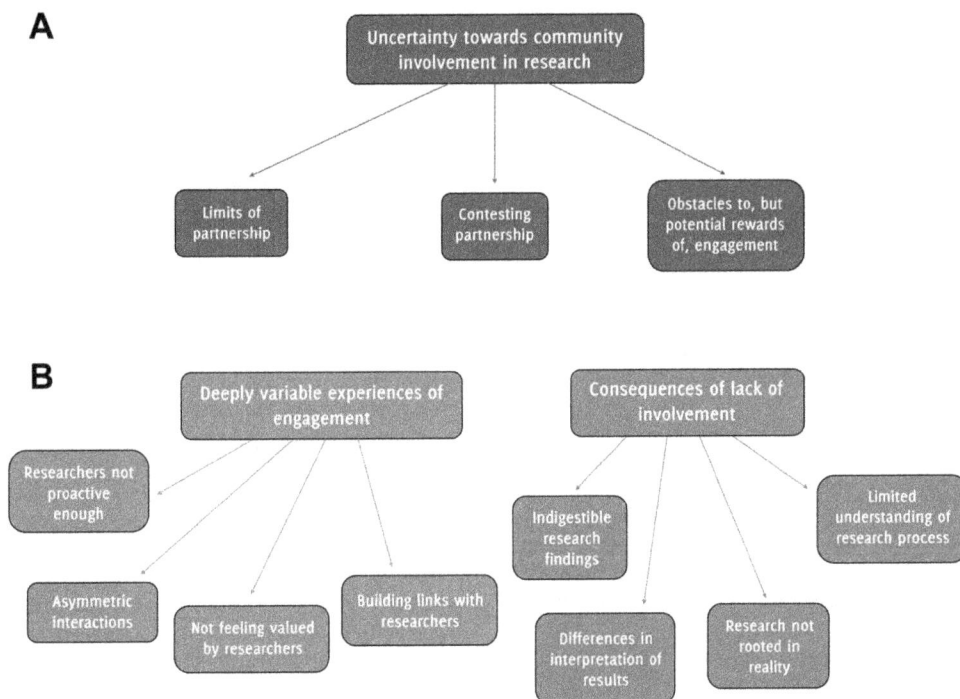

Figure 1. Researchers' (A) and community members' (B) perspectives on involvement in research: themes and subthemes.

maintaining partnerships. Researchers were also concerned about the diversity of views within the autism community and the unlikelihood of any disputes being resolved. Others noted the potential benefits to involvement, including increased awareness of the research process by autistic people, families and practitioners and "a better chance that the research will get translated into practice".

Focus groups/interviews: Community views

The majority of autistic adults, parents of children with autism and professionals wanted to be more involved in the research process. The two themes identified related to their *deeply variable experiences of involvement* and the *consequences of lack of involvement* (see Figure 1B).

Deeply variable experiences of involvement. The nature of participants' experience of involvement in research varied widely but, overall, community members felt that *researchers aren't proactive enough*. Some parents, particularly those whose children had limited spoken communication, commented that they had never been approached by researchers to be part of research: "So I just find it really weird that, as a parent, you aren't approached about doing research, or providing information, that kind of thing, you have to go out and find it yourself." These parents were perplexed that researchers were not "utilizing families" who were "waiting to be tapped into". Practitioners noted the challenges of parental involvement, however, due to the busy nature of their lives: "it is often difficult to round up [parents] and get them involved".

Parents and autistic adults with some experience of research emphasized the largely *asymmetric interactions with researchers*. Parents in particular highlighted that they "never get to find out the outcome." One mother said, "I get a lot of asking for help. And then a bit less [contact] when something's going on, and hardly any results!" They wanted their involvement as participants

to be valued by researchers. Autistic adults' reports were more negative, noting "sometimes we are a bit like monkeys in a zoo." They spoke of the lack of reciprocity in their interactions with researchers: "they only want us as guinea pigs; that's the only contact they want with us."

Autistic adults and parents also reported *not feeling valued by researchers*. Some participants were genuinely unaware that they could have a say in research while others were skeptical of the possibility of actually influencing research: "It's like not anybody is interested" (parent); "Whatever we say, is that really going to influence anyone?" (autistic adult). Some autistic adults reported that even when they had a voice, it was not listened to: "I just think sometimes when we say something we just sort of throw a spanner in the works, it doesn't suit their sort of agenda." Others noted experiences of paternalism: "That's the danger of when someone knows you have a diagnosis, because there suddenly seems to be some sort of ascendency process that goes on and suddenly they have the right then to talk down to you, because you've got a label." These adults stressed the need for researchers to value their expertise (of being autistic: "You have your area of expertise, which is not mine, and we have our area of expertise; you have to look at us on a similar level") and for their involvement in research to extend beyond mere tokenism. Instead, they wanted to see more autistic people involved in research projects because "a lot of things aren't done with the autistic subjective kind of values and wants in mind."

Practitioners were more positive about *building links with researchers* than autistic adults and family members. They highlighted the important links being built between researchers and their schools or clinics: "It's good that the people on the ground are trying to help support academia to come up with questions that are actually pertinent to what we want to find out about."

Consequences of lack of involvement in research. Parents and autistic adults who had been involved as participants in research generally felt that *research findings were indigestible*. They emphasized their interest in research but also noted that they "haven't got the time to read lots of information, absorb it, react to it, go and search for something that links to it" (parent). Many commented that the information they received was not written in a "user-friendly" way, being full of scientific jargon: "when I read stuff that neurotypicals write about autism, for me it just reads like gobbledygook, it just doesn't make any sense" (autistic adult). They suggested that research findings "need to be simplified for them to understand what researchers are actually trying to put across" and needed to be targeted specifically at them, "coming through my door", rather than having to have to find it themselves.

Parents and practitioners spoke of the disconnect between the research that goes on and that research that would actually make a difference to their lives or the lives of those they work with: "Researchers are not interested in social issues or anything like that, all they are interested is in medical issues" (parent). Parents reported feeling "jaded" and "cynical" about "pointless" research that is so far removed from their everyday experiences of autism. One mother said, "I fill in all these questionnaires and do everything I can to help and there's a very nice paper at the end with nice results and it's like "great". But when it comes down to it, it's not real life. It's always missing the next step – great you've done this research, you've listened to my views, you've asked for them I've given them, but now do something with it." Other parents felt as if the people making the decisions about research have probably "never been anywhere near someone with autism." One mother said, "I think [contact with autistic people] would benefit the researchers, because they are kind of getting first hand experience from the people that are living with the children with autism … that I think would help towards the research because it's giving them an idea of what's really happening every single day."

Some parents also felt frustrated with the lack of certainty that research provides; that there were no clear-cut answers or not enough research on the topics about which they needed answers. Their observations suggested that the lack of community involvement potentially resulted in a *limited understanding of the research process*: "I found as well that a lot of the researchers kind of contradict themselves, like one researcher will stand up and sort of say if your child goes on this gluten free diet it will better them, and improve this etc., and then you hear another researcher say no, that's rubbish, absolute rubbish."

Autistic adults specifically spoke of their expertise (of being autistic) and the benefits that an insider autistic view would bring to research. They felt that the lack of community involvement in research led to *differences in interpretation*: "I feel that whoever's doing research is coming from a certain perspective, and you are starting off with an assumption that that person's disabled, and then you are looking at the research on the basis that we are disabled, like a rat in a cage, and if you do research like that you are probably going to end up very far, you know, confirming your own suspicions at the beginning." One autistic adult suggested that, "having more autistic researchers or employing people on teams might guard against the possibility of misinterpretation [of findings]."

Online questionnaire: Frequency ratings

Descriptive statistics for respondents' frequency ratings of engagement are shown in Table 2. With regards to *dissemination*, autistic adults, family members and practitioners reported that they had experienced dissemination of research 'occasionally'

(mode score of '3'), while researchers reported 'frequently' (mode score of '4') participating in dissemination with the broader autism community. With respect to *dialogue*, autistic adults and practitioners indicated that they 'occasionally' experienced dialogue with researchers but family members said that they 'very rarely' (mode score of '1') experienced this sort of engagement. Researchers felt, however, that they 'frequently' participated in a dialogue with members of the autism community. All of the community groups stated that they had 'very rarely' (mode score of '1') experienced *partnership* with researchers while researchers felt that they were 'occasionally' (mode score of '3') involved in partnerships with autism community members.

One-way ANOVAs on participants' mean ratings (see Table 2) with group as a factor (autistic adults, family members, practitioners, researchers) revealed significant group differences for dissemination, $F(3, 1,515) = 22.69$, $p<.001$, dialogue, $F(3, 1,515) = 58.65$, $p<.001$, and partnership, $F(3, 1,515) = 33.28$, $p<.001$. Post-hoc tests (Tukey's HSD) revealed the source of these differences. Note that because of the relatively large number of comparisons conducted, results are not reported as significant unless they reached a p value of less than .01.

Overall, researchers reported being engaged in dissemination, dialogue and partnership significantly more frequently than autistic adults, family members and practitioners reported experiencing such engagement (all ps<.01). There were also some subtle differences between community members' ratings. Autistic adults and family members reported being less involved in dissemination than practitioners (both ps<.005). Family members' mean ratings were significantly lower for dialogue than both autistic adults and practitioners (both ps<.005) but the latter two groups did not differ (p = .95). Finally, family members' ratings of the frequency with which they experienced partnerships with researchers were significantly lower (i.e., less frequent) than practitioners (p<.001) but not autistic adults (p = .22). Autistic adults' and practitioners' ratings did not differ (p = .64).

We then examined the degree to which researchers and non-researchers were satisfied with this level of engagement. A one-way ANOVA on the mean ratings confirmed that the distribution of responses were slightly skewed towards 'dissatisfied' for autistic adults and family members but less so for practitioners and researchers (see Figure 2). There was a main effect of group, $F(3, 1,515) = 14.16$, $p<.001$. Researchers' (M = 3.02; SD = 1.01) and practitioners' (M = 2.96; SD = .90) ratings were significantly higher (reflecting greater satisfaction) than both autistic adults (M = 2.60; SD = 1.26) and family members (M = 2.63; SD = .97) (both ps<.005). There were no other group differences (ps>.90).

Open question: Researcher views

Survey respondents were also asked to specify their reasons for their level of satisfaction with engagement in research (852 responses). Of the 63 researchers who responded to this question (see Table 3 for themes and corresponding quotes), several noted the importance of involving the autism community in the research process: "The perspectives of the population being researched should always be the first starting point." All other comments centred on the *invitation to engage* and the *barriers to engagement* (see Table 3). Several researchers expressed how receptive and supportive the broader autism community had generally been to hearing about, or requests to take part in, research. Others' experiences were less positive, however, noting that involvement often amounted to a "tick-box exercise". With regards to the potential barriers of involvement, some researchers pointed to a lack of a singular voice within the autism community, while others noted that the communication difficulties experienced by autistic

Table 2. Respondents' mean frequency ratings for their experiences of each type of researcher-community engagement.

	Type of Engagement		
	Dissemination	Dialogue	Partnership
	M (SD)	M (SD)	M (SD)
	Range	Range	Range
Autistic adults	2.73 (1.3)	2.50 (1.2)	2.03 (1.2)
(n = 122)	1–5	1–5	1–5
Immediate family members	2.69 (1.3)	2.11 (1.08)	1.84 (1.0)
(n = 849)	1–5	1–5	1–5
Practitioners	3.12 (1.2)	2.42 (1.12)	2.16 (1.1)
(n = 426)	1–5	1–5	1–5
Autism researchers	3.48 (.96)	3.50 (.98)	2.82 (1.1)
(n = 119)	1–5	1–5	1–5

Note: Lower values reflect reduced frequency of involvement in research.

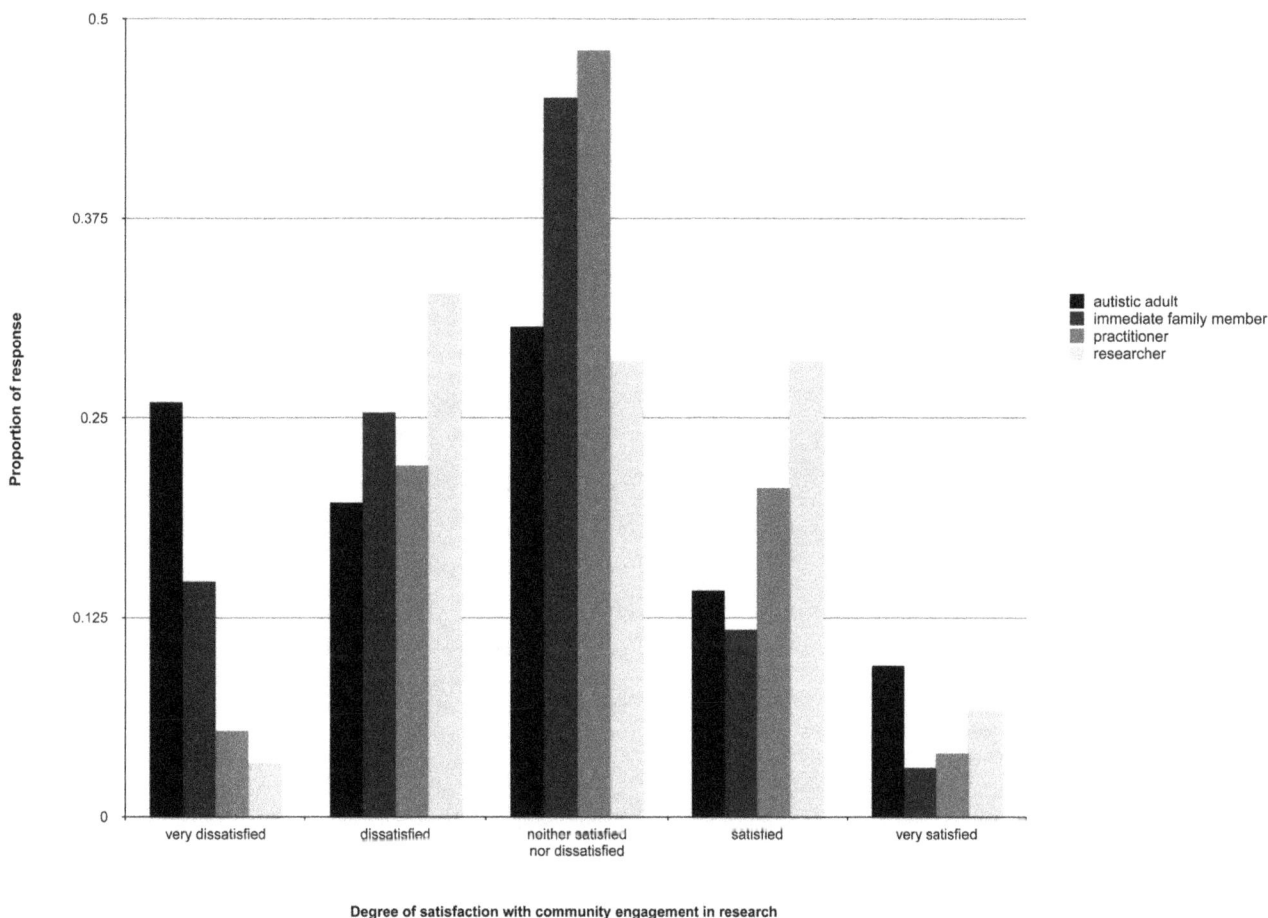

Figure 2. The proportion of responses for each stakeholder group with regards to their degree of satisfaction with community involvement in research.

Table 3. Themes identified from open question in online questionnaire by autism researchers (n = 63).

Themes	Subtheme	Example quotes
Invitation to engage	Positive community attitudes towards research	"The public are very interested to hear about autism research." "Given the huge need for help and support for persons with autism, which is alas, often unmet, the public are very open and willing to take part in research that can go any ways towards this goal."
	Scepticism toward involvement	"I feel that it can often be tokenistic, i.e. asking the same old panel of people with autism to contribute to policy, practice and decision making almost to "tick the box" to say that people with autism have been involved."
Barriers to engagement	No singular voice	"The experiences of individuals with autism and their families are many and varied. Sometimes the most vocal individuals have a completely different experience/agenda than some of the most vulnerable people we engage."
		"Attempts at engagement are very quickly dominated by more able people and people with additional mild to moderate learning disabilities, who could express their views with support, become swamped."
		"Autism charities and groups are disparate and fractious."
	Autistic features make involvement difficult	"Some of the challenges people with autism may face make the interactions quite difficult - trouble taking on board another person's point of view, commenting in a sensitive way that does not cause offense, etc. I would favour more partnership, but very different goals and methods of interaction make this a formidable challenge."
		"It can often be difficult to work with people with autism as their viewpoints may be held very firmly and a 'black and white' thinking style can be a challenge."
		"Due to the nature of autism, inclusion in group discussions/debates and decision making is difficult and time consuming (therefore expensive). I do feel these factors influence the true involvement of people with autism in research."

people posed considerable problems for wider involvement in research.

Open question: Community views

Comments from community members focused on similar themes, including their *experiences of engagement* in research and *barriers to engagement* (see Table 4). With regards to members' experiences of involvement, a common subtheme was the lack of awareness of the research being conducted. All three groups reported receiving few approaches from researchers to participate actively in research and there was uncertainty surrounding how they might come to know about such opportunities. Of those that had participated in research, many community members linked their level of satisfaction with engagement to researchers' attitudes. Respectful attitudes among researchers were often cited for high levels of satisfaction, although community members' experiences were not always so positive, with some highlighting a lack of interest in autistic adults' or practitioners' experience and expertise. Other dissatisfied community members focused on the nature of the often one-sided interactions with researchers. They reported being frustrated with the little or no feedback provided by researchers following participation.

The second theme again centred on *barriers to engagement* in research. For autistic adults and parents, these barriers included their own or their autistic relative's age, gender, and level of functioning; research often excluded adults, especially older adults, girls and women, and those with additional (and severe) intellectual disabilities. Parents also cited the prohibitive time demands of caring for their child with autism and practitioners spoke of difficulties finding the time for involvement in research in their already busy lives. Finally, for some respondents, their experiences of involvement had led to some scepticism about research. Many autistic respondents credited their lack of satisfaction to what they described as "dehumanizing" interactions ("being treated like guinea pigs") and the predominance of a

neurotypical outlook (i.e., one focused on cure and prevention of autism) among researchers.

Some autistic adults, parents and practitioners felt that they had limited access to research and its findings, and were especially critical of the prevalence of prohibitive paywalls and journal subscription requirements. Both parents and practitioners were critical of the language used in research reports, which made it inaccessible to lay audiences, and which caused them to feel "swamped" and "bombarded" with information they did not understand. Community members also commented on researchers' priorities for autism research, which seemed to conflict with their own. They were more likely to feel satisfied by their level of engagement in research if the projects in which they participated had explicit, practical applications. Some members, especially parents and practitioners, reported feeling "let down" by research that had no bearing on their everyday lives.

Discussion

Within traditional models of research, researchers design and implement their studies, and interpret and disseminate the findings, only seeking interaction with the community during the recruitment and participation stages. Yet the need to speed up the translation of basic science findings into practical applications has prompted calls for greater participation in the research process by communities across health-related research [4] (www.invo.org.uk). This study is the first to investigate the degree and nature of community involvement in the field of autism research both from the perspectives of researchers and of members of the autism community. We sought to understand current engagement practices and identify potential barriers and opportunities to engagement in research and, ultimately, to the translational endeavour.

There were competing views between stakeholder groups regarding the degree of engagement in current UK autism research. Overall, researchers perceived themselves to be engaged with the autism community – in terms of the extent to which they

Table 4. Themes identified from open question in online questionnaire by autistic adults (n = 94), immediate family members (n = 476) and practitioners (n = 219).

Themes	Subtheme	Example quotes
Experiences of engagement	Lack of awareness about research	"This is the first time I have heard of any research." *Autistic adult*
		"I have never had any engagement." *Autistic adult*
		"The research is conducted by, in the main, neurotypical researchers looking at, not surprisingly, neurotypically framed problems and questions. There are too many assumptions about what it is like to be autistic, what autistic people want and possibly most important, what autistic people need." *Autistic adult*
		"I feel isolated from any sort of research. I have very little knowledge of any research that may be going on or what its purpose is. Is it purely academic? Does it have practical applications, and if so, how? " *Parent*
		"There is just so little research that I'm aware of. Once diagnosed, you're left to get on with it unless you have the time and inclination to get involved in support groups." *Parent*
		"I have never been approached or asked to take part in research although I would be interested to do so." *Practitioner*
	Experiences depend on researcher attitudes	"The autism researchers that I dealt with personally were always interested in what I had to say, as well as my well-being." *Autistic adult*
		"I find a majority of autism researchers I have managed to speak to unapproachable and more concerned with engaging in academic debates about autism as opposed to speaking to autistics." *Autistic adult*
		"Those I have come into contact with have had a genuine interest and concern for people with autism." *Parent*
		"Some of the researchers have been informative and collaborative, others have no interest in what practitioners need or have to share" *Practitioner*
	Asymmetric interactions	"Despite most research projects claiming that information about the results of these projects will be sent to me upon their completion, I very rarely, if ever, receive any such information. It almost feels like they've got what they need from me by this point, so they don't really need to contact me again with the results, as they won't get anything back by doing so." *Autistic adult*
		"Researchers are more keen on collecting data, but not providing results" *Autistic adult*
		"I would like more detail of the results of research, particularly where I have given time and effort to helping with it. I sometimes only get a very short summary of the research, and often I would welcome more detail." *Parent*
		"Often have not had feedback from the results of a research project and often left thinking... and so? What does that matter, what happens next/what difference does that make?" *Practitioner*
Barriers to engagement	Lack of opportunity to get involved	"I've been turned away from a few studies for being female." *Autistic adults*
		"In my experience researchers are only interested in helping those at the more able end of the spectrum." *Parent*
		"I do get asked for help in research issues but as I work full time and my son is ASD I don't have the time to do them. My son is at respite today and I am having a day off which is the only reason I've been able to complete this." *Parent*
		"Carers don't have much time or energy left over for things that don't directly affect our ability to deal with the day to day issues, however much we want access to latest thinking." *Parent*
		"As a practitioner in the public sector I am overworked and often not able to find time to actively engage with current research, though I like to stay informed on research reports" *Practitioner*
	Skeptical about researcher intentions	"Being used by researchers to further their own career." *Autistic adult*
		"Most autism researchers are engaged in research that I find unacceptable, i.e. looking for 'cures' or which seem to 'objectify' autistic people as odd or freaks or severely flawed." *Autistic adult*
		"I don't think many researchers feel they can talk to autistic people as if they matter, they're too busy studying them like specimens or looking for a 'cure'." *Practitioner*
		"There are pockets of joined up working which are excellent but there are also huge silos within the world of autism research." *Practitioner*
	Absence of accessible, user-friendly research	"Lots of research is not in the public domain and requires subscriptions." *Autistic adult*
		"I have only been involved because I have been proactive myself. Families have lots of information about living with the effects of Autism yet researchers don't seem to be tapping in to this resource." *Parent*
		"It's hard to find out about the research and about what's available publicly. Useful info and links tend to come via word of mouth - other routes are typically time-consuming, material often not user-friendly." *Parent*

Table 4. Cont.

Themes	Subtheme	Example quotes
		"It should be easier to access research papers published in journals. Researchers should be prepared to publish pdfs of their own research papers, since members of the autism community often do not have access to journal subscriptions." *Parent*
		"We live in a society where it can be hard to be sure of who is a credible source of information/ opinion when online, either via blogs or social networking etc. Open access to journals may increase the public's opportunity to find out about the latest autism research from a reliable source." *Practitioner*
		"As an autism professional I have to seek out any information regarding research myself, very rarely is it in a format that is easy to comprehend for a non academic/researcher." *Practitioner*
	Research topics not rooted in reality	"Feels like researchers are working in their own world, with little direct engagement with us. Probably they are following the funding and have become isolated from the practical issues people face." *Parent*
		"Those of us who live and breathe autism and who have to manage daily to support our children can feel left out of the debate. Researchers will look for something of interest TO THEM - and not necessarily useful to the autism community in any practical sense." *Parent*
		"I feel most UK researchers operating from ivory towers with very little contact with real autism." *Parent*
		"Far too interested in causes and cures with intellectual understanding only and no practical application." *Practitioner*
		"It's never about the issues that persons with autism face. It's too airy, too detached from practical application and frankly a waste of time and money. Researchers need to be helping these people, not simply writing papers about them." *Practitioner*

disseminated their findings, consulted the autism community and developed partnerships with its members – but other stakeholders, most notably autistic people and their families, did not share this view to the same degree. Practitioners were more likely to have engaged with researchers either through dialogue or through the building of research-practice networks and were generally satisfied with this degree of engagement. Given that models of translational research have traditionally emphasised knowledge exchange between researchers and practitioners, this finding is perhaps not surprising. Autistic adults and particularly family members were less satisfied with their involvement, however, which ranged widely from non-participation to acting as consultants in research. It is true, of course, that these results may not be representative of the entire autism community – particularly those who cannot communicate well enough to advocate for themselves – but the fact that the findings from the online questionnaire mirrored the findings in the focus groups/interviews give us reason to believe this dissatisfaction is widely shared.

This relative lack of satisfaction by certain community members might be driven by unrealistic expectations of research, in which progress can be frustratingly slow, and for parents in particular, anxieties about the need for "quick fixes" and help in the here-and-now. The challenges surrounding the communication of results and the realities of research to the public are not specific to autism research, but occur across science and humanities [30]. The core skill set of researchers – including experimental design, statistical analysis and communication of results to academic peers – does not involve mechanisms of outreach, especially with potentially vulnerable groups. This issue might well be a problem with researcher training or a lack of clear guidelines [31] but will nevertheless take some time to change.

Beyond better science communication, there were also conflicting views about the nature and extent of involvement in autism research by researchers themselves. Individual researchers had very different conceptions of what engagement in research does – and should – look like. Some researchers felt strongly that the

autism community should be more involved in research, largely in identifying research priorities, which would increase participation and external validity. Others, however, were apprehensive about such involvement, perceiving it as a potential threat to scientific (internal) validity. Notably, all of our researcher respondents implicitly viewed the autism community as relatively passive in the research process, rather than actively involved in knowledge production. Indeed, *no* researcher suggested that community members should be co-producers of research, that is, that the balance of power with regards to key scientific decision-making processes (priority-setting, funding decisions, design, implementation, interpretation or dissemination) should be equal between researchers and members of the autism community, as it is in community-based participatory models of research [32–33], and none mentioned the possibility of user-controlled research (www.invo.org.uk).

This (implicit) resistance to engaging the autism community may be related to the largely negative descriptions of autistic adults' and family members' interactions with researchers. Family members felt disappointed and frustrated at being 'mined' for information and having little or no opportunity to learn about the resulting discoveries and what they might mean for them, while autistic adults reported feeling objectified ("we are a bit like monkeys in a zoo") and their experiential expertise disregarded by researchers. This lack of reciprocity resulted in feelings of distrust and being less motivated to participate in future research.

This pattern is not unique to autism research. Other studies examining researchers' attitudes to user involvement in health research also report feelings of apprehension, particularly with regard to challenges to traditional knowledge production and acquisition [34–35]. Scientific research prizes itself for being impartial, falsifiable and rigorous. For some, the very involvement of those with a vested interest (e.g., patients) potentially introduces bias or reduces objectivity, and is thus seen as less valid and reliable.

Not only does this argument imply that researchers are bias-free (which is not the case; [36–37]), it also suggests that the only people permitted to make decisions about research are researchers themselves. Moreover, in some, possibly many, cases, the benefits of community involvement outweigh the (putative) risks. Community involvement in research theoretically increases the likelihood that research findings will be implemented in communities because their involvement ensures that (i) research findings and interventions are accessible, useful and sustainable, (ii) research addresses issues of real-life practical import, and (iii) services and interventions are tailored to fit the community's needs [14], [38]. Without such involvement, the research findings are at risk of being 'lost in translation'.

Contemporary models of patient involvement have built upon Arnstein's "ladder of citizen participation" [29] in which the rungs of the ladder reflect increasing levels of participation and degree of citizen control in decision making ranging from *non-participation* or manipulation and therapy through to *tokenism*, including informing, consulting and placating, and to the higher rungs of *citizen power* via partnership, delegated power and citizen control. Current policy initiatives, including the UK's Department of Health INVOLVE initiative (www.invo.org.uk), aim to move patient involvement in research "further up the ladder", increasing the degree of involvement – and decision-making power – in the research process. Critics have suggested that the higher rungs of the ladder may not be easily attainable in research because research is often researcher-led [39]. There is, however, a strong literature of successful participatory or emancipatory research with people with intellectual and learning disabilities [41–43] and there are rare exceptions in US autism research [33], [40], providing proof that partnership in research is at least sometimes possible and can be achieved in such a way as to accommodate the fact that the autism community is both diverse in its needs and is geographically widely dispersed. The current findings suggest, however, that the degree of community involvement in UK autism research remains close to the bottom of the ladder.

This lack of involvement in autism research might be one reason for the apparent mismatch between what is currently being researched in the UK and what community members want from such research. A recent survey of the state of current autism research in the UK found that the majority of funded research between 2007 and 2011 focused upon understanding the underlying biology and causes of autism (i.e., basic science) [13]. When consulted about the UK's research profile, there was overwhelming consensus from community members that the imbalance in current research must be addressed, with greater priority on research that has an immediate, practical impact on people's everyday lives [44]. Autistic people, their family members and practitioners are rarely actively engaged in the research process – in deciding how an issue is researched, how it becomes funded, who undertakes the research and so on. Developing ways to involve the autism community both in priority-setting exercises in specific areas and in the research process more broadly is one way to ensure that a greater portion of research has a direct and sustained impact on those who need it most.

How, then, can we support greater community involvement in research? There is no 'one size fits all' approach to community engagement. It will necessarily vary according to the research aims, the project, the target participants, the individual researcher(s) and so on. The process should therefore both be experimental and iterative. Researchers should be encouraged to innovate in a variety of ways as they develop more widespread mechanisms of engagement between researchers and the autism community,

doing so in ways that seem suitable to the particular circumstances and which reflect continuing discussions and debates concerning the right way to represent autistic people and other community members. Researchers need to develop mutually supportive and respectful relationships with members of the autism community – relationships that are both intrinsically valuable and necessary for the transfer of research findings into practice [45–46].

Developing these research-community partnerships takes time, effort and often funding. Indeed, our researcher participants mentioned a lack of supportive infrastructures as a real barrier to community engagement. Others [35], [38] have highlighted many challenges, including lack of time, energy, and resources to build and sustain partnerships, limited funding mechanisms and institutional commitment, and lack of researcher training, especially regarding power-sharing arrangements, raising questions regarding whether such intensive community engagement is suitable for all research. Some of our participants suggested that the degree of engagement in research might differ depending on the area of research. While it is true that basic or laboratory-based scientists might be less likely to interact with, and thus engage, the autism community, or to perceive benefits from such engagement, this distance should not be a rationale for limiting engagement. Many aspects of genetic and biomarker research – the hallmarks of translational research – conducted in basic science laboratories carry complex social and ethical implications related to "risk" (of developing autism) and cure and prevention [25], [47]. These very issues are the ones that often provoke the most unease within the autism community and extra efforts must be taken to ensure that autistic people and their families are involved, not excluded, from basic science research [26]. Engaging with UK community members should be the first step in determining how and to what extent they might shape the research process.

Grant-giving bodies and government agencies should work towards developing supportive infrastructure, actively encouraging researcher-community dialogues at all stages of the translational process, and providing the necessary training. Some research should aim to involve partnerships between researchers and community members, which should be genuinely participatory and not just tokenistic, where autistic people and other key stakeholders are 'co-producers' of the research. Building such institutional mechanisms of engagement requires sustained effort. There are ways, however, in which researchers can act now to develop mutually supportive partnerships with the autism community. Researchers should actively promote their research, ensuring that it reaches community members in an accessible (i.e., jargon-free) manner. They should also listen to the views and perspectives of the autism community to understand – and value – what it is like to be autistic, to care for someone who is autistic, or to work with someone who is autistic – valuing their expertise and thus reducing the epistemological divide [35]. Similarly, the autism community should work towards increasing their 'research literacy', gaining a better understanding of research and the challenges involved.

Conclusion

While the call for greater community involvement in research is not new [48], the current findings suggest that autism researchers have not readily embraced it. The lack of commitment to involving the community in research potentially presents a significant challenge for successful translational autism research. Ensuring that the advances in research impact upon those who need them most requires sustained engagement with the community at all stages of the translation process, however difficult that may seem – from establishing the research priorities and conducting the research, to disseminating and implementing the final products/intervention – while at the same time maintaining scientific rigor. Building and maintaining mutually supportive partnerships is one viable way of achieving this goal [49]. As these partnerships unfold, researchers will need to explore in detail people's experiences of them and, ultimately, to determine their impact.

Acknowledgments

We thank Deepa Korea, Richard Mills and Helen Finch at Research Autism, Erica Salomone and Mark Taylor for help during the focus groups, Dan Sinclair for production of figures and Marc Stears for helpful discussion on a previous version of the manuscript. We are also extremely grateful to all those who took part in all aspects of the research, including the questionnaire, focus groups and interviews.

Author Contributions

Conceived and designed the experiments: EP TC AD. Performed the experiments: EP TC AD. Analyzed the data: EP TC AD. Wrote the paper: EP TC.

References

1. Ioannidis JPA (2004) Materializing research promises: opportunities, priorities and conflicts in translational medicine. J Transl Med 2: 5 doi:10.1186/1479-5876-2-5.
2. Medical Research Council (2008) Research changes lives: Strategic Plan 2009–2014. London, MRC. Available: http://www.mrc.ac.uk/research/strategy/. Accessed 2014 June 2.
3. Cooksey D (2006) A Review of UK Health Research Funding. London: Stationery Office 2006.
4. Insel TR (2009) Translating scientific opportunity into public health impact. A strategic plan for research on mental illness. Arch Gen Psychiatry 66: 128–133.
5. Zerhouni E (2003) The NIH Roadmap. Science 302: 63–72.
6. Fombonne E (2009) Epidemiology of pervasive developmental disorders. Pediatr Res 65: 591–598.
7. Gernsbacher MA, Dawson M, Goldsmith HH (2005) Three reasons not to believe in an autism epidemic. Curr Dir Psychol Sci 14: 55–58.
8. Baird G, Simonoff E, Pickles A, Chandler S, Lucas T, et al. (2006) Prevalence of disorders of the autism spectrum in a population cohort of children in South Thames: the Special Needs and Autism Project (SNAP). Lancet 368: 210–215.
9. Brugha TS, McManus S, Bankart J, Scott F, Purdon S, et al. (2011) Epidemiology of autism spectrum disorders in adults in the community in England. Arch Gen Psychiatry 68: 459–65.
10. Elsabbagh M, Divan G, Koh Y, Kim YS, Kauchali S, et al. (2012) Global prevalence of autism and other pervasive developmental disorders. Autism Res 5: 160–179.
11. Dawson G (2013) Dramatic increase in autism prevalence parallels explosion of research into its biology and causes. Arch Gen Psychiatry 70: 9–10.
12. Office of Autism Research Coordination, National Institute of Mental Health, on behalf of the Interagency Autism Coordinating Committee (IACC) (2010) IACC Autism Spectrum Disorder Research Portfolio Analysis Report 2012. Available: www.iacc.hhs.gov/portfolio-analysis/2010/index.shtml.
13. Pellicano E, Dinsmore A, Charman T (2013) A Future Made Together: Shaping Autism Research in the UK. London: Institute of Education.
14. Callard F, Rose D, Wykes T (2012) Close to the bench as well as at the bedside: Involving service users in all phases of translational research. Health Expect 15: 389–400.
15. Chalmers I (2004) Well informed uncertainties about the effects of treatments: How should clinicians and patients respond? BMJ 328: 475–476.
16. Lloyd K, White J (2011) Democratizing clinical research. Nature 474: 277–278.
17. Partridge N, Scadding J (2004) The James Lind Alliance: Patients and clinicians should jointly identify their priorities for clinical trials. Lancet 364: 1923–1924.
18. van der Laan AL, Boenink M (2012) Beyond bench and bedside: Disentangling the concept of translational research. Health Care Anal 20: 84–102.
19. National Institute for Health Research (2012) INVOLVE Strategy 2012–2015: Putting people first in research. National Institute for Health Research. Available: http://www.invo.org.uk/wp-content/uploads/2012/04/INVOLVEStrategy2012-15.pdf. Accessed 2013 July 15.
20. Bettelheim B (1967) The Empty Fortress: Infantile Autism and the Birth of the Self. New York: The Free Press.
21. Gross L (2009) A broken trust: Lessons from the vaccine-autism wars. PLoS Biol 7: e1000114.
22. Bagatell N (2010) From cure to community: Transforming notions of autism. Ethos 38: 33–55.
23. Dawson M (2004) The misbehavior of behaviourists. Available: http://www.sentex.net/~nexus23/naa_aba.html. Accessed 2013 Aug 2.
24. Sinclair J (1993) Don't mourn for us. First published in the Autism Network International newsletter, Our Voice, 1 1993. Available: http://www.jimsinclair.org/dontmourn.htm. Accessed 2010 Aug 5.
25. Pellicano E, Stears M (2011) Bridging autism, science and society: Moving towards an ethically-informed approach to autism research. Autism Res 4: 271–282.
26. Pellicano E, Ne'eman A, Stears M (2011) Engaging, not excluding: A reply to Walsh et al. Nat Rev Neurosci 12: 769.
27. Braun V, Clarke V (2006) Using thematic analysis in psychology. Qualitative Research in Psychology 3: 77–101.
28. Oliver S, Clarke-Jones L, Rees R, Milne R, Buchanan P, et al. (2004) Involving consumers in research and development agenda setting for the NHS: developing an evidence-based approach. Health Technol Assess 8: 1–148.
29. Arnstein S (1969) A ladder of citizen participation. Journal of the American Institute of Planners 35: 216–224.
30. Lambert R (2003) Lambert Review of Business-University Collaboration: Final Report. Her Majesty's Stationery Office 2003. Available: http://www.hm-treasury.gov.uk/media//EA556/lambert_review_final_450.pdf. Accessed 2013 July 15.
31. Hanley B, Truesdale A, King A, Elbourne D, Chalmers I (2001) Involving consumers in designing, conducting, and interpreting randomized controlled trials: questionnaire survey. BMJ 222: 519–523.
32. Ahmed S, Palermo A (2010) Community engagement in research: Frameworks for education and peer review. Am J Public Health 100: 1380–1387.
33. Nicolaidis C, Raymaker D, McDonald K, Dern S, Ashkenazy E, et al. (2011) Collaboration strategies in nontraditional community-based participatory research partnerships: Lessons from an academic-community partnership with autistic self-advocates. Progress in Community Health Partnerships: Research, Education, and Action, 5: 143–150. doi:10.1353/cpr.2011.0022
34. Thompson J, Ward P, Barber R, Boote JD, Cooper CL, et al. (2009) Health researchers' attitudes towards public involvement in health research. Health Expect 12: 209–220.
35. Ward PR, Thompson J, Barber R, Armitage CJ, Boote JD, et al. (2010) Critical perspectives on 'consumer involvement' in health research: epistemological dissonance and the know-do gap. J Sociol 46: 63–82.
36. Moore K (2008) Disrupting Science: Social Movements, American Scientists, and the Politics of the Military, 1945–1975. Princeton, NJ: Princeton University Press.
37. Pashler H, Wagenmakers EJ (2012) Editors' introduction to the special section on replicability in psychological science: A crisis of confidence? Perspectives Psychol Sci 7: 528.
38. Faridi Z, Grunbaum JA, Sajor Gray B, Franks A, Simoes E (2007) Community-based participatory research: Next steps. Preventing Chronic Disease 4: 1–5.
39. Tritter JQ, McCallum A (2006) The snakes and ladders of user involvement: Moving beyond Arnstein. Health Policy 76: 156–168.
40. Nicolaidis C, Raymaker D, McDonald K, Dern S, Boisclair C, et al. (2013) Comparison of healthcare experiences in autistic and non-autistic adults: A cross-sectional online survey facilitated by an academic-community partnership. J Gen Intern Med 28: 761–769.
41. Ham M, Jones N, Mansell I, Northway R, Price L, et al. (2004) 'I'm a researcher!' Working together to gain ethical approval for a participatory research study. J Learn Disabil 8: 397–407.
42. Powers LE, Garner T, Valnes B, Squire P, Turner A, et al. (2007) Building a successful adult life: Findings from youth-directed research. Exceptionality: A Special Education Journal 15: 45–56.
43. Ward KM, Trigler JS (2001) Reflections on participatory action research with people with developmental disabilities. Mental Retardation 39: 57–59.
44. Pellicano E, Dinsmore A, Charman T (2014) What should autism research focus upon? Community views and priorities from the UK. Autism: doi: 10.1177/1362361314529627
45. Jones L, Wells K (2007) Strategies for academic and clinician engagement in community-participatory partnered research. JAMA 297: 407–410.
46. Tinetti ME, Basch E (2013) Patients' responsibility to participate in decision making and research. JAMA 309: 2331–2332.
47. Yudell M, Tabor HK, Dawson G, Rossi J, Newschaffer C (2013) Priorities for autism spectrum disorders: risk communication and ethics. Autism 17: 701–722.
48. Goodare H, Lockwood S (1999) Involving patients in clinical research. BMJ 319: 724–725.
49. Israel BA, Parker EA, Rowe Z, Salvatore A, Minkler M, et al. (2005) Community-based participatory research: Lessons learned from the centers for children's environmental health and disease prevention research. Environ Health Perspect 113: 1463–1471.
50. Sinclair J (1999) Why I dislike "person first" language. Available: http://www.cafemom.com/journals/read/436505/. Accessed 2013 Jan 19.

## 20

Protein Interaction Networks Reveal Novel Autism Risk Genes within GWAS Statistical Noise

Catarina Correia[1,2,3], Guiomar Oliveira[4,5,6], Astrid M. Vicente[1,2,3]*

1 Departamento de Promoção da Saúde e Doenças não Transmissíveis, Instituto Nacional de Saúde Doutor Ricardo Jorge, 1649-016 Lisboa, Portugal, **2** Center for Biodiversity, Functional & Integrative Genomics, Faculty of Sciences, University of Lisbon, 1749-016 Lisboa, Portugal, **3** Instituto Gulbenkian de Ciência, 2780-156 Oeiras, Portugal, **4** Unidade Neurodesenvolvimento e Autismo, Centro de Desenvolvimento, Hospital Pediátrico (HP) do Centro Hospitalar e Universitário de Coimbra (CHUC), 3000-602 Coimbra, Portugal, **5** Centro de Investigação e Formação Clinica do HP-CHUC, 3000-602 Coimbra, Portugal, **6** Faculdade de Medicina da Universidade de Coimbra, 3000-548 Coimbra, Portugal

Abstract

Genome-wide association studies (GWAS) for Autism Spectrum Disorder (ASD) thus far met limited success in the identification of common risk variants, consistent with the notion that variants with small individual effects cannot be detected individually in single SNP analysis. To further capture disease risk gene information from ASD association studies, we applied a network-based strategy to the Autism Genome Project (AGP) and the Autism Genetics Resource Exchange GWAS datasets, combining family-based association data with Human Protein-Protein interaction (PPI) data. Our analysis showed that autism-associated proteins at higher than conventional levels of significance ($P<0.1$) directly interact more than random expectation and are involved in a limited number of interconnected biological processes, indicating that they are functionally related. The functionally coherent networks generated by this approach contain ASD-relevant disease biology, as demonstrated by an improved positive predictive value and sensitivity in retrieving known ASD candidate genes relative to the top associated genes from either GWAS, as well as a higher gene overlap between the two ASD datasets. Analysis of the intersection between the networks obtained from the two ASD GWAS and six unrelated disease datasets identified fourteen genes exclusively present in the ASD networks. These are mostly novel genes involved in abnormal nervous system phenotypes in animal models, and in fundamental biological processes previously implicated in ASD, such as axon guidance, cell adhesion or cytoskeleton organization. Overall, our results highlighted novel susceptibility genes previously hidden within GWAS statistical "noise" that warrant further analysis for causal variants.

Editor: Branko Aleksic, Nagoya University Graduate School of Medicine, Japan

Funding: The AGP study was funded by Autism Speaks (USA), the Health Research Board (HRB, Ireland; AUT/2006/1, AUT/2006/2, PD/2006/48), The Medical Research Council (MRC, UK), Genome Canada/Ontario Genomics Institute and the Hilibrand Foundation (USA). Additional support for individual groups was provided by the US National Institutes of Health (NIH Grants: HD055751, HD055782, HD055784, MH52708, MH55284, MH061009, MH06359, MH066673, MH080647, MH081754, MH66766, NS026630, NS042165, NS049261), the Canadian Institutes for Health Research (CIHR), Assistance Publique - Hôpitaux de Paris (France), Autism Speaks UK, Canada Foundation for Innovation/Ontario Innovation Trust, Deutsche Forschungsgemeinschaft (Grant: Po 255/17-4) (Germany), EC Sixth FP AUTISM MOLGEN, Fundação Calouste Gulbenkian (Portugal), Fondation de France, Fondation FondaMental (France), Fondation Orange (France), Fondation pour la Recherche Médicale (France), Fundação para a Ciência e Tecnologia (Portugal), the Hospital for Sick Children Foundation and University of Toronto (Canada), INSERM (France), Institut Pasteur (France), the Italian Ministry of Health (convention 181 of 19 October 2001), the John P. Hussman Foundation (USA), McLaughlin Centre (Canada), Ontario Ministry of Research and Innovation (Canada), the Seaver Foundation (USA), the Swedish Science Council, The Centre for Applied Genomics (Canada), the Utah Autism Foundation (USA) and the Wellcome Trust core award 075491/Z/04 (UK). The Autism Genetic Resource Exchange is a program of Autism Speaks and is supported, in part, by grant 1U24MH081810 from the National Institute of Mental Health to Clara M. Lajonchere (PI). Catarina Correia is supported by grant SFRH/BPD/64281/2009 from the Fundação para a Ciência e Tecnologia. The funders had no role in study design, data collection and analysis, decision to publish, or preparation of the manuscript.

Competing Interests: The authors have declared that no competing interests exist.

* Email: astrid.vicente@insa.min-saude.pt

Introduction

Autism Spectrum Disorder (ASD) is a complex neurodevelopmental illness with significant clinical and genetic heterogeneity. Family and twin studies demonstrated that ASD is one of the most heritable neuropsychiatric disorders, but there is yet no consensus on the underlying genetic architecture [1,2]: while single-gene disorders, metabolic disorders and Copy Number Variants (CNVs) account for approximately 30% of the etiology of ASD [1,3–7], the contribution of common risk variants to the remaining heritability is still unclear. Thus far, each large genome-wide association study (GWAS) carried out for ASD highlighted a single, non-overlapping locus [8–11], which frequently was not replicated by subsequent independent replication studies [12].

Devlin et al. (2011) have recently predicted that common variants having an odds ratio of 1.5 or more are very unlikely to exist; few, if any, common variants with an impact on risk exceeding 1.2 may still await discovery, but require much larger sample sizes, while variants with modest impact may range from zero to many thousands [13]. The small effect of common risk variants for ASD represents a challenge for their individual detection using conventional single-marker association analysis, which likely allows many true *loci* to remain hidden within the GWAS statistical "noise". Evidence from classical quantitative genetic analysis further suggests that most of the heritability missing in complex diseases is rather hidden below the threshold for genome-wide significant associations [14,15].

New strategies are therefore needed to increase the power of GWAS analysis. The use of molecular networks, which is not limited by *a priori* sorting the genes into incompletely annotated predefined gene sets, is emerging as an appealing unbiased alternative to pathway analysis. Network-based approaches have been widely applied in the analysis of high-throughput expression data from a wide range of diseases [16] and have proven successful in the identification of subnetwork markers more reproducible and with a higher prediction performance than individual markers [17]. More recent studies incorporated protein networks into the analysis of genome-wide association data, using networks to search for interacting *loci* in human GWAS data [18,19] or to identify genome wide-enriched pathways [20–24]. However, an unsupervised global network analysis of ASD GWAS data that includes all signals without arbitrary significance thresholds has not been performed, and may lead to the identification of many risk variants of small effect below the accepted threshold for statistical significance.

Based on the premise that disease-causing genes are likely to be functionally related, in the present study we applied a network-based approach to two ASD GWAS datasets, the AGP consortium GWAS and the GWAS carried out in the Autism Genetic Resource Exchange (AGRE) dataset [10]. For this purpose we integrated genome wide association data with Human Protein-Protein interaction data and examined topological network properties indicative of connectivity at various levels of association, confirming our hypothesis that genes associated to ASD at a "statistical noise" level are functionally connected beyond random expectation. We compared the enrichment in known ASD candidates of network genes versus top GWAS genes, and the overlap of network genes vs the overlap at gene or SNP level between the two ASD datasets. The network obtained was further tested for ASD specificity using networks derived from six unrelated diseases GWAS, and explored for biological processes associated with ASD.

Materials and Methods

A workflow of the strategy for network definition, validation and identification of the most relevant candidate genes is shown in Figure 1.

Ethics statement

All the data used is previously published and publicly available. Written informed consent has been previously obtained from all families and procedures had approval from institutional review boards from all the institutions involved in recruitment and research, following national and international ethical and legal regulations and the principles of the Declaration of Helsinki.

Datasets

The AGP dataset included 2818 trios consisting of autistic patients and both parents collected as part of the AGP Consortium. Patients were diagnosed and genotyped as previously reported [8]. Written informed consent was obtained from all families and procedures had approval from institutional review boards [8]. A total of 723 423 SNPs meeting the QC criteria [9], genotyped in 8491 individuals, were tested for association using the Transmissions Disequilibrium Test (TDT) implemented in PLINK v1.07 [25].

The GWAS replication dataset from the Autism Genetic Resource Exchange (AGRE) included 943 ASD families (4,444 subjects) from the AGRE cohort [10]. SNP genotyping data was obtained from AGRE [10]. Analysis in this study was limited to

SNPs in common with the AGP GWAS and meeting the same QC criteria (425 587 SNPs).

Summary SNP association results were obtained from the database of Genotype and Phenotype (dbGAP) repository for 6 case-control GWAS for other pathologies, including Parkinson's Disease (PD) [26], Systemic Lupus Erythematosus (SLE) [27], Multiple Sclerosis (MS) [28], Type 1 Diabetes (T1D) [29], Breast Cancer (BC) [30] and Neuroblastoma (NB) [31] (Table S1). All individuals included were of European ancestry and the sample size was as similar as possible to the replication ASD dataset (AGRE).

Integration of gene association data with Protein-Protein interaction data

Genotyped SNPs from the AGP and AGRE GWAS were assigned to specific genes if they were located within or up to 10 kb from the gene, using the GRCh37/hg19 genome build (Step 1). Each gene was assigned a gene score using MAGENTA (Meta-analysis Gene-set Enrichment of variant associations) [32], which allocates to each gene the most significant P-value among the TDT P-values of all individual SNPs mapped to that gene. MAGENTA then uses step-wise multivariate linear regression analysis to regress out of this P-value the confounding effects of gene size, number of SNPs per kilobase (kb), number of independent SNPs, number of recombination hotspots and the number of linkage disequilibrium units per kb.

Genes selected at various gene-wise P-value cutoffs ($0.5 < $-LogP<5) were superimposed onto their corresponding protein on a large human protein-protein interaction (PPI) network, converting Entrez gene IDs to Uniprot IDs (release 2010_04) (Step 2). This PPI network, covering 12372 proteins and 58365 interactions, was previously built compacting data from six public PPI databases: BIND, BioGRID, HPRD, IntAct, MINT and MPPI [33–40].

PPI network analysis

Topological properties from the resulting network were analyzed to select the gene-wise P-value for which corresponding proteins were functionally connected beyond random expectation, thus the lowest gene-wise P-value for which there is still relevant biological data in the GWAS that can be captured through network analysis (step 3). Three metrics indicative of this functional coherence were estimated for various association gene-wise P-value thresholds, for the two ASD datasets, and compared with those determined for 1000 equal size sets of randomly selected proteins from the human PPI network. The metrics evaluated were 1) the percentage of proteins directly interacting; 2) the percentage of isolated nodes, which represents the fraction of selected proteins with no interactions with any other selected protein; and 3) the size of the largest connected component (LCC), the largest group of selected proteins that are reachable from each other in the network. An empirical P-value was obtained computing the fraction of random samples where the value of the network metric is greater (or smaller in the case of isolates) than the observed one. Network analysis was performed using python module Network X.

Performance against a candidate gene list and overlap between datasets

To evaluate the performance of the proteins included in the LCC in retrieving known ASD candidate genes, the precision and recall against a curated list of ASD candidate genes were calculated (step 4). This list was obtained from SFARIGene and

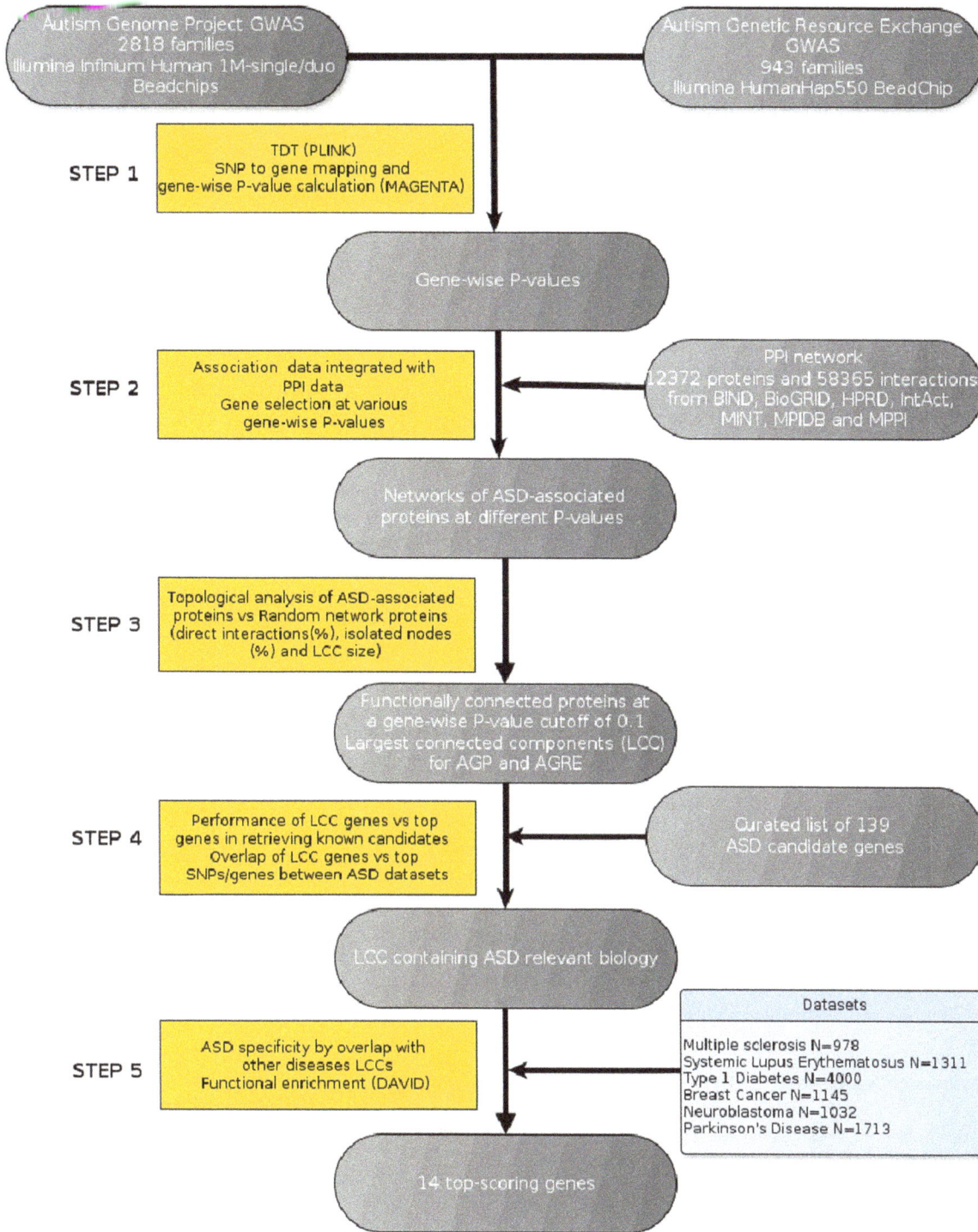

Figure 1. Workflow of the strategy for network definition, validation and identification of most relevant candidate genes.

includes 236 genes having at least minimal evidence of association with ASD (categories 1 to 4) or categorized as syndromic (https://gene.sfari.org/autdb/Welcome.do).

Precision (Positive Predictive value) is the proportion of known candidate genes among the selected genes, while recall (Sensitivity) is the proportion of known candidate genes retrieved by the selection. The precision and recall calculated for the genes encoding LCC proteins were compared to those determined using two other gene selection criteria: a) all genes selected at the same gene *P*-value cutoff used to derive LCC; b) the same number of top genes (ranked according to gene-wise *P*-values) as those included in the LCC.

Overlap between the AGP and AGRE datasets at SNP, gene and LCC levels was determined using the Jaccard index, defined as the size of the intersection divided by the size of the union of the datasets. For comparison purposes the size of each dataset LCC was used to select from each GWAS dataset an equal number of top SNPs (ranked by their TDT *P*-value) and top genes (ranked by their gene-wise *P*-value).

Gene ranking and functional enrichment

To rank ASD-associated proteins included in the AGP LCC by ASD specificity and reproducibility, a prioritization system was created, assigning a score to each protein based on their presence in the LCC derived from the AGRE ASD replication dataset and from each of the six unrelated disease datasets (step 5). Each protein included in the AGP LCC had an initial score of 0.5. If the protein was present in the AGRE ASD dataset LCC, 0.5 was added to the initial protein score, whereas for each unrelated disease dataset LCC where the protein was present, one sixth of 0.5 was subtracted from the score. Therefore, protein scores vary between 0 and 1, with zero representing a protein present in the LCCs of the AGP dataset and the 6 unrelated diseases, while a score of 1 is attributed to a protein present only in the LCCs of both ASD datasets.

Functional enrichment was tested by DAVID (The Database for Annotation, Visualization and Integrated Discovery 2008_version6[th]; http://david.abcc.ncifcrf.gov) [41,42], a publicly available bioinformatics tool that identifies functionally related groups of genes. Overrepresentation of mouse-mutant phenotypes was evaluated using the web tool MamPhea [43]. The complete list of the genes in the PPI network was used as background and *P*-values were corrected by the Benjamini correction. Top-scoring genes were further investigated using NextBio platform (Cupertino, CA, USA), a curated and correlated repository of experimental data derived from an extensive set of public resources (eg. ArrayExpress and GEO) [44]. Protein-protein networks were visualized in Cytoscape [45].

Results

Genes associated to ASD at *P*<0.1 are functionally related

Transmission Disequilibrium Tests were initially carried out in parallel for the AGP and AGRE datasets to identify small effect risk variants. In the sample of 2818 AGP families, single SNP transmission disequilibrium tests of the 723423 SNPs meeting the QC criteria showed no SNPs reaching the threshold for genome-wide significance. Two SNPs showed association signals at $P < 1 \times 10^{-6}$ and very few exceeded $P < 1 \times 10^{-5}$. In the AGRE dataset, after a similar quality control protocol and using only SNPs common to both datasets, three SNPs located in regions with no overlap with the AGP top findings showed association at $P < 1 \times 10^{-6}$. Given the dearth of meaningful results from these two GWAS efforts, we proceeded with a network analysis strategy.

The first step involved calculating gene-wise association *P*-values corrected for gene size and linkage disequilibrium, taking into account only the SNPs mapping within 10kb from each gene (403360 SNPs), followed by the integration of GWAS data onto protein interaction data. Then, we determined the lowest gene-wise *P*-value threshold for which genes encoding the network proteins were functionally related, inferred by their proximity in the network. Statistical noise is expected to have random connections in the network, while disease proteins are more likely to establish direct interactions between them and more rarely be isolated in the network, translating into a larger group of proteins that are all interconnected. For both ASD datasets, proteins encoded by genes selected at a gene-wise $-\text{Log}_{10}P$ cutoff between 0.5 and 1.5 were found to establish significantly more direct interactions than equal sized sets of randomly selected proteins (Empirical *P* values 0.001<*P*<0.043), with the significance maintained up to $-\text{Log}_{10}P = -2.0$ in the case of AGRE dataset (Figure S1, Figure 2A). The number of isolated nodes was found to be significantly smaller in sets of ASD-associated proteins at the same range of gene-wise $-\text{Log}_{10}P$-values than in random sets (Empirical *P* values 0.001<*P*<0.038), again with significant differences maintained for lower gene-wise *P*-values in the AGRE dataset (Figure S1, Figure 2A). When compared to the same number of random proteins from the network, proteins encoded by genes selected at a gene-wise $-\text{Log}_{10}P<1$ from either ASD dataset are interconnected in a significantly larger LCC (Empirical P values 0.001<*P*<0.007) (Figure S1, Figure 2B). The large size of the largest connected components, 416 and 367 proteins for the AGP and AGRE datasets, respectively, indicates the existence of several small effect risk genes reinforcing the high genetic heterogeneity in ASD.

Based on the lowest gene-wise *P*-value for which the percentage of direct interactions was significantly higher, the percentage of isolated nodes significantly smaller and the size of the LCC significantly larger than random expectation (Figure 2A and B), we established gene-wise $-\text{Log}_{10}P = 1$ as the cutoff value to infer functional coherence from the two ASD datasets.

The overall results indicate that, as hypothesized, genes associated with ASD at the range of GWAS statistical noise encode proteins that are functionally related and preferentially directly interact, confirming our expectation that there is indeed unexplored relevant biology at this statistical level.

Functionally coherent sub networks associated with ASD contain relevant ASD biology

To test whether the identified groups of functionally connected proteins captured by the largest connected components indeed contain ASD-relevant biology, we compared the performance of the genes selected through the LCC against a list of known candidates, [5] with the performance of all genes selected from the GWAS at the same gene-wise *P*-value cutoff or the performance of a number of GWAS top genes equal to the number of genes encoding LCC proteins. Genes implicated in ASD are largely unknown, thus low precision values are expectable given the incompleteness and noise in the available knowledge in the field.

Table 1 shows that, for both datasets, genes encoding proteins included in the LCC presented a 2 to 2.5 fold higher precision against the list of known genes than all the GWAS genes selected at the same statistical level cutoff. In other words, genes included in the LCC, and thus encoding functionally related proteins, are enriched in known candidates compared with the set of genes selected from the GWAS at the same statistical level, demonstrating that our filtering approach of association results based on PPIs more specifically captures ASD-relevant genes. A 1.3 to 3.3 fold increase is observed when comparing LCC genes with the same number of GWAS top genes, showing that a protein interaction-based selection was more accurate than selecting only the most strongly associated genes.

A.

B.

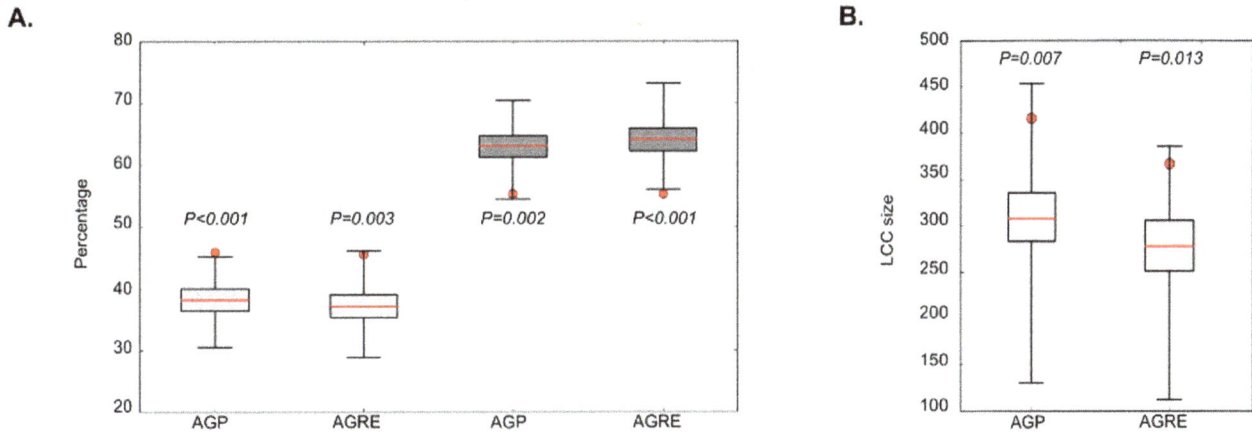

Figure 2. Network properties of proteins selected at gene-wise $P<0.1$ in each ASD. a) Comparison of percentage of direct interactions and isolated nodes between proteins selected at gene-wise $P<0.1$ in each GWAS dataset (red circles) vs 1000 random samples of network proteins (represented by light gray and dark gray box plots, for direct interactions and isolated nodes, respectively). The bottom and top of the box represent the 25th and 75th percentile and the extremity of the whiskers the maximum and minimum of the random samples data. **b)** Same comparison for the largest connected component (LCC) size.

Concerning the proportion of known genes that are retrieved by our selection, or recall, LCC encoding genes had a lower recall compared with all genes selected at the same cutoff, as expected since LCC genes are a subset of this selection (Table 1). However, compared with the top-gene selection, the 1.4 to 3 fold increase in the recall achieved by LCC encoding genes, indicates that additional relevant low effect genes are being captured. Further inspection of the known genes present in the top gene set and the LCC encoding genes confirmed that LCCs capture not only larger effect genes overlapping with top genes, such as *MET* (Uniprot P08581)(in AGP dataset), but additionally capture low effect genes, such as *TSC2* (Uniprot P49815), which single gene association analysis alone does not have the power to detect.

One of the major problems in ASD GWAS and GWAS in general is the low reproducibility of results between different datasets. Indeed, we found only one SNP (rs11837890 in *TBK1* gene) and 10 genes in common between the two datasets, when comparing the same number of SNPs or genes (ranked by *P*-values) than genes included in the LCCs from each dataset. Remarkably, we observed a 25 and 2.5-fold increase in the overlap between the two ASD datasets (AGP and AGRE) at PPI network level when compared to SNP or gene level, respectively (Figure S2).

Taken together, these results showed that our selection of functionally connected genes based on the largest connected component is an effective approach to capture ASD-relevant

disease candidate genes, which might escape detection in an analysis based only on association evidence, even at gene-level.

Functionally connected genes in ASD suggest novel susceptibility genes

Given the observation that the largest connected component contains ASD-relevant proteins, we further explored this network for biological processes implicated in ASD (step 5). The largest connected components generated by genes selected at -$\mathrm{Log}_{10}P<1$ from the AGP and AGRE datasets comprised 416 and 367 proteins, respectively. A first look into the biological processes represented in these networks, using functional enrichment analysis, revealed an enrichment in pathways related to regulation of apoptosis and cell cycle. Additionally, intersection of the protein network data with knockout mice phenotypes from the Mouse Genome Informatics Database, showed that these proteins are primarily involved in aberrant embryogenic and developmental processes and anomalous immune system phenotypes.

A closer inspection of these LCCs at the gene level showed that around 30 (7–8%) of the encoding genes were implicated in neuropsychiatric or neurodegenerative disorders (Table S2). More interestingly, 20 (5–6%) of the LCC encoding genes were found to carry *de novo* mutations in ASD described in at least one of the three whole exome sequencing studies recently published [4,7,46], with 3 genes overlapping between the two datasets (*CSDE1* (Uniprot O75534), *PGD* (Uniprot P52209), *TSC2*). In addition, 80

Table 1. Precision and recall were consistently higher for LCC genes relative to top GWAS genes or genes selected at $P<0.1$.

Gene subset	Precision (%)		Recall (%)	
	AGP dataset	AGRE dataset	AGP dataset	AGRE dataset
LCC genes	2.16	2.74	3.81	4.24
GWAS Top genes	1.68	0.82	1.27	2.97
Genes selected at $P<0.1$	0.96	1,11	8.47	9.43

Precision and Recall (Percentage), by ASD dataset, of three sets of genes (genes selected at a gene wise *P*-value cutoff of 0.1, genes included in the LCC and the same number of GWAS top genes) against a list of known disease candidates.

(~19%) of the AGP LCC-encoding genes were deleted or duplicated by CNVs identified by the AGP whole genome analysis as potentially pathogenic (with less than 50% of length overlap with control datasets) (Table S2).

To further examine the specificity of the proteins in the AGP LCC for ASD, this network was compared with LCCs generated from six unrelated diseases GWAS (MS, SLE, T1D, BC, NB, PD). Based on the presence of each protein in the LCC of each unrelated disease and in the AGRE LCC, we derived a highly stringent ASD-specificity protein score, allowing the prioritization of encoding genes for follow-up. Low scoring proteins were not replicated in the AGRE dataset, and were present in one or more unrelated diseases, whereas the highest scoring proteins were present in both ASD LCCs, but in none of the LCCs generated from the unrelated diseases. This analysis revealed that the majority of proteins (~63%) were present only in the AGP network, while 31% of the proteins were present in at least one additional non-ASD network, and thus were not specific. From the 25 proteins identified in both ASD networks, the majority (56%) was not present in any ASD-unrelated network and 28% were present in one of the ASD-unrelated networks.

Using this gene scoring system, based on gene reproducibility and specificity for ASD, we built a network with the 14 top scoring genes and their first neighbors in the LCC network (Figure 3). The largest component of this network, although approximately 7 times smaller than the original LCCs, showed a similar overlap (~5%) with genes reported to have *de novo* mutations in ASD (*PGD*, *SYNE1* (Uniprot Q8NF91), *TSC2*) and an increased overlap with known candidate genes (*SYNE1*, *TSC2* and *SHANK3* (Uniprot Q9BYB0)) and with genes contained in potentially relevant CNVs identified by the AGP analysis (~26%). Enrichment in mouse phenotypes was also similar but, in addition, an enrichment in abnormal nervous system phenotype became significant, and in abnormal behavior/neurological phenotype borderline significant.

The genes encoding the 14 top scoring proteins were considered the best candidates for harboring common variants associated with ASD risk (Table 2). These genes are involved in various biological processes, such as NGF signaling, axon guidance, cell adhesion and migration, cytoskeleton regulation, apoptosis and DNA repair. A *de novo* mutation in the phosphogluconate dehydrogenase gene (*PGD*) has recently been reported in ASD [4], while potentially pathogenic CNVs deleting or duplicating the *ABL1* (Uniprot P00519), *RPS6KA1* (Uniprot Q15418) and *PPP1CB* (Uniprot P62140) genes were identified in ASD patients from the AGP study. A query of our genes in the NEXTBIO platform, a data mining framework that integrates and correlates global public datasets with several normal and disease phenotypes, revealed correlations of six genes with ASD. For instance, deletions within the *NASP* (Uniprot P49321) gene were identified in ASD patients from the Simons Simplex Collection (SSC) [47]. An altered expression of this gene, as well as of the *NR4A1* (Uniprot P22736), *ABI1* (Uniprot Q8IZP0), *BBS4* (Uniprot Q96RK4), *LMNA* (Uniprot P02545) and *ABL1* genes, was found in postmortem brain tissue [48] or lymphoblastoid cells [49] of ASD patients. Some of the 14 top-scoring genes, namely the *CTSB* (Uniprot P07858), *BBS4*, *LMNA* and *ABL1* genes, were associated with abnormal nervous system phenotypes in animal models. The most strongly associated genes to ASD, using the AGP data, were the peroxiredoxin 1 gene (*PRDX1* (Uniprot Q06830)) and cathepsin B gene (*CTSB*).

Discussion

In this study we have conducted a network-based analysis of two ASD GWAS datasets, hypothesizing that small effect ASD risk

variants hidden at the level of GWAS statistical noise can be discovered from networks of genes with related biological functions. Mapping of association data to a PPI network indeed revealed that, in both datasets, ASD-associated genes at $P<0.1$ encoded proteins that directly interact beyond random expectation, are more rarely found isolated in the network and are connected in significantly larger LCCs than expected by chance, suggesting a functional connection. These results support recent findings from the AGP consortium, showing that stronger association of allele scores with case status was generally achieved when those scores were based on markers associated at significance thresholds higher than 0.2 [8]. The International Schizophrenia GWAS consortium had similar results of optimal discrimination between cases and controls only after the inclusion of markers with P-values as high as 0.2, [14] using this allele scoring approach.

The relevance to ASD of these networks was further illustrated by their higher performance in retrieving known ASD candidates compared to top GWAS genes, and the increased similarity between the two ASD datasets, when compared to SNP or gene level overlap. Remarkably, the AGP and AGRE LCCs included 20 genes, respectively, in which *de novo* mutations have been described in whole-exome sequencing studies of nearly a thousand ASD patients [4,7,50]. A large overlap of our results with the published data of these sequencing studies was not expected, because the LCCs encoding genes are likely to harbor variants transmitted by unaffected parents, whereas these sequencing studies mainly focused, and reported only, *de novo* variants which do not explain the heritability of the disorder, but support recent observations that common and rare variants associated with ASD disturb common neuronal networks [51]. Moreover, around 20% of the AGP LCC encoding genes were deleted or duplicated by potentially pathogenic CNVs detected in the AGP whole genome CNV screening of 2446 ASD patients.

As an additional filter for meaningful ASD biology, we derived an ASD candidate gene prioritization system ranking the genes encoding proteins included in the AGP LCC for ASD reproducibility and specificity. The scoring system used was very stringent, in particular since some of the control disorders are neurological (Parkinson's, multiple sclerosis or neuroblastoma) and may share susceptibility genes and pathways with autism [52–56]. While we may have discarded relevant autism risk genes that are ubiquitous and common to these disorders, we believe that we enriched our list of genes in true positive results with a higher chance of experimental validation. In fact, the enrichment analysis performed with the top-scoring genes and their first neighbors showed a high content in mouse genes associated with nervous system or neurological phenotypes and a similar or higher overlap with candidate genes or genes reported with *de novo* mutations or potentially pathogenic CNVs in ASD.

This approach generated a list of 14 top-scoring genes, present in the two ASD networks and none of the other disorders, which were considered strong candidates to harbor common variants associated with ASD risk. These genes are mostly novel candidates for ASD, and are involved in nervous system pathways or other more fundamental biological processes which have been widely associated to ASD, such as ubiquitination [4,9,57,58], cytoskeleton organization and regulation [5,47,59] and cell adhesion [10,60]. For instance, the *CTSB, BBS4, LMNA* and *ABL1* genes have been associated with neurobiological phenotypes identified in an enrichment analysis of mouse neurobiological phenotypes from a list of 112 ASD candidate genes [61], with *CTSB* and *ABL1* associated with cerebellum morphological and development abnormalities. The AGP genome-wide analysis identified potentially pathogenic CNVs spanning *ABL1, RPS6KA1* and

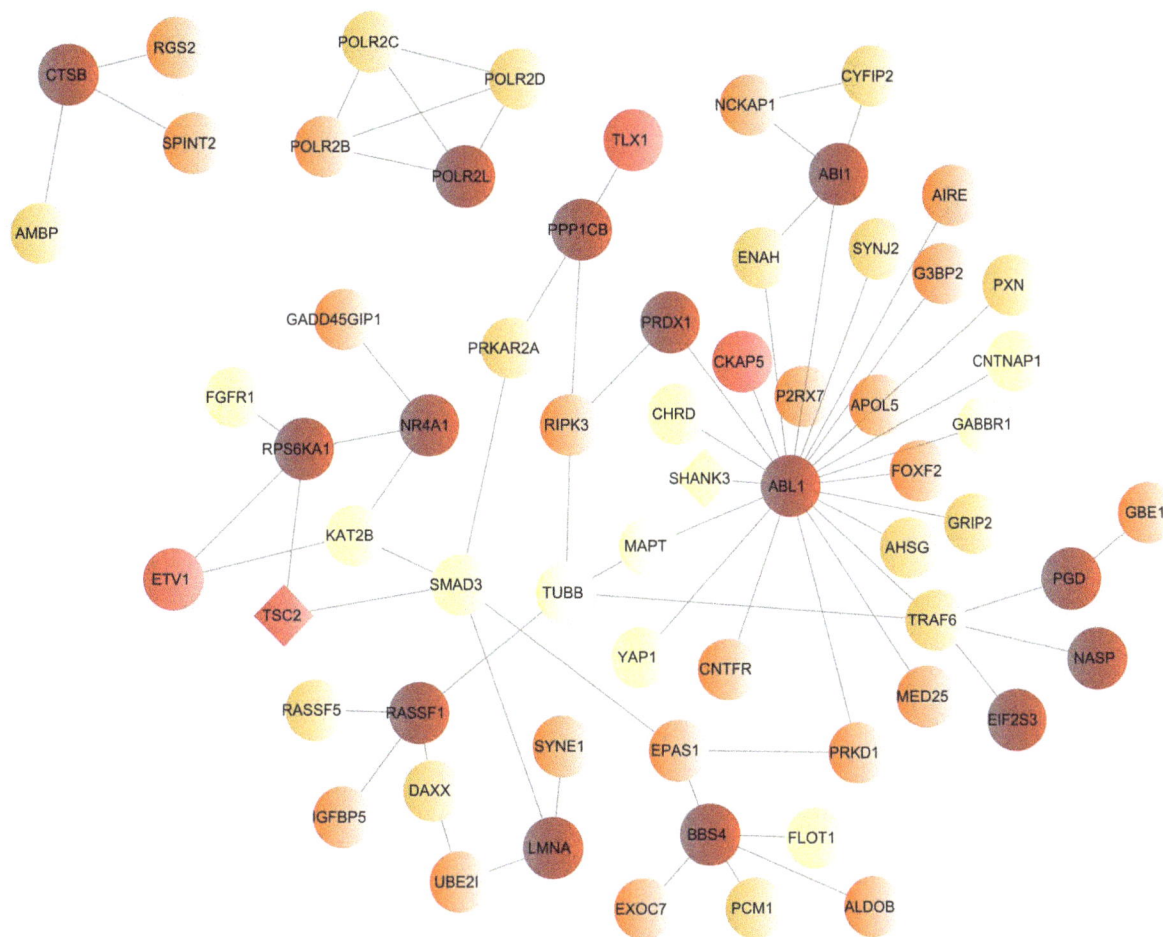

Figure 3. ASD top scoring gene network. This network illustrates the 14 top scoring genes included in the ASD LCC and their first neighbors. Nodes are colored based on a score reflecting their presence in the second ASD dataset and in the 6 unrelated diseases LCCs. A darker color represents a higher score, which means a higher specificity for ASD.

PPP1CB, whose relevance needs to be further established. Likewise, in the phosphogluconate dehydrogenase gene (PGD), a *de novo* mutation has recently been reported in a patient with ASD [4], although with an uncertain deleterious effect. This gene plays a critical role in protecting cells from oxidative stress [62] and, together with *PRDX1*, which also has an important antioxidant protective role in cells [63,64] and shows the strongest association with ASD, supports emerging evidence for a role of oxidative stress in ASD pathophysiology [65,66].

Thus far the use of protein networks to address common risk variants in ASD was limited to enrichment analysis of GWAS top hit genes in co-expressed or differentially expressed networks [51,67]. In contrast, this study incorporated protein interaction data into GWAS analysis, without *a priori* assumptions of association thresholds. The present results have shown that autism-associated genes at higher than conventional levels of significance are functionally related, and were used to extract relevant disease biology and uncover small effect variants contributing to the disorder. The study highlighted a group of novel susceptibility genes relevant for CNS function with a high probability of bearing common variants associated with autism, which have been elusive thus far, and warranting further analysis for identification of causal variants.

Supporting Information

Figure S1   Network properties per gene-wise *P*-value for each ASD dataset. For each $-\text{Log}_{10}$ gene wise association *P*-value cutoff in the x-axis, the percentage of direct interactions (A) and isolated nodes (B) and the logarithm of the LCC size (C) were plotted for proteins encoded by disease-associated genes (red line) and for the mean of 1000 equal sized random samples of proteins (blue line). Dark grey areas represent the range between the 25th and 75th quartiles and light gray areas indicate the range between the minimum and maximum values of the random data. Empirical *P*-values are indicated for each gene wise association *P*-value comparison. Values are plotted until the $-\text{Log}_{10}$ for which the percentage of direct interactions and isolated nodes reaches 0 and 100%, respectively.

Figure S2   Overlap between the two ASD datasets at SNP, gene or network level. Venn diagrams showing the overlap between the two ASD datasets (AGP and AGRE) at SNP, gene or network level.

Table S1   GWAS datasets used in the analysis and genotyping platforms.

Table 2. Top scoring ASD network genes.

Gene (Uniprot ID)	Description	Location	Relevant biological processes	Gene-wise association P-value (MAGENTA)	Published studies in autism	Neurological and behavioral features in mouse models
NASPI(P49321)	nuclear autoantigenic sperm protein (histone-binding)	1p34.1	blastocyst development, cell proliferation, cell cycle	$1.470e^{-02}$	NEXTBIO: deletion in idiopathic females(Sakai et al. 2011), significantly downregulated in brain samples (Chow et al.2011)	NA
PRDX1(Q06830)	peroxiredoxin 1	1p34.1	redox regulation, cell proliferation	$1.760e^{-04}$	-	NA
RPS6KA1(Q15418)	ribosomal protein S6 kinase, 90kDa, polypeptide 1	1p36.11	protein kinase, synaptic transmission, axon guidance, long-term potentiation, toll-like and NGF receptor signaling pathway	$2.422e^{-02}$	-	NNP
PGD(P52209)	phosphogluconate dehydrogenase	1p36.22	cell redox regulation	$7.851e^{-02}$	De novo mutation in autistic patient (O'Roak et al. 2012)	NNP
LMNA(P02545)	lamin A/C	1q22	regulation of cell migration, regulation of apoptotic process, spermatogenesis	$8.226e^{-02}$	Nextbio:altered expression in Lymphoblastoid cells from males with autism (15q11–13 duplication) and brain samples (Chow et al. 2011; Nishimura et al. 2007)	abnormal axon morphology, abnormal myelination
PPP1CB(P62140)	protein phosphatase 1, catalytic subunit, beta isozyme	2p23	regulation of cell cycle, focal-adhesion, long-term potentiation, regulation of actin cytoskeleton	$3.749e^{-02}$	-	NA
RASSF1(Q9NS23)	Ras association (RalGDS/AF-6) domain family member 1	3p21.3	Cell cycle, response to DNA damage stimulus, positive regulation of protein ubiquitination	$1.949e^{-02}$	-	NA
CTSB(P07858)	cathepsin B	8p23.1	regulation of apoptotic process, cellular response to thyroid hormone stimulus	$2.343e^{-03}$		Purkinje cell degeneration, abnormalneuron apoptosis (details)neuron degeneration
ABL1(P00519)	c-abl oncogene 1, non-receptor tyrosine kinase	9q34.1	axon guidance, regulation of cell adhesion, motility, cycle, actin cytoskeleton organization, response to DNA damage stimulus	$9.560e^{-02}$	NextBio:altered expression in autistic brain samples (Chow et al. 2011)	abnormal cerebellum morphology, small cerebellum, abnormal cerebellum development, abnormal cerebellar foliation, ectopic Purkinje cell, abnormal cerebellar lobule formation, absent cerebellar lobules, abnormal neuron differentiation
ABI1(Q8IZP0)	Abl-interactor 1 previously known as spectrin SH3 domain binding protein 1	10p12.1	transmembrane receptor protein tyrosine kinase signaling pathway, negative regulation of cell proliferation	$7.352e^{-02}$	NextBio:downregulation in autistic brain samples (Chow et al. 2011)	NA
POLR2L(P62875)	polymerase (RNA) II (DNA directed) polypeptide L, 7.6kDa	11p15.5	DNA repair, regulation of transcription	$7.821e^{-02}$	-	NNP

Table 2. Cont.

Gene (Uniprot ID)	Description	Location	Relevant biological processes	Gene-wise association P-value (MAGENTA)	Published studies in autism	Neurological and behavioral features in mouse models
NR4A1(P22736)	nuclear receptor subfamily 4, group A, member 1 also known as nerve Growth factor IB (NGFIB)	12q13.13	nuclear transcription factor, epidermal and fibroblast growth factor receptor signaling pathway, nerve growth factor receptor signaling pathway	$4.783e^{-02}$	NextBio:downregulation in autistic brain samples (Chow et al. 2011)	NA
BBS4(Q96RK4)	Bardet-Biedl syndrome 4	15q22.3-q23	centrosome organization, microtubule cytoskeleton organization, neural tube closure, dendrite, striatum, hippocampus, cerebral cortex development	$7.511e^{-02}$	Nextbio:altered expression in lymphoblasts and brain samples (Chow et al. 2011; Nishimura et al. 2007)	abnormal neural tubemorphology/ development, thincerebral cortex, abnormal basal ganglion morphologyabnormal olfactory neuron morphology, small hippocampusenlarged lateral ventriclesenlarged third ventricle
EIF2S3(P41091)	eukaryotic translation initiation factor 2, subunit 3 gamma, 52kDa	Xp22.11	cellular protein metabolic process	$7.322e^{-02}$	-	NNP

List of the 14 top scoring ASD network genes, present in both ASD networks and in none of the other disorders (ASD specificity score = 1), with information on gene-wise association P-value and biological processes relevant for ASD.
NNP - No neurological phenotypes]; NA - No mouse model available.

Table S2   AGP LCC network genes. List of the 416 genes included in the AGP LCC with information on gene-wise association *P*-value, specificity score for ASD and previous findings regarding implication in ASD and other neurological disorders.

Acknowledgments

We gratefully acknowledge the children with ASD and their families enrolling at the AGP and AGRE participating study sites. We are thankful to José Pereira Leal, Yoan Dieckmann and the remaining members of the Computational Genomics group at Instituto Gulbenkian de Ciência for helpful discussions and data sharing. We are grateful to all the AGP investigators, and particularly to Richard Anney, for sharing data, resources and scientific discussions. We gratefully acknowledge the resources provided by the Autism Genetic Resource Exchange (AGRE) Consortium and the participating AGRE families.

We acknowledge the NIH GWAS repository. Public available analysis data for Multiple Sclerosis, Systemic Lupus Erythematosus, Type 1 diabetes, Breast Cancer, Neuroblastoma and Parkinson's Disease were obtained from dbGaP at http://www.ncbi.nlm.nih.gov/gap through dbGaP accession numbers pha002861, pha002848, pha002862, pha002853, pha002845, pha002868, respectively.

Author Contributions

Conceived and designed the experiments: CC AMV. Performed the experiments: CC. Analyzed the data: CC AMV. Contributed reagents/materials/analysis tools: CC GO AMV. Wrote the paper: CC AMV.

References

1. Devlin B, Scherer SW (2012) Genetic architecture in autism spectrum disorder. Curr Opin Genet Dev 22: 229–237.
2. Geschwind DH (2011) Genetics of autism spectrum disorders. Trends Cogn Sci 15: 409–416.
3. Betancur C (2010) Etiological heterogeneity in autism spectrum disorders: more than 100 genetic and genomic disorders and still counting. Brain Res 1380: 42–77.
4. O'Roak BJ, Deriziotis P, Lee C, Vives L, Schwartz JJ, et al. (2012) Exome sequencing in sporadic autism spectrum disorders identifies severe de novo mutations. Nat Genet 44: 471.
5. Pinto D, Pagnamenta AT, Klei L, Anney R, Merico D, et al. (2010) Functional impact of global rare copy number variation in autism spectrum disorders. Nature 466: 368–372.
6. Sanders SJ, Ercan-Sencicek AG, Hus V, Luo R, Murtha MT, et al. (2011) Multiple recurrent de novo CNVs, including duplications of the 7q11.23 Williams syndrome region, are strongly associated with autism. Neuron 70: 863–885.
7. Sanders SJ, Murtha MT, Gupta AR, Murdoch JD, Raubeson MJ, et al. (2012) De novo mutations revealed by whole-exome sequencing are strongly associated with autism. Nature 485: 237–241.
8. Anney R, Klei L, Pinto D, Almeida J, Bacchelli E, et al. (2012) Individual common variants exert weak effects on the risk for autism spectrum disorderspi. Hum Mol Genet 21: 4781–4792.
9. Anney R, Klei L, Pinto D, Regan R, Conroy J, et al. (2010) A genome-wide scan for common alleles affecting risk for autism. Hum Mol Genet 19: 4072–4082.
10. Wang K, Zhang H, Ma D, Bucan M, Glessner JT, et al. (2009) Common genetic variants on 5p14.1 associate with autism spectrum disorders. Nature 459: 528–533.
11. Weiss LA, Arking DE, Daly MJ, Chakravarti A (2009) A genome-wide linkage and association scan reveals novel loci for autism. Nature 461: 802–808.
12. Curran S, Bolton P, Rozsnyai K, Chiocchetti A, Klauck SM, et al. (2011) No association between a common single nucleotide polymorphism, rs4141463, in the MACROD2 gene and autism spectrum disorder. Am J Med Genet B Neuropsychiatr Genet 156B: 633–639.
13. Devlin B, Melhem N, Roeder K (2011) Do common variants play a role in risk for autism? Evidence and theoretical musings. Brain Res 1380: 78–84.
14. Purcell SM, Wray NR, Stone JL, Visscher PM, O'Donovan MC, et al. (2009) Common polygenic variation contributes to risk of schizophrenia and bipolar disorder. Nature 460: 748–752.
15. Yang J, Benyamin B, McEvoy BP, Gordon S, Henders AK, et al. (2010) Common SNPs explain a large proportion of the heritability for human height. Nat Genet 42: 565–569.
16. Barabasi AL, Gulbahce N, Loscalzo J (2011) Network medicine: a network-based approach to human disease. Nat Rev Genet 12: 56–68.
17. Chuang HY, Lee E, Liu YT, Lee D, Ideker T (2007) Network-based classification of breast cancer metastasis. Mol Syst Biol 3: 140.
18. Emily M, Mailund T, Hein J, Schauser L, Schierup MH (2009) Using biological networks to search for interacting loci in genome-wide association studies. Eur J Hum Genet 17: 1231–1240.
19. Pan W (2008) Network-based model weighting to detect multiple loci influencing complex diseases. Hum Genet 124: 225–234.
20. Akula N, Baranova A, Seto D, Solka J, Nalls MA, et al. (2011) A network-based approach to prioritize results from genome-wide association studies. PLoS One 6: e24220.
21. Baranzini SE, Galwey NW, Wang J, Khankhanian P, Lindberg R, et al. (2009) Pathway and network-based analysis of genome-wide association studies in multiple sclerosis. Hum Mol Genet 18: 2078–2090.
22. Jensen MK, Pers TH, Dworzynski P, Girman CJ, Brunak S, et al. (2011) Protein interaction-based genome-wide analysis of incident coronary heart disease. Circ Cardiovasc Genet 4: 549–556.
23. Jia P, Zheng S, Long J, Zheng W, Zhao Z (2011) dmGWAS: dense module searching for genome-wide association studies in protein-protein interaction networks. Bioinformatics 27: 95–102.
24. Lee I, Blom UM, Wang PI, Shim JE, Marcotte EM (2011) Prioritizing candidate disease genes by network-based boosting of genome-wide association data. Genome Res 21: 1109–1121.
25. Purcell S, Neale B, Todd-Brown K, Thomas L, Ferreira MA, et al. (2007) PLINK: a tool set for whole-genome association and population-based linkage analyses. Am J Hum Genet 81: 559–575.
26. Simon-Sanchez J, Schulte C, Bras JM, Sharma M, Gibbs JR, et al. (2009) Genome-wide association study reveals genetic risk underlying Parkinson's disease. Nat Genet 41: 1308–1312.
27. Hom G, Graham RR, Modrek B, Taylor KE, Ortmann W, et al. (2008) Association of systemic lupus erythematosus with C8orf13-BLK and ITGAM-ITGAX. N Engl J Med 358: 900–909.
28. Baranzini SE, Wang J, Gibson RA, Galwey N, Naegelin Y, et al. (2009) Genome-wide association analysis of susceptibility and clinical phenotype in multiple sclerosis. Hum Mol Genet 18: 767–778.
29. Barrett JC, Clayton DG, Concannon P, Akolkar B, Cooper JD, et al. (2009) Genome-wide association study and meta-analysis find that over 40 loci affect risk of type 1 diabetes. Nat Genet 41: 703–707.
30. Hunter DJ, Kraft P, Jacobs KB, Cox DG, Yeager M, et al. (2007) A genome-wide association study identifies alleles in FGFR2 associated with risk of sporadic postmenopausal breast cancer. Nat Genet 39: 870–874.
31. Maris JM, Mosse YP, Bradfield JP, Hou C, Monni S, et al. (2008) Chromosome 6p22 locus associated with clinically aggressive neuroblastoma. N Engl J Med 358: 2585–2593.
32. Segre AV, Groop L, Mootha VK, Daly MJ, Altshuler D (2010) Common inherited variation in mitochondrial genes is not enriched for associations with type 2 diabetes or related glycemic traits. PLoS Genet 6: e1001058.
33. Bader GD, Betel D, Hogue CWV (2003) BIND: the Biomolecular Interaction Network Database. Nucleic Acids Research 31: 248–250.
34. Ceol A, Chatr Aryamontri A, Licata L, Peluso D, Briganti L, et al. (2010) MINT, the molecular interaction database: 2009 update. Nucleic acids research 38: D532–539.
35. Kerrien S, Aranda B, Breuza L, Bridge A, Broackes-Carter F, et al. (2011) The IntAct molecular interaction database in 2012. Nucleic Acids Research 40: D841–D846.
36. Keshava Prasad TS, Goel R, Kandasamy K, Keerthikumar S, Kumar S, et al. (2009) Human Protein Reference Database—2009 update. Nucleic acids research 37: D767–772.
37. Mishra GR, Suresh M, Kumaran K, Kannabiran N, Suresh S, et al. (2006) Human protein reference database—2006 update. Nucleic acids research 34: D411–414.
38. Pagel P, Kovac S, Oesterheld M, Brauner B, Dunger-Kaltenbach I, et al. (2005) The MIPS mammalian protein–protein interaction database. Bioinformatics 21: 832–834.
39. Peri S, Navarro JD, Amanchy R, Kristiansen TZ, Jonnalagadda CK, et al. (2003) Development of human protein reference database as an initial platform for approaching systems biology in humans. Genome Res 13: 2363–2371.
40. Stark C (2006) BioGRID: a general repository for interaction datasets. Nucleic Acids Research 34: D535–D539.
41. Huang DW, Sherman BT, Lempicki RA (2009) Systematic and integrative analysis of large gene lists using DAVID bioinformatics resources. Nat Protoc 4: 44–57.
42. Huang DW, Sherman BT, Lempicki RA (2009) Bioinformatics enrichment tools: paths toward the comprehensive functional analysis of large gene lists. Nucleic Acids Res 37: 1–13.
43. Weng MP, Liao BY (2010) MamPhEA: a web tool for mammalian phenotype enrichment analysis. Bioinformatics 26: 2212–2213.

44. Kupershmidt I, Su QJ, Grewal A, Sundaresh S, Halperin I, et al. (2010) Ontology-based meta-analysis of global collections of high-throughput public data. PLoS One 5.

45. Shannon P, Markiel A, Ozier O, Baliga NS, Wang JT, et al. (2003) Cytoscape: a software environment for integrated models of biomolecular interaction networks. Genome Res 13: 2498–2504.

46. Neale BM, Kou Y, Liu L, Ma'ayan A, Samocha KE, et al. (2012) Patterns and rates of exonic de novo mutations in autism spectrum disorders. Nature 485: 242–245.

47. Sakai Y, Shaw CA, Dawson BC, Dugas DV, Al-Mohtaseb Z, et al. (2011) Protein interactome reveals converging molecular pathways among autism disorders. Sci Transl Med 3: 86ra49.

48. Chow ML, Li HR, Winn ME, April C, Barnes CC, et al. (2011) Genome-wide expression assay comparison across frozen and fixed postmortem brain tissue samples. BMC Genomics 12: 449.

49. Nishimura Y, Martin CL, Vazquez-Lopez A, Spence SJ, Alvarez-Retuerto AI, et al. (2007) Genome-wide expression profiling of lymphoblastoid cell lines distinguishes different forms of autism and reveals shared pathways. Hum Mol Genet 16: 1682–1698.

50. Neale BM, Kou Y, Liu L, Ma'ayan A, Samocha KE, et al. (2012) Patterns and rates of exonic de novo mutations in autism spectrum disorders. Nature 485: 242–245.

51. Ben-David E, Shifman S (2012) Networks of neuronal genes affected by common and rare variants in autism spectrum disorders. PLoS Genet 8: e1002556.

52. Diskin SJ, Hou C, Glessner JT, Attiyeh EF, Laudenslager M, et al. (2009) Copy number variation at 1q21.1 associated with neuroblastoma. Nature 459: 987–991.

53. Eijkelkamp N, Linley JE, Baker MD, Minett MS, Cregg R, et al. (2012) Neurological perspectives on voltage-gated sodium channels. Brain 135: 2585–2612.

54. Hollander E, Wang AT, Braun A, Marsh L (2009) Neurological considerations: autism and Parkinson's disease. Psychiatry Res 170: 43–51.

55. Scheuerle A, Wilson K (2011) PARK2 copy number aberrations in two children presenting with autism spectrum disorder: further support of an association and possible evidence for a new microdeletion/microduplication syndrome. Am J Med Genet B Neuropsychiatr Genet 156B: 413–420.

56. Crespi B (2011) Autism and cancer risk. Autism Res 4: 302–310.

57. Glessner JT, Wang K, Cai G, Korvatska O, Kim CE, et al. (2009) Autism genome-wide copy number variation reveals ubiquitin and neuronal genes. Nature 459: 569–573.

58. Yaspan BL, Bush WS, Torstenson ES, Ma D, Pericak-Vance MA, et al. (2011) Genetic analysis of biological pathway data through genomic randomization. Hum Genet 129: 563–571.

59. Gilman SR, Iossifov I, Levy D, Ronemus M, Wigler M, et al. (2011) Rare de novo variants associated with autism implicate a large functional network of genes involved in formation and function of synapses. Neuron 70: 898–907.

60. Hussman JP, Chung RH, Griswold AJ, Jaworski JM, Salyakina D, et al. (2011) A noise-reduction GWAS analysis implicates altered regulation of neurite outgrowth and guidance in autism. Mol Autism 2: 1.

61. Buxbaum JD, Betancur C, Bozdagi O, Dorr NP, Elder GA, et al. (2012) Optimizing the phenotyping of rodent ASD models: enrichment analysis of mouse and human neurobiological phenotypes associated with high-risk autism genes identifies morphological, electrophysiological, neurological, and behavioral features. Mol Autism 3: 1.

62. He W, Wang Y, Liu W, Zhou CZ (2007) Crystal structure of Saccharomyces cerevisiae 6-phosphogluconate dehydrogenase Gnd1. BMC Struct Biol 7: 38.

63. Hofmann B, Hecht HJ, Flohe L (2002) Peroxiredoxins. Biol Chem 383: 347–364.

64. Immenschuh S, Baumgart-Vogt E (2005) Peroxiredoxins, oxidative stress, and cell proliferation. Antioxid Redox Signal 7: 768–777.

65. Frustaci A, Neri M, Cesario A, Adams JB, Domenici E, et al. (2012) Oxidative stress-related biomarkers in autism: systematic review and meta-analyses. Free Radic Biol Med 52: 2128–2141.

66. Ghanizadeh A, Akhondzadeh S, Hormozi M, Makarem A, Abotorabi-Zarchi M, et al. (2012) Glutathione-related factors and oxidative stress in autism, a review. Curr Med Chem 19: 4000–4005.

67. Voineagu I, Wang X, Johnston P, Lowe JK, Tian Y, et al. (2011) Transcriptomic analysis of autistic brain reveals convergent molecular pathology. Nature 474: 380–384.

Permissions

All chapters in this book were first published in PLOS ONE, by The Public Library of Science; hereby published with permission under the Creative Commons Attribution License or equivalent. Every chapter published in this book has been scrutinized by our experts. Their significance has been extensively debated. The topics covered herein carry significant findings which will fuel the growth of the discipline. They may even be implemented as practical applications or may be referred to as a beginning point for another development.

The contributors of this book come from diverse backgrounds, making this book a truly international effort. This book will bring forth new frontiers with its revolutionizing research information and detailed analysis of the nascent developments around the world.

We would like to thank all the contributing authors for lending their expertise to make the book truly unique. They have played a crucial role in the development of this book. Without their invaluable contributions this book wouldn't have been possible. They have made vital efforts to compile up to date information on the varied aspects of this subject to make this book a valuable addition to the collection of many professionals and students.

This book was conceptualized with the vision of imparting up-to-date information and advanced data in this field. To ensure the same, a matchless editorial board was set up. Every individual on the board went through rigorous rounds of assessment to prove their worth. After which they invested a large part of their time researching and compiling the most relevant data for our readers.

The editorial board has been involved in producing this book since its inception. They have spent rigorous hours researching and exploring the diverse topics which have resulted in the successful publishing of this book. They have passed on their knowledge of decades through this book. To expedite this challenging task, the publisher supported the team at every step. A small team of assistant editors was also appointed to further simplify the editing procedure and attain best results for the readers.

Apart from the editorial board, the designing team has also invested a significant amount of their time in understanding the subject and creating the most relevant covers. They scrutinized every image to scout for the most suitable representation of the subject and create an appropriate cover for the book.

The publishing team has been an ardent support to the editorial, designing and production team. Their endless efforts to recruit the best for this project, has resulted in the accomplishment of this book. They are a veteran in the field of academics and their pool of knowledge is as vast as their experience in printing. Their expertise and guidance has proved useful at every step. Their uncompromising quality standards have made this book an exceptional effort. Their encouragement from time to time has been an inspiration for everyone.

The publisher and the editorial board hope that this book will prove to be a valuable piece of knowledge for researchers, students, practitioners and scholars across the globe.

List of Contributors

Yongxia Zhou
Department of Radiology, University of Pennsylvania, Philadelphia, Pennsylvania, United States of America

Fang Yu
Research Imaging Institute, Departments of Ophthalmology, Radiology, Physiology, University of Texas Health Science Center, South Texas Veterans Health Care System, Department of Veterans Affairs, San Antonio, Texas, United States of America

Timothy Duong
Research Imaging Institute, Departments of Ophthalmology, Radiology, Physiology, University of Texas Health Science Center, South Texas Veterans Health Care System, Department of Veterans Affairs, San Antonio, Texas, United States of America

Yi-Shin Chang
Department of Radiology and Biomedical Imaging, University of California San Francisco, San Francisco, California, United States of America

Julia P. Owen
Department of Radiology and Biomedical Imaging, University of California San Francisco, San Francisco, California, United States of America

Shivani S. Desai
Department of Neurology, University of California San Francisco, San Francisco, California, United States of America

Susanna S. Hill
Department of Neurology, University of California San Francisco, San Francisco, California, United States of America

Anne B. Arnett
Department of Neurology, University of California San Francisco, San Francisco, California, United States of America

Julia Harris
Department of Neurology, University of California San Francisco, San Francisco, California, United States of America

Elysa J. Marco
Department of Neurology, University of California San Francisco, San Francisco, California, United States of America

Pratik Mukherjee
Department of Radiology and Biomedical Imaging, University of California San Francisco, San Francisco, California, United States of America

Jerry Skefos, Christopher Cummings, Katelyn Enzer, Jarrod Holiday, Katrina Weed, Ezra Levy, Tarik Yuce, Thomas Kemper and Margaret Bauman
Department of Anatomy & Neurobiology, Boston University School of Medicine, Boston, Massachusetts, United States of America

Juergen Kornmeier
Institute for Frontier Areas of Psychology and Mental Health, Freiburg, Germany
Eye Center, Albert-Ludwigs-University of Freiburg, Freiburg, Germany

Rike Wö rner
PPD Germany GmbH & Co Kg, Karlsruhe, Germany,

Andreas Riedel
Section for Experimental Neuropsychiatry, Clinic for Psychiatry & Psychotherapy, Albert-Ludwigs-University of Freiburg, Freiburg, Germany

Michael Bach
Eye Center, Albert-Ludwigs-University of Freiburg, Freiburg, Germany

Ludger Tebartz van Elst
Section for Experimental Neuropsychiatry, Clinic for Psychiatry & Psychotherapy, Albert-Ludwigs-University of Freiburg, Freiburg, Germany

Alexandra F. S. Breitenkamp , Jan Matthes , Robert Daniel Nass and Judith Sinzig
Department of Pharmacology, University of Cologne, Cologne, Germany
Department of Child and Adolescent Psychiatry and Psychotherapy, LVR-Klinik Bonn, Bonn, Germany
Department of Child and Adolescent Psychiatry and Psychotherapy, University of Cologne, Cologne, Germany

Gerd Lehmkuhl
Department of Child and Adolescent Psychiatry and Psychotherapy, University of Cologne, Cologne, Germany

Peter Nü rnberg
Cologne Center for Genomics, University of Cologne, Cologne, Germany

Stefan Herzig
Department of Pharmacology, University of Cologne, Cologne, Germany
Center for Molecular Medicine, University of Cologne, Cologne, Germany

Laurence O'Dwyer
Radboud University Medical Center, Donders Institute for Brain, Cognition and Behaviour, Department of Cognitive Neuroscience, Nijmegen, The Netherlands

Colby Tanner
Department of Ecology and Evolution, University of Lausanne, Lausanne, Switzerland

Eelco V. van Dongen
Radboud University Medical Center, Donders Institute for Brain, Cognition and Behaviour, Department of Cognitive Neuroscience, Nijmegen, The Netherlands

Corina U. Greven
Radboud University Medical Center, Donders Institute for Brain, Cognition and Behaviour, Department of Cognitive Neuroscience, Nijmegen, The Netherlands
King's College London, Social, Genetic and Developmental Psychiatry Centre, Institute of Psychiatry, London, United Kingdom

Janita Bralten
Radboud University Medical Center, Donders Institute for Brain, Cognition and Behaviour, Department of Cognitive Neuroscience, Nijmegen, The Netherlands
Department of Human Genetics, Radboud University Medical Center, Nijmegen, The Netherlands

Marcel P. Zwiers
Radboud University Medical Center, Donders Institute for Brain, Cognition and Behaviour, Department of Cognitive Neuroscience, Nijmegen, The Netherlands

Barbara Franke
Department of Human Genetics, Radboud University Medical Center, Nijmegen, The Netherlands
Radboud University Medical Center, Donders Institute for Brain, Cognition and Behaviour, Department of Psychiatry, Nijmegen, The Netherlands

Jaap Oosterlaan
Department of Clinical Neuropsychology, Vrije Universiteit, Amsterdam, The Netherlands

Dirk Heslenfeld
Department of Clinical Neuropsychology, Vrije Universiteit, Amsterdam, The Netherlands
Department of Cognitive Psychology, Vrije Universiteit, Amsterdam, The Netherlands

Pieter Hoekstra
Department of Psychiatry, University Medical Center Groningen, University of Groningen, Groningen, The Netherlands

Catharina A. Hartman
Department of Psychiatry, University Medical Center Groningen, University of Groningen, Groningen, The Netherlands

Nanda Rommelse
Radboud University Medical Center, Donders Institute for Brain, Cognition and Behaviour, Department of Psychiatry, Nijmegen, The Netherlands
Karakter Child and Adolescent Psychiatry University Center Nijmegen, Nijmegen, The Netherlands

Jan K. Buitelaar
Radboud University Medical Center, Donders Institute for Brain, Cognition and Behaviour, Department of Cognitive Neuroscience, Nijmegen, The Netherlands
Karakter Child and Adolescent Psychiatry University Center Nijmegen, Nijmegen, The Netherlands

Daniel P. Kennedy
Department of Psychological and Brain Sciences, Indiana University, Bloomington, Indiana, United States of America
Division of Humanities and Social Sciences, California Institute of Technology, Pasadena, California, United States of America

Ralph Adolphs
Division of Humanities and Social Sciences, California Institute of Technology, Pasadena, California, United States of America
Division of Biology, California Institute of Technology, Pasadena, California, United States of America

Takashi Itahashi
Department of Pharmacognosy and Phytochemistry, Showa University School of Pharmacy, Tokyo, Japan

Takashi Yamada
Department of Psychiatry, Showa University School of Medicine, Tokyo, Japan

Hiromi Watanabe
Department of Psychiatry, Showa University School of Medicine, Tokyo, Japan

Motoaki Nakamura
Department of Psychiatry, Showa University School of Medicine, Tokyo, Japan
Kinko Hospital, Kanagawa Psychiatric Center, Kanagawa, Japan

Daiki Jimbo
Department of Anatomy, Showa University School of Medicine, Tokyo, Japan

Seiji Shioda
Department of Anatomy, Showa University School of Medicine, Tokyo, Japan

Kazuo Toriizuka
Department of Pharmacognosy and Phytochemistry, Showa University School of Pharmacy, Tokyo, Japan

Nobumasa Kato
Department of Psychiatry, Showa University School of Medicine, Tokyo, Japan

Ryuichiro Hashimoto
Department of Psychiatry, Showa University School of Medicine, Tokyo, Japan
Department of Language Sciences, Graduate School of Humanities, Tokyo Metropolitan University, Tokyo, Japan

Andrée-Anne S. Meilleur
The University of Montreal Center of Excellence for Pervasive Developmental Disorders (CETEDUM), Hô pital Rivie`re-des-Prairies, Montreal, Quebec, Canada

Claude Berthiaume
The University of Montreal Center of Excellence for Pervasive Developmental Disorders (CETEDUM), Hô pital Rivière-des-Prairies, Montreal, Quebec, Canada

Armando Bertone
The University of Montreal Center of Excellence for Pervasive Developmental Disorders (CETEDUM), Hô pital Rivière-des-Prairies, Montreal, Quebec, Canada
School Applied Child Psychology, Department of Education and Counselling Psychology, McGill University, Montreal, Quebec, Canada

Laurent Mottron
The University of Montreal Center of Excellence for Pervasive Developmental Disorders (CETEDUM), Hô pital Rivie`re-des-Prairies, Montreal, Quebec, Canada

Hanna B. Cygan
Nencki Institute of Experimental Biology, Department of Neurophysiology, Laboratory of Psychophysiology, Warsaw, Poland

Pawel Tacikowski
Nencki Institute of Experimental Biology, Department of Neurophysiology, Laboratory of Psychophysiology, Warsaw, Poland
Karolinska Institute, Department of Neuroscience, Brain, Body and Self Laboratory, Stockholm, Sweden

Pawel Ostaszewski
University of Social Sciences and Humanities, Department of Psychology, Warsaw, Poland

Izabela Chojnicka
Medical University of Warsaw, Department of Medical Genetics, Warsaw, Poland

Anna Nowicka
Nencki Institute of Experimental Biology, Department of Neurophysiology, Laboratory of Psychophysiology, Warsaw, Poland

Ingrid Kruizinga
Department of Public Health, Erasmus University Medical Center, Rotterdam, the Netherlands

Janne C. Visser
Karakter University Center Nijmegen, Nijmegen, the Netherlands

Tamara van Batenburg-Eddes
Department of Psychology and Education, VU University, Amsterdam, the Netherlands

Alice S. Carter
Department of Psychology, University of Massachusetts Boston, Boston, Massachusetts, United States of America

Wilma Jansen
Department of Youth Policy, Rotterdam Municipal Health Service (GGD Rotterdam-Rijnmond), Rotterdam, the Netherlands

Hein Raat
Department of Public Health, Erasmus University Medical Center, Rotterdam, the Netherlands

Katherine K. M. Stavropoulos and Leslie J. Carver
Psychology Department, University of California San Diego, La Jolla, California, United States of America

Maurizio Marrale
Dipartimento di Fisica e Chimica, Università di Palermo, Palermo, Italy

Nadia Ninfa Albanese
Dipartimento di Fisica e Chimica, Università di Palermo, Palermo, Italy

Francesco Calì
U.O.C. di Genetica Medica Laboratorio di Genetica Molecolare, Associazione Oasi Maria SS. (I.R.C.C.S.), Troina, Italy

Valentino Romano
U.O.C. di Genetica Medica Laboratorio di Genetica Molecolare, Associazione Oasi Maria SS. (I.R.C.C.S.), Troina, Italy

Takeo Fujiwara
Department of Social Medicine, National Research Institute for Child Health and Development, Setagaya-ku, Tokyo, Japan

Ichiro Kawachi
Department of Society and Behavioral Sciences, Harvard School of Public Health, Boston, Massachusetts, United States of America

Yang-Teng Fan
Institute of Neuroscience and Brain Research Center, National Yang-Ming University, Taipei, Taiwan

Yawei Cheng
Institute of Neuroscience and Brain Research Center, National Yang-Ming University, Taipei, Taiwan
Department of Rehabilitation, National Yang-Ming University Hospital, Yilan, Taiwan
Department of Research and Education, Taipei City Hospital, Taipei, Taiwan

Simon Baron-Cohen
Autism Research Centre, Department of Psychiatry, University of Cambridge, Cambridge, United Kingdom
Cambridge Lifespan Asperger Syndrome Service (CLASS)
Clinic, Cambridgeshire and Peterborough National Health Service Foundation Trust, Cambridge, United Kingdom,

Sarah Cassidy
Autism Research Centre, Department of Psychiatry, University of Cambridge, Cambridge, United Kingdom

Bonnie Auyeung
Autism Research Centre, Department of Psychiatry, University of Cambridge, Cambridge, United Kingdom
Department of Psychology, University of Edinburgh, Edinburgh, United Kingdom

Carrie Allison
Autism Research Centre, Department of Psychiatry, University of Cambridge, Cambridge, United Kingdom

Maryam Achoukhi
Autism Research Centre, Department of Psychiatry, University of Cambridge, Cambridge, United Kingdom

Sarah Robertson
Autism Research Centre, Department of Psychiatry, University of Cambridge, Cambridge, United Kingdom

Alexa Poh
Autism Research Centre, Department of Psychiatry, University of Cambridge, Cambridge, United Kingdom

Meng-Chuan Lai
Autism Research Centre, Department of Psychiatry, University of Cambridge, Cambridge, United Kingdom
Cambridge Lifespan Asperger Syndrome Service (CLASS)
Clinic, Cambridgeshire and Peterborough National Health Service Foundation Trust, Cambridge, United Kingdom
Department of Psychiatry, National Taiwan University Hospital and College of Medicine, Taipei, Taiwan

Manoj Kumar
Department of Radiology, Perelman School of Medicine at the University of Pennsylvania, Philadelphia, Pennsylvania, United States of America

Jeffery T. Duda
Department of Radiology, Perelman School of Medicine at the University of Pennsylvania, Philadelphia, Pennsylvania, United States of America

Wei-Ting Hwang
Department of Biostatistics and Epidemiology, Center for Clinical Epidemiology and Biostatistics, Perelman School of Medicine at the University of Pennsylvania, Philadelphia, Pennsylvania, United States of America

Charles Kenworthy
Department of Biology, University of Pennsylvania, Philadelphia, Pennsylvania, United States of America

Ranjit Ittyerah
Department of Radiology, Perelman School of Medicine at the University of Pennsylvania, Philadelphia, Pennsylvania, United States of America

Stephen Pickup
Department of Radiology, Perelman School of Medicine at the University of Pennsylvania, Philadelphia, Pennsylvania, United States of America

Edward S. Brodkin
Center for Neurobiology and Behavior, Department of Psychiatry, Perelman School of Medicine at the University of Pennsylvania, Philadelphia, Pennsylvania, United States of America

James C. Gee
Department of Radiology, Perelman School of Medicine at the University of Pennsylvania, Philadelphia, Pennsylvania, United States of America

Ted Abel
Department of Biology, University of Pennsylvania, Philadelphia, Pennsylvania, United States of America

Harish Poptani
Department of Radiology, Perelman School of Medicine at the University of Pennsylvania, Philadelphia, Pennsylvania, United States of America

Paul R. West, Alan M. Smith, Laura A. Egnash, Mark E. Ross, Jessica A. Palmer, Burr R. Fontaine, Kevin R. Conard, Gabriela G. Cezar, Elizabeth L. R. Donley and Robert E. Burrier
Stemina Biomarker Discovery, Madison, Wisconsin, United States of America

David G. Amaral
The M.I.N.D. Institute and Department of Psychiatry and Behavioral Sciences, University of California Davis, Davis, California, United States of America

Preeti Bais
The Jackson Laboratory for Genomic medicine, University of Connecticut Health Center, Farmington, Connecticut, United States of America

Blythe A. Corbett
Department of Psychiatry, Psychology and Kennedy Center, Vanderbilt University, Nashville, Tennessee, United States of America

Elizabeth Pellicano
Centre for Research in Autism and Education (CRAE), Department of Psychology and Human Development, Institute of Education, University of London, London, United Kingdom

Adam Dinsmore
Centre for Research in Autism and Education (CRAE), Department of Psychology and Human Development, Institute of Education, University of London, London, United Kingdom
Wellcome Trust, Strategic Planning & Policy Unit, London, United Kingdom

Tony Charman
Department of Psychology, King's College London, Institute of Psychiatry, London, United Kingdom

Catarina Correia
Departamento de Promoc,ão da Saúde e Doenças não Transmissíveis, Instituto Nacional de Saúde Doutor Ricardo Jorge, 1649-016 Lisboa, Portugal
Center for Biodiversity, Functional & Integrative Genomics, Faculty of Sciences, University of Lisbon, 1749-016 Lisboa, Portugal
Instituto Gulbenkian de Ciência, 2780-156 Oeiras, Portugal

Guiomar Oliveira
Unidade Neurodesenvolvimento e Autismo, Centro de Desenvolvimento, Hospital Pediátrico (HP) do Centro Hospitalar e Universitário de Coimbra (CHUC), 3000-602 Coimbra, Portugal
Centro de Investigac,ão e Formac,ão Clinica do HP-CHUC, 3000-602 Coimbra, Portugal
Faculdade de Medicina da Universidade de Coimbra, 3000-548 Coimbra, Portugal

Astrid M. Vicente
Departamento de Promoc,ão da Saúde e Doenc,as não Transmissíveis, Instituto Nacional de Saúde Doutor Ricardo Jorge, 1649-016 Lisboa, Portugal
Center for Biodiversity, Functional & Integrative Genomics, Faculty of Sciences, University of Lisbon, 1749-016 Lisboa, Portugal
Instituto Gulbenkian de Ciênncia, 2780-156 Oeiras, Portugal

Index

A

Additional Volumetry Using Mri, 31

Alterations, 20, 26, 28-29, 31, 33, 35, 37, 39-41, 43, 45, 47, 49, 51, 73, 86-87, 90, 92-93, 97, 101-102, 111, 113-114, 117, 156, 189, 194, 203, 206

Altered Network Topologies, 86-87, 89, 91, 93, 95, 97, 99

Animal Housing And Breeding, 185

Asperger Autism, 40

Asymmetric Interactions, 211, 215

Attention-deficit/hyperactivity Disorder (adhd), 63

Attenuation, 174-175, 177, 179, 181, 183

Autism Evaluation, 13

Autism Genome Project (agp), 219

Autism Research, 26, 28-29, 85, 112, 155-156, 174, 182, 206, 208-211, 213-218

Autism Score, 127, 129-130, 132-133

Autism Spectrum Condition (asc), 86

Autism Spectrum Disorder, 1, 3-5, 7, 9-10, 26-27, 39-40, 51, 53, 62-63, 65, 67, 69, 71, 73-77, 79, 81, 83, 85, 99-100, 112, 114-115, 117, 119, 121, 123, 125-126, 130, 133-135, 139, 145, 156-157, 159, 161, 163, 172-173, 182-184, 194-197, 199, 201, 203, 205, 207, 218-219, 228-229

Autism Spectrum Quotient (aq), 174, 177, 182

Autism-specific Covariation, 101, 103, 105, 107, 109, 111, 113

B

Behavioral Data Analysis, 121

Behavioral Measures, 12, 28, 31-32, 34, 135, 137, 139-140, 142, 172

Biomolecular Targets, 195

Blood Plasma, 195-197, 199, 201, 203, 205-207

Brain Volumetric, 63, 65, 67, 69, 71, 73, 75

C

Caucasians, 54, 150

Chromatogram, 56, 198

Chromosome, 74, 148-151, 154-156, 228

Classification Modeling, 198-200, 203

Cognitive Characteristics, 65, 70, 182

Cognitive Social Capital, 157, 160-162

Copy Number Variants, 147, 149-153, 155, 205, 219

Current Source Density Analyses, 168

D

Demographic Variables, 129

E

Electroencephalography Apparatus, 166, 172

Electrophysiological Studies, 136

Electrophysiology, 45, 55, 125, 136-137

Emotional Assessment, 127-129, 131, 133-134

Event-related Brain Potentials (erps), 164

Experimental Paradigm, 41, 44, 117

Experimental Procedure, 121, 124

F

Functional Magnetic Resonance Imaging (fmri), 86, 114

Functional Neuroimaging Studies, 136

G

Gas Chromatography, 198

General Cognition, 12

General Demographics, 12

Genetic Factors, 63, 147, 157

Genome-wide Association Studies (gwas), 219

Graph Theory, 1-3, 5-7, 9, 99

H

High Functioning Autism, 40, 50, 52, 75, 99, 172, 175, 182

Homogenous Autistic Subcategory, 40

Hub Organization, 86-87, 89-93, 95-97, 99

Hyperactivity Disorder, 63, 65-67, 69, 71, 73-75, 99, 175

I

Image Acquisition, 14, 69

Independent Validation Sets, 198

Institutional Review Board (irb), 12

Intracranial Volume, 67-68, 71-72

L

Liquid Chromatography, 197, 206

Low-level Auditory Task, 106

Low-level Visual Task, 105

M

Magnetic Resonance Imaging (mri), 29, 184

Maternal Social Networks, 157-159, 161, 163

Metabolite Chemical Structure, 198

Metabolomics, 195-197, 199, 201, 203, 205-207

Mismatch Negativity (mmn), 164

Monte Carlo Simulation, 147, 149, 151, 153, 155

Mri Characterization, 1, 3, 5, 7, 9

Multiparametric, 1-3, 5, 7-9

Multisensory Integration (msi), 11

N

Network Metrics, 87, 89-90, 96, 98

Neural Correlates, 10, 72, 99, 114-115, 117, 119, 121, 123, 125-126, 136-137, 145-146, 173

Neuroligin, 100, 184-185, 187, 189, 191, 193-194

Neurophysiological Measures, 166

Novel Autism Risk Genes, 219, 221, 223, 225, 227, 229

P

Perceptual Performances, 101-103, 105, 107, 109-111, 113

Phenotypic Information, 2

Plurimodal Co-variation, 107

Positive Chromosomes, 148, 150-151

Purkinje Cell Density, 28-29, 31, 33-35, 37, 39

S

Schematic Representation, 102, 104, 151

Screening Accuracy, 127-133

Sensory Processing Disorders, 11, 13, 15, 17, 19, 21, 23, 25-27

Sensory Processing Evaluation, 13

Site-directed Mutagenesis, 55

Social Approach, 184-187, 189, 191, 193

Social Responsiveness Scale, 2, 77, 85, 138, 146

Social-emotional Pathways, 11

Spn Amplitude, 137, 144

Statistical Noise, 219-225, 227, 229

Stereological Methodology, 30

Stimuli And Procedure, 105

T

Threshold Selection, 89

Tissue Preparation, 29

Tract Delineation, 14

Typical Sex Differences, 174-175, 177, 179, 181, 183

U

Univariate Filtering Of Mass Features, 198

V

Volumetry Analysis, 3, 5

W

White Matter Disruption, 11, 13, 15, 17, 19, 21, 23, 25, 27

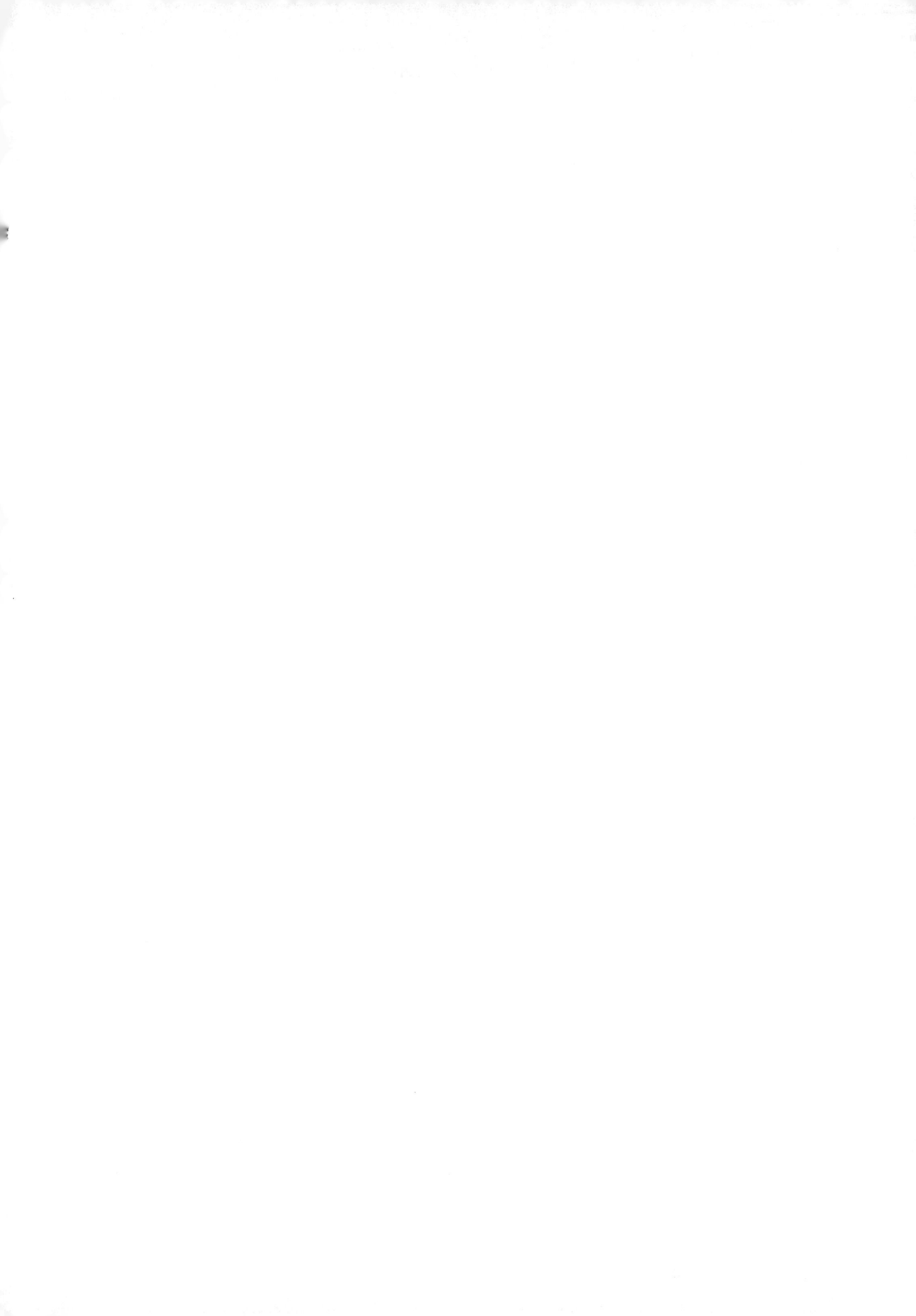

www.ingramcontent.com/pod-product-compliance
Lightning Source LLC
Chambersburg PA
CBHW061258190326
41458CB00011B/3707